Molecular Medicine: Beyond the Basics

Molecular Medicine:
Beyond the Basics

Editor: Jim Remington

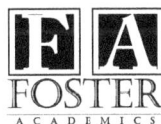

FA FOSTER ACADEMICS

www.fosteracademics.com

www.fosteracademics.com

FA
FOSTER
ACADEMICS

Cataloging-in-Publication Data

Molecular medicine : beyond the basics / edited by Jim Remington.
 p. cm.
Includes bibliographical references and index.
ISBN 978-1-63242-904-9
1. Medical genetics. 2. Molecular Biology. 3. Pathology, Molecular. I. Remington, Jim.
RB155 .M65 2020
616.042--dc23

Foster Academics,
118-35 Queens Blvd., Suite 400,
Forest Hills, NY 11375, USA

ISBN 978-1-63242-904-9 (Hardback)

Contents

            surgery in female mice..183
            Mary K. Herrick, Kristin M. Favela, Richard B. Simerly, Naji N. Abumrad and
            Nathan C. Bingham

Chapter 19   **MicroRNAs 143 and 150 in whole blood enable detection of T-cell**
            immunoparalysis in sepsis 193
            P Möhnle, S Hirschberger, L C Hinske, J Briegel, M Hübner, S Weis,
            G Dimopoulos, M Bauer, E J Giamarellos-Bourboulis and S Kreth

            Permissions

            List of Contributors

            Index

Preface

In my initial years as a student, I used to run to the library at every possible instance to grab a book and learn something new. Books were my primary source of knowledge and I would not have come such a long way without all that I learnt from them. Thus, when I was approached to edit this book; I became understandably nostalgic. It was an absolute honor to be considered worthy of guiding the current generation as well as those to come. I put all my knowledge and hard work into making this book most beneficial for its readers.

An emerging approach to the study of diseases is through an examination of molecular structures and mechanisms, identification of the molecular and genetic errors of disease, and the formulation of molecular interventions to correct these. This approach is what characterizes the field of molecular medicine. An understanding of disease pathogenesis at the molecular level and normal body functioning is crucial for the development of the field. It integrates the domains of molecular genetics and molecular biology for a comprehension of human health and disease. Some of its key focuses are cancer research, immunology, gene expression, proteins, biotechnology, etc. This book covers in detail some existing theories and innovative concepts revolving around molecular medicine. The various advancements in molecular medicine are glanced at and their applications as well as ramifications are looked at in detail. With state-of-the-art inputs by acclaimed experts of this field, this book targets students and professionals.

I wish to thank my publisher for supporting me at every step. I would also like to thank all the authors who have contributed their researches in this book. I hope this book will be a valuable contribution to the progress of the field.

Editor

Metformin suppresses UHMWPE particle-induced osteolysis in the mouse calvaria by promoting polarization of macrophages to an anti-inflammatory phenotype

Zhao Yan[1†], Xiaoxi Tian[2†], Jinyu Zhu[1†], Zifan Lu[3], Lifeng Yu[1], Dawei Zhang[1], Yanwu Liu[1], Chongfei Yang[1], Qingsheng Zhu[1*] and Xiaorui Cao[1*]

Abstract

Background: Implant failure remains a major obstacle to successful treatment via TJA. Periprosthetic osteolysis and aseptic loosening are considered as proof of wear debris-induced disruption of local regulatory mechanisms related to excessive bone resorption associated with osteolysis and the damage at the bone-prosthesis interface. Therefore, there is an immediate need to explore strategies for limiting and curing periprosthetic osteolysis and aseptic loosening.

Methods: We analyzed the in vitro cytokine production by primary mouse bone marrow macrophages (BMMs) that were exposed to ultra-high molecular weight polyethylene (UHMWPE) particles and treated with metformin at different concentrations with or without 5-aminoimidazole-4-carboxamide ribonucleoside to activate or inhibit AMPK. A mouse calvarial model was used to examine the in vivo effects of metformin on UHMWPE particle-induced osteolysis.

Results: With particles, primary mouse BMMs secreted more pro-inflammatory cytokines tumor necrosis factor-α and interleukin (IL)-6. Treatment with metformin inhibited these variations and promoted the release of cytokine IL-10 with anti-inflammatory capability. In vivo, metformin reduced the production of pro-inflammatory cytokines, osteoclastogenesis, and osteolysis, increasing IL-10 production. Metformin also promoted the polarization of macrophages to an anti-inflammatory phenotype in vivo via AMPK activation.

Discussion: A crucial point in limiting and correcting the periprosthetic osteolysis and aseptic loosening is the inhibition of inflammatory factor production and osteoclast activation induced by activated macrophages. The ability of metformin to attenuate osteolysis induced in mouse calvaria by the particles was related to a reduction in osteoclast number and polarization of macrophages to an anti-inflammatory functional phenotype.

Conclusions: Metformin could limit the osteolysis induced by implant debris. Therefore, we hypothesized that metformin could be a potential drug for osteolysis induced by implant debris.

Keywords: Inflammation, Osteoclasts, AMPK, Macrophage, Osteolysis

---

* Correspondence: zhuqsh@fmmu.edu.cn; caoxiaorui.810428@aliyun.com
†Equal contributors
[1]PLA Institute of Orthopaedics, Xijing Hospital, Fourth Military Medical University, Xi'an 710032, China
Full list of author information is available at the end of the article

Background

Total joint arthroplasty (TJA) is a widely performed surgery for reducing the pain and restoring the mobility of patients with major joint damage or severe arthritis. Implant failure remains a major obstacle to successful treatment via TJA. Osteolysis induced by implant wear debris is the dominant cause of implant failure, causing ~ 50,000 revision surgeries per year in the United States alone (Kurtz et al. 2007). Long-range data regarding TJA outcomes are insufficient, and osteolysis continues to be a common complication. Therefore, there is an immediate need to explore strategies for limiting and curing periprosthetic osteolysis and aseptic loosening.

Osteolysis begins with the activation of macrophages in addition to foreign-body giant cells and the phagocytosis of particulate wear debris. These events stimulate the release of cytokines with pro-inflammatory capability and mediators and reduce the phosphorylation of AMP-activated protein kinase (AMPK) (Vasamsetti et al. 2015), promoting the production of osteoclasts that are differentiated from phagocyte precursors and in turn facilitating the periprosthetic osteolysis and corresponding implant loosening (Glant et al. 1993). Osteoblast activity is hampered by exposure to prosthetic particles. For example, osteoblasts expressed a catabolic phenotype upon exposure to polyethylene particles (Atkins et al. 2009). Periprosthetic osteolysis and aseptic loosening, thus, are considered as proof of wear debris-induced disruption of local regulatory mechanisms related to excessive bone resorption associated with osteolysis and the damage at the bone-prosthesis interface (Purdue et al. 2006). A crucial point in limiting and correcting the periprosthetic osteolysis and aseptic loosening, thus, is the inhibition of inflammatory factor production and osteoclast activation induced by activated macrophages.

As an anti-hyperglycemic agent, metformin is widely used in treating type II diabetes to improve insulin resistance (Inzucchi et al. 2014). Metformin has a bone-protective property (La Fontaine et al. 2016) and enhances the mineralization and differentiation of osteoblasts (Kanazawa et al. 2008), negatively regulating RANKL in osteoclast differentiation (Lee et al. 2010). The reason is related to the activation of a serine/threonine protein kinase of AMP-activated protein kinase (AMPK), which is critical in maintaining metabolic homeostasis in eukaryotic cell types (Kudo et al. 1995). The anti-inflammatory effect of metformin is associated with AMPK phosphorylation. In addition, AMPK promoted the polarization of macrophages to an anti-inflammatory functional phenotype (Sag et al. 2008). Therefore, we hypothesized that metformin could limit the osteolysis induced by implant debris. Here, how metformin affects the in vitro production of inflammatory factors in primary mouse bone marrow macrophages (BMMs) in response to ultra-high molecular weight polyurethane (UHMWPE) particles was investigated. The ability of metformin to attenuate osteolysis induced in mouse calvaria by the particles was examined and found to be related to a reduction in osteoclast number and polarization of macrophages to an anti-inflammatory functional phenotype.

Methods

Preparation of UHMWPE-coated coverslips

The average diameter of the UHMWPE particles (provided by Mr. Ernst Krendlinger of Clariant, Gersthofen, Germany) was 1.74 ± 1.43 μm (range, 0.05–11.06 μm), with 90% particles smaller than 9 μm. (The particle diameter in membranes around total joint prostheses ranged from approximately 0 to 1 μm.) Notably, this particle diameter is within the range considered biologically active and differs from the diameter of particles isolated from the periprosthetic membranes. All particles were rinsed to remove the endotoxins using ethanol before desiccation in drying oven, and correspondingly, tests for endotoxins using the Limulus assay (Sigma-Aldrich, St. Louis, MO, USA) were negative. Before use in cell culture, the particles were disinfected under γ-irradiation in air (2.5 MR) and kept at 4 °C. The particles were exposed to UV light for 1 h immediately before use.

Glass coverslips were coated with UHMWPE particles. Previously characterized UHMWPE particles were placed in dimethyl sulfoxide (DMSO; 1 mg particles in 0.5 mL DMSO) in a sterile quartz pestle and mortar. Subsequently, the materials were suspended in 14.5 mL of collagen type-I monomer (0.01%) solution prepared from calf skin (C-8919; Sigma-Aldrich) and maintained at 4 °C. The final particle concentration was set at 10^7 particle/mL. The microscope coverslips with dimensions of 22×22 mm (Dingjie Biological Technology Co., Ltd., Shanghai, China) were disinfected for 2 h at 200 °C. Aliquots of collagen-suspended particles (10^5 particles/ 10 μL) were distributed onto the coverslip uniformly, before collagen polymerization was allowed to occur at room temperature. Coverslips not coated with UHMWPE were also created and used in control samples. The coverslips were placed into 6-well tissue culture plates before irradiation with ultraviolet light overnight in a sterile tissue culture hood. The plates were placed in PE packages and covered with aluminum foil. The storage temperature was 5 °C. Another 1 h exposure was performed immediately before usage of the coverslips (Nich et al. 2011).

Cell culture and IL-6, and TNF-α measurements

Dulbecco's Modified Eagle Medium (DMEM) supplemented with 10% fetal bovine serum (FBS; Gibco) and penicillin (100 U/mL) was used for primary mouse

BMM culture, and the cells were obtained from mouse femurs as described previously (Shah et al. 2010). RPMI-1640 supplemented with streptomycin (100 mg/mL), 10% FBS (Gibco), penicillin (100 U/mL), 10% heat-inactivated fetal calf serum, and L-glutamine (2 mM) was used for RAW264.7 cell culture, and the cells were obtained from American Type Culture Collection (Rockville, MD, USA).

The cells were seeded at 1×10^6 cells/2 mL/well and exposed to UHMWPE particles on the coated coverslips for 24 h in 6-well tissue culture plates. To examine how the particles affected both cells, the cells were treated with metformin at a concentration of 0.05, 0.5, or 5 mM with or without various concentrations of compound C (Sigma-Aldrich), a chemical inhibitor of AMPK, as well as 5-aminoimidazole-4-carboxamide1-β-D-ribofurano-side (AICAR, Sigma-Aldrich), which stimulates AMPK activity. The control samples were exposed to deionized water and incubated for 24 h. After each incubation period, the media samples were collected for cytokine measurement. Enzyme-linked immunosorbent assay (ELISA) kits from R&D Systems (Minneapolis, MN, USA) were used to measure the concentrations of tumor necrosis factor (TNF)-α, IL-6, and IL-10. Cells were lysed and centrifuged at 1000 g at 4 °C for 5 min and then at 10,000 g at 4 °C for 10 min. After the supernatants were collected, ARG-1 in the supernatants was quantified using an ELISA kit (Life-Span BioSciences) according to the manufacturer's instructions.

Animals and surgical procedure

Ninety 12-week-old C57BL/J6 male mice were utilized to establish the calvarial model of particle-induced osteolysis. All experiments involving animals were approved by the Institutional Review Board of Xijing Hospital (permit No. 20161003). All methods were performed in accordance with National Institute of Health Guide for the Care and Use of Laboratory Animals. The mice were divided into four groups randomly ($n = 22$/group). Five mice in each group were used to collect calvaria for tissue culture, five for RNA extraction and qRT-PCR, five for Western blot analysis, and the other seven for histologic evaluation after micro-computed tomography scanning. For surgery, mice were placed under general anesthesia via inhalation of isoflurane. An area (0.5×0.5 cm^2) of the periosteum was exposed via a midline sagittal incision of 10 mm on the calvaria. The incision in the sham control was sutured without further procedure. In the experimental groups in which UHMWPE particles were implanted, a sterile sharp surgical spoon was used to uniformly distribute 20 μg of particles over the intact periosteum. A simple, interrupted 4-0 Ethicon suture was utilized to close the incision. The mice were subsequently placed into cages and provided food and water ad libitum. All animals were given metformin (80 mg/kg, once a day for 2 weeks in a row), alendronate (ALN, Sigma-Aldrich, as positive control, 50 μg/kg, once a day for 2 weeks as previously described as anti-osteoporosis use), or normal saline as negative control via intragastric administration immediately after surgery. The animals were sacrificed 14 days after the operation via an overdose of intraperitoneal sodium pentobarbital.

Characterizations

The detailed descriptions of micro-CT analyses, histologic evaluation of osteolysis, quantitative real-time polymerase chain reaction (qRT-PCR), calvaria culture, and western blot analysis are provided in Additional file 1: Supporting Information S3.

Statistical analysis

All experiments were performed at least three times. All data are presented as mean ± standard deviation (SD). The SPSS software package (SPSS 11.0, Chicago, IL, USA) was used for statistical analyses. One-way analysis of variance (ANOVA) was performed to compare the different groups. Post-hoc testing of discrepancies among groups was performed via Duncan's test when the ANOVA results were significant. All P values < 0.05 were considered indicative of significance.

Results

Effects of metformin on TNF-α, IL-6 and IL-10 production and macrophage transition in primary mouse BMMs

Production of IL-6 and TNF-α as pro-inflammatory mediators, as well as IL-10 as an anti-inflammatory mediator by primary mouse BMMs exposed to UHMWPE particles for 24 h was measured using ELISA kits. Within the incubation period of 24 h, the TNF-α and IL-6 levels in the media increased significantly ($P < 0.05$), greater than those in the control cultures not exposed to particles (Fig. 1a–b). In contrast, the IL-10 levels in the culture media did not differ obviously between the groups (Fig. 1c). Treatment with metformin significantly reduced the increase in production of both TNF-α and IL-6, but enhanced the release of IL-10 after exposure to the particles for 24 h in a dose-dependent manner (Fig. 1a–c). ALN is widely used for the prevention and treatment of osteoporosis in postmenopausal women and has been shown to increase bone mass in men with osteoporosis (Kostenuik et al. 2015). ALN is used here as a positive control to facilitate the understanding of the mechanisms of metformin's action. ALN cannot inhibit the production of TNF-α and IL-6, nor can it enhance the release of IL-10 (Fig. 1d–f; $P < 0.05$). We also investigated RAW264.7 cells and obtained similar results (see Additional file 1: Supporting Information S1 and Figure S1). Moreover, flow cytometric results showed polarization of macrophages to

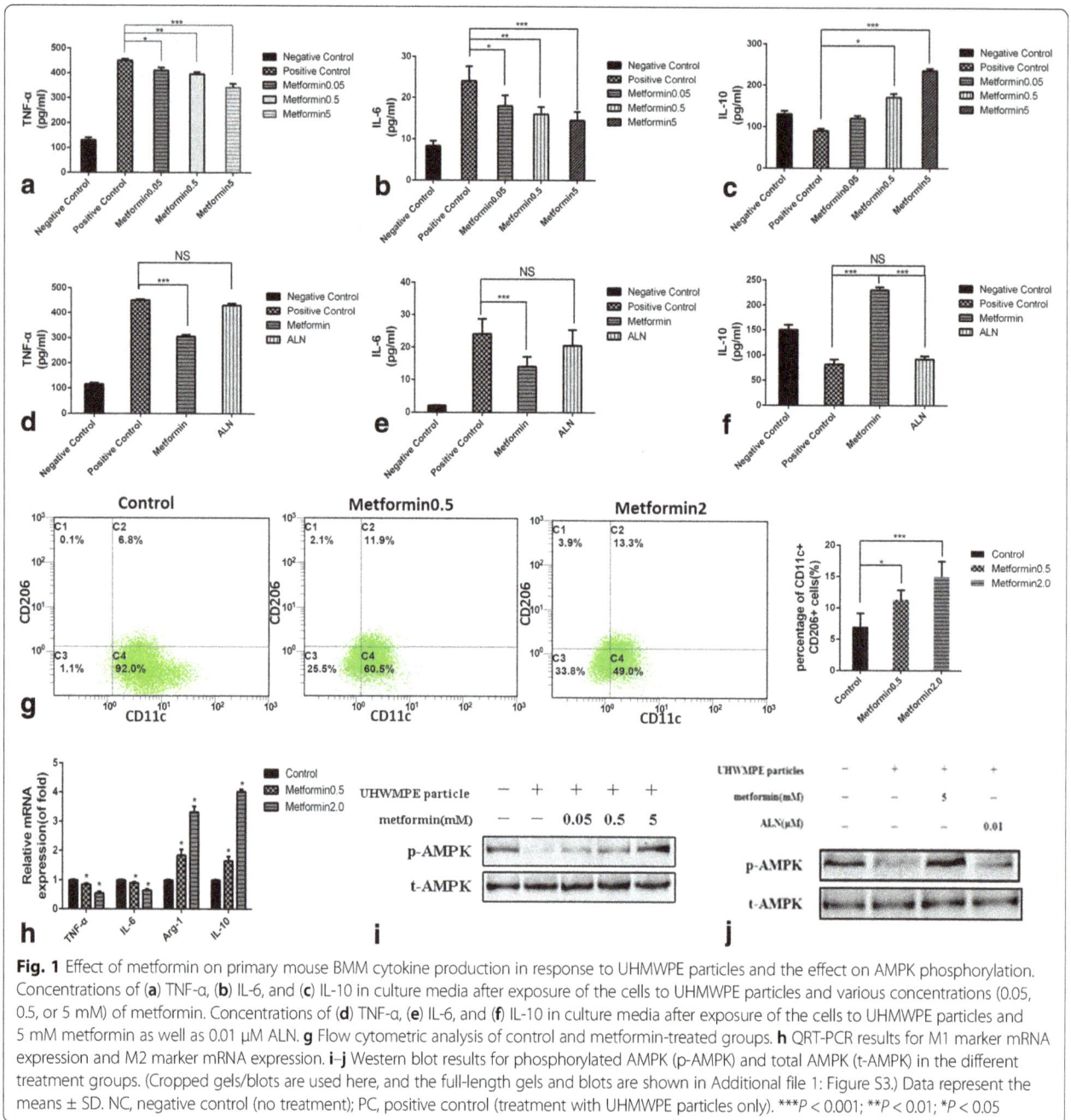

Fig. 1 Effect of metformin on primary mouse BMM cytokine production in response to UHMWPE particles and the effect on AMPK phosphorylation. Concentrations of (a) TNF-α, (b) IL-6, and (c) IL-10 in culture media after exposure of the cells to UHMWPE particles and various concentrations (0.05, 0.5, or 5 mM) of metformin. Concentrations of (d) TNF-α, (e) IL-6, and (f) IL-10 in culture media after exposure of the cells to UHMWPE particles and 5 mM metformin as well as 0.01 μM ALN. g Flow cytometric analysis of control and metformin-treated groups. h QRT-PCR results for M1 marker mRNA expression and M2 marker mRNA expression. i–j Western blot results for phosphorylated AMPK (p-AMPK) and total AMPK (t-AMPK) in the different treatment groups. (Cropped gels/blots are used here, and the full-length gels and blots are shown in Additional file 1: Figure S3.) Data represent the means ± SD. NC, negative control (no treatment); PC, positive control (treatment with UHMWPE particles only). ***P < 0.001; **P < 0.01; *P < 0.05

the M2 phenotype upon treatment with UHMWPE particles and metformin (Fig. 1g). QRT-PCR results also showed reduced M1 marker mRNA expression and increased M2 marker mRNA expression (Fig. 1h).

Role of AMPK activation in the effect of metformin on the exposed primary mouse BMMs

Metformin inhibition of inflammatory cytokine by lipopolysaccharide (LPS)-treated macrophages depended on the AMPK phosphorylation (Musi et al. 2002; Tsoyi et al. 2011). Whether AMPK activation played a role in the effect of metformin on cytokine release by primary mouse

BMMs exposed to UHMWPE particles was examined. Immunoblot analysis demonstrated negative regulation of phosphorylated AMPK with particle exposure, whereas the expression of total AMPK was not significantly altered upon exposure to the particles (Fig. 1i). The inhibition of AMPK phosphorylation in primary mouse BMMs with particles was recovered by metformin also in a dose-dependent manner. This effect was similar to that observed in relation to cytokine release. However, AMPK phosphorylation was not affected by ALN (Fig. 1j). Metformin thus stimulated the activation of AMPK in macrophages exposed to UHMWPE particles.

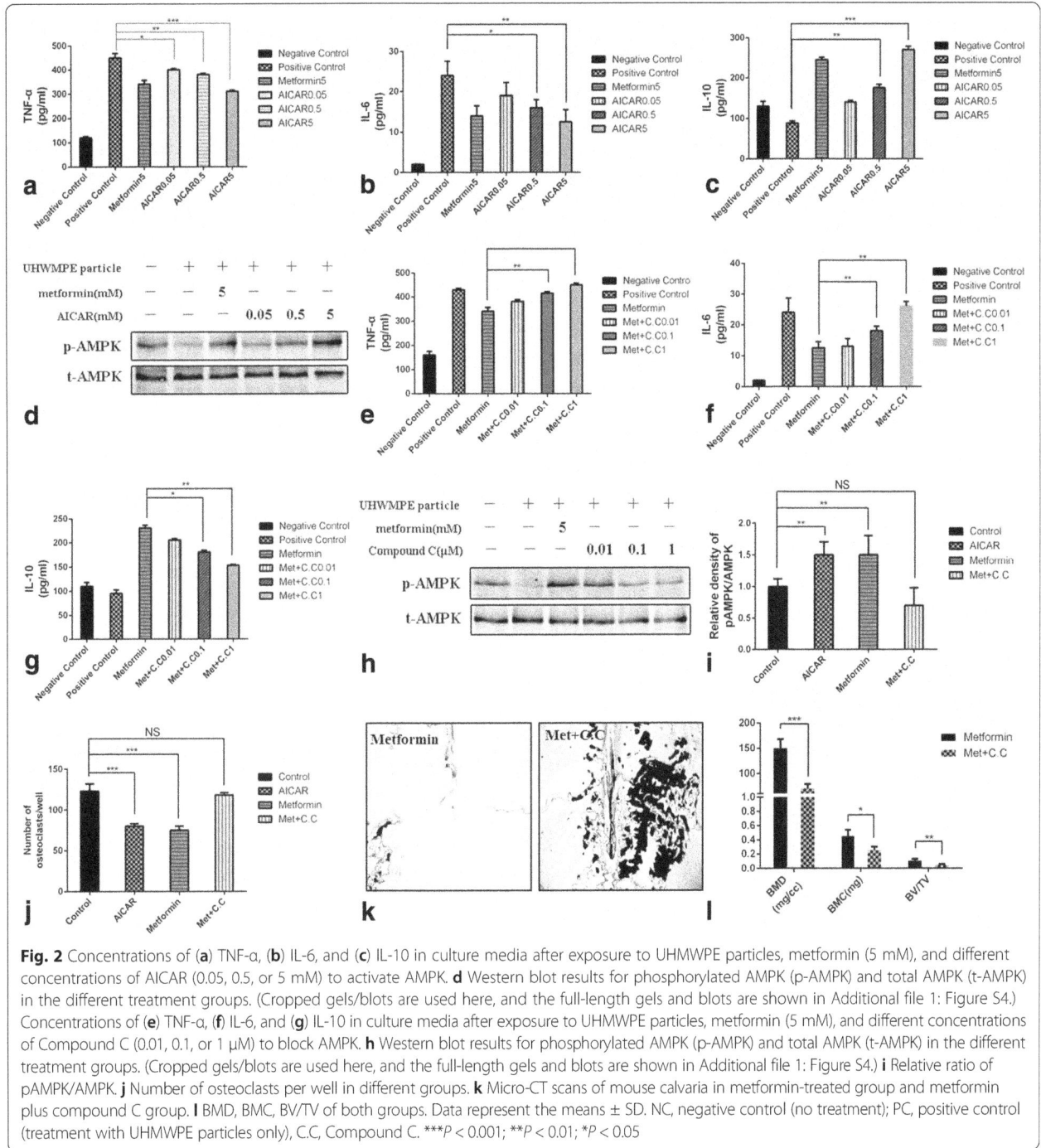

Fig. 2 Concentrations of (**a**) TNF-α, (**b**) IL-6, and (**c**) IL-10 in culture media after exposure to UHMWPE particles, metformin (5 mM), and different concentrations of AICAR (0.05, 0.5, or 5 mM) to activate AMPK. **d** Western blot results for phosphorylated AMPK (p-AMPK) and total AMPK (t-AMPK) in the different treatment groups. (Cropped gels/blots are used here, and the full-length gels and blots are shown in Additional file 1: Figure S4.) Concentrations of (**e**) TNF-α, (**f**) IL-6, and (**g**) IL-10 in culture media after exposure to UHMWPE particles, metformin (5 mM), and different concentrations of Compound C (0.01, 0.1, or 1 μM) to block AMPK. **h** Western blot results for phosphorylated AMPK (p-AMPK) and total AMPK (t-AMPK) in the different treatment groups. (Cropped gels/blots are used here, and the full-length gels and blots are shown in Additional file 1: Figure S4.) **i** Relative ratio of pAMPK/AMPK. **j** Number of osteoclasts per well in different groups. **k** Micro-CT scans of mouse calvaria in metformin-treated group and metformin plus compound C group. **l** BMD, BMC, BV/TV of both groups. Data represent the means ± SD. NC, negative control (no treatment); PC, positive control (treatment with UHMWPE particles only), C.C, Compound C. ***P < 0.001; **P < 0.01; *P < 0.05

To investigate the dependence of cytokine production on AMPK activation by metformin, primary mouse BMMs were treated with AICAR to induce AMPK activation. In the same culture conditions, AICAR inhibited the particle-induced increases in TNF-α and IL-6 production and promoted IL-10 release in a concentration-dependent manner (Fig. 2a–c). Furthermore, as expected, AICAR treatment was associated with increased AMPK phosphorylation in a dose-dependent manner.

The changes in AMPK phosphorylation with AICAR treatment mirrored those observed with metformin treatment (Fig. 2d). AMPK was blocked next using compound C as a chemical inhibitor (Li et al. 2015). Compound C not only limited the AMPK phosphorylation in a concentration-dependent manner, but clearly neutralized the effect of metformin on cytokine production (Fig. 2e–h). The effect of metformin on cytokine release, thus, was highly related to AMPK activation in primary mouse BMMs exposed to the particles. We next examined the effects of metformin on osteoclastic differentiation. Primary mouse BMMs were treated with PBS, metformin, AICAR, or metformin plus compound C and then stimulated with soluble recombinant RANKL (100 ng/ml) and M-CSF (30 ng/ml). After 7 days, we observed elevated pAMPK activity in the metformin- and AICAR-treated groups (Fig. 2i). Similarly, we observed reduced OC numbers in these two groups (Fig. 2j). Therefore, we inferred that metformin inhibited the differentiation of BMMs into osteoclasts by activating AMPK phosphorylation.

We also investigated in vitro cytokine production by RAW246.7 cells exposed to UHMWPE particles and treated with metformin at different concentrations with or without 5-aminoimidazole-4-carboxamide ribonucleoside to activate or inhibit AMPK (see Additional file 1: Supporting Information S2 and Figure S2). Similar results were obtained, which confirmed the influence of metformin.

Metformin attenuated particle-induced mouse calvarial osteolysis without changing the blood glucose level

Mouse calvaria harvested 14 days after surgical implantation of UHMWPE particles were qualitatively and quantitatively analyzed by micro-CT (Fig. 3). The low signal area represents the sagittal suture area with neighboring bone resorption. Four groups were used to investigate the metformin effect. The area of bone resorption observed following implantation of the UHMWPE particles was reduced by treatment with metformin and ALN compared with that in mice that received no further treatment (Fig. 3a). From 3D reconstruction imaging, bone quantity and quality were evaluated according to the BMD, BMC, and BV/TV of ROIs (Fig. 3b). All three parameters were the lowest in the mice calvaria implanted with UHMWPE particles and given no further treatment, and the bone resorption reaction was evident. With daily metformin or ALN treatment, the BMD, BMC, and BV/TV of the calvaria were higher than those without additional treatment following particle implantation, whereas no significant differences were observed between the groups treated with metformin and ALN (Fig. 3c–e). At the same time, the metformin-treated group exhibited an age-related reduction in body mass but a stable glucose level compared with the control group (Fig. 3f–g).

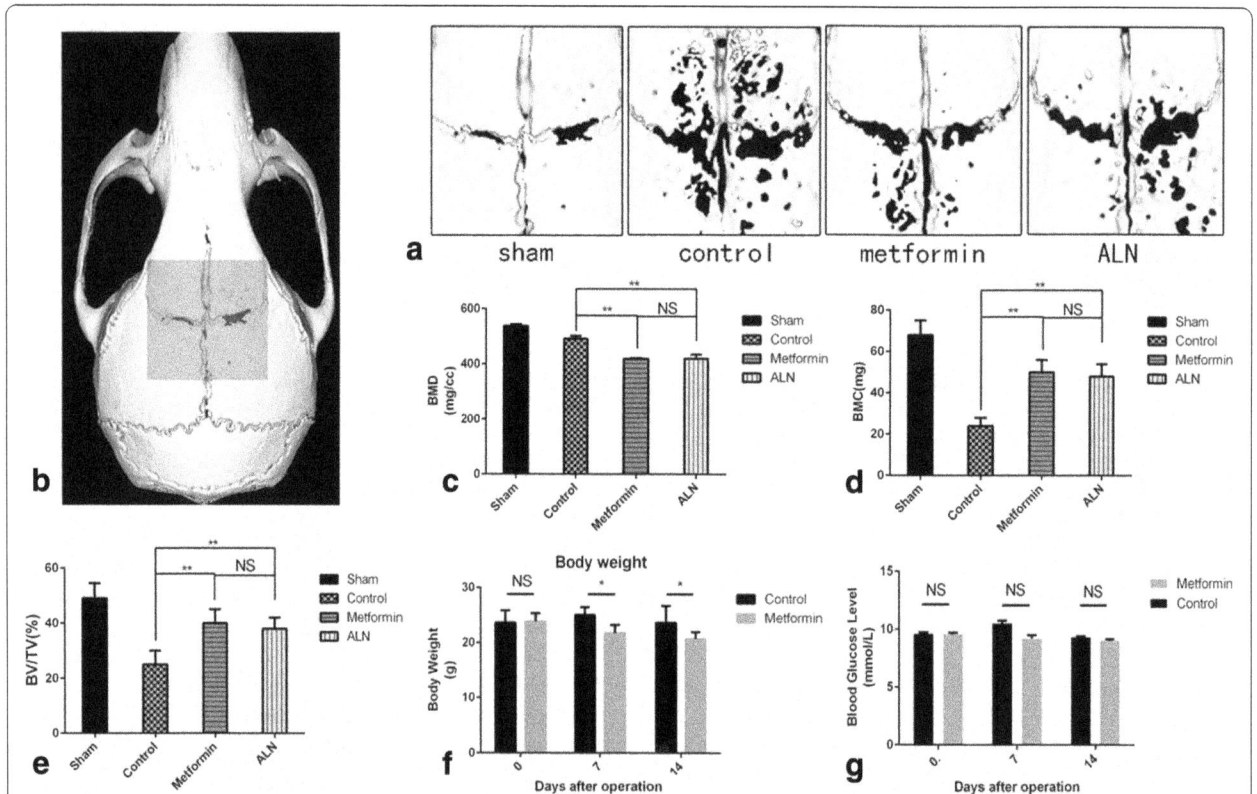

Fig. 3 Metformin attenuated particle-induced mouse calvarial osteolysis without changing the blood glucose level. **a** Three-dimensional images from micro-CT scans of mouse calvaria, showing evidence of resorption pits along the suture lines in mice in which UHMWPE particles were implanted in comparison with representative images from the metformin- and ALN-treated groups. **b** ROI selected for quantitative analysis of BMD (**c**), BMC (**d**), and BV/TV (**e**) in each group. **f** Changes in body weight after operation at days 0, 7 and 14. **g** Comparison of blood glucose levels between groups ***$P < 0.001$; **$P < 0.01$; *$P < 0.05$; NS, not significant, $P > 0.05$

Metformin inhibited particle-induced osteoclastogenesis in association with a reduction in the expression of osteoclastic genes

After particle implantation, histological staining of the harvested calvaria revealed an intense inflammatory infiltrate associated with osteolysis. Infiltrate resulting from an intense inflammatory response was revealed by histological staining of harvested calvaria with implanted particles. Fig. 4a shows the H&E stained tissue sections of the sham group. The osteolysis and fibrous tissue laden with the particles were observed in the H&E stained tissue sections (Fig. 4b). The histomorphometric data also suggested that the suture and osteolysis area increased from 0.082 ± 0.012 (sham group) to 0.406 ± 0.080 mm^2 (particle-implanted group; $P < 0.01$) after particle implantation. The inflammation area decreased to 0.117 ± 0.010 mm^2 with metformin treatment ($P < 0.01$) and 0.117 ± 0.010 mm^2 with ALN treatment ($P < 0.01$; Fig. 4c, d). Via TRAP staining, osteoclasts were identified in the cytoplasm of multinuclear giant cells as purplish to dark red granules. TRAP staining confirmed the presence

of osteoclasts in resorptive lacunae (Fig. 4e–h). Bone histomorphometric analysis showed reduced bone volume, bone surface area and increased erosion area in the control group. Metformin treatment reversed these changes (Fig. 4i–j, l). In the metformin- and ALN-treated groups, the mean numbers of osteoclasts per section (12.80 ± 3.03 and 18.60 ± 2.07, respectively) were significantly less than that in the particle-implantation group (22.7 ± 5.0, $P < 0.01$; Fig. 4k). One-way ANOVA revealed that the osteolysis area or the average number of osteoclasts were almost the same between the metformin- and ALN-treated groups. A considerable increase in the expression of osteoclastic genes in the metformin- and ALN-treated groups was observed (Fig. 4m). Immunohistochemical staining for CD11b showed more positive cells in the control group than in the metformin-treated group (Fig. 4n–o). Overall, the variation in osteolysis observed in the two-dimensional histological analysis was consistent with that observed by micro-CT, suggesting that metformin treatment decreased the osteolysis induced by the particles.

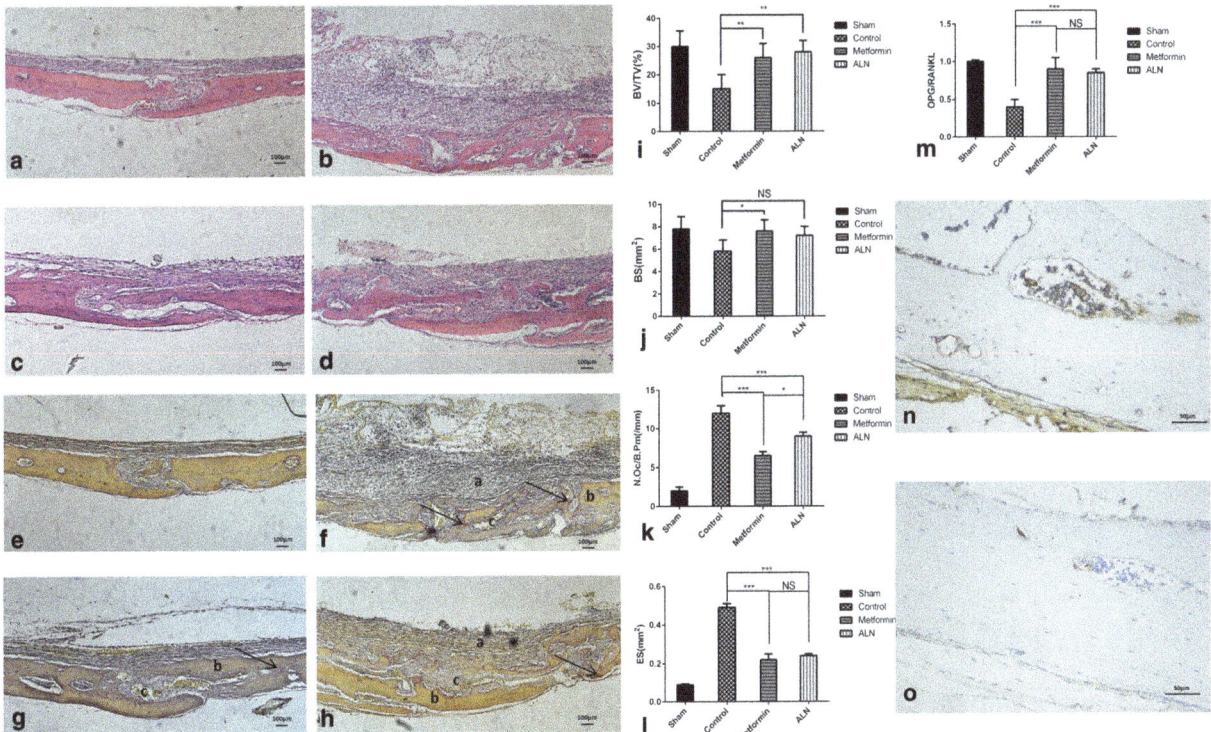

Fig. 4 Representative images of histological sections of harvested calvaria for evaluation of inflammatory infiltration and associated osteolysis after implantation of UHMWPE particles. Compared to the sham control group (a), inflammatory infiltrate and osteolysis was observed in calvaria implanted with UHMWPE particles (b). The inflammatory response was suppressed by treatment with metformin (c) or ALN (d). Representative images of TRAP staining of mouse calvarial tissue from the different groups (e–h). a, inflammatory tissue, b, bone tissue, c, erosion area, arrow, osteoclasts. Quantitated bone histomorphometric analysis including BV/TV (i), bone surface area (j), average numbers of osteoclasts (k), and erosion surface area (l). m Expression of osteoclastic genes. Immunohistochemical staining for CD11b in control (n) and metformin-treated groups (o). Data are presented as means ± SD. ***$P < 0.001$; **$P < 0.01$; *$P < 0.05$; NS, $P > 0.05$

Metformin inhibited UHMWPE particle-induced osteoclastogenenic cytokine production in vivo

To study the mechanisms of the inhibitory effect of metformin on particle-induced osteolysis, the ability of metformin to suppress osteoclastogenic cytokine production induced by particle implantation was examined. The qRT-PCR results showed that particle implantation stimulated IL-6, TNF-α, and RANKL mRNA expression and suppressed IL-10 mRNA expression in calvaria. However, both metformin and ALN treatment inhibited these effects on cytokine production. Metformin presented potent effects on inflammatory cytokine release, whereas

ALN strongly inhibited RANKL expression as compared to controls ($P = 0.047$; Fig. 5a, c, e, g). Analysis of the cytokine production in organ culture suggested that TNF-α, IL-6, and RANKL production were greatly increased upon exposure to particles. However, metformin and ALN treatment again significantly suppressed the particle's effect on osteoclastogenic cytokine production. In addition, metformin treatment increased release of IL-10, whereas IL-10 secretion remained considerably lower in the ALN-treated group ($P = 0.002$ and $P = 0.002$, respectively; Fig. 5b, d, f, h). Consistent with the results of qRT-PCR, the results of calvaria culture also suggested that

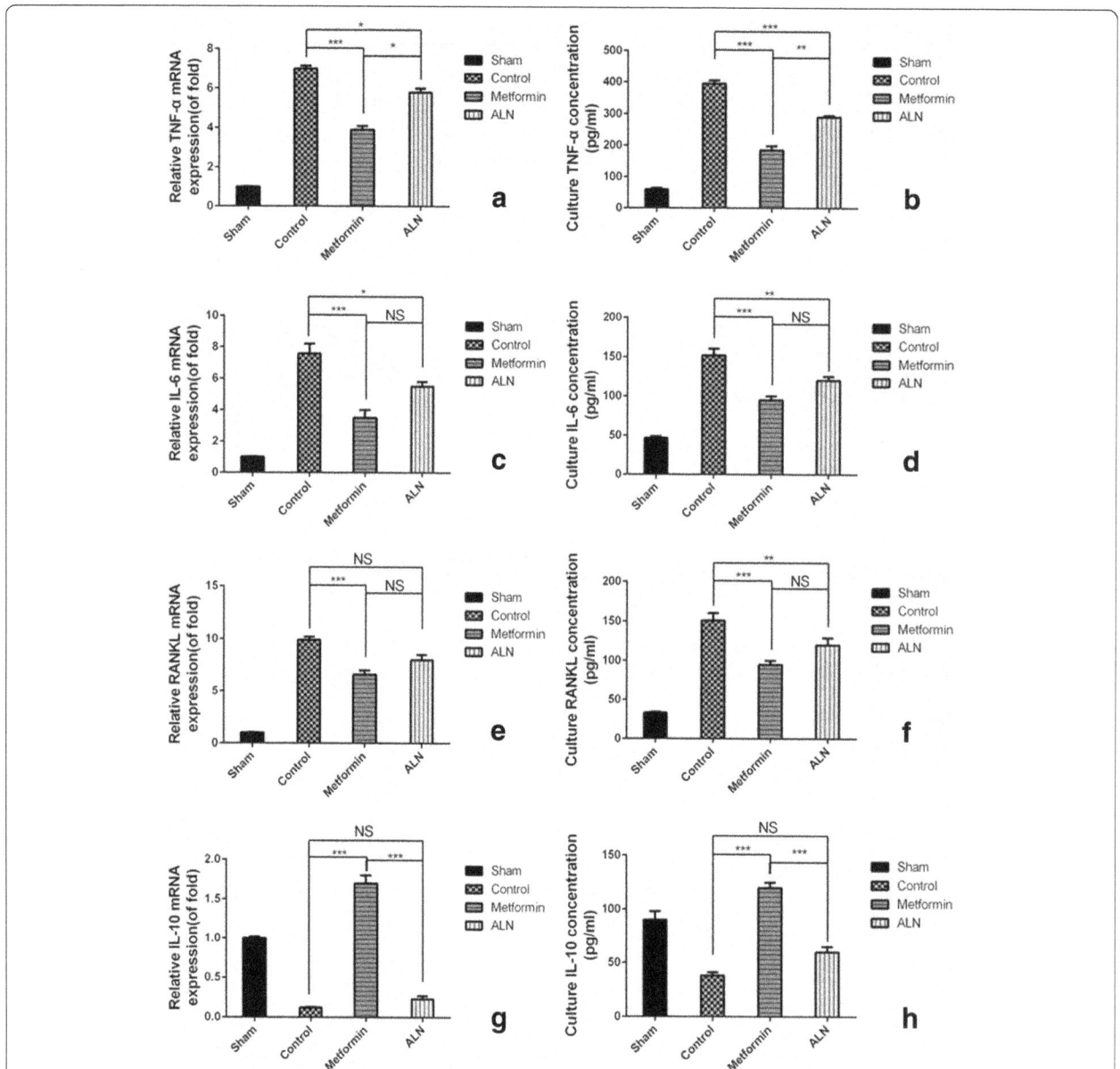

Fig. 5 mRNA expression and secretion of cytokines by mouse calvarial tissue after implantation of UHMWPE particles and treatment with saline (control), metformin, or ALN. Relative (to that in the sham group) expression of TNF-α, IL-6, RANKL, and IL-10 (**a, c, e, g**, respectively) and secretion of TNF-α, IL-6, RANKL, and IL-10 (**b, d, f, h**, respectively) among the different treatment groups. ***$P < 0.001$; **$P < 0.01$; *$P < 0.05$; NS, $P > 0.05$

that metformin had a potent effect on inflammatory cytokine production.

Inhibitory effect of metformin on mouse calvarial osteolysis is dependent on promotion of macrophage polarization to M2 phenotype by AMPK activation

To determine whether metformin could promote macrophage polarization to an anti-inflammatory phenotype from a pro-inflammatory phenotype via AMPK activation, the effect of metformin on the expression of proteins related to macrophage functional phenotypes was investigated. The qRT-PCR results showed that particle implantation stimulated COX-2 and iNOs mRNA expression in calvaria (Fig. 6a–b). However, both metformin and ALN treatment inhibited these effects. Western blot analysis indicated that particle implantation caused increased expression of COX-2 from a relative expression ratio (relative to expression in the control group) of 0.594 to 1 and iNOS from 0.156 to 1, while metformin reduced the respective protein expression ratios from 1 and 0.799 to 1 and 0.308 (Fig. 6d). The increased COX-2 expression can be induced by inflammatory cytokines, and iNOS is expressed by M1 macrophages (Minghetti 2007). These results suggest that metformin inhibited the inflammation induced upon particle implantation in the mouse calvarial model. The qRT-PCR results and Western blot analysis also showed that metformin increased the expression of Arg-1, which is usually expressed by M2 macrophages (Fig. 6c–d). Moreover, the effect of metformin on the expression of proteins related to macrophage functional

phenotypes depended on AMPK activation, as demonstrated by the increased expression of anti-inflammatory cytokines and the changes in the expression of phosphorylated AMPK. Double-labelling immunofluorescence of p-AMPK and CD68 showed more pAMPK and less CD68 positive cells in the metformin-treated group (Fig. 6e–f). These data imply that metformin inhibited mouse calvarial osteolysis by promoting macrophage polarization to the M2 phenotype via AMPK activation.

Discussion

Osteolysis around orthopedic implants can develop via the formation of an inflamed periprosthetic membrane containing high levels of inflammatory cytokines, macrophages, and implant wear debris. Implant-derived wear particles can induce a unique immune response based on the particle size and concentration. The chemotactic cytokines secreted in response to UHMWPE particles can activate macrophages located in the tissues surrounding joint replacements (Frokjaer et al. 1995), creating an environment conducive to osteoclastogenesis and osteolysis. Bone marrow-derived macrophages may play dual roles in the osteolysis associated with TJA. One role is as the major cell type responsible for cytokine production in the host defense against UHMWPE particles, and the other is as the precursor cells for osteoclasts responsible for subsequent bone resorption. An additional study reported that the immune response to UHMWPE wear particles is characterized by cells of monocytic or osteoclastogenic lineage (Ren et al. 2011).

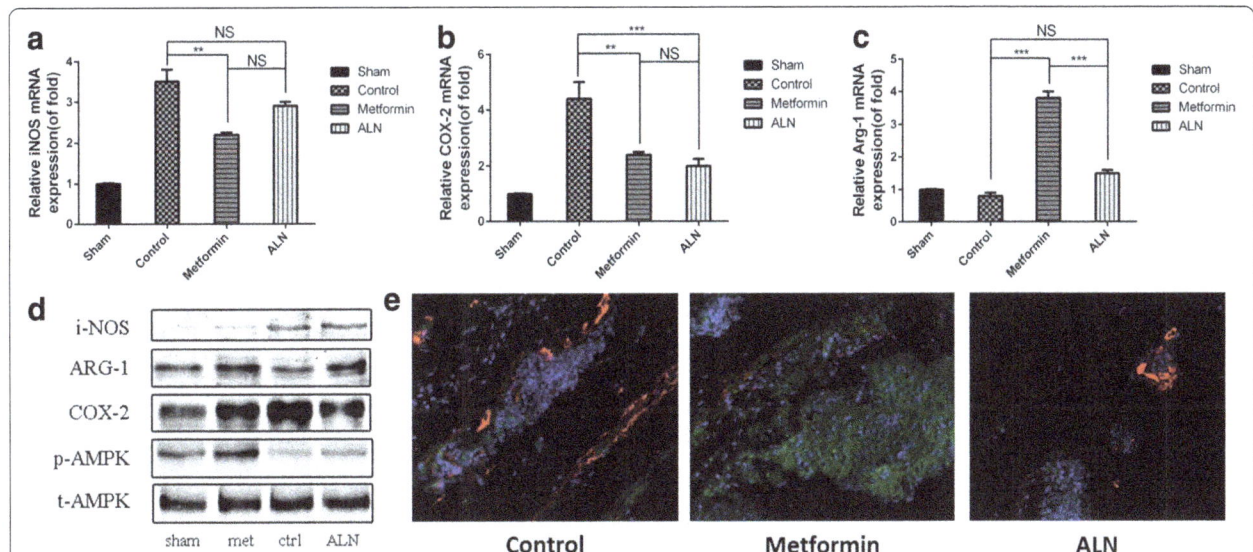

Fig. 6 mRNA expression of proteins associated with macrophage phenotype and changes of protein expression according to western blot analysis in mouse calvarial tissue after implantation of UHMWPE particles and treatment with saline (control), metformin, or ALN. Relative mRNA expression of iNOS (a), COX-2 (b), and Arg-1 (c) among tissues from the different groups. d Protein expression of iNOS, COX-2, Arg-1, p-AMPK, and t-AMPK among tissues from the different treatment groups. e Double-labelling immunofluorescence of p-AMPK (green) and macrophage marker CD68 (red) in control group, metformin-treated group and ALN-treated group. (Cropped gels/blots are used here, and the full-length gels and blots are shown in Additional file 1: Figure S5.) ***$P < 0.001$; **$P < 0.01$; *$P < 0.05$; NS, $P > 0.05$

Macrophages produce varied arrays of mediators with pro- and anti-inflammatory capabilities in response to different tissue environments or stimuli (Malyshev and Malyshev 2015; Martinez et al. 2008). Macrophages expressing a pro-inflammatory versus an anti-inflammatory functional profile are distinguished using the designations M1 and M2 (Davies and Taylor 2015) . IL-10 is a regulating factor in macrophage polarization that inhibits the UHMWPE particle-induced increase in phospho-STAT1 and phospho-nuclear factor (NF)-κB p65 production and promotes phospho-STAT3 expression (Jiang et al. 2016). Therefore, manipulation of macrophage functional phenotypes can represent a potential therapeutic target for some diseases (Singh et al. 2014).

The AMPK pathway has emerged recently as a critical sensing mechanism in regulating cellular energy homeostasis and maintaining normal bone physiology (Patel et al. 2015; Wang et al. 2016). The bone mass in mice is decreased with deletion of the α or β subunit of AMPK (Shah et al. 2010; Quinn et al. 2010). Activation of AMPK stimulates bone formation in vitro (Kanazawa et al. 2008; Wang et al. 2016) and negatively regulates RANKL expression in the differentiation of osteoclasts (Kang et al. 2013). In addition, AMPK can promote macrophage polarization to an anti-inflammatory functional phenotype (Sag et al. 2008). Many studies have reported that AMPK phosphorylation was reduced in cells under the condition of inflammation or exposed to cytokines such as TNF-α (Vasamsetti et al. 2015). Activation of macrophages by UHMWPE particles induced inflammation and secretion of TNF-α, which reduced AMPK phosphorylation. Metformin has been discovered as a potent AMPK agonist that can suppress inflammatory cytokine production and osteoclast activation. Therefore, we hypothesized that it may be an effective drug against osteolysis induced by particles representing implant wear debris.

The effects of metformin on UHMWPE particle-induced production of inflammatory cytokines by primary mouse BMMs in vitro were examined. Incubation with the particles increased IL-6 and TNF-α production. Metformin not only inhibited the elevated production of IL-6 and TNF-α induced by UHMWPE particles, but promoted the release of the anti-inflammatory cytokine IL-10 and shifted polarization to M2 type in a dose-dependent manner. More importantly, the suppressed production of inflammatory cytokines was associated with phosphorylation of AMPK. Given the effects of metformin on both primary mouse BMMs and RAW264.7 cells as well as the fact that AMPK plays a significant role in the metabolism of both cell types, the results indicate that the effect of metformin on the production of macrophage-derived cytokines is dependent on AMPK activation.

Metformin attenuated the particle-induced mouse calvarial osteolysis, in association with a reduction in the severity of inflammation and osteoclast numbers. Consistent with in vitro results, activation of AMPK was involved in the protective effect of metformin against UHMWPE particle-induced osteolysis, via the promotion of macrophage polarization to an anti-inflammatory phenotype.

The anti-osteolysis effects of metformin and ALN as well-established leading drugs for treating osteoporosis (Black and Rosen 2016) show no significant difference, but their mechanisms are different. The classical pharmacological effects of ALNs are attributed to two key properties: the affinity for bone mineral and the ability to slow the activities of osteoclasts (Russell et al. 2008; Cantatore et al. 1999). Metformin, on the other hand, inhibited pro-inflammatory cytokine production, osteoclastogenesis, and osteolysis via the AMPK pathway. ALN cannot fundamentally inhibit osteolysis due to its limited capacity to inhibit the production of inflammatory cytokines and RANKL. For example, Zhang et al. (Zhang et al. 2005) reported that high local levels of TNF-α produced during periprosthetic inflammation prevented ALN-induced apoptosis among osteoclasts in vivo. Therefore, metformin should be more effective and useful than ALN in the treatment of periprosthetic osteolysis after TJA.

Oral administration of metformin hydrochloride (0.5–1.5 g) is routinely prescribed for the treatment of type II diabetes and has protective actions on the skeletal system (Monami et al. 2008; Hamann et al. 2012). According to our study, administration of 100 mg/kg metformin had a significant protective effect against the osteolysis induced by wear particles in the mouse calvarial osteolysis model. According to standard drug dose conversion between humans and animals, the dose of metformin used in this study is within the physiologically acceptable range. Since metformin can enhance insulin sensitivity and improve metabolic syndrome, it has been used not only for treating diabetes patients, but also for treating osteoporosis patients and individuals with metabolic syndromes barely affecting glucose levels. Many TJA patients are elderly and suffer from diabetes, which can cause osteoporosis (Voronov et al. 1998). Based on our results, we propose that long-term usage of metformin for treating type II diabetes might lessen the symptoms related to type II diabetes-related osteoporosis and offer some degree of protection against wear particle-derived periprosthetic osteolysis as well.

In summary, as shown in Fig. 7, metformin remarkably inhibited the UHMWPE particle-induced polarization of mouse macrophages to the M1 phenotype, which is pro-inflammatory and characterized by iNos expression as a

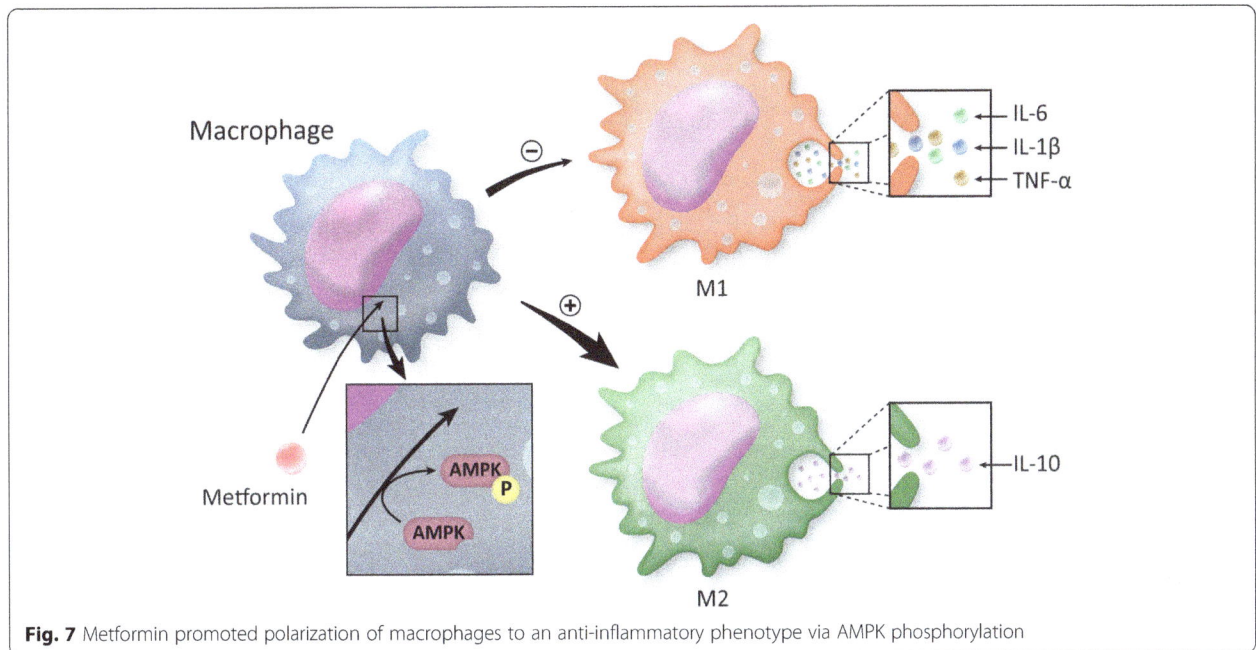

Fig. 7 Metformin promoted polarization of macrophages to an anti-inflammatory phenotype via AMPK phosphorylation

surface marker, and instead promoted the polarization of mouse macrophages to the M2 phenotype, which is anti-inflammatory and characterized by Arg-1 expression as a surface marker. As a result, the anti-diabetic drug inhibited the elevated production of IL-6 and TNF-α induced by UHMWPE particles and promoted the release of the anti-inflammatory cytokine IL-10 via the activation of AMPK in a dose-dependent manner. The results of the present study indicate that metformin inhibited the osteolysis in vivo induced by UHMWPE particles. These effects were found to be related to potent activation of AMPK.

The mechanism by which UHMWPE particles reduced the AMPK phosphorylation was not explored in our study, and the long-term effects of metformin administration on bone metabolism remain to be explored in our future experiments. Despite of the limitations of the present study, our work still indicates that metformin may represent a promising therapeutic agent for preventing or correcting periprosthetic osteolysis and implant loosening.

Conclusion

Periprosthetic osteolysis and aseptic loosening are considered as proof of wear debris-induced disruption of local regulatory mechanisms related to excessive bone resorption associated with osteolysis and the damage at the bone-prosthesis interface. A crucial point in limiting and correcting the periprosthetic osteolysis and aseptic loosening is the inhibition of inflammatory factor production and osteoclast activation induced by activated macrophages. Metformin could limit the osteolysis induced by implant debris. The ability of metformin to attenuate osteolysis induced in mouse calvaria by the particles was related to a reduction in osteoclast number and polarization of macrophages to an anti-inflammatory functional phenotype.

Additional file

Additional file 1: Supporting Information S1. Effects of Metformin on TNF-α, IL-6 and IL-10 production in RAW264.7. **Supporting Information S2.** Role of AMPK activation in the effect of metformin on the exposed in RAW264.7. **Supporting Information S3.** Characterizations. **Figure S1.** Effect of metformin on RAW264.7 cytokine production in response to UHMWPE particles and the effect on AMPK phosphorylation. **Figure S2.** Effect of metformin on RAW264.7 cytokine production with AICAR or Compound C in response to UHMWPE particles and the effect on AMPK phosphorylation. **Figure S3.** Full-length gels and blots of western blot results for phosphorylated AMPK (p-AMPK) and total AMPK (t-AMPK) in the different treatment groups. **Figure S4.** Full-length gels and blots of western blot results for phosphorylated AMPK (p-AMPK) and total AMPK (t-AMPK) in the different treatment groups with AICAR or Compound C. **Figure S5.** Full-length gels and blots of protein expression of iNOS, COX-2, Arg-1, p-AMPK, and t-AMPK among tissues from the different treatment groups. (DOC 1902 kb)

Acknowledgments
This work was supported by the Project of Natural Science Foundation of Shaanxi Province (2014JQ4142) and the National Natural Science Foundation of China (81501936) and (31571215). The authors thank Xiaorui Cao and Qingsheng Zhu from the PLA Institute of Orthopaedics, Xijing Hospital, and the Fourth Military Medical University, China as well as Zifan Lu of the State Key Laboratory of Cancer Biology, Fourth Military Medical University, China, for their technical help and advice.

Authors' contributions

ZY, XC and QZ wrote the main manuscript text; XT, JZ and ZL contributed to the design the experiments. ZY and LY performed all the experiments. DZ, YL and CY prepared Figs. 1, 2, 3, 4, 5 and 6. ZY designed Fig. 7. All authors reviewed the manuscript. All authors read and approved the final manuscript.

Competing interests

The authors declare they have no competing interests as defined by Molecular Medicine, or other interests that might be perceived to influence the results and discussion reported in this paper.

Author details

[1]PLA Institute of Orthopaedics, Xijing Hospital, Fourth Military Medical University, Xi'an 710032, China. [2]Emergency department of Tangdu Hospital, Fourth Military Medical University, Xi'an 710038, China. [3]State Key Laboratory of Cancer Biology, Department of Pharmacogenomics, Fourth Military Medical University, Xi'an 710032, China.

References

Atkins GJ, Welldon KJ, Holding CA, Haynes DR, Howie DW, Findlay DM. The induction of a catabolic phenotype in human primary osteoblasts and osteocytes by polyethylene particles. Biomaterials. 2009;30:3672–81.

Black DM, Rosen CJ. Clinical Practice. Postmenopausal Osteoporosis. N Engl J Med. 2016;374:254–62.

Cantatore FP, Acquista CA, Pipitone V. Evaluation of bone turnover and osteoclastic cytokines in early rheumatoid arthritis treated with alendronate. J Rheumatol. 1999;26:2318–23.

Davies LC, Taylor PR. Tissue-resident macrophages: then and now. Immunology. 2015;144:541–8.

Frokjaer J, Deleuran B, Lind M, Overgaard S, Soballe K, Bunger C. Polyethylene particles stimulate monocyte chemotactic and activating factor production in synovial mononuclear cells in vivo. An immunohistochemical study in rabbits. Acta Orthop Scand. 1995;66:303–7.

Glant TT, Jacobs JJ, Molnar G, Shanbhag AS, Valyon M, Galante JO. Bone resorption activity of particulate-stimulated macrophages. J Bone Miner Res. 1993;8:1071–9.

Hamann C, Kirschner S, Gunther KP, Hofbauer LC. Bone, sweet bone—osteoporotic fractures in diabetes mellitus. Nat Rev Endocrinol. 2012;8:297–305.

Inzucchi SE, Lipska KJ, Mayo H, Bailey CJ, McGuire DK. Metformin in patients with type 2 diabetes and kidney disease: a systematic review. JAMA. 2014;312:2668–75.

Jiang J, Jia T, Gong W, Ning B, Wooley PH, Yang SY. Macrophage polarization in IL-10 treatment of particle-induced inflammation and Osteolysis. Am J Pathol. 2016;186:57–66.

Kanazawa I, Yamaguchi T, Yano S, Yamauchi M, Sugimoto T. Metformin enhances the differentiation and mineralization of osteoblastic MC3T3-E1 cells via AMP kinase activation as well as eNOS and BMP-2 expression. Biochem Biophys Res Commun. 2008;375:414–9.

Kang H, Viollet B, Wu D. Genetic deletion of catalytic subunits of AMP-activated protein kinase increases osteoclasts and reduces bone mass in young adult mice. J Biol Chem. 2013;288:12187–96.

Kostenuik PJ, Smith SY, Samadfam R, Jolette J, Zhou L, Ominsky MS. Effects of denosumab, alendronate, or denosumab following alendronate on bone turnover, calcium homeostasis, bone mass and bone strength in ovariectomized cynomolgus monkeys. J Bone Miner Res. 2015;30:657–69.

Kudo N, Barr AJ, Barr RL, Desai S, Lopaschuk GD. High rates of fatty acid oxidation during reperfusion of ischemic hearts are associated with a decrease in malonyl-CoA levels due to an increase in 5'-AMP-activated protein kinase inhibition of acetyl-CoA carboxylase. J Biol Chem. 1995;270:17513–20.

Kurtz S, Ong K, Lau E, Mowat F, Halpern M. Projections of primary and revision hip and knee arthroplasty in the United States from 2005 to 2030. J Bone Joint Surg Am. 2007;89:780–5.

La Fontaine J, Chen C, Hunt N, Jude E, Lavery L. Type 2 diabetes and metformin influence on fracture healing in an experimental rat model. J Foot Ankle Surg. 2016;55:955–60.

Lee YS, Kim YS, Lee SY, Kim GH, Kim BJ, Lee SH, Lee KU, Kim GS, Kim SW, Koh JM. AMP kinase acts as a negative regulator of RANKL in the differentiation of osteoclasts. Bone. 2010;47:926–37.

Li DJ, Huang F, Lu WJ, Jiang GJ, Deng YP, Shen FM. Metformin promotes irisin release from murine skeletal muscle independently of AMP-activated protein kinase activation. Acta Physiol (Oxf). 2015;213:711–21.

Malyshev I, Malyshev Y. Current concept and update of the macrophage plasticity concept: intracellular mechanisms of reprogramming and M3 macrophage "switch" phenotype. Biomed Res Int. 2015;2015:341308.

Martinez FO, Sica A, Mantovani A, Locati M. Macrophage activation and polarization. Front Biosci. 2008;13:453–61.

Minghetti L. Role of COX-2 in inflammatory and degenerative brain diseases. Subcell Biochem. 2007;42:127–41.

Monami M, Cresci B, Colombini A, Pala L, Balzi D, Gori F, Chiasserini V, Marchionni N, Rotella CM, Mannucci E. Bone fractures and hypoglycemic treatment in type 2 diabetic patients: a case-control study. Diabetes Care. 2008;31:199–203.

Musi N, Hirshman MF, Nygren J, Svanfeldt M, Bavenholm P, Rooyackers O, Zhou G, Williamson JM, Ljunqvist O, Efendic S, Moller DE, Thorell A, Goodyear LJ. Metformin increases AMP-activated protein kinase activity in skeletal muscle of subjects with type 2 diabetes. Diabetes. 2002;51:2074–81.

Nich C, Langlois J, Marchadier A, Vidal C, Cohen-Solal M, Petite H, Hamadouche M. Oestrogen deficiency modulates particle-induced osteolysis. Arthritis Res Ther. 2011;13:R100.

Patel VA, Massenburg D, Vujicic S, Feng L, Tang M, Litbarg N, Antoni A, Rauch J, Lieberthal W, Levine JS. Apoptotic cells activate AMP-activated protein kinase (AMPK) and inhibit epithelial cell growth without change in intracellular energy stores. J Biol Chem. 2015;290:22352–69.

Purdue PE, Koulouvaris P, Nestor BJ, Sculco TP. The central role of wear debris in periprosthetic osteolysis. HSS J. 2006;2:102–13.

Quinn JM, Tam S, Sims NA, Saleh H, McGregor NE, Poulton IJ, Scott JW, Gillespie MT, Kemp BE, van Denderen BJ. Germline deletion of AMP-activated protein kinase beta subunits reduces bone mass without altering osteoclast differentiation or function. FASEB J. 2010;24:275–85.

Ren PG, Irani A, Huang Z, Ma T, Biswal S, Goodman SB. Continuous infusion of UHMWPE particles induces increased bone macrophages and osteolysis. Clin Orthop Relat Res. 2011;469:113–22.

Russell RG, Watts NB, Ebetino FH, Rogers MJ. Mechanisms of action of bisphosphonates: similarities and differences and their potential influence on clinical efficacy. Osteoporos Int. 2008;19:733–59.

Sag D, Carling D, Stout RD, Suttles J. Adenosine 5'-monophosphate-activated protein kinase promotes macrophage polarization to an anti-inflammatory functional phenotype. J Immunol. 2008;181:8633–41.

Shah M, Kola B, Bataveljic A, Arnett TR, Viollet B, Saxon L, Korbonits M, Chenu C. AMP-activated protein kinase (AMPK) activation regulates in vitro bone formation and bone mass. Bone. 2010;47:309–19.

Singh A, Talekar M, Raikar A, Amiji M. Macrophage-targeted delivery systems for nucleic acid therapy of inflammatory diseases. J Control Release. 2014;190:515–30.

Tsoyi K, Jang HJ, Nizamutdinova IT, Kim YM, Lee YS, Kim HJ, Seo HG, Lee JH, Chang KC. Metformin inhibits HMGB1 release in LPS-treated RAW 264.7 cells and increases survival rate of endotoxaemic mice. Br J Pharmacol. 2011;162:1498–508.

Vasamsetti SB, Karnewar S, Kanugula AK, Thatipalli AR, Kumar JM, Kotamraju S. Metformin inhibits monocyte-to-macrophage differentiation via AMPK-mediated inhibition of STAT3 activation: potential role in atherosclerosis. Diabetes. 2015;64:2028–41.

Voronov I, Santerre JP, Hinek A, Callahan JW, Sandhu J, Boynton EL. Macrophage phagocytosis of polyethylene particulate in vitro. J Biomed Mater Res. 1998;39:40–51.

Wang YG, Qu XH, Yang Y, Han XG, Wang L, Qiao H, Fan QM, Tang TT, Dai KR. AMPK promotes osteogenesis and inhibits adipogenesis through AMPK-Gfi1-OPN axis. Cell Signal. 2016;28:1270–82.

Zhang Q, Badell IR, Schwarz EM, Boulukos KE, Yao Z, Boyce BF, Xing L. Tumor necrosis factor prevents alendronate-induced osteoclast apoptosis in vivo by stimulating Bcl-xL expression through Ets-2. Arthritis Rheum. 2005;52:2708–18.

2

Reversal of angiotensin II-induced β-cell dedifferentiation via inhibition of NF-κb signaling

Hong Chen[1†], Wenjun Zhou[1†], Yuting Ruan[1], Lei Yang[2], Ningning Xu[1], Rongping Chen[1], Rui Yang[1], Jia Sun[1*] and Zhen Zhang[1*] 🅾

Abstract

Background: Type 2 diabetes mellitus (T2DM) is characterized by pancreatic β-cell failure, which arises from metabolic stress and results in β cell dedifferentiation, leading to β-cell death. Pathological activation of the renin–angiotensin system (RAS) contributes to increase cell stress, while RAS intervention reduces the onset of T2DM in high-risk populations and promotes insulin secretion in rodents. In this study, we investigated whether and how RAS induces β-cell dedifferentiation and the mechanism underlying this process.

Methods: In vitro, with the methods of quantitative real-time reverse transcriptase-PCR (qRT-PCR) and western blotting, we examined the change of cell identity-related gene expression, progenitor like gene expression, cellular function, and nuclear factor kappa b (NF-κb) signaling activity in β cell lines after exposure to angiotensin II (AngII) and disruption of RAS. In vivo, parallel studies were performed using db/db mice. Related protein expression was detected by Immunofluorescence analysis.

Result: Activation of RAS induced dedifferentiation and impaired insulin secretion, eventually leading to β-cell failure. Mechanistically, AngII induced β-cell dedifferentiation via NF-κb signaling, while treatment with Irbesartan and sc-514 reversed the progenitor state of β cells.

Conclusion: The present study found that RAS might induce β-cell dedifferentiation via angiotensin II receptor type 1 activation, which was promoted by NF-κb signaling. Therefore, blocking RAS or NF-κb signaling efficiently reversed the dedifferentiated status of β cells, suggesting a potential therapy for patients with type 2 diabetes.

Keywords: β-Cell dedifferentiation, Renin-angiotensin system, Angiotensin II, Type 2 diabetes, NF-κb

Background

Pancreatic β-cell failure underlies the progressive development of type 2 diabetes, accompanied by the functional decline of β cells which commonly arises from metabolic stress and dedifferentiation (Swisa et al., 2017; Weir et al., 2013). Increasing evidence shows that the pathological stimulation of the renin–angiotensin system (RAS) is associated with type 2 diabetes and that RAS inhibitors, either Angiotensin (Ang) II type 1 receptor blockers (ARBs) or AngII-converting enzyme inhibitors (ACEi), delay new onset-type 2 diabetes in high-risk populations (Abuissa et al., 2005; Prisant 2004). The local components of RAS have been detected in many tissues and organs, including the pancreas, adipose tissue, skeletal muscle, and brain, suggesting an important physiological role of systemic RAS (Chan et al., 2017; Grobe and Rahmouni 2012; Jones and Woods 2003; Mateos et al., 2011). AngII, a powerful RAS component, not only diminishes islet blood flow, but also is involved in increased oxidative stress, proinflammatory cytokines, and islet fibrosis (Ihoriya et al., 2014; Xu et al., 2011). Furthermore, studies show that AngII contributes to impaired β-cell function in AngII-infused mice, while the detrimental effect is independent of vasoconstriction, implying a complex mechanism underlying AngII-induced β-cell dysfunction (Sauter et al., 2015).

* Correspondence: sunjia@smu.edu.cn; zzhen311@163.com
†Hong Chen and Wenjun Zhou contributed equally to this work.
[1]Department of Endocrinology, Zhujiang Hospital, Southern Medical University, 253, Gongyedadao Middle, Guangzhou, Guangdong 510282, People's Republic of China
Full list of author information is available at the end of the article

Mechanistically, inhibition of RAS promotes insulin secretion and β-cell function in diabetic mice (Huang et al., 2007; Saitoh et al., 2009). However, although previous studies have shed some light on the relationship between RAS and type 2 diabetes, the underlying role of RAS remains incompletely understood.

Emerging evidence shows that β-cell failure can develop through different mechanisms, including oxidative stress, endoplasmic reticulum stress, hypoxic stress, and the induction of proinflammatory cytokines (Sauter et al., 2015; Chan et al., 2017; Cnop et al., 2017). In response to the stressors, β cells become dedifferentiated, reverting to a progenitor-like stage or converting into other types of pancreatic cells, such as α, δ, and pancreatic polypeptide cells (Pp cells) (Talchai et al., 2012a). Hence, it has been recognized recently that loss of the fully differentiated state is a potential mechanism underlying compromised β-cell function in type 2 diabetes (Spijker et al., 2015; Steven et al., 2016).

In *Foxo1* knockout mice, metabolic stress triggers the loss of β cells-related transcription factors PDX1 and MAFA, and increases the expression of endocrine progenitor markers NGN3 and OCT4. These changes lead to the loss of mature β cell identity (Talchai et al., 2012a). Consistently, multiple studies have found β-cell dedifferentiation and increased progenitor cell marker expression in patients with type 2 diabetes (Cinti et al., 2016; Guo et al., 2013b). Conversely, RAS blockers preserve β-cell function and attenuate oxidative stress and NADPH oxidase activation in pancreatic β cells (Saitoh et al., 2009).

Recently, clinical trial and experimental evidence have shown that nuclear factor kappa b (NF-κb)-mediated inflammation is associated with the cardioprotective effects of RAS inhibitors (Huynh et al., 2014; Thomas et al., 2013), and AngII has been reported to stimulate NF-κb activity in different types of cells (Pandey et al., 2015; Xu et al., 2011). NF-κB was reported to be a major transcription factor that positively regulates angiotensin II type 1 receptor (*AT1R*) gene expression (Daniluk et al., 2012; Wolf et al., 2002). The inactivated NF-κB complex is localized in the cytoplasm and includes the DNA binding p65 subunits and an inhibitory subunit, IκBα, which is bound to p65. In response to stimulation, phosphorylation of the IκB kinase (IKK) complex releases IkBα from the complex and promotes the nuclear translocation of p65, which regulates gene transcription (Gilmore 2006). Moreover, inhibition of IκB-kinase prevents AngII-induced upregulation of proinflammatory cytokines (interleukin (IL)-1b and IL-6) in human islets (Sauter et al., 2015). Taken together, this evidence suggests an interaction between RAS and NF-κB in the development of diabetes.

In summary, these findings allowed us to formulate a hypothesis that RAS activation plays an important role in β cell dedifferentiation, while interference with RAS or NF-κb signaling could be an efficient way to reverse β-cell dedifferentiation.

Methods

Pancreatic β-cell line culture

The pancreatic β-cell line Min6 (Mouse insulinoma 6) (Miyazaki et al., 1990) and INS-1 (rat insulinoma cells) (Zhang et al., 2014a) were cultured in Roswell Park Memorial Institute (RPMI) 1640 (Invitrogen) medium containing 11.1 mmol/L glucose, supplemented with 10% fetal bovine serum (FBS), 10 mmol/L HEPES, 2 mmol/L L-Glutamine, 50 U/mL penicillin, 50 mg/mL streptomycin and 50 mmol/L 2-mercaptoethanol at 37 °C in a humidified atmosphere of 95% air and 5% CO_2. We conducted experiments when the cells reach 70% confluence. For the experiments, we subcultured the cells in a 6-well plate when the cells reached 70% confluence. Cells were cultured in 1640 medium containing 11.1, 22.2, or 33.3 mM glucose and were treated with or without 10 μmol/L irbesartan for 24 h. For AngII-treatment experiments, pancreatic β cells were cultured with or without 1 μmol/L AngII in the presence or absence of 20 μmol/L sc-514, an NF-κb signaling inhibitor, or 10 μmol/L Irbesartan for 48 h. The effect of Ang II on NF-κb signaling in β cells was determined at 0.1, 1, and 10 mol/L of Ang II.

Glucose-stimulated insulin secretion (GSIS)

Glucose-starved cell preparation was conducted in Krebs–Ringer bicarbonate HEPES (KRBH) buffer (115 mM NaCl, 5 mM KCl, 1 mM $MgCl_2$, 24 mM $NaHCO_3$, 2.5 mM $CaCl_2$, 10 mM HEPES supplemented with 0.5% bovine serum albumin (BSA)) for 45 min. The cells were incubated in basal glucose conditioned KRBH buffer containing 3 mM glucose for 1 h and then incubated in glucose stimulation KRBH buffer containing 25 mM glucose for 1 h (Tuo et al., 2011). Before treatment with different media, the cells were washed twice with phosphate-buffered saline (PBS), and the media were collected for ultra-sensitive enzyme-linked immunosorbent assay (ELISA) analysis (Mercodia, Sweden).

Animals and treatments

Eight-week-old male C57BL/KsJ-db/db mice and wild-type littermate controls (C57BL/KsJ-db/m mice) were purchased from the Model Animal Research Center of Nanjing University. All the animal protocols were approved by the Ethics Committee for the use of Experimental Animals at Southern Medical University. All mice were maintained in a specific pathogen-free environment and housed in clean cages in groups of two animals per cage, with appropriate temperature and humidity and 12 h/12 h light/dark cycles. After 1 week of acclimatization, non-fasting blood glucose levels in 9-week-old db/db mice were > 16.7 mmol/L, with symptoms of polyuria, polydipsia, and polyphagia. The mice at 9 weeks of age were randomly divided into five groups: (1) Normal group [db/m mice injected with PBS subcutaneously; $n = 8$], (2) vehicle control [db/db mice were injected with PBS subcutaneously; $n = 8$], mice in remaining three groups were injected with human AngII (60 μg/kg; A9525; Sigma) subcutaneously twice a day for 4 weeks, (3) AngII [AngII injection; $n = 8$], (4) AngII+IRB [AngII injection and Irbesartan (IRB; 50 mg/kg; S1507; Sellect) was administered through oral gavage for 4 weeks; $n = 8$], (5) AngII+sc-514 [AngII injection and sc-514 (IRB; 30 mg/kg; S4907; Sellect) was administered through oral gavage for 4 weeks; $n = 8$]. The body weight and blood glucose (the sample for which was withdrawn from the tail vein) were measured and recorded two times weekly during the experiment.

Glucose tolerance test and insulin measurement

For intraperitoneal glucose tolerance tests (2.5 g glucose/ kg body weight), mice were fasted for 5 h, in the indicated groups, before obtaining the blood samples at various time points (0–120 min) from orbital sinus; the blood glucose concentration was determined using a glucometer (Roche, Indianapolis, IN). For insulin measurements, blood samples were centrifuged (2000 rpm for 2 min at 4 °C) and the plasma insulin concentrations were measured using a mouse insulin ELISA kit (Mercodia, Sweden), according to the manufacturer's instructions.

Quantitative real-time reverse transcription PCR

Total RNA was extracted from β cells using the TRIzol reagent (Takara Biotechnology, Japan), after which the RNA quantity and purity were evaluated using an NanoDrop 2000 apparatus (Thermo Scientific) and then reverse-transcribed into cDNA using a Reverse Transcription Kit (Takara). For quantitative PCR, the real-time PCR system 7500 (Applied Biosystems) and primers were used to detect gene expression. Gene expression was determined by relative gene expression using the $2^{-\Delta\Delta Ct}$ method.

Western blotting analysis

Western blotting and immunohistochemistry. Sodium dodecyl sulfate polyacrylamide gel electrophoresis and western blotting were performed as previously described (Zhang et al., 2014a, b) using primary antibodies against Insulin, NGN3, FOXO1, PDX-1, OCT4, phospho-IκBα (p-IκBα), IκBα, phospho-p65 (p-p65), p65, β-actin, and the horseradish peroxidase-labeled secondary antibodies were goat anti-rabbit IgG and goat anti-mouse IgG (Table 1).

Immunofluorescence analysis

The pancreatic samples were obtained without saline perfusion (Cheng et al., 2017) and processed for paraffin embedding. Pancreatic sections (5 mm) were dewaxed in dimethylbenzene and rehydrated through graded ethanol series (100, 95, 80, and 70%). Heat-mediated antigen retrieval with citrate buffer was performed and sections were blocked in a 2% BSA solution for 30 min at room temperature. The following primary antibodies were used: anti-insulin, anti-glucagon anti-PDX1, anti-FOXO1 (the primary antibodies were purchased from Cell Signaling), and anti-NGN3 (LifeSpan Biosciences). Sections were incubated with primary antibodies overnight at 4 °C. After washing with PBS, sections were incubated for 40 min at room temperature with secondary antibodies: Alexa Fluor 594 donkey anti-mouse immunoglobulin IgG and Alexa Fluor 488 donkey anti-rabbit IgG (Proteintech). The double staining was captured using a Nikon Y-TV55 fluorescent microscope. Numbers of cells or areas of interest were measured from 3 to 5 mice per group, or 4–5 pancreas sections per mouse for 20 islets. We then measured the positive stained area divided by total islet area (to calculate the staining index) using Image-Pro analyzer software (version 6.0, Media Cybernetics, USA).

Statistical analysis

Data are expressed as means ± standard error. Statistical analyses were performed using Prism7.0 (GraphPad). For statistical significance of different experimental groups, we used one-way, or repeated measures, analysis of variance (ANOVA). $P < 0.05$ indicated a statistically significant difference.

Results

RAS inhibition reverses glucotoxicity-induced compromised β-cell identity

To investigate the effect of RAS blockade on glucose-induced β-cell dysfunction, mouse pancreatic β-cell lines were exposed to increased concentrations of glucose in the presence or absence of Irbesartan (10 μmol/L) for 24 h (Additional file 1: Table S1). β-cell dysfunction was closely related to glucose levels, and exposure to a high glucose environment resulted in a sharp decrease in glucose-stimulated insulin secretion and the stimulatory index in β cells (Fig. 1a-d). By contrast, we observed a slight increase in basal secretion of β cells under 22.2 mmol/L glucose conditions. Furthermore, impaired GSIS was not only associated with decreased mRNA expression of *Pdx1* and *Ins1* in β cells cultured in 33.3 mmol/L glucose, but also was related to upregulated dedifferentiated cells markers NGN3 and OCT4 (Fig. 1e-l), indicating a significant correlation between impaired GSIS and compromised β-cell identity. Subsequently, we found that a high glucose concentration triggered RAS signaling, which could be inhibited by Irbesartan, an AT1R blocker. Insulin secretion from β-cell stimulated with 25 mmol/L of glucose in the IRB-treated group was slightly improved compared with that in β cells cultured in the high glucose environment (22.2 mmol/L or 33.3 mmol/L, Fig. 1a-b). In addition, IRB

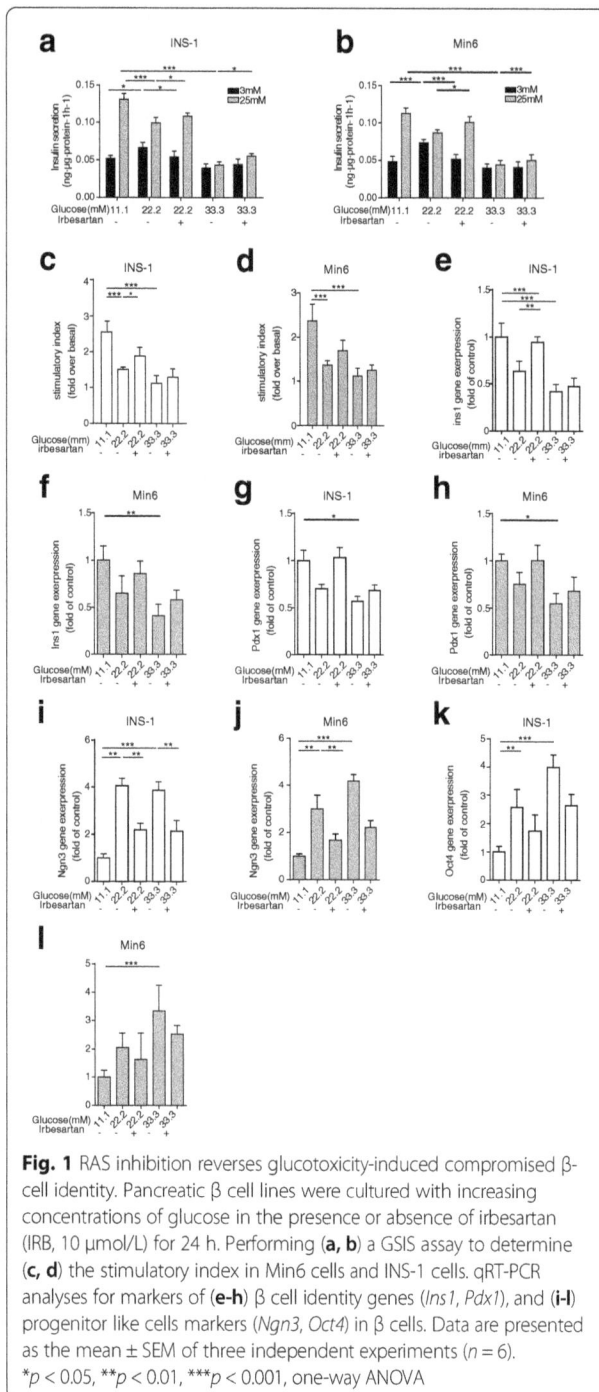

Fig. 1 RAS inhibition reverses glucotoxicity-induced compromised β-cell identity. Pancreatic β cell lines were cultured with increasing concentrations of glucose in the presence or absence of irbesartan (IRB, 10 μmol/L) for 24 h. Performing (a, b) a GSIS assay to determine (c, d) the stimulatory index in Min6 cells and INS-1 cells. qRT-PCR analyses for markers of (e-h) β cell identity genes (Ins1, Pdx1), and (i-l) progenitor like cells markers (Ngn3, Oct4) in β cells. Data are presented as the mean ± SEM of three independent experiments (n = 6). *p < 0.05, **p < 0.01, ***p < 0.001, one-way ANOVA

The deleterious effect of AngII is dependent on NF-κb signaling in β cells

To identify the role of RAS activation in β-cell dedifferentiation, we cultured INS-1 and Min6 cells with or without AngII (1 μmol/L) in the presence with Irbesartan or with sc-514. As observed in β cells, AngII obviously increased the gene expression of Ngn3, Oct4, and IL6 compared with that in the control group (Fig. 2a-f). Meanwhile, the dedifferentiation and proinflammatory effects of AngII on β cells were significantly attenuated by Irbesartan. Similarly, sc-514, an IkB-kinase-2 inhibitor, markedly decreased the AngII-induced dedifferentiation level. Furthermore, we investigated the protein expression levels of dedifferentiation markers NGN3, OCT4, and insulin in the indicated groups, to examine the differentiation stage of β cells (Fig. 2g, h). As expected, AngII increased the levels of NGN3 and OCT4, while Irbesartan and sc-514 both efficiently blocked NGN3 and OCT4, especially in Min6 cells. Meanwhile, Irbesartan and sc-514 restored the expression of Insulin. Therefore, inhibiting IkB-kinase reversed the dedifferentiation effect of AngII, which provided evidence that compromised β-cells identity is associated with NF-κb signaling.

AngII induces the activation of NF-κb, leading to dedifferentiation and dysfunction in β cells

We further investigated the relationship between NF-κb signaling and AngII-dependent β-cell dedifferentiation. Pancreatic β cells treated with increasing doses of AngII showed a remarkable increase in basal insulin secretion and a dose-dependent decline in the stimulatory index (Fig. 3a-d). We also found that AngII activated NF-κb signaling via the phosphorylation of p65 and IκBα, in a dose-dependent manner. Meanwhile, β cells that had lost their identity displayed decreased expression of PDX1 and FOXO1, and increased NGN3 expression (Fig. 3o, p). Moreover, consistent with the change in protein expression, we found that the mRNA expression levels of p65, IκBα, Ngn3, and Oct4 were positively correlated with the AngII dose in β cells (Fig. 3e-l). Interestingly, we found that IL6 was significantly increased when the cells were incubated with 10 μm/L AngII, indicating the proinflammatory effect of AngII (Fig. 3m, n).

AngII treatment of diabetic mice potentiated impaired glucose tolerance and compromised β-cell identity

Next, type 2 diabetic mice models (db/db mice) and wild-type controls (db/m mice) were used to identify the role of AngII in the deterioration of β-cell function in vivo. The mice were randomly divided into five groups. The diabetic mice were injected with AngII (60 μg/kg) or vehicle subcutaneously twice a day for 4 weeks and orally administered with sc-514 (30 mg/kg) or Irbesartan (50 mg/kg) at the same time. After 4 weeks, an intraperitoneal glucose tolerance test (IPGTT) showed elevated blood glucose and

enhanced the stimulatory index in INS1 cells under 22.2 mmol/L glucose conditions (Fig. 1c). The inhibitor improved GSIS and markedly reduced the mRNA expression of Ngn3, especially in 22.2 mmol/L glucose. We observed an increasing trend of the stimulatory index in min6 cells, although there was no significant change, and the basal, as well as stimulated, insulin secretion was significantly promoted by Irbesartan in the high glucose environment (22.2 mmol/L or 33.3 mmol/L).

Table 1 Antibodies used in this study

Primary Antibody; Monoclonal or Polyclonal	Manufacturer	Reactivity	Dilution	Identifier
Rabbit anti-Neurog3; polyclonal	LifeSpan BioSciences	H, M, R	1:200 1:50	LS-C97692; RRID: AB_2282494
Rabbit anti-glucagon; polyclonal	Cell Signaling	H, M, R	1:400	Cat# 2760S RRID:AB_10698611
Mouse anti-insulin; monoclonal	Cell Signaling	H, M, R	1:200	Cat# 8138S, RRID:AB_10949314
Rabbit anti-Pdx; polyclonal	Cell Signaling	H, M, R	1:500 1:200	Cat# 5679, RRID:AB_10706174
Rabbit anti-FoxO1; polyclonal	Cell Signaling	H, M, R	1:500 1:200	Cat# 2880, RRID:AB_2106495
Mouse anti-p-NF-κBp65; Monoclonal	Cell Signaling	H, M, R	1:500	Cat# 3033 RRID:AB_331284
Mouse anti- NF-κBp65; Monoclonal	Cell Signaling	H, M, R	1:500	Cat# 6956, RRID:AB_10828935
Rabbit anti-Oct-4A polyclonal	Cell Signaling	H,M	1:500	Cat# 2890, AB_10841298
Mouse anti- IκBα; monoclonal	Cell Signaling	H, M, R	1:500	Cat# 4814, RRID:AB_390781
Rabbit anti-Phospho-IκBα polyclonal	Cell Signaling	H,M,R	1:250	Cat# 2859, RRID:AB_561111
β-actin	Cell Signaling	H,M	1:1000	Cat# 12262, RRID:AB_2566811

H human, *M* mouse, *R* rat

reduced plasma insulin concentration in db/db mice treated with Ang II alone compared with that in control db/db mice, suggesting impaired glucose tolerance induced by Ang II (Fig. 4a-b). The body weight of db/db mice at 9 weeks of age was significantly higher than that of wild-type littermates. Meanwhile, we did not observe significant difference between the db/db control group and db/db treatment groups (Additional file 2: Figure S1). In addition, we observed increasing release of cytokine IL6 in the AngII-treated mice, suggesting an AngII-induced proinflammatory effect that can be attenuated by an IkB-kinase-2 inhibitor (Fig. 4c). Irbesartan or sc-514 slightly restored the impaired glucose tolerance caused by AngII and thus decreased blood sugar levels. Moreover, progressive loss of islet β cells during AngII treatment resulted in a significantly low β-cell ratio, which decreased by 12% per islet, as well as an increased glucagon-positive islet ratio. Conversely, the loss of insulin positive cells could be reversed by Irbesartan. (Fig. 4d-f). Intriguingly, mice treated with AngII alone had comparably increased numbers of cells co-expressing both glucagon and insulin to that in the control db/db mice (Fig. 4g), suggesting that AngII induced β cells to convert into α cells.

Sc-514 reversed the β-cell dedifferentiated state and dysfunction in db/db mice
We further assessed whether AngII-induced β-cell failure is associated with the activation of NF-κb signaling. The proportion of PDX1 (Fig. 5a, b) positive cells markedly decreased by 17% and the percentage of Ngn3 (Fig. 5c) positive cells increased to 53% in mice with chronic activation of RAS compared with that in the control db/db mice Meanwhile, the number of PDX1 or NGN3 positive

cells was consistent with their ratio change (Fig. 5g, h). In addition, FOXO1 was mainly localized in the cytoplasm of β cells in normal control mice, whereas it was translocated into the nucleus in db/db mice (Fig. 5e). In db/db mice treated with AngII, we found a loss of expression of FOXO1 (Fig. 5f) and increased nuclear-localized FOXO1 protein compared with control db/db mice (Fig. 5i). Furthermore, blocking RAS with Irbesartan partially reversed β-cell failure and marginally increased the islet PDX1-positive ratio by 12% (Fig. 5b). Meanwhile, in the sc-514 treated group, there was an upward trend in the islet PDX1-positive ratio compared with that in the control db/db group, although we observed no detectable differences in the ratio between these two groups. In addition, we observed that sc-514 decreased the NGN3 positive ratio by 20% (Fig. 5d), which was 7% higher than that in mice treated with Irbesartan. The results indicated that Irbesartan rescues the loss of β cells and restores β-cell identity; largely depend on enhanced key β-cell transcription factors. Moreover, sc-514 improves β-cell function mainly by suppressing the expression of NGN3, and thus reverses β-cell dedifferentiation.

Discussion
Growing evidence suggests that activation of RAS increases oxidative stress and impairs insulin secretion in islets (Chan et al., 2017; Sauter et al., 2015). Accordingly, blocking RAS helps to protect β cells from glucotoxicity and leads to functional improvement (Wang et al., 2011). Studies have shown that metabolic stress is a potential underlying cause of β-cell dedifferentiation (Guo et al., 2013a; Talchai et al., 2012a), which is an important contributory factor to β-cell

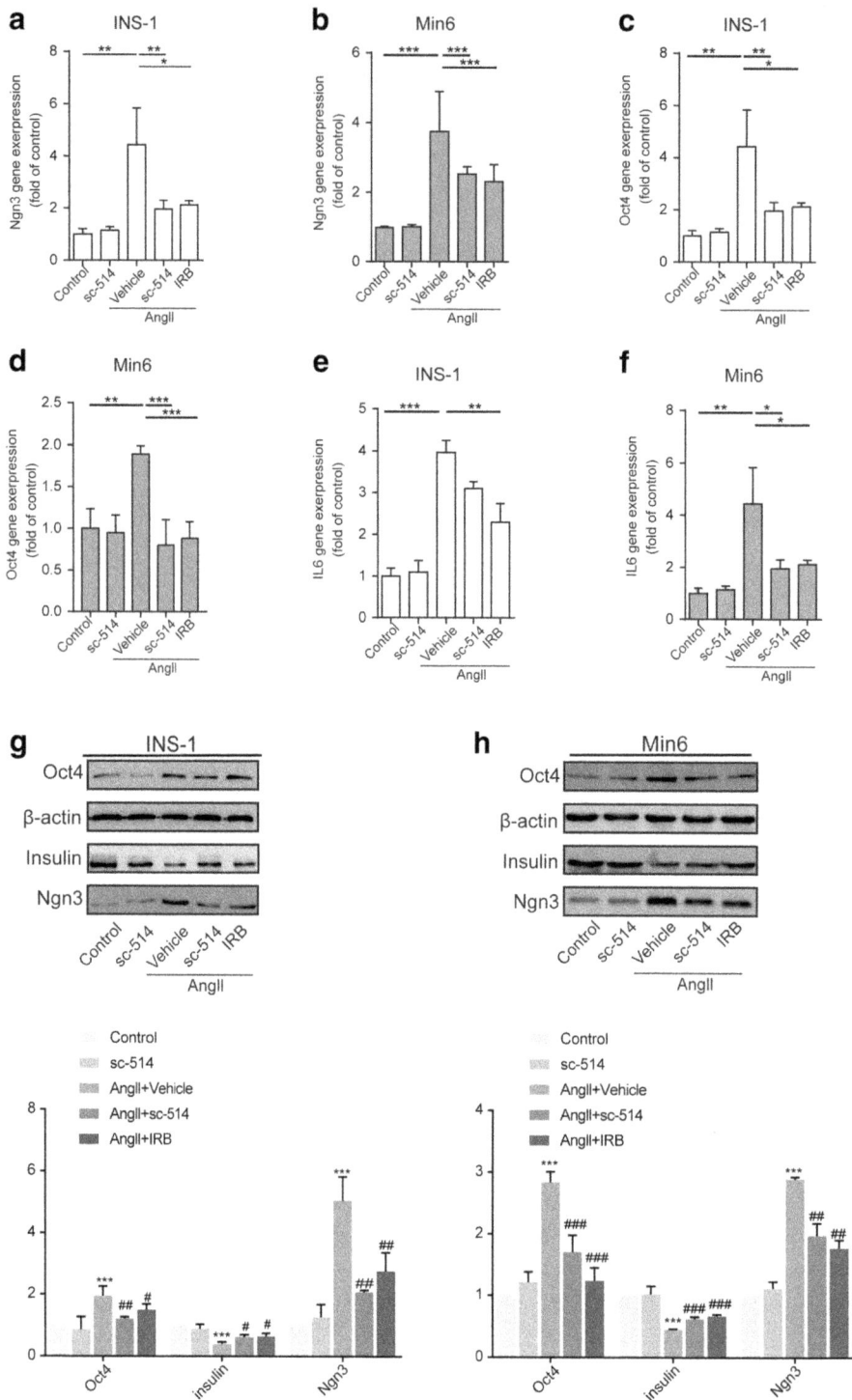

Fig. 2 The deleterious effect of AngII is dependent on NF-κb signaling in β cells. Pancreatic β cell lines were cultured with or without AngII (1 μmol/L) in the presence or absence of sc-514, an IκB-kinase-2 inhibitor (20 μmol/L), or Irbesartan (IRB) (10 μmol/L) for 48 h. qRT-PCR analyses for (**a-d**) progenitor likes cell markers (*Ngn3, Oct4*) and (**e, f**) proinflammatory cytokine *Il6*. Data are presented as the mean ± SEM of three independent experiments (*n* = 6), *$p < 0.05$, **$p < 0.01$, ***$p < 0.001$, one-way ANOVA. **g, h** Western blotting for NGN3, OCT4, and insulin in Min6 cells and INS-1 cells. β-actin was used as a loading control. Densitometric analyses of the western blotting results are presented below. Data are presented as the mean ± SEM of three independent experiments(*n* = 6). **$p < 0.01$, ***$p < 0.001$ vs Control group, #$p < 0.05$, ##$p < 0.01$, ###$p < 0.001$ vs Vehicle group, one-way ANOVA

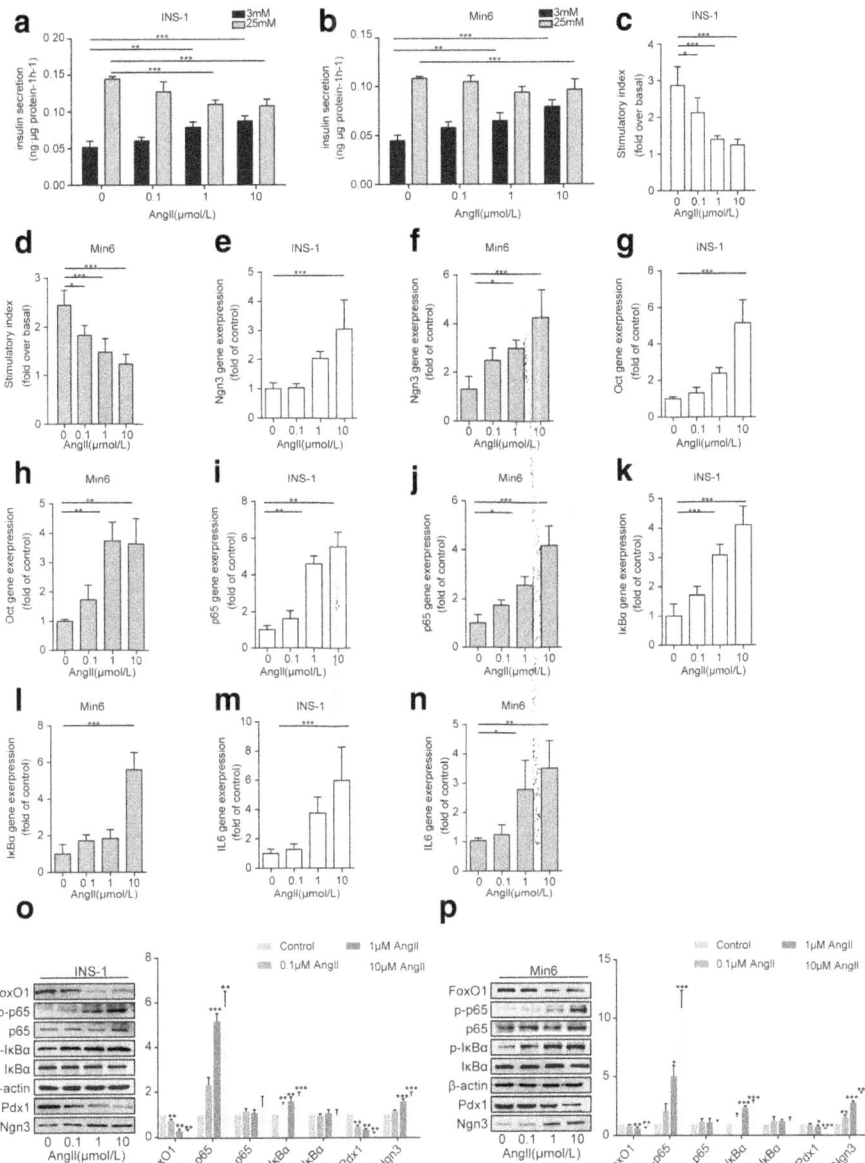

Fig. 3 AngII induces the activation of NF-κb, leading to dedifferentiation and dysfunction in β cells. Pancreatic β cell lines were cultured with increasing doses of AngII for 48 h. Performing (**a, b**) a GSIS assay to determine (**c, d**) the stimulatory index in Min6 cells and INS-1 cell. qRT-PCR analyses for (**e-h**) progenitor like cells markers (Ngn3, Oct4), (**i-l**) NF-κb signaling (IκBα, p65) and (**m, n**) proinflammatory cytokines Il6 in Min6 cells and INS-1 cell. Data are presented as the mean ± SEM of three independent experiments (n = 6), *p < 0.05, **p < 0.01, ***p < 0.001, one-way ANOVA. **o, p** Western blotting for P65, IκBα, PDX1, NGN3, FOXO1, and the phosphorylated forms of P65 (p-P65) and IκBα (p-IκBα) in Min6 cells and INS-1 cells. β-actin was used as a loading control. Densitometric analyses of the western blotting results are presented. Data are presented as the mean ± SEM of three independent experiments. (n = 6) *p < 0.05, **p < 0.01, ***p < 0.001 vs control group, one-way ANOVA

failure (Cinti et al., 2016; White et al., 2013). However, the relationship between RAS and the dedifferentiated status of β cells remains elusive. Our study, for the first time, found that AngII contributes to β-cell dedifferentiation via AT1R activation in diabetic mice. Moreover, this contribution is strengthened by NF-κb signaling (Fig. 6).

High glucose levels are known to be closely associated with β-cell dysfunction in type 2 diabetes, and abnormal glucose-stimulated insulin secretion (GSIS) can explain

the mechanism. In addition, High glucose levels can cause glucotoxicity, which reduces β-cell-identity markers, including MAFA, PDX1, and lNS1 (Jonas et al., 1999; Kondo et al., 2009), and triggers RAS. In our study, we confirmed that lrbesartan, a RAS inhibitor, markedly reversed impaired GSIS, and downregulated dedifferentiated cells markers in a high glucose environment. Subsequently, we identified the role of RAS in β-cell dedifferentiation.

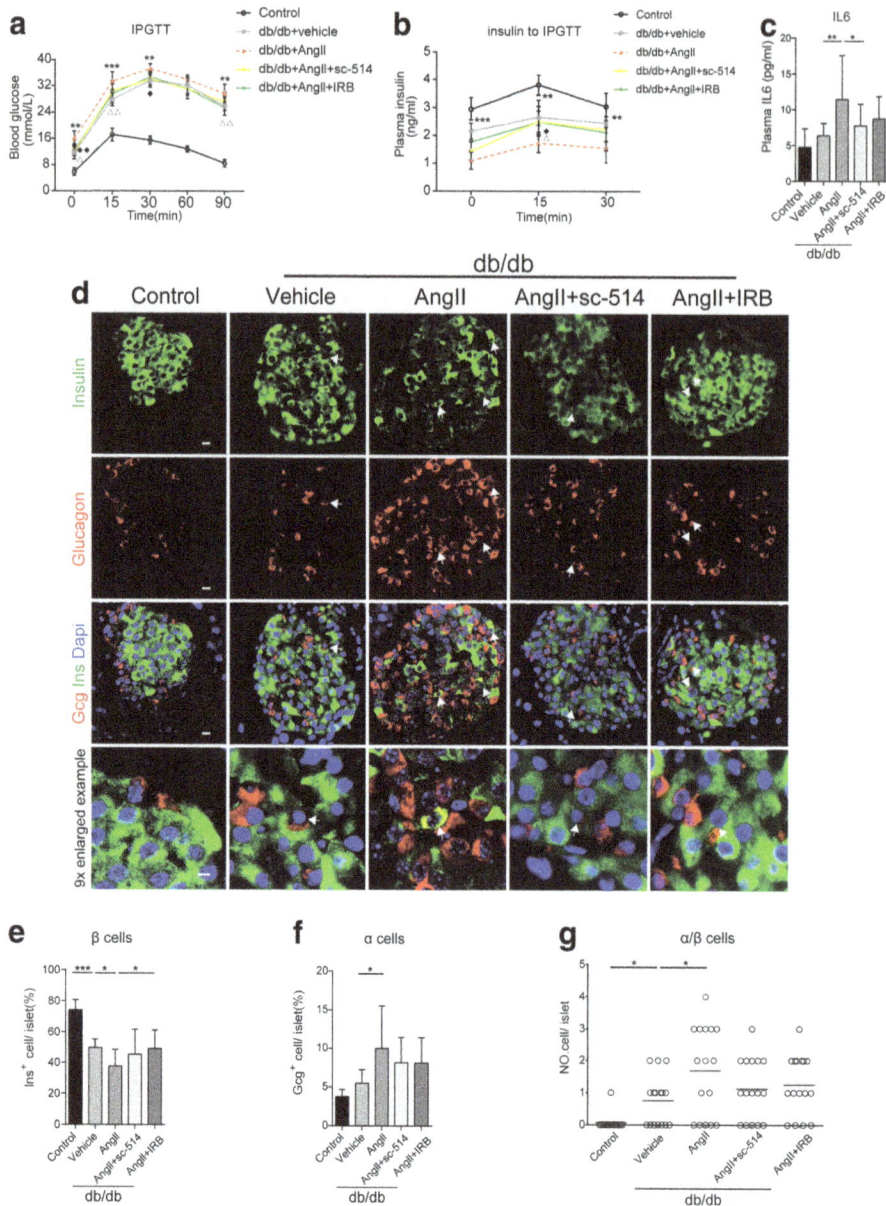

Fig. 4 (color; online only) AngII treatment of diabetic mice potentiates impaired glucose tolerance and compromised β-cell identity. db/db mice were injected with AngII (60 μg/kg) subcutaneously twice a day for 4 weeks. Where indicated, either sc-514 (30 mg/kg) or Irbesartan (IRB) (50 mg/kg) was also administered. **a** Glucose levels in homeostasis and intraperitoneal glucose tolerance tests (IPGTTs) for the indicated groups ($n \geq 6$ for each group). **b** Levels of circulating insulin during IPGTT ($n = 6$ for each group). Data (**a, b**) are presented as the mean ± SEM, *$p < 0.05$, **$p < 0.01$, ***$p < 0.001$ (AngII treated vs. db/db control); ♦$p < 0.05$, ♦♦$p < 0.01$ (AngII treated vs. sc-514 treated); △$p < 0.05$, △△$p < 0.01$, (AngII treated vs. IRB treated), as assessed using repeated measures ANOVA (**c**) Plasma IL-6 measurements ($n \geq 6$ for each group). Mean ± SEM, *$p < 0.05$, **$p < 0.01$, ***$p < 0.001$, one-way ANOVA (**d**) Paraffin embedded sections from the indicated groups were immunolabeled for insulin (green), glucagon (red), and DAPI (blue). Scale bar (10 μm). Arrow in the 9× enlarged example image indicates a typical insulin⁺glucagon⁺ (Ins + Gcg+) cell. Scale bar (5 μm) in the 9× enlarged example image. **e, f** Quantification of labeled insulin or glucagon positive cells per islet. **g** Numbers (NO.) of insulin⁺glucagon⁺ cells. For Immunofluorescence analysis (e-g): $n \geq 4$ mice per group, $n \geq 20$ islets per marker. Mean ± SEM *$p < 0.05$, **$p < 0.01$, ***$p < 0.001$, one-way ANOVA

Recent studies have reported that pancreatic β cells become dedifferentiated and convert to other endocrine cells under certain circumstances (Chakravarthy et al., 2017; Thorel et al., 2010) Consistently, we demonstrated that AngII efficiently induces the conversion of β cells into glucagon-producing α-like cells in db/db mice, which might explain the phenomenon that patients with type 2 diabetes are more likely to have elevated plasma glucagon levels and a glucagon-to-insulin ratio (Dunning and Gerich 2007). Although we did not observe a significant effect of treatment

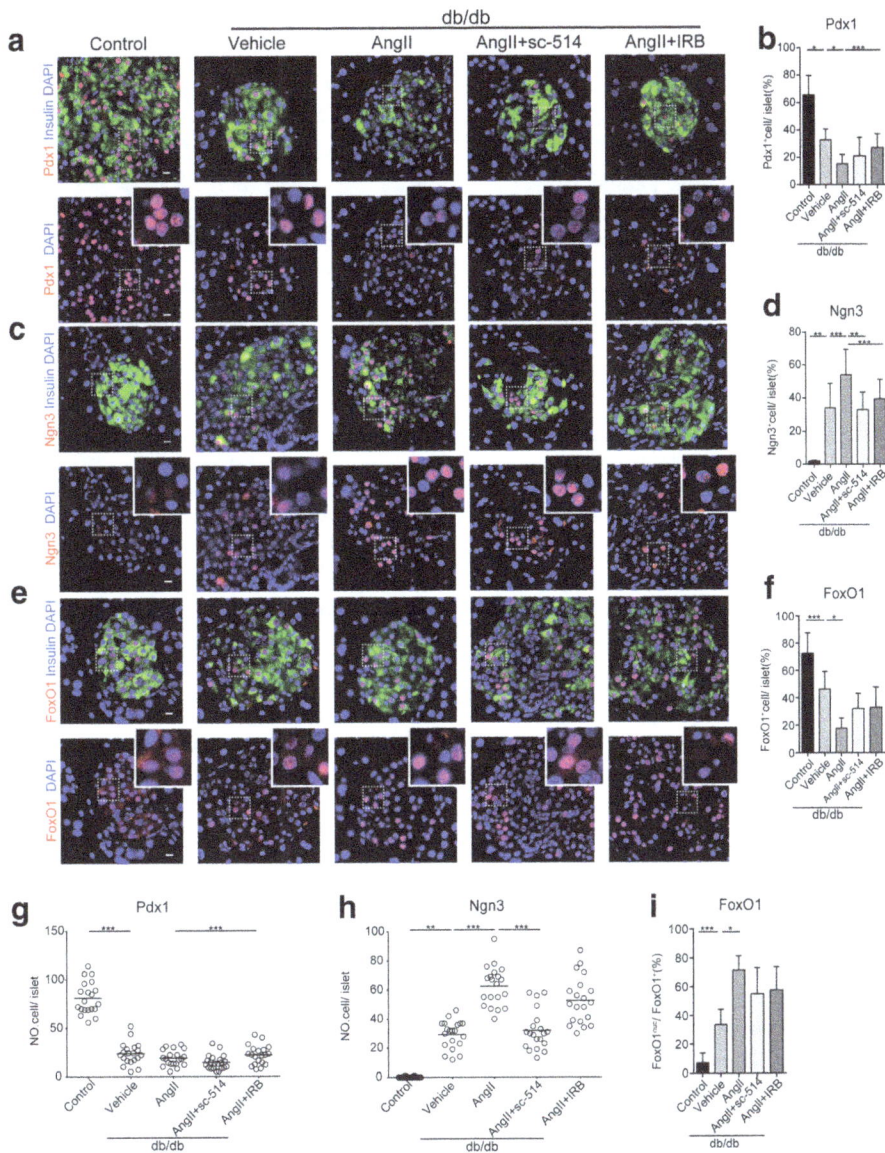

Fig. 5 (color; online only) sc-514 reversed β-cell dedifferentiation and dysfunction in db/db mice. **a, c, e** paraffin-embedded sections from the indicated groups were immunolabeled for insulin (green), PDX1 (red), insulin (green), NGN3 (red), insulin (green), FOXO1 (red), and DAPI (blue) (**b, d, f**) Quantification of labeled PDX1 or NGN3 or FOXO1 positive cells per islet. The squares (dashed white lines) show regions 9× enlarged and depicted as inserts at the top right of the corresponding images. **g, h** Numbers (NO.) of PDX1 or NGN3 positive cells. Scale bar (10 μm). (**i**) Quantification of FOXO1 translocated to the nuclei of FOXO1-positive cells. For the immunofluorescence analysis: $n \geq 4$ mice per group, $n \geq 20$ islets per marker. Mean ± SEM *$p < 0.05$, **$p < 0.01$, ***$p < 0.001$, one-way ANOVA

(sc-514 or IRB) on the number of α/β cells, there was a decreasing trend of α/β cells compared with that in the AngII-treated db/db group. In addition, we found a reversed insulin-positive ratio and a decreasing trend in glucagon-positive cells in the Irbesartan-treated group, which both indicate the reversible identity of β cells, as well as the potential conversion of other types of pancreatic cell into β-cells. However, the specific types of pancreatic cell involved need to be clarified. On the basis of previous studies, we investigated AngII, a RAS signaling component that functions as a promoter of inflammation, fibrosis, and

apoptosis via the angiotensin II type 1 receptor (AT1R) in many tissues (Miyazaki and Takai 2006; Paul et al., 2006). Consistently, we observed increased serum IL6 and loss of insulin positive cells in AngII-treated diabetic mice, which suggested the proinflammatory effect of AngII. In addition, several studies have demonstrated the possible vasoconstrictive effect of AngII on glucose and insulin kinetics. Recently, Sauter et al. (2015) found that AngII induced impaired glucose tolerance and insulin secretion, independent of its vasoconstrictive effects. The authors ruled out the vasoconstrictive effect of AngII by treatment

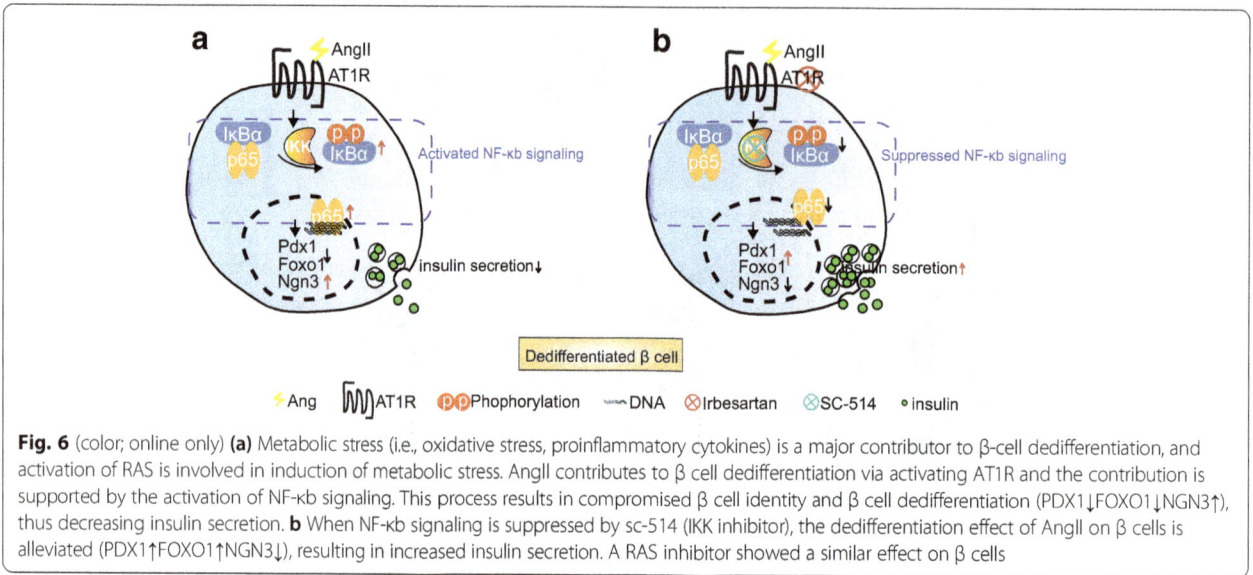

Fig. 6 (color; online only) **(a)** Metabolic stress (i.e., oxidative stress, proinflammatory cytokines) is a major contributor to β-cell dedifferentiation, and activation of RAS is involved in induction of metabolic stress. AngII contributes to β cell dedifferentiation via activating AT1R and the contribution is supported by the activation of NF-κb signaling. This process results in compromised β cell identity and β cell dedifferentiation (PDX1↓FOXO1↓NGN3↑), thus decreasing insulin secretion. **b** When NF-κb signaling is suppressed by sc-514 (IKK inhibitor), the dedifferentiation effect of AngII on β cells is alleviated (PDX1↑FOXO1↑NGN3↓), resulting in increased insulin secretion. A RAS inhibitor showed a similar effect on β cells

with hydralazine, a direct-acting vasodilator. Furthermore, the study suggested that AngII leads to islet dysfunction via induction of inflammation; however, they did not conduct further experiments to determine the status of β cells. Therefore, the study shed a light on the vasoconstrictive effect of AngII, which might not be a confounding factor in impaired glucose tolerance, and the underlying mechanism of AngII dysfunction was not fully clarified. The present study might be considered as a hypothesis to observe the effect of direct activation of RAS induced by AngII on the state of β cells. We detected the differentiation effect of AngII in β cell lines, manifested by downregulation of β-cell identity markers and a decrease in glucose-stimulated insulin secretion. We then examined the dedifferentiation effect of directly triggering RAS on β cells in diabetic mice. The results showed a loss of positive areas for PDX1 and FOXO1 and high expression of NGN3, indicating the development of dedifferentiation in β cells, although we failed to identify the possible vasoconstrictive effect of AngII on glucose and insulin in db/db mice. The loss of mature status of β cells is detrimental to their identity, ultimately leading to β-cell dysfunction.

The expression pattern of FOXO1 during pancreatic organogenesis is identical to that of PDX1 (Kitamura et al., 2009). FOXO1 increases the expression of transcription factor HES-1, which is a repressor of NGN3. Consequently, in *FoxO1* knockout mice, *Ngn3* expression is upregulated in gut endocrine cells (Talchai et al., 2012a, b), suggesting that FOXO1 essentially prevents β-cell differentiation. Meanwhile, we found that FOXO1 translocates from the cytoplasm to the nucleus in response to AngII, which was consistent with previous reports that FOXO1 is a malfunctional protein involved in insulin signaling and translocation in β cells when faced with oxidative stress (Kitamura 2013; Kitamura et al., 2005). Irbesartan slightly

promoted these effects and rescued the loss of insulin positive cells by increasing the numbers of insulin positive cells in AngII-infused db/db mice. Importantly, these data suggested that AngII-induced RAS activation is a major contributor to dedifferentiation, which can be reversed by RAS inhibitors, resulting in restoration of β-cell function.

Studies have reported that activation of NF-κb occurs through AT1R (Luo et al., 2015; Thomas et al., 2014). In a diabetic mice model treated with AngII, Sauter et al. (2015) found that NF-κb signaling meditated inflammation and participated in AngII-induced deterioration of glucose metabolism, suggesting an interaction between RAS and NF-κb in hypertension and diabetes. The present study showed that blockade of NF-κb using sc-514 reversed dedifferentiation by decreasing the NGN3-positive area by 20%. Consequently, we proved that sc-514 promotes glucose metabolism by reversing the differentiated state of β cells, without affecting the number of β cells. In the present study, we observed a strong inhibitory effect of Irbesartan and sc-514 on the suppression of dedifferentiation of β cells in AngII-treated db/db mice. Additionally, NGN3 levels increased significantly in the db/db control group compared with those in the control group. This corresponded with the compromised β-cell identity in patients with type 2 diabetes. It would be interesting to determine whether IRB or NF-κb inhibition also result in an improvement in the identity of β cells in the db/db control group. Considering the notable effect we observed in vivo and the potential clinical significance, this is a direction worthy of further study.

Recently, Cinti et al. (2016) hypothesized that β-cell dedifferentiation could be a mechanism to protect β cells from undergoing apoptosis, enabling them to redifferentiate under more favorable circumstances. In support of this, we showed that β cells lose their differentiated characteristics under metabolic stress, eventually leading to compromised function. However, the progressive impairment of β cells is reversible. Taken together, this evidence suggests that dedifferentiation-driven β-cell failure can be reversed under certain circumstances. Meanwhile, amelioration of insulin secretion by residual cells, such as differentiated cells, is likely to be a rapid way to restore β-cell function.

Conclusions

In summary, we propose a pathway lead from chronic RAS accumulation to NF-κb signaling that eventually causes β-cell dedifferentiation. Our findings prove that RAS induces pancreatic β-cell dedifferentiation and provide pharmacological strategies to reverse dedifferentiation by suppressing NF-κb signaling.

Additional files

Additional file 1: Table S1. Body weight development in each group. Data are presented as the mean ± SEM (n = 8 each) ***p < 0.001 vs control group, one-way ANOVA. DM, db/db mice; Age (weeks). (PDF 183 kb)

Additional file 2: Figure S1. Related to Fig. 1. Pancreatic β cell lines were cultured in the presence or absence of irbesartan (IRB, 10 μmol/L) for 24 h. Performing a GSIS assay to determine the stimulatory index in Min6 cells and INS-1 cells. qRT-PCR analyses for markers of β cell identity genes, and progenitor like cells markers in β cells. Data are presented as the mean ± SEM of three independent experiments (n = 6). (TIF 1669 kb)

Abbreviations
ACEi: AngII-converting enzyme inhibitors; AngII: Angiotensin II; ARBs: Angiotensin II type 1 receptor blockers; AT1R: Angiotensin II type 1 receptor; GSIS: Glucose-stimulated insulin secretion; IKK: IκB kinase; IL-1b: Interleukin-1b; IL6: Interleukin-6; IRB: Irbesartan; KRBH: Krebs–Ringer bicarbonate HEPES; RAS: Renin–angiotensin system

Acknowledgements
All authors sincerely thank Taotao at the Southern Medical School for his excellent secretarial assistance. The authors appreciate the Guangdong Provincial Key Laboratory of Molecular Tumor Pathology, Southern Medical University, Guangdong, China for their technical support.

Funding
This work was supported by the National Natural Science Foundation of China [grant numbers 81500623, 81770804].

Authors' contributions
WZ performed most of the experiments and analyzed the data. HC, YR, LY, NX, RY, and RC performed some of the experiments. WZ and NX wrote the draft of the manuscript. HC, and JS designed the experiments and provided technical support. ZZ provided funding and wrote the manuscript. All authors approved the final version of the manuscript.

Competing interests
The authors declare that they have no competing interests.

Author details
[1]Department of Endocrinology, Zhujiang Hospital, Southern Medical University, 253, Gongyedadao Middle, Guangzhou, Guangdong 510282, People's Republic of China. [2]Department of Nephrology, Zhujiang Hospital, Southern Medical University, 253, Gongyedadao Middle, Guangzhou, Guangdong 510282, People's Republic of China.

References
Abuissa H, Jones PG, Marso SP, et al. Angiotensin-converting enzyme inhibitors or angiotensin receptor blockers for prevention of typetab 2 diabetes: a meta-analysis of randomized clinical trials. J Am Coll Cardiol. 2005;46(5):821–6.

Chakravarthy H, Gu X, Enge M, et al. Converting adult pancreatic islet alpha cells into beta cells by targeting both Dnmt1 and Arx. Cell Metab. 2017;25(3):622–34.

Chan SMH, Lau YS, Miller AA, et al. Angiotensin II causes beta-cell dysfunction through an ER stress-induced Proinflammatory response. Endocrinology. 2017;158(10):3162–73.

Cheng CW, Villani V, Buono R, et al. Fasting-mimicking diet promotes Ngn3-driven beta-cell regeneration to reverse diabetes. Cell. 2017;168(5):775–88. e12

Cinti F, Bouchi R, Kim-Muller JY, et al. Evidence of beta-cell dedifferentiation in human type 2 diabetes. J Clin Endocrinol Metab. 2016;101(3):1044-54.

Cnop M, Toivonen S, Igoilloesteve M, et al. Endoplasmic reticulum stress and eIF2α phosphorylation: the Achilles heel of pancreatic β cells. Mol Metab. 2017;6(9):1024–39.

Daniluk J, Liu Y, Deng D, et al. An NF-κB pathway-mediated positive feedback loop amplifies Ras activity to pathological levels in mice. J Clin Investig. 2012; 122(4):1519–28.

Dunning BE, Gerich JE. The role of α-cell dysregulation in fasting and postprandial hyperglycemia in type 2 diabetes and therapeutic implications. Endocr Rev. 2007;28(3):253–83.

Gilmore TD. Introduction to NF-|[kappa]|B: players, pathways, perspectives. Oncogene. 2006;25(51):6680.

Grobe JL, Rahmouni K. The adipose/circulating renin-angiotensin system cross-talk enters a new dimension. Hypertension. 2012;60(6):1389–90.

Guo S, Dai C, Guo M, et al. Inactivation of specific beta cell transcription factors in type 2 diabetes. J Clin Invest. 2013a;123(8):3305–16.

Guo S, Dai C, Guo M, et al. Inactivation of specific β cell transcription factors in type 2 diabetes. J Clin Investig. 2013b;123(8):3305–16.

Huang Z, Jansson L, Sjoholm A. Vasoactive drugs enhance pancreatic islet blood flow, augment insulin secretion and improve glucose tolerance in female rats. Clin Sci (Lond). 2007;112(1):69–76.

Huynh K, Bernardo BC, Mcmullen JR, et al. Diabetic cardiomyopathy: mechanisms and new treatment strategies targeting antioxidant signaling pathways. Pharmacol Ther. 2014;142(3):375–415.

Ihoriya C, Satoh M, Kuwabara A, et al. Angiotensin II regulates islet microcirculation and insulin secretion in mice. Microcirculation. 2014;21(2):112–23.

Jonas JC, Sharma A, Hasenkamp W, et al. Chronic hyperglycemia triggers loss of pancreatic beta cell differentiation in an animal model of diabetes. J Biol Chem. 1999;274(20):14112–21.

Jones A, Woods DR. Skeletal muscle RAS and exercise performance. Int J Biochem Cell Biol. 2003;35(6):855–66.

Kitamura T. The role of FOXO1 in beta-cell failure and type 2 diabetes mellitus. Nat Rev Endocrinol. 2013;9(10):615–23.

Kitamura T, Kitamura Y, Kobayashi M, et al. Regulation of pancreatic Juxtaductal endocrine cell formation by FoxO1. Mol Cell Biol. 2009;29(16):4417–30.

Kitamura Y, Kitamura T, Kruse J, et al. FoxO1 protects against pancreatic β cell failure through NeuroD and MafA induction. Cell Metab. 2005;2(3):153–63.

Kondo T, El KI, Nishimura W, et al. p38 MAPK is a major regulator of MafA protein stability under oxidative stress. Mol Endocrinol. 2009;23(8):1281.

Luo H, Wang X, Wang J, et al. Chronic NF-kappaB blockade improves renal angiotensin II type 1 receptor functions and reduces blood pressure in Zucker diabetic rats. Cardiovasc Diabetol. 2015;14:76.

Mateos L, Ismail MAM, Gilbea FJ, et al. Upregulation of brain renin angiotensin system by 27-hydroxycholesterol in Alzheimer's disease. J Alzheimers Dis. 2011;24(4):669–79.

Miyazaki J, Araki K, Yamato E, et al. Establishment of a pancreatic β cell line that retains glucose-inducible insulin secretion: special reference to expression of glucose transporter isoforms*. Endocrinology. 1990;127(1):126–32.

Miyazaki M, Takai S. Tissue angiotensin II generating system by angiotensin-converting enzyme and Chymase. J Pharmacol Sci. 2006;100(5):391–7.

Pandey A, Goru SK, Kadakol A, et al. Differential regulation of angiotensin converting enzyme 2 and nuclear factor-kappaB by angiotensin II receptor subtypes in type 2 diabetic kidney. Biochimie. 2015;118:71–81.

Paul M, Poyan Mehr A, Kreutz R. Physiology of local renin-angiotensin systems. Physiol Rev. 2006;86(3):747–803.

Prisant LM. Preventing type II diabetes mellitus. J Clin Pharmacol. 2004;44(4):406–13.

Saitoh Y, Hongwei W, Ueno H, et al. Telmisartan attenuates fatty-acid-induced oxidative stress and NAD(P)H oxidase activity in pancreatic beta-cells. Diabetes Metab. 2009;35(5):392–7.

Sauter NS, Thienel C, Plutino Y, et al. Angiotensin II induces intaerleukin-1beta-mediated islet inflammation and beta-cell dysfunction independently of vasoconstrictive effects. Diabetes. 2015;64(4):1273–83.

Spijker HS, Song H, Ellenbroek JH, et al. Loss of β-cell identity occurs in type 2 diabetes and is associated with islet amyloid deposits. Diabetes. 2015;64(8): 2928–38.

Steven S, Hollingsworth KG, Small PK, et al. Weight loss decreases excess pancreatic triacylglycerol specifically in type 2 diabetes. Diabetes Care. 2016; 39(1):158–65.

Swisa A, Glaser B, Dor Y. Metabolic stress and compromised identity of pancreatic Beta cells. Front Genet. 2017;8:21.

Talchai C, Xuan S, Lin HV, et al. Pancreatic beta cell dedifferentiation as a mechanism of diabetic beta cell failure. Cell. 2012a;150(6):1223–34.

Talchai C, Xuan S, Kitamura T, et al. Generation of functional insulin-producing cells in the gut by Foxo1 ablation. Nat Genet. 2012b;44(4):406–12.

Thomas CM, Yong QC, Rosa RM, et al. Cardiac-specific suppression of NF-kappaB signaling prevents diabetic cardiomyopathy via inhibition of the renin-angiotensin system. Am J Physiol Heart Circ Physiol. 2014;307(7):H1036–45.

Thomas CM, Yong QC, Seqqat R, et al. Direct renin inhibition prevents cardiac dysfunction in a diabetic mouse model: comparison with an angiotensin receptor antagonist and angiotensin-converting enzyme inhibitor. Clin Sci. 2013;124(8):529–45.

Thorel F, Nepote V, Avril I, et al. Conversion of adult pancreatic alpha-cells to beta-cells after extreme beta-cell loss. Nature. 2010;464(7292):1149–54.

Tuo Y, Wang D, Li S, et al. Long-term exposure of INS-1 rat insulinoma cells to linoleic acid and glucose in vitro affects cell viability and function through mitochondrial-mediated pathways. Endocrine. 2011;39(2):128–38.

Wang HW, Mizuta M, Saitoh Y, et al. Glucagon-like peptide-1 and candesartan additively improve glucolipotoxicity in pancreatic beta-cells. Metabolism. 2011;60(8):1081–9.

Weir GC, Aguayo-Mazzucato C, Bonnerweir S. β-cell dedifferentiation in diabetes is important, but what is it? Islets. 2013;5(5):233–7.

White MG, Marshall HL, Rigby R, et al. Expression of mesenchymal and α-cell phenotypic markers in islet β-cells in recently diagnosed diabetes. Diabetes Care. 2013;36(11):3818–20.

Wolf G, Wenzel U, Burns KD, et al. Angiotensin II activates nuclear transcription factor-[[kgr]]B through AT1 and AT2 receptors1. Kidney Int. 2002;61(6):1986.

Xu S, Zhi H, Hou X, et al. IκBβ attenuates angiotensin II–induced cardiovascular inflammation and fibrosis in mice. Hypertension. 2011;58(2):310–6.

Zhang Z, Li J, Jiang X, et al. GLP-1 ameliorates the proliferation activity of INS-1 cells inhibited by intermittent high glucose concentrations through the regulation of cyclins. Mol Med Rep. 2014a;10(2):683.

Zhang Z, Li J, Yang L, et al. The cytotoxic role of intermittent high glucose on apoptosis and cell viability in pancreatic beta cells. J Diabetes Res. 2014b; 2014(1):712781.

3

Dysequilibrium of the PTH-FGF23-vitamin D axis in relapsing remitting multiple sclerosis

Mark Simon Stein[1,2,3*] [iD], Gregory John Ward[4], Helmut Butzkueven[1,5,6,7], Trevor John Kilpatrick[1,5,6] and Leonard Charles Harrison[1,3,6]

Abstract

Background: Parathyroid glands of people with relapsing remitting multiple sclerosis (RRMS) fail to respond to low serum 25-hydroxyvitamin D (25OHD) and low serum calcium, which are stimuli for parathyroid hormone (PTH) secretion. This led us to hypothesise: that there is suppression of PTH in RRMS due to higher than normal serum concentrations of fibroblast growth factor 23 (FGF23). We therefore sought evidence for dysregulation of the PTH-FGF23-vitamin D axis in RRMS.

Methods: Longitudinal study (winter to summer) with fasting venepunctures. For RRMS subjects who recruited a healthy control (HC) friend, pairs analyses were performed. For each pair, the within-pair difference of the variable of interest was calculated (RRMS minus HC). Then, the median of the differences from all pairs was compared against a median of zero (Wilcoxon) and the 95% confidence interval of that median difference (CI) was calculated (Sign Test).

Results: RRMS had lower winter PTH than HC, $P = 0.005$, (CI -2.4 to 0.5 pmol/L, $n = 28$ pairs), and lower summer PTH, $P = 0.04$, (CI -1.8 to 0.5, $n = 21$ pairs). Lower PTH associates physiologically with lower intact FGF23 (iFGF23), yet RRMS had higher iFGF23 than HC in winter, $P = 0.04$, (CI -3 to 15 pg/mL, $n = 28$ pairs) and iFGF23 levels comparable to HC in summer, $P = 0.14$, (CI -5 to 13, $n = 21$ pairs). As PTH stimulates and FGF23 reduces, renal 1-alpha hydroxylase enzyme activity, which synthesises serum 1,25-dihydroxyvitamin D (1,25(OH)$_2$D) from serum 25OHD, we examined the ratio of serum 1,25(OH)$_2$D to serum 25OHD. In winter, this ratio was lower in RRMS versus HC, $P = 0.013$, (CI -1.2 to - 0.3, $n = 28$ pairs).

Conclusions: This study revealed a dysequilibrium of the PTH-FGF23-vitamin D axis in RRMS, with lower plasma PTH, higher plasma iFGF23 and a lower serum 1,25(OH)$_2$D to 25OHD ratio in RRMS compared with HC subjects. This dysequilibrium is consistent with the study hypothesis that in RRMS there is suppression of the parathyroid glands by inappropriately high plasma concentrations of iFGF23. Studying the basis of this dysequilibrium may provide insight into the pathogenesis of RRMS.

Keywords: Multiple sclerosis, Vitamin D, Parathyroid hormone, Fibroblast growth factor 23

Background

Vitamin D is synthesised in skin upon exposure to ultraviolet light and converted in the liver to 25-hydroxyvitamin D (25OHD), the main vitamin D metabolite in serum and the clinical indicator of vitamin D nutrition (Parfitt et al. 1982; Hollis 1996). Serum 25OHD is converted in the kidney tubules and immune cells (macrophages, dendritic cells, and potentially B and T lymphocytes) to a very potent form of vitamin D, 1,25-dihydroxyvitamin D (1,25(OH)$_2$D), by 1-alpha hydroxylase (Tanaka and DeLuca 1981; Reichel et al. 1987a; Reichel et al. 1987b; Bacchetta et al. 2013; Shimada et al. 2004; Shimada et al. 2005; Enioutina et al. 2009; Carvalho et al. 2017), which is increased by parathyroid hormone (PTH) and reduced by fibroblast growth factor-23 (FGF23) (Tanaka and DeLuca 1981; Bacchetta et al. 2013; Shimada et al. 2004; Shimada et al. 2005; Gattineni et al. 2011). Serum 1,25(OH)$_2$D is

* Correspondence: mark.stein@mh.org.au
[1]The Royal Melbourne Hospital, Parkville, Australia
[2]Department of Diabetes and Endocrinology, The Royal Melbourne Hospital, Parkville, VIC 3050, Australia
Full list of author information is available at the end of the article

degraded by renal 24-hydroxylase, which is reduced by PTH and increased by FGF23 (Tanaka and DeLuca 1981; Shimada et al. 2004; Gattineni et al. 2011). PTH and FGF23 thus regulate serum $1,25(OH)_2D$ concentrations through opposite effects on synthetic and degradative hydroxylases.

These regulatory pathways include serum $1,25(OH)_2D$ itself, which feeds back both on the enzymes 1-alpha-hydroxylase and 24-hydroxylase (Colston et al. 1977) and on the hormones PTH and FGF23. $1,25(OH)_2D$ directly stimulates the synthesis of FGF23 by osteoblasts and osteocytes (Shimada et al. 2004; Nguyen-Yamamoto et al. 2017). It can increase the absorption of dietary calcium and phosphate, and higher serum concentrations of calcium and phosphate may feedback to stimulate FGF23 secretion (Shimada et al. 2005; Nguyen-Yamamoto et al. 2017; Quinn et al. 2013). Serum $1,25(OH)_2D$ also feeds back directly on the parathyroid glands to reduce PTH synthesis (Silver et al. 1986) and also indirectly by its action to increase serum concentrations of FGF23, which may then further reduce PTH synthesis and secretion (Ben-Dov et al. 2007; Lavi-Moshayoff et al. 2010). Completing another feedback loop, PTH, the secretion of which is reduced by FGF23, in turn stimulates FGF23 synthesis by osteoblasts and osteocytes (Ben-Dov et al. 2007; Lavi-Moshayoff et al. 2010).

FGF23 circulates as an intact molecule (iFGF23), which is cleaved to release a C-terminal fragment (cFGF23) (Razzaque and Lanske 2007; Blau and Collins 2015). FGF23 binds a variety of FGF receptor subtypes, either directly or in conjunction with the Klotho receptor (Gattineni et al. 2011; Razzaque and Lanske 2007; Blau and Collins 2015; Kurosu et al. 2006). A soluble alpha fragment of the Klotho receptor may also circulate and may serve to stimulate FGF23 synthesis (Smith et al. 2012).

In winter, a decrease in sunlight exposure and vitamin D synthesis is associated with an increase in serum PTH, which maintains the serum calcium concentration. In people with relapsing remitting multiple sclerosis (RRMS), Soilu-Hänninen et al. (Soilu-Hänninen et al. 2008) observed that the winter rise in serum PTH was blunted and was associated with lower serum calcium, compared to healthy controls (HC). It appeared that the parathyroid glands of people with RRMS failed to respond to two stimuli for PTH secretion, namely lower concentrations of vitamin D and serum calcium. This led us to hypothesise that there is suppression of PTH in RRMS due to higher than normal serum concentrations of FGF23. In the present study, we sought evidence for dysregulation of the PTH-FGF23-vitamin D axis in RRMS, in a longitudinal study from winter to summer.

Methods

Subjects

People with RRMS (aged ≥18 years) were recruited from hospital clinics and through publicity on the MS Australia Victoria website in July–August 2011. They were asked to bring one or more healthy friends (aged ≥18 years) to serve as healthy controls (HC).

The study was approved by the Human Research Ethics Committees of Melbourne Health and Eastern Health, Victoria. All subjects provided written informed consent.

Exclusions to filter out conditions affecting mineral metabolism were:

Pregnancy, breast-feeding, fracture, bone/joint surgery, treatment with raloxifene, alendronate, risedronate, zoledronate, strontium ranelate or teriparetide in the previous 6 months.

Except for the oral contraceptive, treatment with estrogen or progesterone, testosterone, phenytoin, valproate or levetiracetam in the previous 3 months.

Treatment with oral or systemic glucocorticoid in the previous month.

Treatment with furosemide or thiazide diuretic in the previous week.

Inability to ambulate 300 m without assistance of another person.

HC were excluded if a 1st- or 2nd-degree relative had a history of demyelination.

The following were permitted: oral contraceptives, asthma inhalers, over-counter vitamin/mineral supplements.

We sought to enrol at least 20 individuals with RRMS and 20 HC based on the sample size used to report that people with RRMS failed to increase their serum PTH concentrations in winter (Soilu-Hänninen et al. 2008).

Between August 19th-September 28th 2011 subjects had fasting 'winter' venepuncture at collection centres of Melbourne Pathology (Sonic Healthcare, Collingwood, Victoria). Venepuncture was performed between 7:30 am–10 am to control for circadian variation in PTH. Subjects were asked to avoid alcohol for at least 24 h before venepuncture. Each RRMS-HC friend pair attended the same centre at the same time and was randomised (via central computer) as to within-pair venepuncture order. They completed questionnaires regarding anthropometrics, personal and family health. Body mass index (BMI) was calculated as weight (kg)/[height (m)]^2.

Subjects with serum 25OHD < 50 nM were advised that their vitamin D nutrition was suboptimal. They were given their serum 25OHD result to take to their primary care physician with the recommendation that they commence vitamin D3 (1000 IU daily). We did not mandate or monitor such supplementation as we planned to directly measure serum 25OHD on repeat venepuncture.

Subjects were invited to return February 2012 for identical 'summer' collections, preserving within-pair venepuncture order.

Laboratory assays

EDTA blood tubes were centrifuged immediately, as were serum separator tubes after blood had clotted. Plasma for PTH assay was transported at ambient temperature (Glendenning et al. 2002). Remaining plasma and sera were frozen on site then transported for same day general biochemistry analysis or for storage at -80 C. Melbourne Pathology Central Laboratory (Collingwood, Melbourne) measured serum biochemistry (Modular c701 chemistry analyser; Roche, Mannheim, Germany), plasma human intact PTH (Modular e602 immunoassay analyser; Roche, Mannheim, Germany) with coefficient of variation (CV) = 4.0% (2–50 pmol/L) and serum 25OHD (Liaison analyser in winter, Liaison XL analyser in summer; DiaSorin, Turin, Italy), with CV = 7.5% (40–280 nmol/L). Calcium corrected for albumin (Cacorr) was calculated as total calcium (mmol/L) + (40-albumin [g/L]) × 0.02.

Sullivan Nicolaides Pathology, (Sonic Healthcare, Brisbane, Australia) measured plasma intact FGF23 (iFGF23) by ELISA (CY4000; Kainos Laboratories, Tokyo, Japan) (Yamazaki et al. 2002 and see also Imel et al. 2006 and Smith et al. 2013), with interassay CV = 3% (at mean 71.8 pg/mL) and 4% (at mean 203.3 pg/mL), plasma C-terminal FGF23 peptide (FGF23c) by ELISA (Immunotopics, San Clemente, USA) with interassay CV = 9% (at mean 32.3) and 1% (at mean 293) and plasma soluble alpha klotho (Klotho) by ELISA (IBL, Hamburg Germany), with interassay CV = 4% (at mean 1130.8 pg/mL) and 4% (at mean 1322.3 pg/mL). Serum ferritin was assayed with the Architect kit, (Abbott, Abbott Park, Illinois, USA). Serum $1,25OH_2D$ was measured by immunoassay (IDS iSYS, Tyne and Wear, UK).

For ELISAs, summer and winter specimens from each RRMS-HC pair were measured in the same assay (within the same ELISA plate). Laboratory personnel were blind to source of specimens.

Statistics

The frequencies of characteristics of RRMS and HC subjects were compared by Fisher's exact test. Cohort median values for biochemical analytes of RRMS and HC subjects were compared by Mann-Whitney test. The 95% confidence intervals (CIs) for differences between cohort medians were calculated by Moods Median Test.

For RRMS subjects who had recruited an HC friend, pairs analyses were performed. For each pair, the within-pair difference of the variable of interest was calculated (RRMS minus HC). Then, the median of the differences from all pairs was compared against a median

of zero (Wilcoxon) and the 95% CI of that median difference was calculated (Sign Test).

Modelling (general linear modelling/multiple regression/path analysis) was not performed as bi-directional causality (Ben-Dov et al. 2007) renders such approaches invalid (personal communication, Professor Terry Speed, Bioinformatics Division, Walter and Eliza Hall Institute of Medical Research, Melbourne).

Statistical analyses were performed on Minitab 13.1 and 17 (http://www.minitab.com). Outliers were defined by the Minitab definition, i.e. > 1.5 x interquartile range (IQR) outside the IQR. $P < 0.05$ was considered significant. Hypotheses with an a priori direction, viz. lower PTH, higher FGF23 (RRMS versus HC), were tested one-tailed (Armitage and Berry 1994). Other hypotheses were tested two-tailed.

Results

55 RRMS and 35 HC subjects were recruited in winter. Their median (IQR) ages were 46.5 (36.5–52.5) and 49.5 (38.5–56.0) years, respectively ($P = 0.2$). RRMS and HC were 71% and 43% female (F), respectively, ($P = 0.007$). Subjects were excluded for non-return of the questionnaire (3 RRMS, 2 HC) and confounding medication (2 HC), leaving 83 winter subjects. Of RRMS, 14 (27%) were on no therapy, 6 (12%) took glatiramer acetate, 26 (50%) interferon-beta, 2 (4%) natalizumab and 4 (8%) fingolimod; 38% were taking vitamin D compared to 16% HC ($P = 0.02$), and 12% were taking calcium compared to 6% HC ($P = 0.4$).

Median (IQR) BMIs were: RRMS 23.9 (21.2–29.2) and HC 26.2 (22.8–29.0) kg/m^2 ($P = 0.4$). Two RRMS females with outlier BMIs (43.3, 43.0) and 1 RRMS female with BMI 16.9 (not clinically consistent with normal mineral metabolism) were excluded. One female HC had a failed winter venepuncture. This left 79 subjects (49 RRMS, 30 HC) for whom winter plasma PTH and other analytes were studied for cohort analyses. Of these, 61 (38 RRMS, 23 HC) agreed to return for summer venepuncture for measurement of plasma PTH and other analytes. After the above exclusions, 28 RRMS-HC pairs remained for winter analyses and 23 RRMS-HC pairs for summer analyses. We did not ascertain the reasons why some subjects declined to return in summer.

25OHD and 1,25(OH)$_2$D

Serum 25OHD increased from winter to summer in both RRMS and HC ($P < 0.01$). However, for serum $1,25(OH)_2D$ a significant seasonal rise was detected only in the HC ($P = 0.02$) (Fig. 1, Table 1).

PTH and iFGF23

Pairs analysis revealed that subjects with RRMS had lower plasma PTH than HC in winter and summer

(Fig. 2, Table 2). For example, the median winter within-pair difference (RRMS-HC) in plasma PTH was − 1.6 pmol/L ($P = 0.005$). To put the magnitude of this difference in context, it is over half the magnitude of the HC IQR for winter plasma PTH (Table 1).

In subjects with RRMS, plasma iFGF23 was the same as or higher than in HC (Fig. 3, Table 2). For example, the median winter within-pair difference (RRMS-HC) in plasma iFGF23 was 5 pg/mL ($P = 0.04$). To put the magnitude of this difference in context, it approximates one third the magnitude of the HC IQR for winter plasma iFGF23 (Table 1).

Ratio of serum 1,25(OH)2D to 25OHD

As PTH increases and iFGF23 reduces the activity of renal 1-alpha hydroxylase, which synthesises serum $1,25(OH)_2D$ from serum 25OHD, (and as PTH reduces and iFGF23 increases the activity of renal 24-hydroxylase which degrades serum $1,25(OH)_2D$) we compared the ratio of the serum concentrations of $1,25(OH)_2D$ and 25OHD between RRMS and HC. Subjects with RRMS had a lower ratio of serum $1,25(OH)_2D$ (pmol/L) to serum 25OHD (nmol/L). The median winter within-pair difference (RRMS-HC) in this ratio was − 0.7 ($P = 0.013$, 95% CI -1.2 to − 0.3, $n = 28$ pairs) (Fig. 4). To put the magnitude of this difference in context, it is over one third the magnitude of the HC IQR for the winter ratio of serum $1,25(OH)_2D$ (pmol/L) to serum 25OHD (nmol/L); as the median (IQR) HC winter ratio was 3.1 (2.0–3.8).

In the smaller sample of summer pairs, the median within-pair difference (RRMS-HC) of the ratio of serum $1,25(OH)_2D$ to serum 25OHD was − 0.3, which did not reach significance ($P = 0.07$, 95% CI -0.9 to 0.1, $n = 22$ pairs) (Fig. 4), potentially because of the smaller sample size.

Examination of potential confounders

The RRMS cohort contained a higher proportion of females, and plasma PTH may vary with renal function and plasma FGF23 with serum magnesium and ferritin (Takeda et al. 2011; Braithwaite et al. 2012; Durham et al. 2007). Therefore, we explored post-hoc whether the lower plasma PTH and paradoxically similar or higher plasma iFGF23 in subjects with RRMS could be due to confounding by sex or serum creatinine, magnesium, ferritin or 25OHD.

Either for all subjects combined, or within the separate RRMS and HC cohorts, plasma PTH and plasma iFGF23 did not differ by sex and in winter neither was associated with serum creatinine, which itself did not differ between RRMS and HC.

The median within-pair difference (RRMS-HC) in serum magnesium was not significantly different from zero (both in winter and summer). The median within-pair difference (RRMS-HC) in serum ferritin was not significantly different from zero (both in winter and summer). Furthermore, there was no correlation between within-pair differences in plasma iFGF23 and within-pair differences in serum ferritin.

The bivariate relationship between serum 25OHD and plasma PTH was weak (Fig. 5). Winter serum 25OHD correlated inversely with winter plasma PTH for all subjects combined ($r = -0.27$, $P = 0.02$) and within the RRMS ($r = -0.32$, $P = 0.03$) but not the HC cohort ($r = -0.06$, $P = 0.7$). In summer, serum 25OHD did not correlate with plasma PTH. Furthermore, serum 25OHD did not correlate with plasma iFGF23, plasma FGF23c, plasma klotho or serum ferritin.

In summary, lower plasma PTH and similar or higher plasma iFGF23 in RRMS compared with HC subjects was not due to confounding by sex or serum creatinine, magnesium, ferritin or 25OHD.

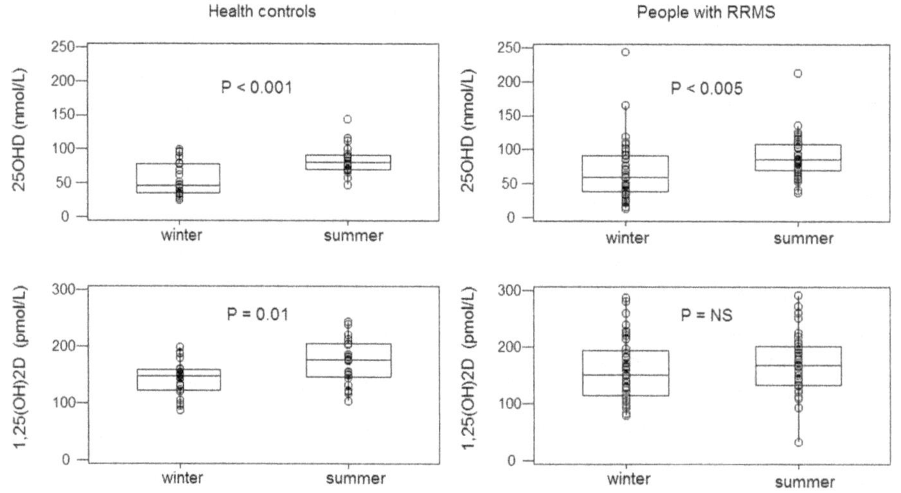

Fig. 1 Serum 25OHD and serum $1,25(OH)_2D$ Individual values (open circles), cohort medians and interquartile ranges (boxes) are plotted for those subjects who had both winter and summer measurement of serum $1,25(OH)_2D$. Serum 25OHD increased from winter to summer in both HC and RRMS subjects. However, only HC demonstrated a significant seasonal rise in serum $1,25(OH)_2D$

Table 1 Cohort analyses

Chemical	RRMS median (IQR)	HC median (IQR)	95% CI for difference (RRMS-HC) in medians	P value
For 25OHD and PTH, $n = 49$ for RRMS and 30 for HC.				
For all other analytes below, $n = 38$ for RRMS and $n = 25$ for HC				
Winter 25OHD	58 (40–89)	43 (36–71)	-3 to 32	0.09
Summer 25OHD	87 (70–108)[***]	81 (70–92)[***]	−6 to 18	0.4
Winter PTH	4.5 (3.7–6.0)	5.8 (4.1–6.6)	−1.6 to −0.3	0.02
Summer PTH	4.7 (3.9–5.7)	5.0 (4.0–6.0)	− 1.5 to 0.5	0.2
Winter iFGF	43 (36–56)	41 (35–49)	−5 to 8	0.14
Summer iFGF	46 (40–60)	47 (38–52)	−6 to 6	0.3
Winter FGFc	95 (76–136)	85 (73–112)	− 12 to 38	0.08
Summer FGFc	93 (77–114)	90 (72–124)	− 15 to 18	0.3
Winter Klotho	682 (517–817)	677 (553–964)	− 182 to 134	0.6
Summer Klotho	588 (491–743)	732 (571–976)	− 257 to 16	0.08
Winter Ferritin	103 (58–214)	73 (24–170)	−34 to 75	0.2
Summer Ferritin	98 (44–185)	90 (35–148)	−32 to 67	0.5
Winter 125(OH)$_2$D	148 (116–181)	139 (121–155)	−19 to 25	0.4
Summer 125(OH)$_2$D	168 (133–201)[+]	176 (147–204)[**]	−27 to 27	0.7
Restricted to subjects who provided both a winter and summer specimen,				
For all analytes below $n = 38$ for RRMS and $n = 23$ for HC				
Winter 25OHD	59 (38–91)	47 (37–79)	−17 to 32	0.4
Summer 25OHD	87 (70–108)[**]	81 (70–92)[**]	−6 to 18	0.4
Winter PTH	4.5 (3.8–6.1)	5.8 (4.0–6.6)	−1.7 to 0.3	0.09
Summer PTH	4.7 (3.9–5.7)	5.0 (4.0–6.0)	−1.5 to 0.5	0.3
Winter iFGF	45 (36–59)	45 (35–50)	−6 to 9	0.3
Summer iFGF	46 (40–60)	49 (40–52)	−6 to 5	0.4
Winter FGFc	93 (77–134)	96 (76–123)	− 23 to 24	0.4
Summer FGFc	93 (77–114)	90 (75–134)	− 15 to 17	0.5
Winter Klotho	681 (523–749)	677 (569–1034)	− 154 to 104	0.5
Summer Klotho	588 (491–743)	725 (563–984)	− 231 to 27	0.1
Winter Ferritin	108 (60–224)	62 (21–153)	−4 to 87	0.06
Summer Ferritin	98 (44–188)	89 (32–134)	−25 to 67	0.4
Winter 125(OH)$_2$D	150 (114–193)	148 (126–160)	−16 to 31	0.5
Summer 125(OH)$_2$D	168 (133–201)[++]	177 (145–204)[*]	−27 to 27	0.7

Abbreviations: *IQR* interquartile range

P: [*] < 0.05, [**] < 0.005, [***] < 0.0005, [+] 0.07, [++] 0.23 for within-cohort, winter versus summer values for 25OHD and 1,25(OH)$_2$D tabulated above

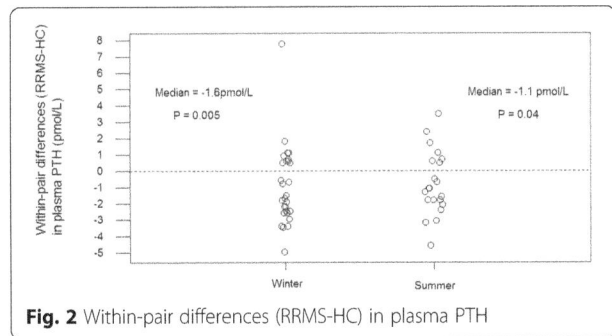

Fig. 2 Within-pair differences (RRMS-HC) in plasma PTH

Discussion

We present evidence for dysequilibrium of the PTH-FGF23-vitamin D axis in RRMS. Subjects with RRMS had lower plasma PTH concentrations than HC, yet their plasma iFGF was the same as or higher than HC. In winter, when vitamin D nutrition was lowest, they had a lower serum 1,25(OH)$_2$D to 25OHD ratio and in summer they failed to demonstrate a rise in serum 1,25(OH)$_2$D, as observed in HC. These findings are consistent with our initial hypothesis that there is suppression of PTH in RRMS, associated with higher serum FGF23. The magnitude of this dysequilibrium was

Table 2 Pairs analyses (subject with RRMS minus HC friend)

Chemical	Median difference (IQR)	95% CI for median difference	P value
Analyses of all pairs: n = 28 pairs (winter) 21–23 (summer)			
Winter 25OHD	17 (–8 to 48)	–5 to 37	0.03
Summer 25OHD	11 (– 12 to 41)	–9 to 35	0.09
Winter PTH	– 1.6 (– 2.6 to 0.6)	–2.4 to 0.5	0.005
Summer PTH	–1.1 (–2.0 to 0.7)	–1.8 to 0.5	0.04
Winter iFGF	5 (–6 to 18)	–3 to 15	0.04
Summer iFGF	4 (–6 to 15)	–5 to 13	0.14
Winter FGFc	7 (–25 to 49)	–15 to 45	0.15
Summer FGFc	–4 (–34 to 29)	–26 to 19	0.7
Winter Klotho	–58 (– 314 to 147)	– 252 to 88	0.4
Summer Klotho	– 206 (– 469 to 117)	– 386 to 40	0.05
Winter Ferritin	50 (–58 to 89)	–45 to 63	0.3
Summer Ferritin	27 (–57 to 90)	–36 to 79	0.4
Winter 125(OH)$_2$D	6 (–20 to 29)	–9 to 18	0.4
Summer 125(OH)$_2$D	–4 (–50 to 18)	–42 to 15	0.5
BMI	–1.4 (–5.6 to 4.4)	–4.5 to 2.4	0.8
Restricted to pairs who provided winter and summer specimens: n = 21–23 pairs			
Winter 25OHD	7 (–8 to 51)	–6 to 46	0.08
Summer 25OHD	11 (–12 to 41)	–9 to 35	0.09
Winter PTH	–1.5 (–2.6 to 0.6)	–2.5 to 0.6	0.02
Summer PTH	–1.1 (–2.0 to 0.7)	– 1.8 to 0.5	0.04
Winter iFGF	6 (–4 to 16)	–3 to 15	0.05
Summer iFGF	4 (–6 to 15)	–5 to 13	0.14
Winter FGFc	3 (–36 to 47)	–25 to 42	0.4
Summer FGFc	–4 (–34 to 29)	–26 to 19	0.7
Winter Klotho	–81 (– 349 to 96)	– 297 to 88	0.2
Summer Klotho	–206 (–469 to 117)	–386 to 40	0.05
Winter Ferritin	52 (–54 to 164)	–21 to 87	0.13
Summer Ferritin	27 (–57 to 90)	–36 to 79	0.4
Winter 125(OH)$_2$D	2 (–32 to 30)	–19 to 22	0.7
Summer 125(OH)$_2$D	–4 (–50 to 18)	–42 to 15	0.5

No significant differences were detected across season

Abbreviations: *IQR* interquartile range

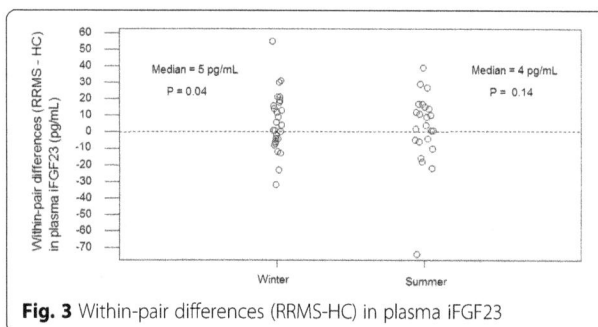

Fig. 3 Within-pair differences (RRMS-HC) in plasma iFGF23

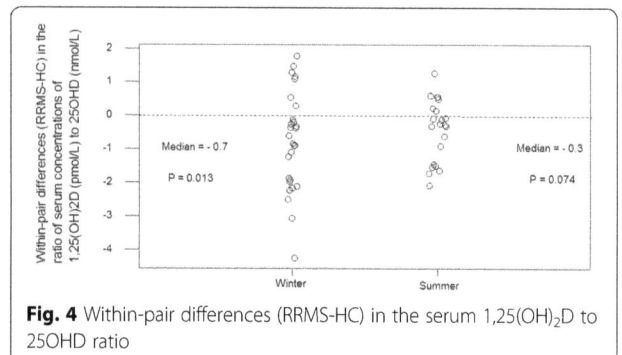

Fig. 4 Within-pair differences (RRMS-HC) in the serum 1,25(OH)$_2$D to 25OHD ratio

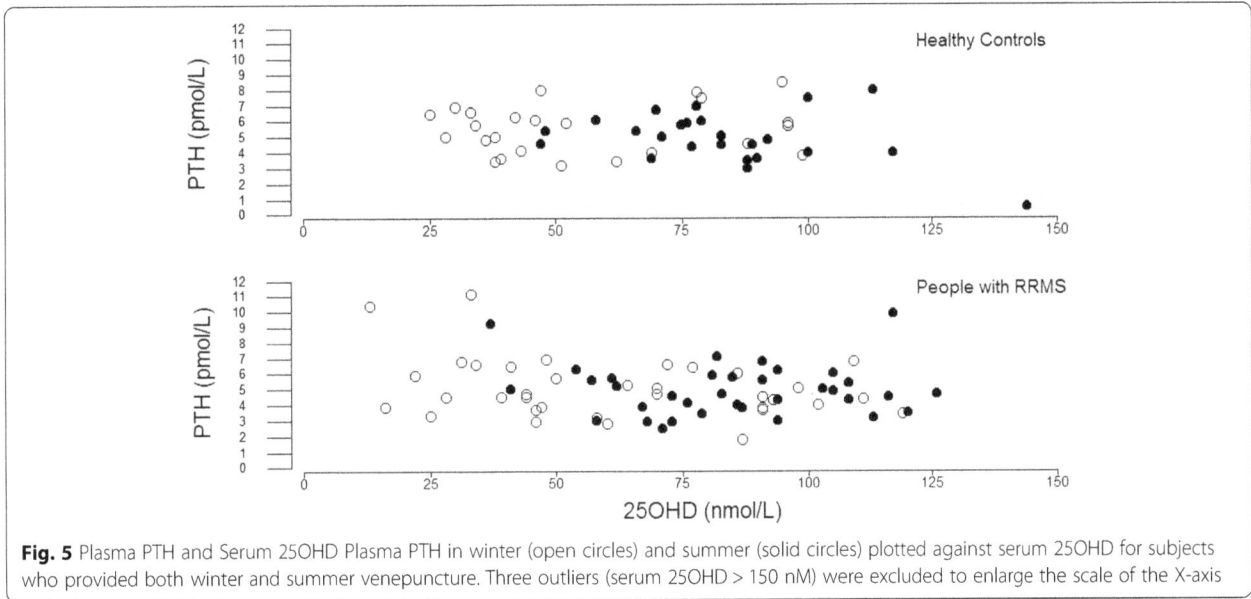

Fig. 5 Plasma PTH and Serum 25OHD Plasma PTH in winter (open circles) and summer (solid circles) plotted against serum 25OHD for subjects who provided both winter and summer venepuncture. Three outliers (serum 25OHD > 150 nM) were excluded to enlarge the scale of the X-axis

large. The median winter RRMS-HC difference in plasma PTH exceeded half the HC IQR for winter plasma PTH and the median winter RRMS-HC difference in plasma iFGF23 approximated a third of the HC IQR for winter iFGF23. Similarly, the median winter RRMS-HC difference in the ratio of serum 1,25(OH)$_2$D to 25OHD exceeded a third of the HC IQR for the winter value of this ratio.

Dysequilibrium of the PTH-FGF23-vitamin D axis data exhibited internal consistency. Thus, lower plasma PTH and higher plasma iFGF23 observed in RRMS would be expected to lead to lower renal 1-alpha hydroxylase activity in RRMS and thus decreased synthesis of serum 1,25(OH)$_2$D from 25OHD (Tanaka and DeLuca 1981; Bacchetta et al. 2013; Shimada et al. 2004; Shimada et al. 2005). Lower plasma PTH and higher plasma iFGF23 in RRMS would also be expected to lead to higher renal 24-hydroxylase activity in RRMS with increased degradation of serum 1,25(OH)$_2$D (Tanaka and DeLuca 1981; Bacchetta et al. 2013; Shimada et al. 2004; Shimada et al. 2005). Accordingly, the winter serum 1,25(OH)$_2$D to 25OHD ratio was lower in RRMS than HC and subjects with RRMS did not demonstrate the expected summer rise in serum 1,25(OH)$_2$D observed in HC. Unlike the Finnish study of Soilu-Hänninen et al. (Soilu-Hänninen et al. 2008), we did not find a lower winter serum calcium concentration in RRMS, which might be explained by the fact that the winter serum 25OHD was higher in the Australian subjects. Irish researchers examined PTH at low levels of 25OHD (Lonergan et al. 2011; McKenna et al. 2018). In one study (Lonergan et al. 2011) a significant inverse correlation of PTH with 25OHD was present in controls but not in people with MS. Those studies, however, did not report plasma calcium and

their MS cohort grouped primary progressive and secondary progressive MS together with RRMS (Lonergan et al. 2011; McKenna et al. 2018). Blau and Collins (Blau and Collins 2015) wrote "The action of FGF23 on the parathyroid gland has been reported to suppress PTH secretion in vitro and in rodent models, but demonstration of a similar effect in humans is lacking." Although our findings are correlative they are consistent with a physiological effect of FGF23 to suppress the parathyroid glands in RRMS.

We were not able to determine if dysequilibrium of the PTH-FGF23-vitamin D axis precedes or follows the pathophysiology of RRMS. It is interesting, however, that while we find differences (RRMS vs HC) in the levels of hormones (PTH and iFGF23) that regulate the activity of the enzymes 1-alpha hydroxylase and 24-hydroxylase, which respectively synthesise and degrade the potent vitamin D metabolite 1,25(OH)$_2$D, others find differences between people with MS versus HC in the genes coding for these same enzymes (Pierrot-Deseilligny and Souberbielle 2017). This certainly raises the possibility that dysequilibrium of the PTH-FG23-vitamin D axis could have a pathogenic role. In addition, because PTH and FGF23 also regulate extra-renal 1-alpha hydroxylase in innate and adaptive immune cells, (for example see Ref Bacchetta et al. 2013) this dysequilibrium has the potential to modify immune-inflammatory processes in MS via autocrine as well as endocrine vitamin D metabolism, in keeping with evidence that impaired vitamin D nutrition is associated with MS (Pierrot-Deseilligny and Souberbielle 2017; Munger et al. 2006; van der Mei et al. 2007; Simpson Jr et al. 2010).

It will be important to determine whether plasma PTH and plasma iFGF23 could be used as biomarkers to identify individuals at risk for RRMS or predict disease course and response to therapy. It will also be important to determine whether there is dysequilibrium in the PTH-FGF23-vitamin D axis in other autoimmune diseases such as type 1 diabetes, systemic lupus erythematosus and rheumatoid arthritis that exhibit an incidence or disease activity which correlates with vitamin D nutrition (Munger et al. 2013; Watad et al. 2017).

This study has several limitations. Not all of the differences between RRMS and HC demonstrated by within-pair analysis were seen in comparison of RRMS and HC cohort medians. Furthermore, not all subjects with RRMS recruited a HC friend to the study. While cohort analyses have the advantage of larger sample size, analysis of RRMS-HC pairs may be more sensitive as it controls for pre-analytical specimen handling measurement error (each RRMS-HC friend pair attended the same specimen collection centre at the same time), which may contribute up to 50% of total analyte measurement error (Plebani 2006). To reduce analytical laboratory error, winter and summer specimens from each RRMS-HC pair were analysed within the same ELISA plate. In addition, we deliberately recruited HC from friends of the people with RRMS to minimise bias from unmeasured lifestyle, social and demographic variables that could potentially mask disease-specific differences. A further potential limitation is that we did not measure markers of inflammation, which could confound the interpretation of serum ferritin concentrations, if people with RRMS had more inflammation than HC. Lower serum ferritin concentrations have been associated with higher serum concentrations of FGF23c and iFGF23 (Braithwaite et al. 2012; Durham et al. 2007), but this relationship appears to be assay specific (Durham et al. 2007). In particular, the Kainos iFGF23 assay used in this study was not affected by low concentrations of serum ferritin (Durham et al. 2007). Hence, potential confounding of serum ferritin by inflammation in the RRMS cohort would not explain higher RRMS plasma concentrations of iFGF23 in this study. Finally, the fact that some subjects chose not to return for summer venepuncture may have introduced bias into the study. However, subjects were recruited both from hospital MS clinics and from the community, supporting the generalizability of the results.

Conclusions

This study revealed a dysequilibrium of the PTH-FGF23-vitamin D axis in RRMS, with lower plasma PTH, higher plasma iFGF23 and a lower serum 1,25(OH)$_2$D to 25OHD ratio in RRMS compared with HC subjects. This dysequilibrium is consistent with the study hypothesis that in RRMS there is suppression of the parathyroid glands by inappropriately high plasma concentrations of iFGF23. The

basis of this dysequilibrium may provide insight into the pathogenesis of RRMS and requires further investigation.

Abbreviations
1,25(OH)$_2$D: 1,25-dihydroxyvitamin D; 25OHD: 25-hydroxyvitamin D; CI: Confidence interval; FGF23: Fibroblast growth factor 23; FGFc: c-terminal fibroblast growth factor 23; HC: Healthy control(s); iFGF23: Intact fibroblast growth factor 23; IQR: Interquartile range; Klotho: Soluble alpha klotho; PTH: Parathyroid hormone; RRMS: Relapsing remitting multiple sclerosis

Acknowledgements
Professor TJ Martin (St Vincent's Institute of Medical Research, Melbourne) and Professor Seiji Fukumoto (University of Tokyo) gave helpful advice on the iFGF23 assay. Professor Terry Speed (Walter and Eliza Hall Institute of Medical Research) and Professor Ian Gordon (Statistical Consulting Centre, University of Melbourne) provided statistical advice and review. Mary Tanner (Royal Melbourne Hospital), Kelly-Jane Lazarus (Box Hill Hospital) and Elizabeth McDonald (Medical Director, MS Australia Victoria) helped with recruitment. Bob Hutton (Royal Melbourne Hospital Information Technology Department) assisted with the study website. Dr. Ken Sikaris (Pathologist, Melbourne Pathology and Chair, International Federation Clinical Chemistry Committee on Analytical Quality) advised and supervised general biochemistry. Hayley Tacon, Eliza Ticknell and Marzi DeGaris (Melbourne Pathology) advised and assisted with specimen collection. Melissa Gresle (University of Melbourne) helped with sample storage. Karen Young, Michael Freemantle, Melissa Nelson, Eric Simons (Sullivan Nicolaides Pathology) performed the iFGF, FGFc, klotho, ferritin and 1,25(OH)2D assays. Advanced Professional Systems Pty Ltd. assisted with Medilink software to remind subjects of venepuncture arrangements.

Funding
This study was funded by charitable research grants from The Myer Foundation Australia (Martyn Myer [President], Christine Edwards [then CEO]) and Multiple Sclerosis Research Australia (Professor Bill Carroll [then Director], Heather Cato [then MS Grants Research Co-ordinator]). These funding bodies gave generous support and encouragement but had no role in the design of the study, in the collection, analysis, and interpretation of data or in writing the manuscript.

Authors' contributions
Study concept and design: All authors. Acquisition, analysis, or interpretation of data: All authors. Drafting of the manuscript: MS, LCH. Critical revision of the manuscript for important intellectual content: All authors. Statistical analysis: MS. Obtained funding: All authors. Administrative, technical, or material support: All authors. Study supervision: All authors. All authors read and approved the final manuscript.

Competing interests
The authors declare that they have no competing interests.

Author details
[1]The Royal Melbourne Hospital, Parkville, Australia. [2]Department of Diabetes and Endocrinology, The Royal Melbourne Hospital, Parkville, VIC 3050, Australia. [3]Walter and Eliza Hall Institute of Medical Research, Parkville, Australia. [4]Sullivan Nicolaides Pathology, Brisbane, Australia. [5]Florey Neuroscience Institutes, Parkville, Australia. [6]University of Melbourne, Parkville, Australia. [7]Monash University, Melbourne, Australia.

References

Armitage P, Berry G. Statistical Methods in Medical Research. 3rd ed. London: Blackwell Scientific Publications; 1994. p. 96–7.

Bacchetta J, Sea JL, Chun RF, Lisse TS, Wesseling-Perry K, Gales B, et al. FGF23 inhibits extra-renal synthesis of 1,25-dihydroxyvitamin D in human monocytes. J Bone Miner Res. 2013;28:46–55.

Ben-Dov IZ, Galitzer H, Lavi-Moshayoff V, Goetz R, Kuro-o M, Mohammadi M, et al. The parathyroid is a target organ for FGF23 in rats. J Clin Invest. 2007;117: 4003–8.

Blau JE, Collins MT. The PTH-vitamin D-FGF23 axis. Rev Endocr Metab Disord. 2015;16:165–74.

Braithwaite V, Prentice AM, Doherty C, Prentice A. FGF23 is correlated with iron status but not with inflammation and decreases after iron supplementation: a supplementation study. Int J Pediatr Endocrinol. 2012;2012:27.

Carvalho JTG, Schneider M, Cuppari L, Grabulosa CC, Aoike DT, Redublo BMQ, et al. Cholecalciferol decreases inflammation and improves vitamin D regulatory enzymes in lymphocytes in the uremic environment: a randomized controlled pilot trial. PLoS One. 2017;12:e0179540. https://doi.org/10.1371/journal.pone.0179540.eCollection 2017.

Colston KW, Evans IM, Spelsberg TC, MacIntyre I. Feedback regulation of vitamin D metabolism by 1,25-dihydroxycholecalciferol. Biochem J. 1977;164:83–9.

Durham BH, Joseph F, Bailey LM, Fraser WD. The association of circulating ferritin with serum concentrations of fibroblast growth factor-23 measured by three commercial assays. Ann Clin Biochem. 2007;44:463–6.

Enioutina EY, Bareyan D, Daynes RA. TLR-induced local metabolism of vitamin D3 plays an important role in the diversification of adaptive immune responses. J Immunol. 2009;182:4296–305.

Gattineni J, Twombley K, Goetz R, Mohammadi M, Baum M. Regulation of serum 1,25(OH)2 vitamin D3 levels by fibroblast growth factor 23 is mediated by FGF receptors 3 and 4. Am J Physiol Renal Physiol. 2011;301:F371–7.

Glendenning P, Laffer LAL, Weber HK, Musk AA, Vasikaran SD. Parathyroid hormone is more stable in EDTA plasma than in serum. Clin Chem. 2002;48: 766–7.

Hollis BW. Assessment of vitamin D nutritional and hormonal status: what to measure and how to do it. Calcif Tissue Int. 1996;58:4–5.

Imel EA, Peacock M, Pitukcheewanont P, Heller HJ, Ward LM, Shulman D, et al. Sensitivity of fibroblast growth factor 23 measurements in tumor-induced osteomalacia. J Clin Endocrinol Metab. 2006;91:2055–61.

Kurosu H, Ogawa Y, Miyoshi M, Yamamoto M, Nandi A, Rosenblatt KP, et al. Regulation of fibroblast growth factor-23 signaling by klotho. J Biol Chem. 2006;281:6120–3.

Lavi-Moshayoff V, Wasserman G, Meir T, Silver J, Naveh-Many T. PTH increases FGF23 gene expression and mediates the high-FGF23 levels of experimental kidney failure: a bone parathyroid feedback loop. Am J Physiol Renal Physiol. 2010;299:F882–9.

Lonergan R, Kinsella K, Fitzpatrick P, Brady J, Murray B, Dunne C, et al. Multiple sclerosis prevalence in Ireland: relationship to vitamin D status and HLA genotype. J Neurol Neurosurg Psychiatry. 2011;82:317–22.

McKenna MJ, Murray B, Lonergan R, Segurado R, Tubridy N, Kilbane MT. Analysing the effect of multiple sclerosis on vitamin D related biochemical markers of bone remodelling. J Steroid Biochem Mol Biol. 2018;177:91–5.

Munger KL, Levin LI, Hollis BW, Howard NS, Ascherio A. Serum 25-hydroxyvitamin D levels and risk of multiple sclerosis. JAMA. 2006;296:2832–8.

Munger KL, Levin LI, Massa J, Horst R, Orban T, Ascherio A, et al. Preclinical serum 25-hydroxyvitamin D levels and risk of type 1 diabetes in a cohort of US military personnel. Am J Epidemiol. 2013;177:411–9.

Nguyen-Yamamoto L, Karaplis AC, St-Arnaud R, Goltzman D. Fibroblast growth factor 23 regulation by systemic and local osteoblast-synthesized 1,25-dihydroxyvitamin D. J Am Soc Nephrol. 2017;28:586–97.

Parfitt AM, Gallagher JC, Heaney RP, Johnston CC, Neer R, Whedon GD. Vitamin D and bone health in the elderly. Am J Clin Nutr. 1982;36:1014–31.

Pierrot-Deseilligny C, Souberbielle JC. Vitamin D and multiple sclerosis: an update. Mult Scler Relat Disord. 2017;14:35–45.

Plebani M. Errors in clinical laboratories or errors in laboratory medicine? Clin Chem Lab Med. 2006;44:750–9.

Quinn SJ, Thomsen AR, Pang JL, Kantham L, Brauner-Osborne H, Pollak M, et al. Interactions between calcium and phosphorus in the regulation of the production of fibroblast growth factor 23 in vivo. Am J Physiol Endocrinol Metab. 2013;304:E310–20.

Razzaque MS, Lanske B. The emerging role of the fibroblast growth factor-23–klotho axis in renal regulation of phosphate homeostasis. J Endocrinol. 2007;194:1–10.

Reichel H, Koeffler HP, Barbers R, Norman AW. Regulation of 1,25-dihydroxyvitamin D3 production by cultured alveolar macrophages from normal human donors and from patients with pulmonary sarcoidosis. J Clin Endocrinol Metab. 1987b;65:1201–9.

Reichel H, Koeffler HP, Norman AW. 25-Hydroxyvitamin D3 metabolism by human T-lymphotropic virus-transformed lymphocytes. J Clin Endocrinol Metab. 1987a;65:519–26.

Shimada T, Hasegawa H, Yamazaki Y, Muto T, Hino R, Takeuchi Y, et al. FGF-23 is a potent regulator of vitamin D metabolism and phosphate homeostasis. J Bone Miner Res. 2004;19:429–35.

Shimada T, Yamazaki Y, Takahashi M, Hasegawa H, Urakawa I, Oshima T, et al. Vitamin D receptor-independent FGF23 actions in regulating phosphate and vitamin D metabolism. Am J Physiol Renal Physiol. 2005;289:F1088–95.

Silver J, Naveh-Many T, Mayer H, Schmelzer HJ, Popovtzer MM. Regulation by vitamin D metabolites of parathyroid hormone gene transcription in vivo in the rat. J Clin Invest. 1986;78:1296–301.

Simpson S Jr, Taylor B, Blizzard L, Ponsonby AL, Pittas F, Tremlett H, et al. Higher 25-hydroxyvitamin D is associated with lower relapse risk in multiple sclerosis. Ann Neurol. 2010;68:193–203.

Smith ER, McMahon LP, Holt SG. Method-specific differences in plasma fibroblast growth factor 23 measurement using four commercial ELISAs. Clin Chem Lab Med. 2013;51:1971–81.

Smith RC, O'Bryan LM, Farrow EG, Summers LJ, Clinkenbeard EL, Roberts JL, et al. Circulating αKlotho influences phosphate handling by controlling FGF23 production. J Clin Invest. 2012;122:4710–5.

Soilu-Hänninen M, Laaksonen M, Laitinen I, Erälinna JP, Lilius EM, Mononen I. A longitudinal study of serum 25-hydroxyvitamin D and intact parathyroid hormone levels indicate the importance of vitamin D and calcium homeostasis regulation in multiple sclerosis. J Neurol Neurosurg Psychiatry. 2008;79:152–7.

Takeda Y, Komaba H, Goto S, Fujii H, Umezu M, Hasegawa H, et al. Effect of intravenous saccharated ferric oxide on serum FGF23 and mineral metabolism in hemodialysis patients. Am J Nephrol. 2011;33:421–6.

Tanaka Y, DeLuca HF. Measurement of mammalian 25-hydroxyvitamin D3 24R- and 1α-hydroxylase. Proc Natl Acad Sci USA. 1981;78:196–9.

van der Mei IA, Ponsonby AL, Dwyer T, Blizzard L, Taylor BV, Kilpatrick T, et al. Vitamin D levels in people with multiple sclerosis and community controls in Tasmania, Australia. J Neurol. 2007;254:581–90.

Watad A, Azrielant S, Bragazzi NL, Sharif K, David P, Katz I, et al. Seasonality and autoimmune diseases: the contribution of the four seasons to the mosaic of autoimmunity. J Autoimmun. 2017;82:13–30.

Yamazaki Y, Okazaki R, Shibata M, Hasegawa Y, Satoh K, Tajima T, et al. Increased circulatory level of biologically active full-length FGF-23 in patients with hypophosphatemic rickets/osteomalacia. J Clin Endocrinol Metab. 2002;87:4957–60.

4

Changes in the process of alternative RNA splicing results in soluble B and T lymphocyte attenuator with biological and clinical implications in critical illness

Sean F. Monaghan[1]*, Debasree Banerjee[2], Chun-Shiang Chung[1], Joanne Lomas-Neira[1], Kamil J. Cygan[3], Christy L. Rhine[3], William G. Fairbrother[3], Daithi S. Heffernan[1], Mitchell M. Levy[2], William G. Cioffi[1] and Alfred Ayala[1]

Abstract

Background: Critically ill patients with sepsis and acute respiratory distress syndrome have severely altered physiology and immune system modifications. RNA splicing is a basic molecular mechanism influenced by physiologic alterations. Immune checkpoint inhibitors, such as B and T Lymphocyte Attenuator (BTLA) have previously been shown to influence outcomes in critical illness. We hypothesize altered physiology in critical illness results in alternative RNA splicing of the immune checkpoint protein, BTLA, resulting in a soluble form with biologic and clinical significance.

Methods: Samples were collected from critically ill humans and mice. Levels soluble BTLA (sBTLA) were measured. Ex vivo experiments assessing for cellular proliferation and cytokine production were done using splenocytes from critically ill mice cultured with sBTLA. Deep RNA sequencing was done to look for alternative splicing of BTLA. sBTLA levels were fitted to models to predict sepsis diagnosis.

Results: sBTLA is increased in the blood of critically ill humans and mice and can predict a sepsis diagnosis on hospital day 0 in humans. Alternative RNA splicing results in a premature stop codon that results in the soluble form. sBTLA has a clinically relevant impact as splenocytes from mice with critical illness cultured with soluble BTLA have increased cellular proliferation.

Conclusion: sBTLA is produced as a result of alternative RNA splicing. This isoform of BTLA has biological significance through changes in cellular proliferation and can predict the diagnosis of sepsis.

Keywords: BTLA, ARDS, RNA splicing, Critical illness

Background

Patients with severe critical illness, such as sepsis and acute respiratory distress syndrome, have severely modified physiology resulting in organ dysfunction. The current definition of sepsis utilizes the SOFA score to standardize the organ dysfunction that results (Singer et al., 2016). As there is more focus on organ dysfunction, more effort is needed to understand basic molecular mechanisms that may influence critical illness and the subsequent organ dysfunction.

It is known that physiologic conditions seen in critical illness, such as hypoxia and acidosis, influence the normal process of RNA splicing (Elias & Dias, 2008). Preliminary data also suggests that models of critical illness result in multiple instances of statistically significant changes in the alternative RNA splicing process and/or the nature/levels of gene products transcribed into mRNA/protein (Monaghan et al., 2017). A better understanding of alternative RNA splicing as it pertains to immune modulating proteins is needed as not only are many of these proteins proposed to be central mediators of pathological process that

* Correspondence: smonaghan@lifespan.org
[1]Division of Surgical Research, Department of Surgery, Alpert School of Medicine at Brown University and Rhode Island Hospital, 593 Eddy Street, Providence, RI 02903, USA
Full list of author information is available at the end of the article

Changes in the process of alternative RNA splicing results in soluble B and T lymphocyte attenuator...

35

contribute to organ dysfunction, but as these proteins become therapeutic targets in critical illness more needs to be understood about the impact of alternative splicing impact on their pharmacological impact. In this respect RNA splicing is the proposed mechanism for processing of message for the soluble form of the immune cell-surface co-inhibitory receptor, a.k.a., a checkpoint protein, <u>B</u> and <u>T</u> lymphocyte <u>a</u>ttenuator (sBTLA).

Lack of the gene for BTLA has been shown to improve mortality in animal models of sepsis (Shubin et al., 2012; Cheng et al., 2016). In addition, humans with increased leukocyte cell surface expression of BTLA are more likely to have sepsis, are at an increased risk of subsequent infections, and have longer hospital lengths of stay (Shubin et al., 2013). In addition, the soluble form has recently been shown to be elevated in sepsis and predict mortality and disease severity (Lange et al., 2017) and alternative RNA splicing is the proposed mechanism for the generation of sBTLA (Elias & Dias, 2008; Kasim et al., 2014). Soluble BTLA has also been implicated in enhanced vaccine response to cancer (Han et al., 2009; Han et al., 2014).

However, although previous work has suggested an important role in critical illness for sBTLA, there was no mention of how this isoform is produced or its biologic relevance. In this respect, PD-1 is a similar immune cell-surface co-inhibitory molecule/checkpoint protein inhibitor with similar effects in critical illness (Huang et al., 2009; Monaghan et al., 2012a; Monaghan et al., 2012b). PD-1 also has a soluble form that is increased with a biologic impact and this isoform is due to alternative RNA splicing (Monaghan et al., 2016). Here we propose that sBTLA is produced as a result of alternative RNA splicing and the soluble isoform has both biologic and clinical importance.

Methods

Collection of samples from humans
Samples from humans were collected from patients admitted to the medical intensive care unit (MICU) at Rhode Island Hospital. Patients were considered to have sepsis if they had corresponding ICD-10 coding on admission, attending physician documentation of sepsis, septic shock in their problem list with evidence of hypo-perfusion (lactate > 2 mmol/L, systolic blood pressure < 90 mmHg, mean arterial pressure < 65 after 30 cm^3/kg crystalloid bolus within 3 h of identification), suspected or documented infection with evidence of at least one organ failure as defined by the SOFA score. (Singer et al., 2016) Patients were excluded due to malignancy, trauma within 30 days, pulmonary fibrosis, known recent antibiotic use (within last week of admission), prisoners, pregnancy, age less than 18 years old and immune-compromised state. Patients were enrolled

upon arrival to the ICU or within 24 h of developing sepsis in the ICU. Consent was obtained and the IRB approved this study (IRB# 4159–14).

Collection of samples from mice with critical illness
C57BL/6 male mice (The Jackson Laboratory, Bar Harbor, ME) between 10 and 12 weeks of age were used. Critical illness was induced in the mice by hemorrhage (non-lethal shock) followed by cecal ligation and puncture (CLP) (Monaghan et al., 2012a; Ayala et al., 2002; Lomas-Neira et al., 2006; Perl et al., 2007; Thakkar et al., 2011). The control group was sham hemorrhage followed by sham CLP (Sham-Sham). All experiments were done according to guidelines from the National Institutes of Health (Bethesda, MD) and were approved by the Rhode Island Hospital animal use committee (AWC#: 0206–15).

Measurement of sBTLA
Blood from mice and humans was centrifuged at 10,000×g at 4°C for 10 min, the serum layer was isolated, and red blood cells were lysed with 1 mL double distilled water with 0.037 g EDTA (Invitrogen, Carlsbad, CA), 8.26 g NH_4Cl (Sigma, St. Louis, MO), and 1 g $KHCO_3$ (Sigma, St. Louis, MO). In humans sBTLA was measured using a multiplex analysis with the Thermo Fischer multiplex kit (Waltham, MA). In mice the soluble level of BTLA was measured in the serum using the BTLA ELISA kit (Cusabio, College Park, MD). A bronchial alveolar lavage (BAL) sample was collected from the mice after euthanasia as previously done (Monaghan et al., 2016). These samples were tested for BTLA using the same kit for the serum (Cusabio, College Park, MD). The detection of soluble BTLA was done in samples that were free of cellular components to minimize the amount of membrane bound BTLA that may be detected in the samples and this is in line with previous work regarding soluble immune modulating proteins (Lange et al., 2017; Monaghan et al., 2016).

Ex vivo experiments
Splenocytes were harvested from either mice with severe critical illness (hemorrhage/CLP) or sham controls as previously described (Monaghan et al., 2016). In brief, after the mice were euthanized with CO_2 the spleens were harvested and then crushed between two slides to liberate the cells into 10 mL sterile PBS. Red blood cells were lysed with sodium chloride. Splenocytes were cultured with DMEM (ThermoScientific, Waltham, MA) with 10% fetal calf serum (Atlantic Biologicals, Miami, FL) and 0.1% gentamycin (Sigma, St. Louis, MO).

BTLA fusion protein (R&D Systems, Minneapolis, MN) at 1000 ng/mL or 10,000 ng/mL or control was then used as an additive to the culture of splenocytes (as above) from mice with critical illness compared to mice who underwent sham hemorrhage and sham CLP as previously described (Monaghan et al., 2016). This fusion protein was selected as it mimics the binding of the extracellular portion of BTLA and will be added to culture in conditions similar to the soluble form. All cells were cultured for 72 h. At that point, proliferation was assessed using the CyQuant assay (ThermoScientific, Waltham, MA). Supernatants were collected and analyzed for the production of cytokines using a multiplex analysis with the Mouse Th 1/2/9/17 panel 17 multiplex kit (Thermo Fischer, Waltham, MA) per the manufacturer instructions on a Luminex machine (Austin, TX).

Isolation of RNA and RNA sequencing
Samples were collected as whole blood from mice with critical illness induced by hemorrhagic shock followed by sepsis via CLP (IACUC approved) as described above. RNA was extracted using the MasterPure Complete DNA/RNA Purification kit (epicenter, Madison WI) followed by the Globin Clear Kit (ThermoScientific, Waltham, MA). RNA was then sent to Gene Wiz for sequencing as 1400 ng RNA in 40uL of fluid.

Assessment of RNA splicing
The raw RNA sequencing data first underwent quality control with MultiQC (Ewels et al., 2016). Using rMATS, alternative RNA splicing events were identified, in addition to an assessment of gene transcription (Li et al., 2017; Shen et al., 2012; Shen et al., 2014). Significant alternative RNA splicing events in the BTLA gene were then further studied to predict the protein outcome for those events.

Statistical analysis
Data was analyzed using SigmaPlot 10.0 (Systat Software, San Jose, CA) or code contained within rMATS. Paired t-tests or rank sum analysis were done when two groups are compared. Multiple groups were compared by or two-way ANOVA with Holm-Sidak correction. Receiver operator characteristic curves were fit to use sBTLA level to predict sepsis diagnosis. Graphs are displayed as mean or median with error bars representing the standard deviation. Alpha was set to 0.05.

Results
Soluble BTLA levels were assessed in the lungs, BAL fluid and serum of mice with severe critical illness induced by hemorrhagic shock followed by septic shock. Mouse sBTLA increased in the serum in critical illness as compared to controls (2.66 ng/mL vs 1.208 ng/mL, $p = 0.0037$, Fig. 1a), but no differences were seen in the BAL fluid (0.371 ng/mL vs. 0.227, $p = 0.476$, Fig. 1c) or the lung samples (40.077 ng/mL vs. 43.086 ng/mL, $p = 0.519$).

Humans were recruited from a medical intensive care unit after consent was obtained, 30 had a diagnosis of sepsis (Singer et al., 2016) and 30 were non-sepsis ICU controls. 5 patients in the sepsis group and 1 patient in the control group died during the hospital stay despite similar ages between the groups (sepsis 60, control 56). Human sBTLA in the blood increased in sepsis vs ICU controls (557.030 pg/mL (255.370–1485.693) vs 158.350 (33.233–284.831), $p < 0.001$, Fig. 1b). In addition the level of sBTLA can predict sepsis on hospital day 0 (ROC curve area 0.7598, 95% CI 0.6326 To 0.8869, $p = 0.0006111815643966$, Fig. 1d).

In order to assess the potential mechanism by which sBTLA is produced, RNA from the blood of mice with critical illness and controls was sent for deep RNA sequencing to look for alternative RNA splicing. From this sequencing it was found that the while the extent of overall gene expression of BTLA was similar between the two groups, there were changes in two significant splicing events noted. A skipped exon event was noticed in which exon 3 is skipped (Fig. 2). Exon three encodes much of the extracellular domain of BTLA, and as a result, this event leads to the loss of 70% of the extracellular domain. In the control mice, the exon is skipped 19% of the time, but in critical illness, the exon is never skipped (FDR =0.0000471413836931). A second significant splicing event predicts the production of sBTLA. In this event there is an alternative 3′ splice site before exon 4 (Fig. 3). This alternative 3′ splice site results in a premature stop codon so only exons 1–3 are translated. This protein with exons 1–3 could be the soluble form as the transmembrane and intracellular portions are not translated with this isoform. In the control mice the alternative 3′ splicing site occurs 40% of the time, but in critically ill mice, this level increases to 53% (FDR =0.0000429857901449).

Since sBTLA is increased in sepsis/critical illness and results from the alternative RNA splicing analysis implied that nature of the process had changed, experiments were undertaken to assess a biological significance of sBTLA. Splenocytes from mice with critical illness or controls were cultured with a BTLA fusion protein and cytokines and cellular proliferation were assessed. In the supernatant of the cells there was no significant difference in the levels of granulocyte-monocyte colony stimulating factor (GM-CSF), interferon (IFN)-gamma, interleukin (IL)-1beta, IL-2, IL-4, IL-5, IL-12p70, IL-13, IL-18, IL-10, IL-17a, IL-22, IL-23, or tumor necrosis factor (TNF)-alpha based upon the source of the cells (critically ill mice or control) or level of BTLA (1000 ng/mL vs 10,000 ng/mL). Cells from mice with critical illness produced significantly more IL-6 (Diff of means 5.919, $p = 0.41$, Fig. 4a), IL-9 (Diff of means 5.410, $p = 0.019$, Fig. 4b) and IL-27 (Diff of means 0.549, $p = 0.044$, Fig. 4c), but there was no influence on the sBTLA fusion protein. Cellular proliferation was increased in cells from

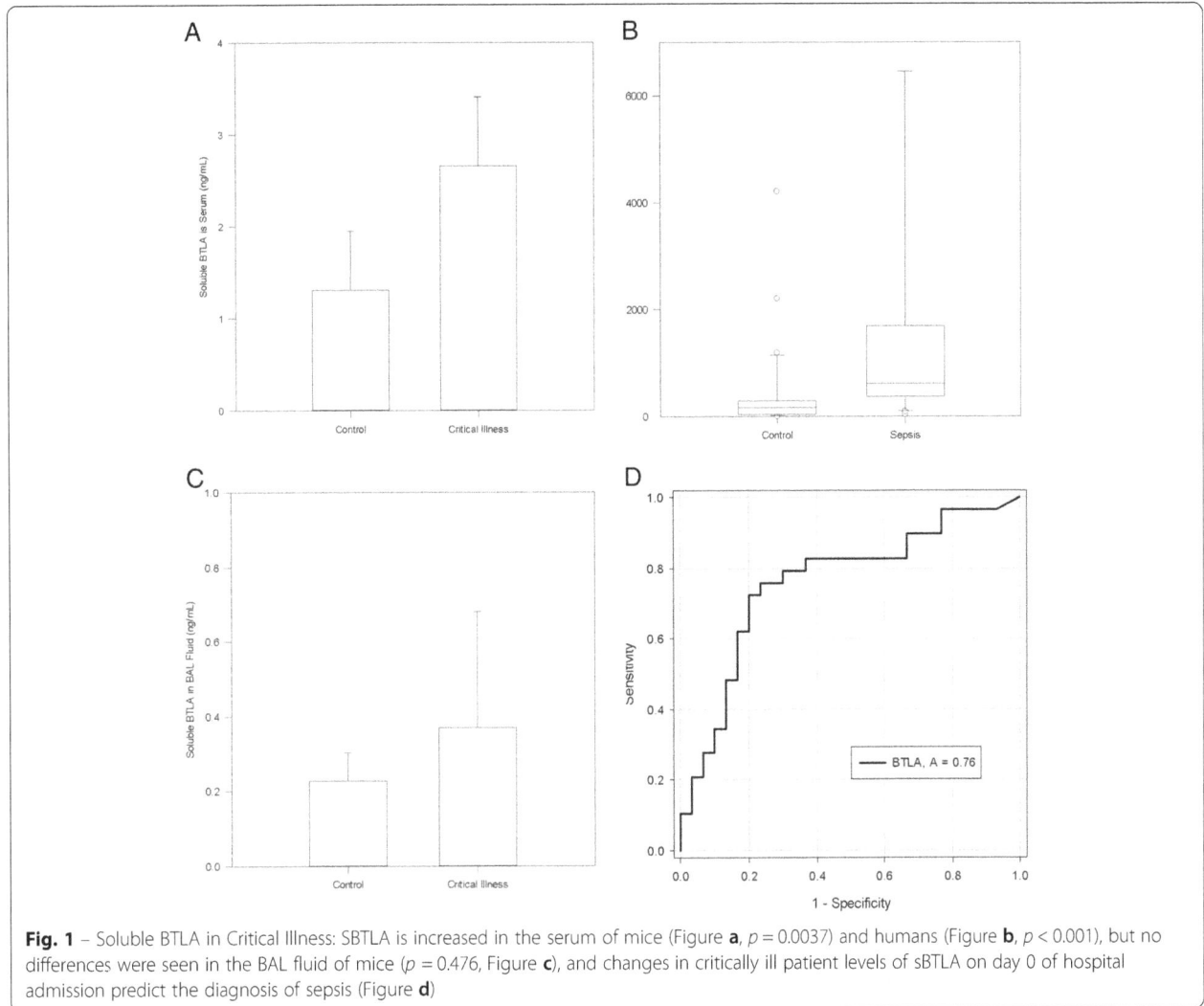

Fig. 1 – Soluble BTLA in Critical Illness: SBTLA is increased in the serum of mice (Figure **a**, $p = 0.0037$) and humans (Figure **b**, $p < 0.001$), but no differences were seen in the BAL fluid of mice ($p = 0.476$, Figure **c**), and changes in critically ill patient levels of sBTLA on day 0 of hospital admission predict the diagnosis of sepsis (Figure **d**)

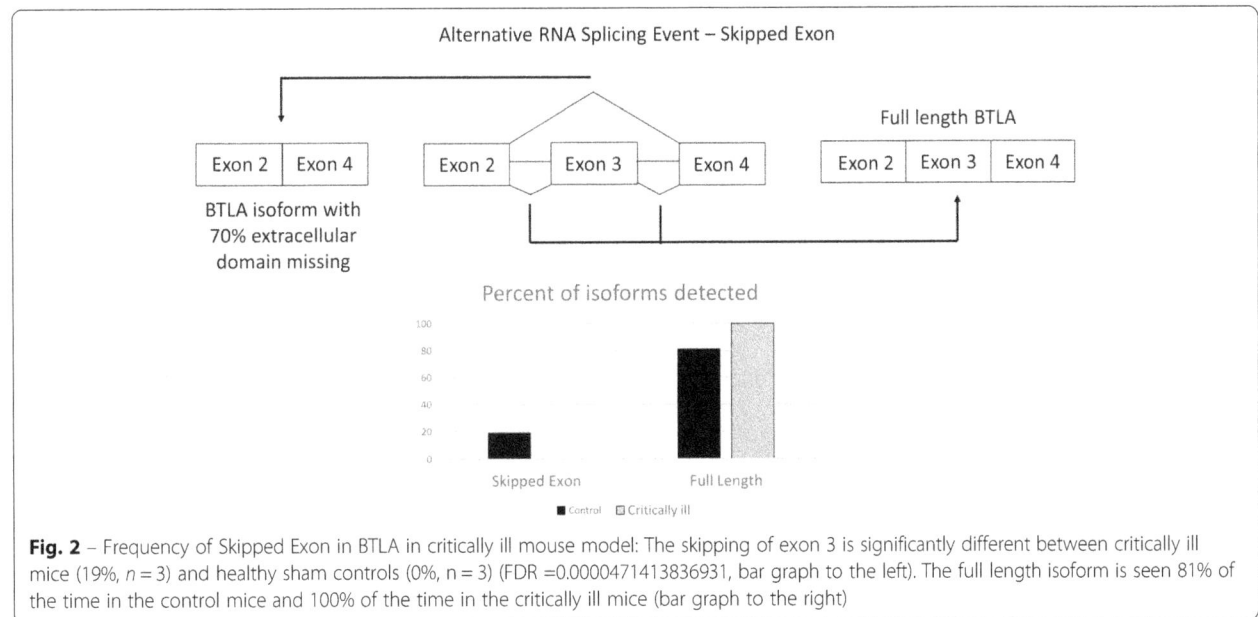

Fig. 2 – Frequency of Skipped Exon in BTLA in critically ill mouse model: The skipping of exon 3 is significantly different between critically ill mice (19%, $n = 3$) and healthy sham controls (0%, n = 3) (FDR =0.0000471413836931, bar graph to the left). The full length isoform is seen 81% of the time in the control mice and 100% of the time in the critically ill mice (bar graph to the right)

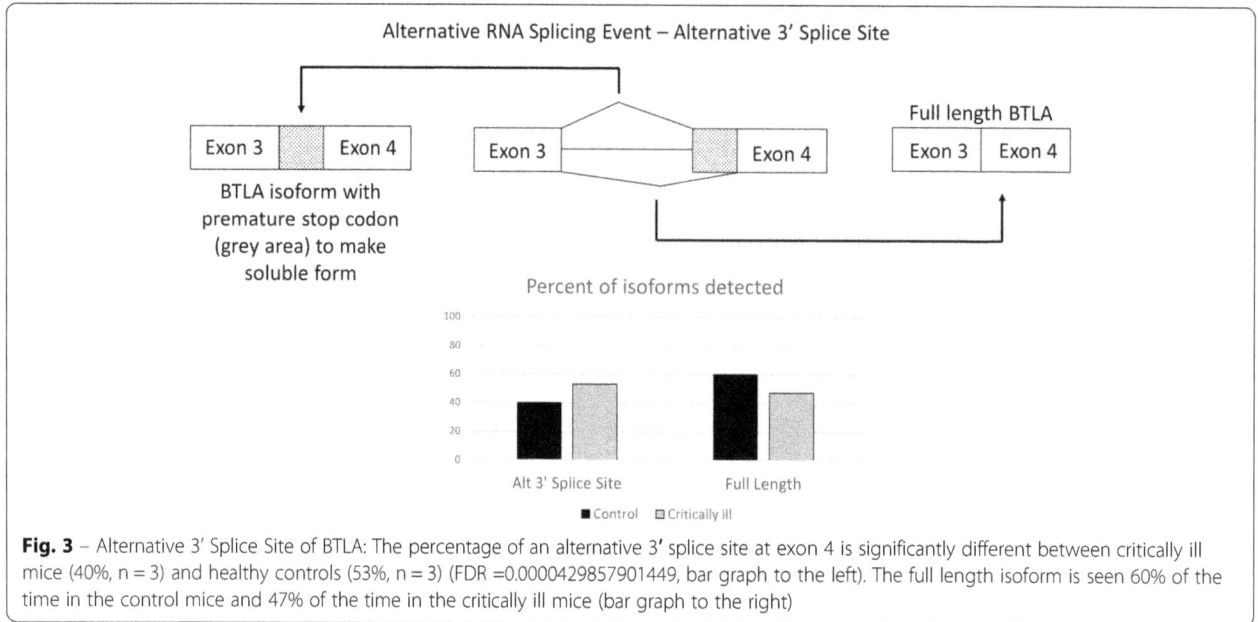

Alternative RNA Splicing Event – Alternative 3' Splice Site

Full length BTLA

Exon 3 | | Exon 4   Exon 3 | | Exon 4   Exon 3 | Exon 4

BTLA isoform with premature stop codon (grey area) to make soluble form

Percent of isoforms detected

Alt 3' Splice Site   Full Length

■ Control   □ Critically ill

Fig. 3 – Alternative 3' Splice Site of BTLA: The percentage of an alternative 3' splice site at exon 4 is significantly different between critically ill mice (40%, n = 3) and healthy controls (53%, n = 3) (FDR =0.0000429857901449, bar graph to the left). The full length isoform is seen 60% of the time in the control mice and 47% of the time in the critically ill mice (bar graph to the right)

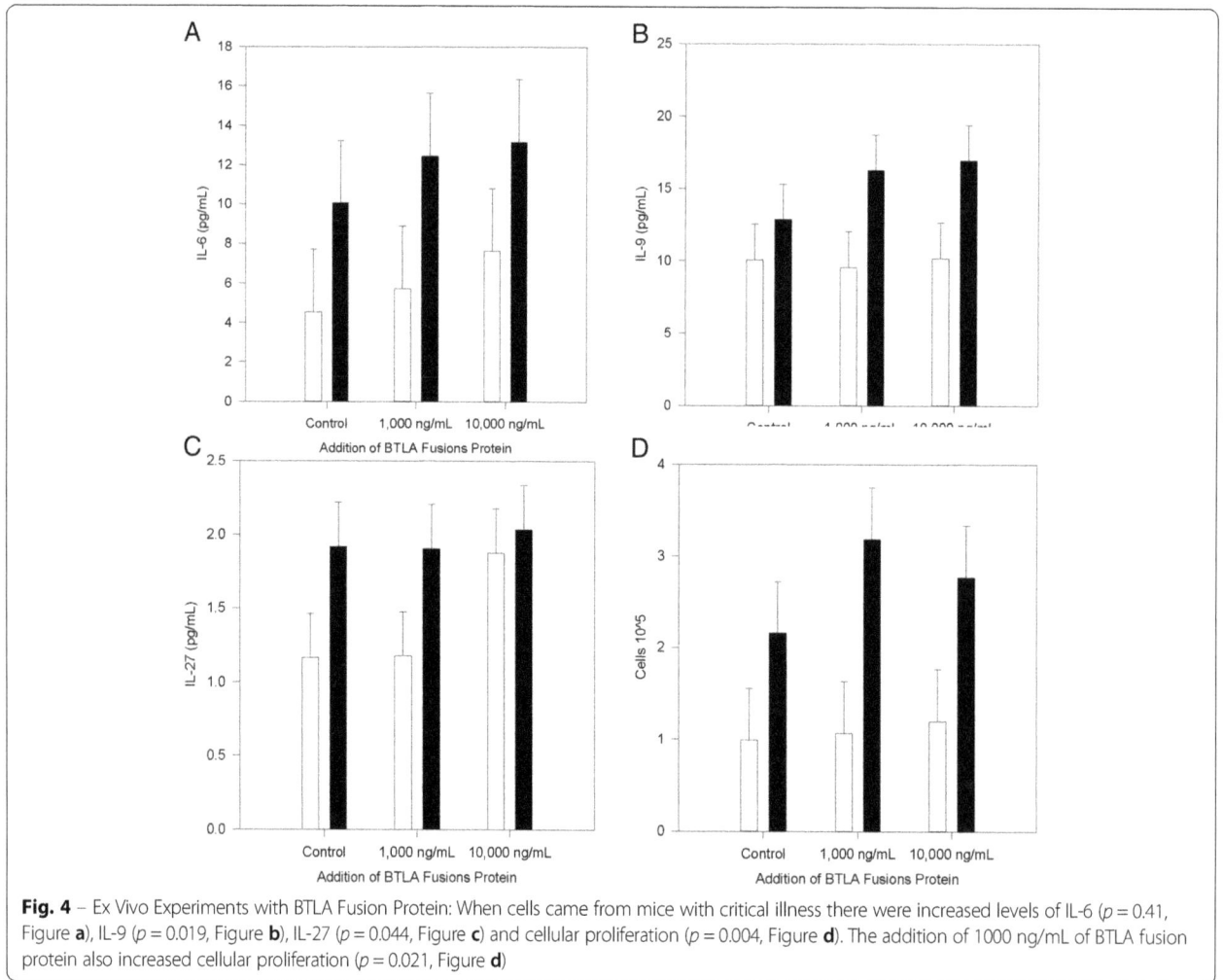

Fig. 4 – Ex Vivo Experiments with BTLA Fusion Protein: When cells came from mice with critical illness there were increased levels of IL-6 ($p = 0.41$, Figure **a**), IL-9 ($p = 0.019$, Figure **b**), IL-27 ($p = 0.044$, Figure **c**) and cellular proliferation ($p = 0.004$, Figure **d**). The addition of 1000 ng/mL of BTLA fusion protein also increased cellular proliferation ($p = 0.021$, Figure **d**)

mice with critical illness (Diff of Means 1.615, $p = 0.004$, Fig. 4d). Although there were no changes in cytokine production during the co-culture with the BTLA fusion protein across the two cell groups (critically ill and controls), the 1000 ng sBTLA/mL resulted in increased proliferation when comparing cells from mice with critical illness (Diff of means 2.112, $p = 0.021$) to controls.

Discussion

In this study we have again found that sBTLA levels are increased in humans with sepsis, but also in a murine model of critical illness (Fig. 1a and b) and this is inline with previous clinical studies of sBTLA (Lange et al., 2017). Further, we show that the rise sBTLA, on hospital day 0, was able to predict the diagnosis of sepsis (Fig. 1d) with prognostic capacity close to SOFA and other soluble co-inhibitory receptors/checkpoint proteins recently reported (Singer et al., 2016; Banerjee et al., 2018). Previous work has focused on the influence of membrane bound BTLA relative to outcomes in the murine model and ICU patients (Shubin et al., 2012; Shubin et al., 2013; Shubin et al., 2011) as assessed by flow cytometry. Assessing sBTLA is easier as it can be accomplished via ELISA of the serum and as such could be a novel biomarker for sepsis with a quicker throughput compared to flow cytometry or bacterial cultures (Shao et al., 2015; Sherwood & Hotchkiss, 2013).

However, for a truly impactful, beyond its potential merits as a biomarker, an understanding of the mechanism by which it is not only produced, but its ultimate function is essential in order to gain insight into pathological potential as well as into clinical/pharmacological scenarios where the levels are not in line with expectations or if BTLA is to be a therapeutic target (Patil et al., 2017). This study has showed that sBTLA is likely the result of changes in the nature but not the extent of the alternative RNA splicing process in response the combined insults of shock and sepsis in mice (Figs. 2 and 3). Importantly, alternative RNA splicing can also explain why previous work has shown an increase in membrane bound levels (Shubin et al., 2012; Shubin et al., 2013; Shubin et al., 2011), but we detected no difference in level of gene expression in our samples. Fig. 2 demonstrates how skipping an exon in the control animal's results in a relative decrease in the membrane bound BTLA identified because 70% of the extracellular portion is removed, and therefore this protein may not be seen by antibodies directed to the extracellular portion. In addition, alternative splicing has been shown to result in lack of translation to a protein without the creation of a new premature stop codon and this isoform may be degraded (Martinez-Nunez & Sanford, 2016).

Again, alternative RNA splicing can explain how more sBTLA is observed despite similar levels of gene expression. Alternative RNA splicing has been suggested as a mechanism for the production of other membrane bound immune checkpoint proteins such as PD-1 and CTLA-4 (Monaghan et al., 2016; Rossille et al., 2014; Ward et al., 2014). In the current study, the soluble form is created as a result of a premature stop codon from an alternative 3′ splice site (Fig. 3). Although previously stated mechanisms of degradation are possible (Martinez-Nunez & Sanford, 2016), the protein levels seen in fig. 1a and b support the production of the soluble form. However, in order to truly know if an alternatively spliced isoform is translated to a gene advanced techniques utilizing mass spectroscopy (Ivanov et al., 2018) would be needed since the antibodies to proteins may not detect the novel isoform.

The creation of sBTLA via alternative splicing would be novel; however, sBTLA also has some biological function. Despite the testing for numerous cytokines in the supernatant of splenocytes from critically ill mice or controls, few were influenced by critical illness (Fig. 4a, b, c) and none were influenced by the presence of the BTLA fusion protein in the media. Despite no changes in cytokine production from the BTLA fusion protein, it did cause an increase in cellular proliferation at the 1000 ng/mL level; this is the level most in line with the in vivo level detected here. Increase in proliferation shows a biological significance of this protein, but its mechanism is not completely clear. However, sBTLA may explain some differences seen in experiments conducted previously. Lack of BTLA gene expression has reported to reduce septic mortality in murine models (Shubin et al., 2012; Shubin et al., 2013), however, addition of BTLA antibody did not improve septic mouse survival (Cheng et al., 2016). The lack of survival benefit from antibody addition may be due to interference of sBTLA, which we have shown to be increased in this model, particularly if the antibody is directed against the extra-cellular portion. In addition a thorough understanding of the soluble/membrane bound interaction and target of potential antibodies is critical as these checkpoint inhibitors are therapeutic targets (Patil et al., 2017). Another potential reason for limited results as it pertains to cytokine production is the heterogeneous nature of splenocytes. BTLA and its ligand HVEM are located on many cells and results could be minimized due to this heterogeneous cell populations.

Conclusions

sBTLA is increased in human and murine models of critical illness, is produced as a result of a change in the nature but not the extent of alternative RNA splicing, has biological significance in altering cellular proliferation, and can predict the development of sepsis in in critical ill patients.

Abbreviations
BAL: bronchial alveolar lavage; BTLA: B and T Lymphocyte Attenuator;
CLP: cecal ligation and puncture; Interferon: IFN; Interleukin: IL;
MICU: medical intensive care unit

Funding
This work was funded in part by NIH P20GM103652-Pilot (S.F.M.); NIH-NIGMS
R35GM118097 (A.A.), NIH P20GM103652 (J.L.N.), NIH K08GM110495 (D.S.H.), NIH
P20GM103652-Pilot (D.B.); the C. James Carrico, MD, FACS, Faculty Research
Fellowship for the Study of Trauma and Critical Care from the American College
of Surgeons (S.F.M.); the Deans Emerging Area of New Science (DEANS) Award
from Brown University (S.F.M. and W.G.F.).

Authors' contributions
SFM, DB, DSH, MML, WGC analyzed and interpreted the patient data regarding
BTLA. SFM, CSC, JLN, AA performed the experiments pertaining to the mouse
model. SFM, KJC, CLR, and WGF performed work as it related to RNA splicing.
SFM wrote the majority of the paper with edits from DB, DSH, MML, WGC, WGF,
and AA. All authors read and approved the final manuscript.

Competing interests
The authors declare that they have no competing interests.

Author details
[1]Division of Surgical Research, Department of Surgery, Alpert School of
Medicine at Brown University and Rhode Island Hospital, 593 Eddy Street,
Providence, RI 02903, USA. [2]Division of Pulmonary and Critical Care,
Department of Medicine, Alpert School of Medicine at Brown University and
Rhode Island Hospital, Providence, RI 02903, USA. [3]MCB Department, Brown
University, Providence, RI 02903, USA.

References
Ayala A, et al. Shock-induced neutrophil mediated priming for acute lung injury
in mice: divergent effects of TLR-4 and TLR-4/FasL deficiency. Am J Pathol.
2002;161:2283–94.

Banerjee D, et al. Soluble programmed cell death protein-1 and programmed cell
death ligand-1 in sepsis. Crit Care. 2018;22:146.

Cheng T, et al. Enhanced innate inflammation induced by anti-BTLA antibody in
dual insult model of hemorrhagic shock/Sepsis. Shock (Augusta, Ga). 2016;45:
40–9.

Elias AP, Dias S. Microenvironment changes (in pH) affect VEGF alternative
splicing. Cancer microenvironment : official journal of the International
Cancer Microenvironment Society. 2008;1:131–9.

Ewels P, Magnusson M, Lundin S, Kaller M. MultiQC: summarize analysis results
for multiple tools and samples in a single report. Bioinformatics (Oxford,
England). 2016;32:3047–8.

Han L, et al. (2009) Soluble B and T lymphocyte attenuator possesses antitumor
effects and facilitates heat shock protein 70 vaccine-triggered antitumor
immunity against a murine TC-1 cervical cancer model in vivo. Journal of
immunology (Baltimore, Md.: 1950) 183: 7842–7850.

Han L, et al. AAV-sBTLA facilitates HSP70 vaccine-triggered prophylactic
antitumor immunity against a murine melanoma pulmonary metastasis
model in vivo. Cancer Lett. 2014;354:398–406.

Huang X, et al. PD-1 expression by macrophages plays a pathologic role in
altering microbial clearance and the innate inflammatory response to sepsis.
Proc Natl Acad Sci U S A. 2009;106:6303–8.

Ivanov MV, Lobas AA, Levitsky LI, Moshkovskii SA, Gorshkov MV. Brute-force
approach for mass spectrometry-based variant peptide identification in
Proteogenomics without personalized genomic data. J Am Soc Mass
Spectrom. 2018;

Kasim M, et al. Shutdown of achaete-scute homolog-1 expression by
heterogeneous nuclear ribonucleoprotein (hnRNP)-A2/B1 in hypoxia. J Biol
Chem. 2014;289:26973–88.

Lange A, Sunden-Cullberg J, Magnuson A, Hultgren O. Soluble B and T
lymphocyte attenuator correlates to disease severity in Sepsis and high levels

are associated with an increased risk of mortality. PLoS One. 2017;12:
e0169176.

Li Z, Zhao K, Tian H. Integrated analysis of differential expression and alternative
splicing of non-small cell lung cancer based on RNA sequencing. Oncol Lett.
2017;14:1519–25.

Lomas-Neira J, et al. Role of alveolar macrophage and migrating neutrophils in
hemorrhage-induced priming for ALI subsequent to septic challenge.
American journal of physiology Lung cellular and molecular physiology.
2006;290:L51–8.

Martinez-Nunez RT, Sanford JR. Studying isoform-specific mRNA recruitment to
polyribosomes with Frac-seq. Methods in molecular biology (Clifton, NJ).
2016;1358:99–108.

Monaghan SF, et al. Mechanisms of indirect acute lung injury: a novel role for
the coinhibitory receptor, programmed death-1. Ann Surg. 2012a;255:158–64.

Monaghan SF, et al. Programmed death 1 expression as a marker for immune
and physiological dysfunction in the critically ill surgical patient. Shock
(Augusta, Ga.). 2012b;38:117–22.

Monaghan SF, et al. Soluble programmed cell death receptor-1 (sPD-1): a potential
biomarker with anti-inflammatory properties in human and experimental acute
respiratory distress syndrome (ARDS). J Transl Med. 2016;14:312.

Monaghan SF, et al. Modes of alternative RNA splicing: divergent changes in
response to critical illness. But Similarity Across Two Tissues Shock (Augusta,
Ga). 2017;47:100.

Patil NK, Guo Y, Luan L, Sherwood ER. Targeting immune cell checkpoints during
Sepsis. Int J Mol Sci. 2017;18

Perl M, et al. Fas-induced pulmonary apoptosis and inflammation during indirect
acute lung injury. Am J Respir Crit Care Med. 2007;176:591–601.

Rossille D, et al. High level of soluble programmed cell death ligand 1 in blood
impacts overall survival in aggressive diffuse large B-cell lymphoma: results
from a French multicenter clinical trial. Leukemia. 2014;28:2367–75.

Shao R, Li CS, Fang Y, Zhao L, Hang C. Low B and T lymphocyte attenuator
expression on CD4+ T cells in the early stage of sepsis is associated with the
severity and mortality of septic patients: a prospective cohort study. Critical
care (London, England). 2015;19:308.

Shen S, et al. MATS: a Bayesian framework for flexible detection of differential
alternative splicing from RNA-Seq data. Nucleic Acids Res. 2012;40:e61.

Shen S, et al. (2014) rMATS: robust and flexible detection of differential
alternative splicing from replicate RNA-Seq data. Proc Natl Acad Sci of the
United States of America 111: E5593–E5601.

Sherwood ER, Hotchkiss RS. BTLA as a biomarker and mediator of sepsis-induced
immunosuppression. Critical care (London, England). 2013;17:1022.

Shubin NJ, Monaghan SF, Ayala A. Anti-inflammatory mechanisms of sepsis.
Contrib Microbiol. 2011;17:108–24.

Shubin NJ, Monaghan SF, Heffernan DS, Chung CS, Ayala A. (2013) B and T
lymphocyte attenuator expression on CD4+ T-cells associates with sepsis and
subsequent infections in ICU patients. Critical care (London, England) 17: R276.

Shubin NJ, et al. BTLA expression contributes to septic morbidity and mortality by
inducing innate inflammatory cell dysfunction. J Leukoc Biol. 2012;92:593–603.

Singer M, et al. The third international consensus definitions for Sepsis and septic
shock (Sepsis-3). Jama. 2016;315:801–10.

Thakkar RK, et al. Local tissue expression of the cell death ligand, fas ligand, plays
a central role in the development of extrapulmonary acute lung injury.
Shock (Augusta, Ga.). 2011;36:138–43.

Ward FJ, Dahal LN, Khanolkar RC, Shankar SP, Barker RN. Targeting the
alternatively spliced soluble isoform of CTLA-4: prospects for
immunotherapy? Immunotherapy. 2014;6:1073–84.

5

Circular RNA CEP128 acts as a sponge of miR-145-5p in promoting the bladder cancer progression via regulating *SOX11*

Zhun Wu, Wei Huang, Xuegang Wang, Tao Wang, Yuedong Chen, Bin Chen, Rongfu Liu, Peide Bai and Jinchun Xing[*]

Abstract

Background: This study aimed to investigate the effect of over-expressing circular RNA CEP128 (circCEP128) on cell functions and explore the molecular mechanism of which in bladder carcinoma.

Methods: The differentially expressed circRNAs and mRNAs in bladder carcinoma cells and cells in adjacent tissues were screened out using microarray analysis. Expression levels of circRNAs and mRNAs in tissues and cells were determined by qRT-PCR. Expression of *SOX11* was detected by western blot. Luciferase reporter assay and RNA pull-down assay were used to investigate the interactions between the specific circRNA, miRNA and mRNA. Cell cycle and apoptosis were measured using flow cytometry after transfection. MTT assay was also performed to detect the cell proliferation.

Results: In present study, circCEP128 and *SOX11* were observed significantly up-regulated in bladder cancer tissues, while the expression of miR-145-5p was decreased in cancer samples compared to normal samples. Cytoscape was used to visualize circCEP128-miRNA-target gene interactions based on the TargetScan and circular RNA interactome, which revealed that circCEP128 served as a sponge of miR-145-5p and indirectly regulated *SOX11*. Knockdown of circCEP128 induced the inhibition of cell proliferation and the increased bladder cancer cell apoptosis rate.

Conclusions: CircCEP128 functions as a ceRNA for miR-145-5p, which could up regulates *SOX11* and further promotes cell proliferation and inhibits cell apoptosis of bladder cancer.

Keywords: Bladder cancer, Circle RNA, circCEP128, miR-145-5p, *SOX11*

Background

Global Cancer Statistics alarms that bladder cancer, a tumor in urinary system, caused 130,000 deaths each year (Li et al., 2017). In China, the mortality and morbidity of bladder cancer ranked first among all the tumors in urinary system (Huang et al., 2016). Especially for the patients suffer from muscle-invasive bladder cancer, the occurrence of metastasis is more frequently and the prognosis is poorer than other kinds of bladder cancers (Zhong et al., 2017). Besides, most clinical trials of chemotherapy for advanced bladder carcinoma displayed limited benefits. Therefore, it is urgent for us to identify novel molecular targets for inhibiting the tumorigenesis of bladder cancer (Zhong et al., 2016).

MicroRNAs (miRNAs) are endogenous small non-coding RNA molecules (19–22 nucleotides in length) that negatively modulate protein-coding genes expression through binding to the specific sequence of genes (Enokida et al., 2016). Increasing evidences have demonstrated that miRNAs usually expressed abnormally in bladder cancer and resulted in multiple alterations during the development of cancer, such as promoting or inhibiting carcinogenesis (Li et al., 2017). MicroRNA-145 (miR-145) has been frequently reported to be down-regulated in various human cancers, including prostate cancer, bladder cancer and colon cancer, as well as in B-cell

* Correspondence: xibuliadi@163.com
Department of Urology, the First Affiliated Hospital of Xiamen University, No.55 Zhenhai Road, Xiamen 361003, Fujian, China

malignancies (Noguchi et al., 2013). Exogenous miR-145 has also been speculated as tumor inhibitor when being administrated intravesically (Minami et al., 2017).

Circular RNAs (circRNAs), without cap and polyA tails, forms covalently closed continuous loops by non-sequential back-splicing of pre-mRNA transcripts. They generally expressed in eukaryotic cells, but the biological function of them remains unclear (Zhong et al., 2017). CircRNAs are less prone to degrade since they are resistant to exonuclease, the property of which makes circRNAs superior than linear RNAs in terms of biological markers (Huang et al., 2016). Multiple properties of circRNAs have been identified in recent years, among which "miRNA sponges" role was most frequently discussed (Shang et al., 2016). Zhong et al., 2017 investigated competing endogenous RNA mechanism in bladder cancer, among which circRNA MYLK was profoundly discussed but circCEP128 was neglected (Zhong et al., 2017). CircTCF25 and circHIPK3 have been fully illustrated in other studies about ceRNA network and variant pathways (Li et al., 2017; Huang et al., 2016; Zhong et al., 2016). However, this speculation refers to cirCEP128 as a new bio-functional marker which has a close interaction with miR-145-5p in bladder cancer.

SOX11, as an intronless gene regulates cell fate, functions in tumorigenesis and adult neurogenesis. It is known to promote tissue remodeling, progenitor cell expansion and differentiation of a number of cell types, including neural progenitor cells (Oliemuller et al., 2017). *SOX11* is a diagnostic and prognostic antigen in B cell lymphomas and has recently been demonstrated to have tumor suppressor functions (Sernbo et al., 2011). It was found that miR-223-3p inhibitor restrains ovarian cancer development by increasing *SOX11* expression (Fang et al., 2017). Therefore, we hypothesized that *SOX11* might be regulated by miR-145-5p in human bladder cancer.

In present study, the expression profiles of circRNA and miRNA in cells of bladder tumor and adjacent tissues were illustrated clearly. The expression of SOX11 was also detected. The directly interactions among circRNA, miRNA and SOX11 were confirmed by luciferase assay. We hypothesized that circCEP128 might function as a competing endogenous RNA (ceRNA) for miR-145-5p in regulating *SOX11*, which might further inhibit cell proliferation and promote cell apoptosis of bladder cancer. The study might be of biological and clinical importance.

Methods
Clinical specimens
Ten pairs of bladder tumor tissues and adjacent bladder tissues were obtained from patients who suffered from radical cystectomy at the First Affiliated Hospital of Xiamen University. The normal bladder urothelium samples were collected with a distance of ≥3 cm from the edge of cancer

Table 1 SiRNA sequences

	sense	anti-sense
si-circCEP128	5'-GAGAGCUUGAACAG GAAUU-3'	3'-AAUUCCUGUUCAAG CUCUC-5'
si-CEP128	5'-GCGCTACACCAAAT ACAAA-3'	3'-UUUGUAUUUGGUGU AGCGC-5'
si-SOX11	5'-GCGAGAAGATCCCG TTCAT-3'	3'-AUGAACGGGAUCUU CUCGC-5'

tissues in the resected bladder. All the specimens for histological and pathological detections were snap-frozen in liquid nitrogen and stored at − 80 °C after surgical removal. Samples were obtained from the patients with proper informed consent and approved by the Institutional Review Board of the First Affiliated Hospital of Xiamen University.

Cell culture and treatment
Human bladder cancer cells lines (RT-112, 5637, BIU-87 and TCCSUP) and human embryonic kidney cells lines (HEK293T) were all purchased from the BNCC cell bank (Beijing, China). Cells were inoculated in Dulbecco's modified Eagle's medium (DMEM) supplemented with 10% FBS (GIBCO BRL, NY, USA), 1% Glutamax (35,050, Invitrogen, Carlsbad, CA, USA), 1% Non-essential Amino Acids1 (111,401, Invitrogen) and 1% Sodium Pyruvate 100 mM Solution (113,600,070, Invitrogen). Cultured cells were stored at 37 °C in a humidified atmosphere (5% CO_2 and 95% O_2).

Microarray analysis
Microarray datasets GSE92675 at platform GPL19978 were used. Four pairs of matched bladder tumor tissues and adjacent tissues were prepared for analyzing the expression level and biological functions of circRNAs.

Table 2 Primer sequences

Genes	Primers
circCEP128	F: 5'-ACCCACATCGCTGGTTAGC-3'
	R: 5'-TCGATCACCTTCTGCTTTCGT-3'
SOX11	F: 5'-GCCTCTTTTCTGCTGGGTCT-3'
	R: 5'-ACTGAAAACCTCCTCCGCTG-3'
hsa-miR-155-5p	F: 5'-TGCCTCCAACTGACTCCTAC-3'
	R: 5'-GCGAGCACAGAATAATACGAC-3'
hsa-miR-223-3p	F: 5'-GGGGTGTCAGTTTGTCAAA-3'
	R: 5'-CAGTGCGTGTCGCGTGGAGT-3'
hsa-miR-145-5p	F: 5'-CTCACGGTCCAGTTTTCCCA-3'
	R: 5'-ACCTCAAGAACAGTATTTCCAGG-3'
GAPDH	F: 5'-GGAAAGCTGTGGCGTGAT-3'
	R: 5'-AAGGTGGAAGAATGGGAGTT-3'
U6	F: 5'-GCTTCGGCAGCACATATACTAAAAT-3'
	R: 5'-CGCTTCACGAATTTGCGTGTCAT-3'

Differentially expressed genes were identified using *t*-test (*P* < 0.05) combined with fold change (FC > 2). As for mRNA analysis, 19 pairs of tumor tissues and adjacent tissues obtained from TCGA (https://cancergenome.nih.gov/) were screened by R programme (Fold change> 2, *P* < 0.001).

MiRNA targets prediction of circCEP128

We predicted the miRNA-binding sites of circCEP128 and *SOX11* using TargetScan (http://www.targetscan.org/) and circular RNA interactome (https://circinteractome.nia.nih.gov/), respectively.

Cell transfection

TCCSUP and BIU-87 cells were transfected with corresponding plasmids using the Lipofectamine 2000 (Invitrogen) in the light of the manufacturer's recommendations. And the cells were harvested at 48 h after transfection. Cells were generally assigned to different groups as follows: (1) negative control (NC) group: bladder cancer cells transfected with pCDNA3.1 (GenePharma, Shanghai, China). (2) mimics group: bladder cancer cells transfected with miR-145-5p mimic. (3) inhibitor group: bladder cancer cells transfected with miR-145-5p inhibitor. (4)

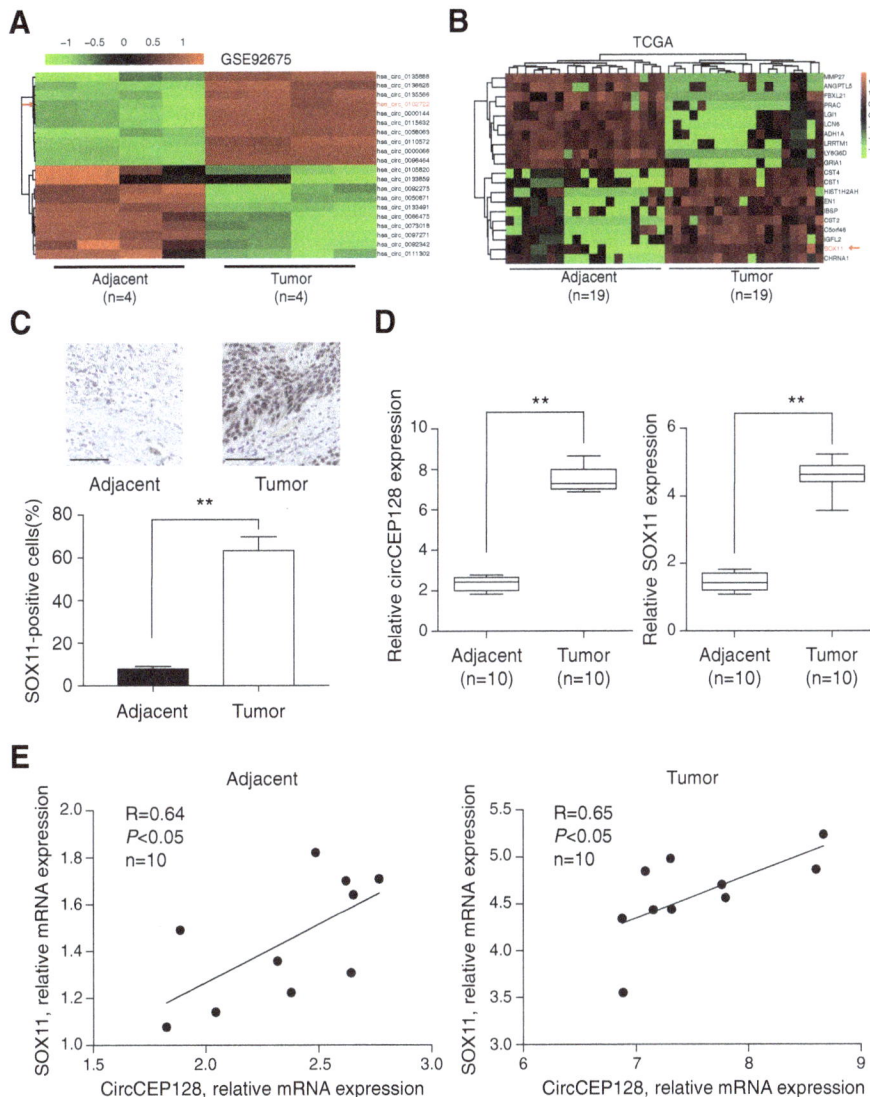

Fig. 1 CircCEP128 and *SOX11* are up-regulated in bladder cancer. **a** The cluster heatmap showed some of the differentially expressed circRNAs over 2-fold change between tumor tissues and adjacent normal tissues. Red color indicates high expression level, and green color indicates low expression level. The red arrow indicates hsa_circ_0102722 (circCEP128). **b** The cluster heat map showed some of the differentially expressed mRNAs over 2-old change in tumor tissues and adjacent normal tissues. The red arrow indicates *SOX11*. **c** Immunochemistry staining showed more *SOX11*-positive cells in tumor tissues than in adjacent normal tissues. Scale bar, 50 μm. **P* < 0.01, compared with adjacent tissues. **d** CircCEP128 and *SOX11* were highly expressed in tumor tissues. **P* < 0.01, compared with adjacent tissues. **e** According to the results of qRT-PCR, circCEP128 and *SOX11* were positively related in cancer tissues and in cancer adjacent tissues

si-circRNA group: bladder cancer cells transfected with si-circCEP128. (5) si-CEP128 group: bladder cancer cells transfected with si-CEP128. (6) si-*SOX11* group: bladder cancer cells transfected with si-*SOX11*. (7) si-circRNA and inhibitor group: bladder cancer cells transfected with si-circCEP128 and miR-145-5p inhibitor. (8) si-*SOX11* and inhibitor group: bladder cancer cells transfected with si-*SOX11* and miR-145-5p (Thermo Fisher, Waltham, MA, USA). Si-circCEP128 and siCEP128 were designed on Thermo Fisher (https://rnaidesigner.thermofisher.com/) and produced by Sangon Biotech (Shanghai, China) which were shown in Table 1.

qRT-PCR assay

The reverse transcription of RNA was developed using Prime Script RT Master Mix (Takara, Japan). PCR reaction was performed with PCR Master Mix (2×) (ThermoFisher Scientific, Waltham, Ma, USA). For the quantitative determination of circRNA, miRNA and mRNA, real-time PCR analysis was performed using SYBRremix Ex TaqTM kit (Takara, Tokyo, Japan) with GAPDH and U6 as internal controls. All analyses were performed using the StepOne-Plus Real-Time PCR System (Applied Biosystems, Carlsbad, CA, USA). The primer sequence was listed in Table 2.

Immunohistochemistry

Bladder tissues were immunostained by anti-*SOX11* (1:200, Abcam, Cambridge, MA, USA) and HRP-conjugated goat anti-rabbit IgG (1:1000, Abcam), respectively. The resultant immunostaining images were captured using the AxioVision Rel.4.6 computerized image analysis system (Carl Zeiss, Oberkochen, Germany). Proteins expression levels were analyzed using Image-Pro Plus version 6.0 (Media Cybernetics, MD) by calculating the integrated optical density in each stained area (IOD/area).

Western blot

Cell lysates were prepared with RIPA buffer (Thermo Scientific). The concentration was determined using a bicinchoninic acid (BCA) protein assay kit (Pierce, Thermo Scientific). Immunoreactive bands were detected by using the Immobilon ECL substrate kit (Millipore, Merck KGaA, Germany). The images were acquired by using BioSpectrum 600 Imaging System (UVP, CA, USA). Antibodies used included primary and secondary antibodies, primary antibodies including anti-*SOX11* (1:1000, Abcam), Bcl-2 (1:500, Abcam), Bax (1:500, Abcam), Cleaved-caspase3 (Anti-active Caspase-3, 1:500, Abcam) and anti-GAPDH (1:10000, Abcam); secondary antibody was HRP-conjugated secondary goat anti-rabbit IgG (1:2000, Abcam).

Table 3 Log_2 (Fold Change) of ten increased circular RNA and ten decreased circular RNA

Circular RNA	Log_2(Fold Change)
hsa_circ_0135888	4.88
hsa_circ_0136628	4.93
hsa_circ_0135566	4.97
hsa_circ_0102722	5.06
hsa_circ_0000144	5.71
hsa_circ_0115632	4.64
hsa_circ_0058063	4.85
has_circ_0110572	5.30
hsa_circ_0000066	5.62
hsa_circ_0096464	5.30
hsa_circ_0105820	− 3.03
hsa_circ_0133859	−2.63
hsa_circ_0092275	−2.71
hsa_circ_0050871	−2.63
hsa_circ_0133491	−2.89
hsa_circ_0066475	−4.10
hsa_circ_0073018	−3.41
hsa_circ_0097271	−3.44
hsa_circ_0092342	−3.83
hsa_circ_0111302	−3.24

The positive number means circular RNA was increased in tumor samples, the minus means circular RNA was decreased in tumor samples

Table 4 Log_2 (Fold Change) of ten increased mRNA and ten decreased mRNA

mRNA	Log_2 (Fold Change)
MMP27	−14.42
ANGPTL5	−12.50
FBXL21	−13.47
PRAC	−14.15
LGI1	−12.83
LCN6	−13.61
ADH1A	−12.92
LRRTM1	−13.19
LY6G6D	−14.23
GRIA1	−12.39
CST4	10.29
CST1	10.75
HIST1H2AH	10.68
EN1	10.96
IBSP	11.36
CST2	12.33
C5orf46	13.47
IGFL2	11.94
SOX11	11.56
CHRNA1	10.61

The positive number means mRNA was increased in tumor samples, the minus means mRNA was decreased in tumor samples

Fluorescence in situ hybridization (FISH)

TCCSUP and BIU-87 cells were performed with cytospin, the collected cells were fixed with Carnoy's fixative (3:1 methanol (ThermoFisher Scientific, Leicestershire, UK): acetic acid (Sigma-Aldrich, Bornem, Belgium) and then air dried for 5 min. CircCEP128 was localized in bladder cells by FISH using CEP Y SpectrumGreen DNA probe (ACCB Biotech, Beijing, China) under the manufacturer's instructions. After that, the slides with collected cells were mounted with Fluorescence Mounting Medium (Antifade) (Abace Biology, Beijing, China) to counterstain all nucleic on the slide. Subsequently, the slide was scanned at 20-fold magnification using Carl Zeiss Short Distance Plan- Apochromat® objective.

Flow cytometry (FCM) assay

Transfected cells were subjected to PI staining for detection with Cell Cycle assay Kit (ab112116, Abcam). Then they were subjected to FITC-Annexin V and PI double staining for flow cytometry detection (EPICS, XL-4, Beckman, CA, USA) according to manufacturer's instructions. Cells were trypsinized, resuspended and incubated with 1.0 μl of PI and 5.0 μl of Annexin V-fluorescein and the apopotosis rate was determined by flow cytometry (FACScan; Becton Dickinson, MountainView, CA, USA) and analyzed with analyzed using Flowjo 7.6 software (BD Bioscience, San Jose, CA, USA).

MTT assay

Well transfected cells were seeded into 96-well plates at 2×10^4 cells/ml in a 5% CO_2 atmosphere and incubated overnight. 20 μl MTT reagent (Sigma-Aldrich, Bornem, Belgium) was added to each well respectively at 0, 24, 48 and 72 h. at an absorbance of 490 nm, cell viability was detected with an automatic enzyme-linked immune detector. The experiment was repeated in triplicate.

Luciferase reporter assay

Dual-luciferase reporter assay system (Promega, Madison, WI, USA) was operated for the co-transfection of HEK293T cells. Mutagens were used to mutate the sequence in 3'UTR of circCEP128 and SOX11. The mutant circCEP128 was transfected with miR-145-5p or empty vector as negative control. The mutant SOX11 was also transfected with miR-145-5p and empty control for two groups. The luciferase results were detected by Luc-Pair™ Duo-Luciferase Assay Kit (Yeasen, Shanghai, China) and the luciferase activity in empty vector cells was normalized as 1.

RNA pull-down assay

Cells transfected with biotinylated miR-145-5p or mutant miR-145-5p mimics (50 nM) using Lipofectamine RNAiMax (Life Technologies) were harvested and sonicated 48 h after transfection. Remaining cell lysates were incubated with C-1 magnetic beads (Life Technologies) at 4 °C for 2 h and then purified using RNeasy Mini Kit (QIAGEN, Duesseldorf, Germany) for analysis, following detected RNA enrichment by qRT-PCR.

Table 5 The relationship between circCEP128/SOX11 expression and clinicopathological characteristics in bladder cancer patients

Items	Patients ($N = 10$)	circCEP128 RNA (X ± SD)	P value	SOX11 mRNA (X ± SD)	P value
N	10	0.00563 ± 0.00235	0.0038[b]	3.2565 ± 2.0583	0.0032[b]
T	10	0.02568 ± 0.01897		6.0354 ± 1.5568	
Gender			0.7704		0.4643
Male	4	0.02258 ± 0.01989		3.3564 ± 3.0254	
Female	6	0.01897 ± 0.01765		4.8697 ± 3.0658	
Age (years)			0.3785		0.463
< 60	2	0.00897 ± 0.00458		2.7856 ± 1.8975	
> =60	8	0.02305 ± 0.02035		5.6578 ± 4.9876	
Tumor size			0.0291[a]		0.0168[a]
< 10	5	0.01756 ± 0.00968		1.8756 ± 0.9873	
> =10	5	0.03457 ± 0.01057		5.5893 ± 4.5760	
TNM stage			0.0361[a]		0.0263[a]
I-II	3	0.01687 ± 0.00952		3.8976 ± 1.0687	
III-IV	7	0.04356 ± 0.01689		6.3654 ± 1.3873	
Lymphatic metastasis			0.0313[a]		0.0343[a]
NO	3	0.00897 ± 0.00563		1.7056 ± 0.9856	
Yes	7	0.03056 ± 0.01347		6.0325 ± 2.7846	

N: Adjacent normal tissues; T: Bladder cancer tissues; Student-t test
[a]$P < 0.05$, [b]$P < 0.01$ was recognized as a significant difference

Tunnel staining

TCCSUP were cultured on coverslips after transfected with miR-145-5p mimics, miR-145-5p inhibitor, si-circRNA, or si-SOX11. 48 h after, cells were harvested and fixed with 4% paraformaldehyde. Cell apoptosis analysis was performed using a tunnel staining kit (Abcam, USA). Cell nuclei were stained with DAPI. All fluorescent images were examined using a Leica DM3000 microscope and photographed using a DFC 420 camera (Leica, Germany).

EdU incorporation

At the last 18 h of cell culture, Edu-labeling reagent (Invitrogen) (1:1000 dilution) was added into medium.

EdU was detected using the Click-iT kit (Invitrogen) following the manufacturer's protocol. The slides were counterstained with DAPI (4′,6-diamidino-2-phenylindole). Images were captured and analyzed using OpenLab software, and cells were quantitated using ImageJ software.

Statistical analysis

All data were shown as mean ± standard error of the mean (SEM). Statistical analyses were performed using Graphpad Prism statistical software (Version 6.0; La Jolla, CA, USA). Statistical significance ($P < 0.05$) was determined by Student's t-test (unpaired) for two-group compared and chi-square test was used to assess the RNA correlation.

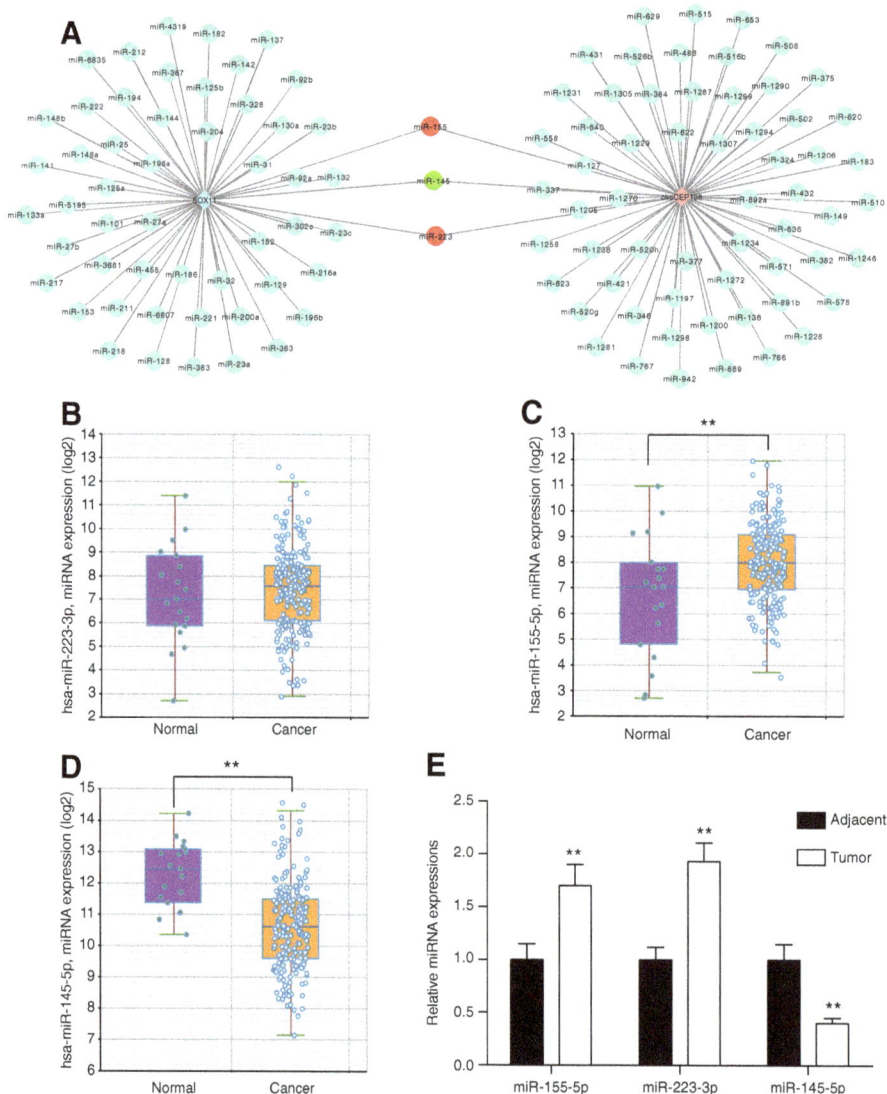

Fig. 2 CeRNA analysis for circCEP128. **a** Cytoscope was used to visualize circCEP128-miRNA-target gene interactions based on the TargetScan and circular RNA interactome. Red color indicates high expression level in bladder cancer and green color indicates low expression level in bladder cancer. **b-d** TCGA bladder cancer patients' data analysis was that miR-223-3p expression had no significant difference, miR-155-5p expression increased but miR-145-5p expression decreased in tumor samples. $^{**}P < 0.01$, compared with adjacent samples. **e** QRT-PCR results showed that miR-155 and miR-223 was up-regulated in tumor tissues while miR-145 was down-regulated in tumor tissues. $^{**}P < 0.01$, compared with adjacent tissues

Results

CircCEP128 (hsa_circ_0102722) and *SOX11* are significantly up-regulated in bladder cancer

A total of 433 circRNAs were differentially expressed (Fold change> 2 and $P < 0.05$) with the analysis of circRNA microarray from GEO database. 169 circRNAs were significantly down-regulated, and 264 circRNAs were up-regulated in 4 bladder cancer samples. The top ten up- and down-regulated circRNAs were chosen by fold change to draw the cluster heat map (Fig. 1a). CircCEP128 was up-regulated in bladder tumor tissues with a fold change value of 5.06 (Table 3). Data of 19 pairs sample (tumor and adjacent tissue of patients) were obtained from TCGA and analyzed by R software, the cluster heat map was drawn (Fig. 1b). *SOX11* was up-regulated in bladder tumor tissues with a fold change value of 11.56 (Table 4). Immunochemistry staining showed more *SOX11*-positive cells in tumor tissues than that of adjacent normal tissues (Fig. 1c, $P < 0.01$). The

highly expressions of circCEP128 and SOX11 were validated in 10 paired of bladder tissues by RT-PCR (Fig. 1d, $P < 0.01$). Analysis of clinicopathologic features, circCEP128 and *SOX11* showed significant higher expressions in bladder cancer tissues compared with adjacent normal tissue (Table 5). Gender and age had no relationships with the expression of circCEP128 or *SOX11*except for tumor size, TNM stage and lymphatic metastasis. CircCEP128 and *SOX11* had a positively related dependency both in cancer tissues and in adjacent normal tissues (Fig. 1e, $P < 0.05$). Thus we hypothesized that circCEP128 may function as a ceRNA (competing endogenous RNAs) and promote the expression of *SOX11*.

CeRNA analysis for circCEP128 according to the database

In Fig. 2a, miR-155, miR-223 and miR-145 were found to have the same targeting relations with circCEP128 and *SOX11* by using circular RNA interactome (https://

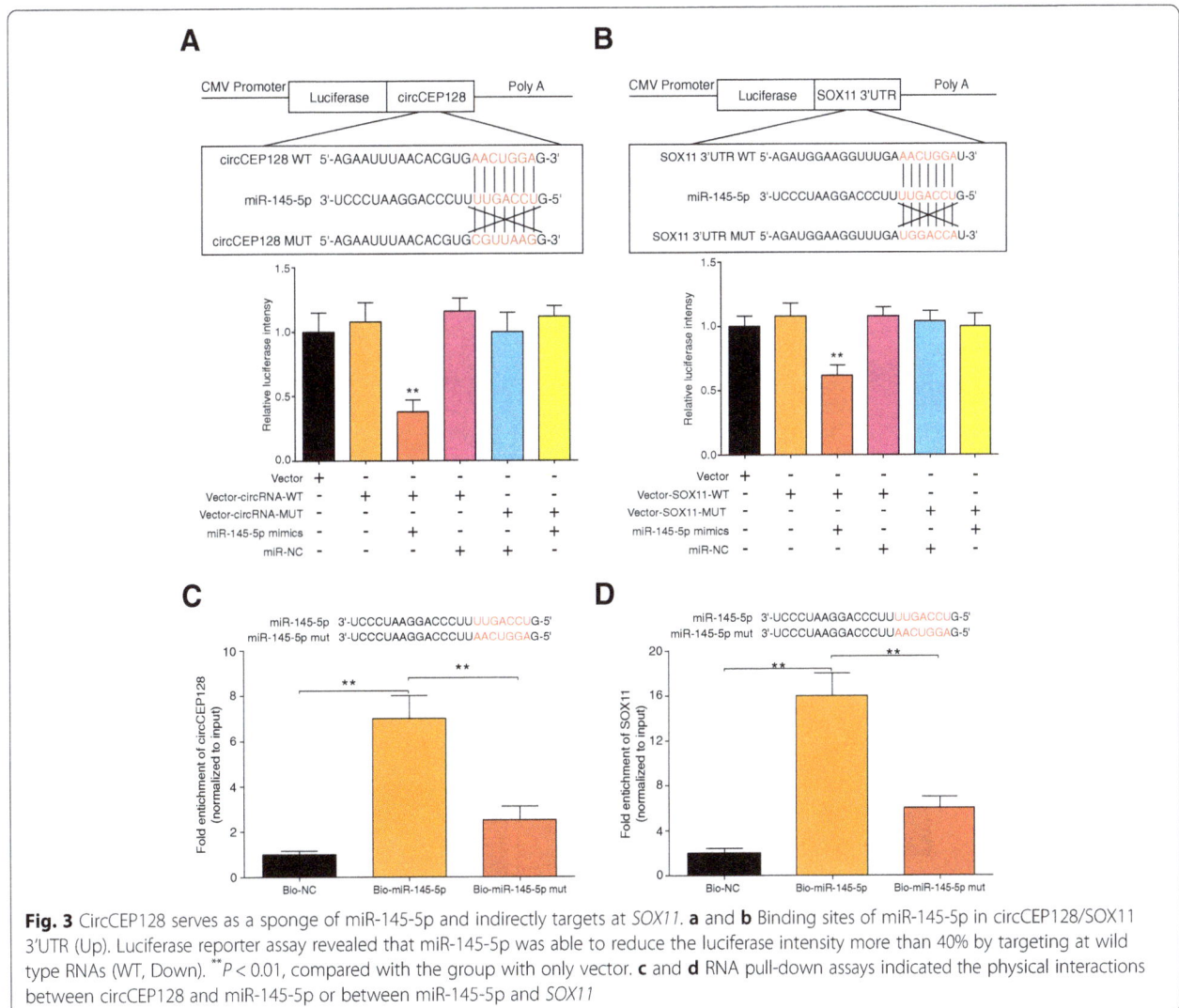

Fig. 3 CircCEP128 serves as a sponge of miR-145-5p and indirectly targets at *SOX11*. **a** and **b** Binding sites of miR-145-5p in circCEP128/SOX11 3'UTR (Up). Luciferase reporter assay revealed that miR-145-5p was able to reduce the luciferase intensity more than 40% by targeting at wild type RNAs (WT, Down). **P < 0.01, compared with the group with only vector. **c** and **d** RNA pull-down assays indicated the physical interactions between circCEP128 and miR-145-5p or between miR-145-5p and *SOX11*

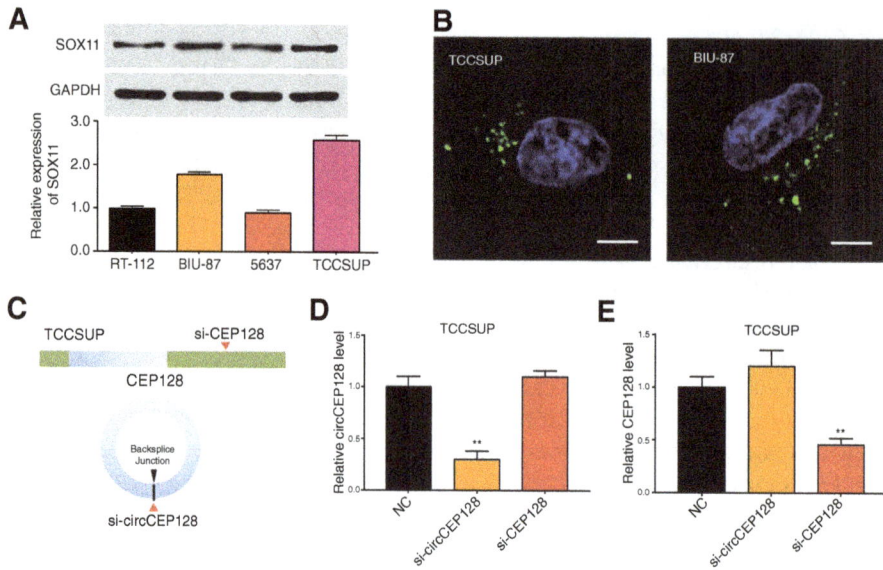

Fig. 4 Si-circCEP128 inhibits the expression of circCEP128 not CEP128. **a** SOX11detection of 4 bladder cancer cells was conducted by qRT-PCR. **b** Cellar locations of circCEP128 were in TCCUSP and BIU-87 cytoplasm. Scale bar, 2 μm. **c** Schematic model of the si-circRNAs. si-CEP128 targets the CEP128 linear transcript, si-circCEP128 targets the back-splice junction of circCEP128. **d** and **e** Si-circCEP128 knocked down only the circular transcript and did not affect the expression of linear species. Si-CEP128 knocked down only the CEP128 linear transcript but not the circular transcript. $^{**}P < 0.01$, compared with NC

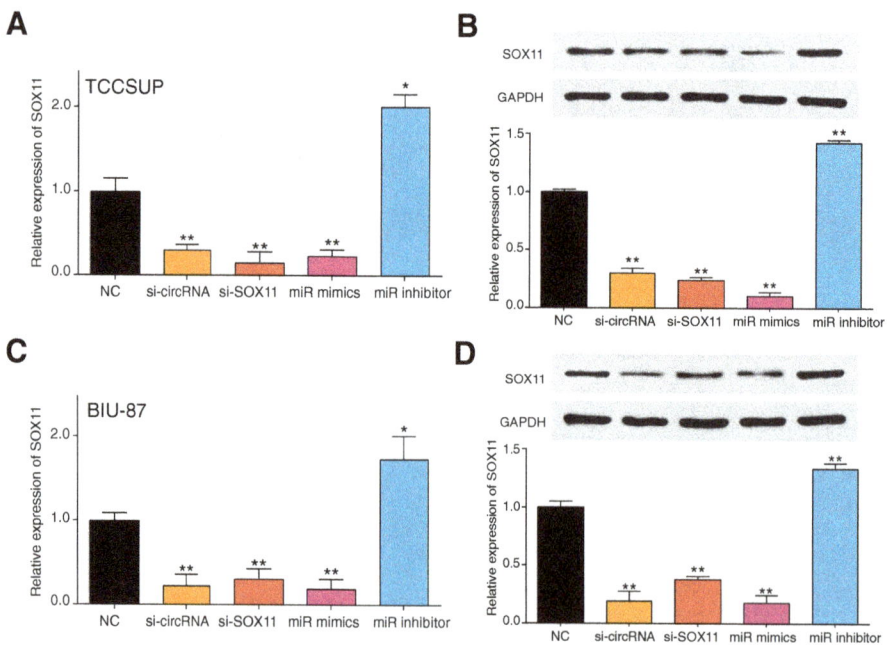

Fig. 5 Knockdown of circCEP128 inhibits expression of *SOX11*. The expression levels of *SOX11* were detected following knockdown of circCEP127 using si-circCEP128, miR-145-5p inhibitor, co-transfection with si-circCEP128 and the miR-145-5p inhibitor or si-*SOX11* (**a**) in TCCSUP and (**c**) in BIU-87. $^{**}P < 0.01$, compared with NC. *SOX11* protein relative expression levels were analyzed by western blotting (**b**) in TCCSUP and (**d**) in BIU-87. $^{**}P < 0.01$, compared with NC

circinteractome.nia.nih.gov/Circular_RNA/circular_r-na.html) and TargetScan (http://www.targetscan.org/). Firstly, the analysis results had been verified in database of starBase v2.0 (http://starbase.sysu.edu.cn/) with TCGA data in bladder cancers, which showed that miR-155-5p obviously up-regulated while miR-145-5p obviously down-regulated in tumor cells ($P < 0.01$, Fig. 2c and d), miR-223-3p expression had no statistically change between normal and tumor cells ($P > 0.05$, Fig. 2b). Subsequently, the experiments of qRT-PCR were conducted in 10 bladder cancer tissues (Fig. 2e). It showed that miR-155-5p, miR-233-3p were upregulated and miR-145-5p was downregulated in tumor cells ($P < 0.01$). The down-regulation of miR-145-5p was speculated as a competitive target of circCEP128 and SOX11 in bladder cancer.

CircCEP128 serves as a sponge of miR-145-5p which directly regulates *SOX11*

StarBase v2.0 predicted the binding relationship between CircCEP128 and miR-145-5p. Luciferase reporter assay showed that the luciferase intensity of HEK293T cells transfected with circCEP128 wild type or miR-145-5p mimics were significantly reduced, but the luciferase intensity of cells transfected with circCEP128 muted type or miR-145-5p mimics were hardly changed ($P > 0.05$, Fig. 3a). Similarly, with the targetScan prediction of the binding sequences of miR-145-5p and *SOX11*, it showed that the luciferase activity was significantly reduced in *SOX11* wild type + miR-145-5p mimics co-transfection group ($P < 0.01$, Fig. 3b). After RNA pull-down assay, the circCEP128 level of the miR-145-5p group was 6.73 times as much as NC group and 2.28 times

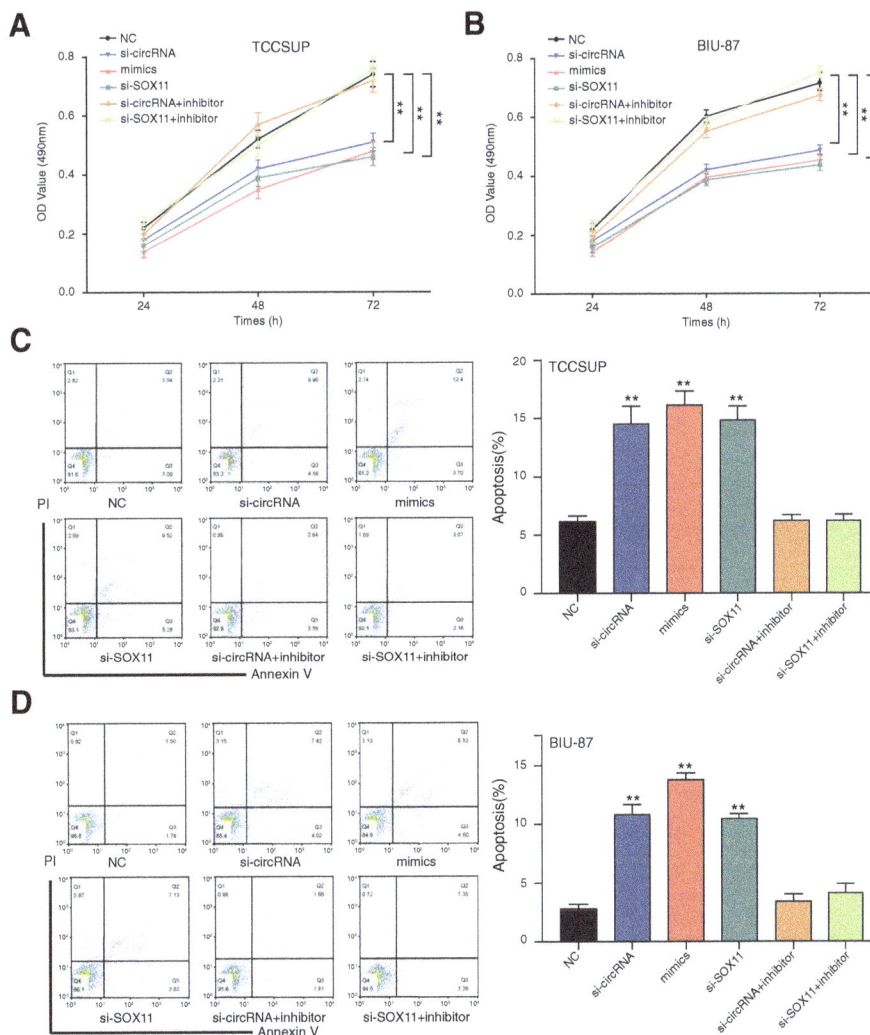

Fig. 6 Effects of circCEP128 on cell proliferation. MTT assay was also performed to assess cell proliferation after transfection with si-circRNA of circCEP128, miR-145-5p mimics, si-*SOX11*, co-transfection with si-circRNA and the miR-145-5p inhibitor and co-transfection with si-*SOX11* and the miR-145-5p inhibitor (**a**) in TCCSUP and (**b**) in BIU-87. Knockdown of circCEP128 inhibited cell proliferation. *$P < 0.05$, compared with NC. Cell apoptosis was analyzed using flow cytometry (**c**) in TCCSUP and (**d**) in BIU-87 with double staining of PI and Annexin V-FITC. Knockdown of circCEP128 induced the increased cell apoptosis rate. **$P < 0.05$, compared with NC

as much as miR-145-5p-mut group ($P < 0.01$, Fig. 3c) and the miR-145-5p group was found high *SOX11* level which was 16.69 times as much as NC group ($P < 0.01$, Fig. 3d).

Knockdown of circCEP128 inhibits expression of *SOX11*

In bladder cancer cell lines, SOX11 expressed higher in BIU-87 and TCCSUP compared with RT-112 and 5637 (Fig. 4a). TSSCP showed the highest expression level of SOX11. Experiments of fluorescent probe localized circCEP128 in the plasma of bladder cell lines (Fig. 4b). Si-circCEP128 (Fig. 4c) could knockdown the expression of circCEP128 while si-CEP128 had no effect on altering the expression of circCEP128 ($P > 0.05$, Fig. 4d). Similarly, Si-circCEP128 had no effect on regulating the expression of CEP128, while si-CEP128 could knockdown the expression of CEP128 ($P < 0.01$, Fig. 4e). Expression of *SOX11* was detected by qRT-PCR ($P < 0.01$, Fig. 5a and c) and western blot ($P < 0.01$, Fig. 5b and d) in TCCSUP and BIU-87 cells. Expression of SOX11 was increased greatly in miRNA inhibitor group while decreased dramatically in si-SOX11 group. The results verified that knockdown of circCEP128 inhibited expression of *SOX11* and it could be guessed that knockdown of circCEP128 promotes expression of miR-145-5p to inhibit expression of *SOX11*.

The effect of circCEP128 on bladder tumor cell proliferation, apoptosis and cell cycle

Knockdown of circCEP128 inhibited cell proliferation ($P < 0.05$, Fig. 6a and b) but promoted cell apoptosis ($P < 0.05$, Fig. 6c and d). Cell cycle induced bladder cancer cell G1/S arrest in si-cirRNA, miR-145-5p mimics and si-*SOX11* group ($P < 0.01$, Fig. 7a and b). Similar results were generated after improving expression of miR-145-5p or knocking down *SOX11* ($P < 0.01$, Fig. 6a-Fig. 7b). Cell cycle, cell apoptosis rate and cell proliferation were recovered with the addition of miR-145-5p inhibitor after knocking down the circCEP128 ($P > 0.05$, Fig. 6a-Fig. 7b). Similarly, Cell cycle, cell apoptosis rate and cell proliferation were recovered with si-*SOX11* after the inhibition of miR-145-5p ($P > 0.05$, Fig. 6a-Fig. 7b). As a result, knockdown of circCEP128 induced the inhibition of cell proliferation and increased bladder cancer cell apoptosis rate.

Knockdown of circCEP128 promoted TCCSUP cells damage and apoptosis

Damaged TCCSUP cells marked Edu and Tunnel staining, a strong positive cells presented in si-cirRNA, miR-145-5p mimics and si-*SOX11* group ($P < 0.01$, Fig. 8a and b). The effects of si-circRNA and si-SOX11 on TCCSUP had been recovered by miR-145-5p inhibitor. The expression levels of three apoptosis relative proteins were detected (Fig. 8c), the results showed that the expression of Bcl-2 was significantly

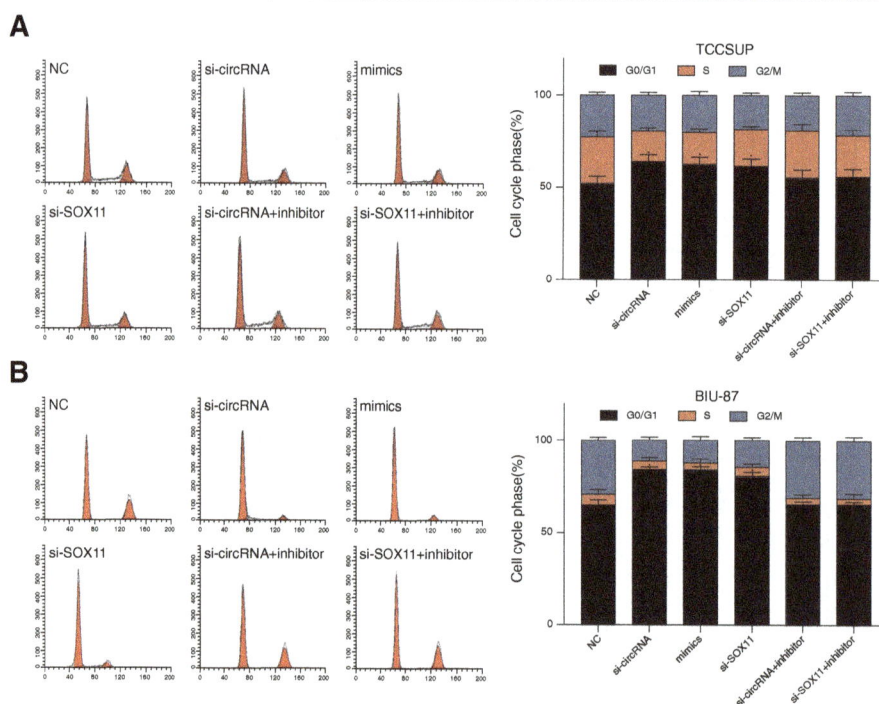

Fig. 7 Effects of circCEP128 on cell cycle. Cell cycle was analyzed using flow cytometry after transfection with si-circRNA of circCEP128, miR-145-5p mimics, si-*SOX11*, co-transfection with si-circRNA and the miR-145-5p inhibitor and co-transfection with si-*SOX11* and the miR-145-5p inhibitor (a) in TCCSUP and (b) in BIU-87. Knockdown of circCEP128 induced G1/S arrest. *$P < 0.05$, compared with NC

decreased in si-circRNA group, mimics group as well as si-SOX11 group ($P < 0.01$). However, the expression levels of bax and cleaved caspase3 were increased obviously in si-circRNA group, mimics group and si-SOX11 group ($P < 0.01$). All in all, inhibition of circCEP128 induced TCCSUP cell damage and apoptosis through the regulation of miR-145-5p/SOX11.

Discussion

In this study, circCEP128 and *SOX11* were found highly expression and positively related in bladder cancer tissues.

The relation could be regulated by miR-145-5p, a down-regulated miRNA in bladder cancer samples. CircCEP128 served as a sponge of miR-145-5p and indirectly regulated *SOX11*. Knockdown of circCEP128 could induce the inhibition of cell proliferation and increase bladder cancer cell apoptosis rate.

Many studies have confirmed that stable transcripts with a host of miRNA-binding sites or miRNA response elements (MREs) could function as miRNA sponges (Memczak et al., 2013) and circular RNAs are found to be enriched in functional miRNA binding sites (Huang et al., 2016). For

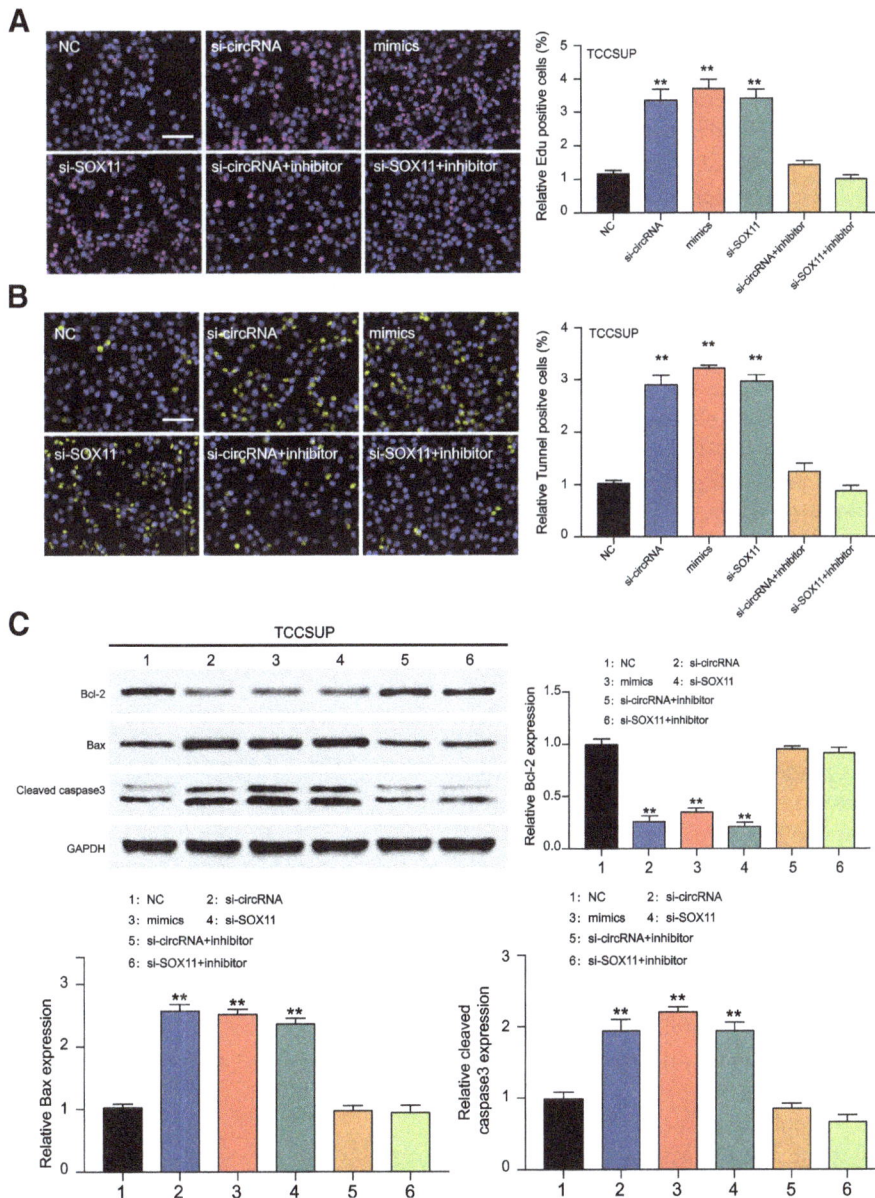

Fig. 8 Effects of circCEP128 on TCCSUP cell damage and apoptosis. After transfected with corresponding siRNA or mimics/inhibitor, higher DNA damage happened in si-circRNA, miR-145-5p mimics and si-*SOX11* with the experiments of **a** Edu staining **b** Tunnel staining. **$P < 0.01$, compared with NC. Scale bar, 20 μm. c Western blot showed the result of apoptosis related proteins bax and caspase3 were higher but bcl-2 was lower in si-circRNA, miR-145-5p mimics and si-*SOX11* groups compared with NC group. **$P < 0.01$, compared with NC

example, Li et al. found that circHIPK3 inhibited migration, invasion and angiogenesis of human invasive bladder cancer by targeting miR-558 (Markopoulos et al., 2017). In addition, other studies indicated that circRNA-MYLK could function as an endogenous sponge for miR-29a in bladder cancer (Zhong et al., 2017). What is more, circRNA CDR1as was reported to negatively regulate miR-7 and increase the levels of miR-7 targets (Xu et al., 2015; Hansen et al., 2013). These conclusions coincide with the results of our study, which indicate that circCEP128 is able to function as a ceRNA for miR-145-5p.

Recently, studies about circular RNA mainly focus on its interactions with miRNA and miRNA targets. For example, it is revealed that circRNA-MYLK functions as a ceRNA for miR-29a, thus boosting *VEGF/VEGFR2* expressions and activating downstream Ras/ERK signaling pathway in bladder cancer progression (Zhong et al., 2017). Li et al. demonstrated that cir-ITCH increased the expression of the miRNA target gene *ITCH* in esophageal squamous cell carcinoma (Li et al., 2015). Other studies showed that the over-expression of circHIPK3 induced efficiently interaction with miR-558 and then down-regulated the expression of *HPSE* and its downstream targeted *MMP-9* and *VEGF* to attenuate the promoting effect of miR-558 on bladder cancer cell migration, invasion, and angiogenesis (Li et al., 2017). Also, it was speculated that circTCF25 may competitively bind with miR-103a-3p and miR-107 and relieve their suppression on associated target genes (Zhong et al., 2016). Similarly, in our study, we found that circCEP128 served as a sponge of miR-145-5p and indirectly regulated *SOX11*.

SOX11 have been proved to promote invasive growth and progression of DCIS cells (Oliemuller et al., 2017) and prevent cell differentiation in mantle cell lymphoma (Meggendorfer et al., 2013). However, Sernbo et al. demonstrated that the overexpression of *SOX11* could induce growth arrest in ovarian cancer cells (Sernbo et al., 2011). Varied findings may result from differential populations and cancer types (Fang et al., 2017). In this study, *SOX11* was a contributor to bladder cancer in terms of proliferation and apoptosis. Therefore, it was verified that circCEP128 acted as a ceRNA for miR-145-5p to regulate *SOX11*, which further promoted cell proliferation and suppressed cell apoptosis of bladder cancer.

In this study, siRNA could only specifically target the circular form but not the linear form of CEP128; thus the off-target effect have to be considered. Therefore, more effective, accurate and specific methods of RNA interference remain to be exploited. Additionally, further research on functions and mechanisms underlying circCEP128 are required.

Conclusion

In conclusion, the results of our study demonstrate that circCEP128 is up-regulated in human bladder cancer, and is able to sponge miR-145-5p for promoting *SOX11* expression with high efficiency. We also demonstrate that knockdown of circCEP128 can effectively inhibit cell proliferation and promote cell apoptosis rate of bladder cancer cells through targeting miR-145-5p/*SOX11* axis. Our findings provide novel evidences that circRNAs might act as "microRNA sponges" and provide a new therapeutic target for the treatment of bladder cancer.

Abbreviations
BCA: Bicinchoninic acid; ceRNA: Competing endogenous RNA; circCEP128: Circular RNA CEP128; circRNAs: Circular RNAs; FCM: Flow cytometry; FISH: Fluorescence in situ hybridization; miR-145: MicroRNAs; miRNAs: MicroRNAs; MREs: MiRNA response elements; NC: Negative control; SEM: Standard error of the mean

Funding
This project was supported by Natural Science Foundation of Fujian Province of China (Grant No.2016D009, Grant No.2017 J01355, Grant No.2011–2-60).

Authors' contributions
Research conception and design: ZW & WH; Data analysis and interpretation: XW, TW, YC & BC; Statistical analysis: ZW, RL & PB; Drafting of the manuscript: ZW; Critical revision of the manuscript: JX; Receiving grant: JX; Approval of final manuscript: all authors.

Competing interests
The authors declare that they have no competing interests.

References
Enokida H, Yoshino H, Matsushita R, Nakagawa M. The role of microRNAs in bladder cancer. Investigative and Clin Urology. 2016;57(Suppl 1):S60–76.

Fang G, Liu J, Wang Q, Huang X, Yang R, Pang Y, et al. MicroRNA-223-3p regulates ovarian Cancer cell proliferation and invasion by targeting SOX11 expression. Int J Mol Sci. 2017;18(6):1208.

Hansen TB, Jensen TI, Clausen BH, Bramsen JB, Finsen B, Damgaard CK, et al. Natural RNA circles function as efficient microRNA sponges. Nature. 2013;495:384–8.

Huang M, Zhong Z, Lv M, Shu J, Tian Q, Chen J. Comprehensive analysis of differentially expressed profiles of lncRNAs and circRNAs with associated co-expression and ceRNA networks in bladder carcinoma. Oncotarget. 2016;7:47186–200.

Li F, Zhang L, Li W, Deng J, Zheng J, An M, et al. Circular RNA ITCH has inhibitory effect on ESCC by suppressing the Wnt/beta-catenin pathway. Oncotarget. 2015;6:6001–13.

Li Y, Zheng F, Xiao X, Xie F, Tao D, Huang C, et al. CircHIPK3 sponges miR-558 to suppress heparanase expression in bladder cancer cells. EMBO Rep. 2017;18:1646–59.

Markopoulos GS, Roupakia E, Tokamani M, Chavdoula E, Hatziapostolou M, Polytarchou C, et al. A step-by-step microRNA guide to cancer development and metastasis. Cell Oncol (Dordr). 2017;40:303–39.

Meggendorfer M, Kern W, Haferlach C, Haferlach T, Schnittger S. SOX11 overexpression is a specific marker for mantle cell lymphoma and correlates with t (11;14) translocation, CCND1 expression and an adverse prognosis. Leukemia. 2013;27:2388–91.

Memczak S, Jens M, Elefsinioti A, Torti F, Krueger J, Rybak A, et al. Circular RNAs are a large class of animal RNAs with regulatory potency. Nature. 2013;495:333–8.

Minami K, Taniguchi K, Sugito N, Kuranaga Y, Inamoto T, Takahara K, et al. MiR-145 negatively regulates Warburg effect by silencing KLF4 and PTBP1 in bladder cancer cells. Oncotarget. 2017;8:33064–77.

Noguchi S, Yamada N, Kumazaki M, Yasui Y, Iwasaki J, Naito S, et al. socs7, a target gene of microRNA-145, regulates interferon-beta induction through STAT3 nuclear translocation in bladder cancer cells. Cell Death Dis. 2013;4:e482.

Oliemuller E, Kogata N, Bland P, Kriplani D, Daley F, Haider S, et al. SOX11 promotes invasive growth and ductal carcinoma in situ progression. J Pathol. 2017;243:193–207.

Sernbo S, Gustavsson E, Brennan DJ, Gallagher WM, Rexhepaj E, Rydnert F, et al. The tumour suppressor SOX11 is associated with improved survival among high grade epithelial ovarian cancers and is regulated by reversible promoter methylation. BMC Cancer. 2011;11:405.

Shang X, Li G, Liu H, Li T, Liu J, Zhao Q, et al. Comprehensive circular RNA profiling reveals that hsa_circ_0005075, a new circular RNA biomarker, is involved in hepatocellular Crcinoma development. Medicine. 2016;95:e3811.

Xu H, Guo S, Li W, Yu P. The circular RNA Cdr1as, via miR-7 and its targets, regulates insulin transcription and secretion in islet cells. Sci Rep. 2015;5:12453.

Zhong Z, et al. Circular RNA MYLK as a competing endogenous RNA promotes bladder cancer progression through modulating VEGFA/VEGFR2 signaling pathway. Cancer Lett. 2017;403:305–17.

Zhong Z, Lv M, Chen J. Screening differential circular RNA expression profiles reveals the regulatory role of circTCF25-miR-103a-3p/miR-107-CDK6 pathway in bladder carcinoma. Sci Rep. 2016;6:30919.

6

Ligation of free HMGB1 to TLR2 in the absence of ligand is negatively regulated by the C-terminal tail domain

Hannah Aucott[1,3]* , Agnieszka Sowinska[1], Helena Erlandsson Harris[1] and Peter Lundback[2]

Abstract

Background: High mobility group box 1 (HMGB1) protein is a central endogenous inflammatory mediator contributing to the pathogenesis of several inflammatory disorders. HMGB1 interacts with toll-like receptors (TLRs) but contradictory evidence regarding its identity as a TLR2 ligand persists. The aim of this study was to investigate if highly purified HMGB1 interacts with TLR2 and if so, to determine the functional outcome.

Methods: Full length or C-terminal truncated (Δ30) HMGB1 was purified from *E.coli*. Binding to TLR2-Fc was investigated by direct-ELISA. For the functional studies, proteins alone or in complex with peptidoglycan (PGN) were added to human embryonic kidney (HEK) cells transfected with functional TLR2, TLR 1/2 or TLR 2/6 dimers, macrophages, whole blood or peripheral blood mononuclear cells (PBMCs). Cytokine levels were determined by ELISA.

Results: In vitro binding experiments revealed that Δ30 HMGB1, lacking the acidic tail domain, but not full length HMGB1 binds dose dependently to TLR2. Control experiments confirmed that the interaction was specific to TLR2 and could be inhibited by enzymatic digestion. Δ30 HMGB1 alone was unable to induce cytokine production via TLR2. However, full length HMGB1 and Δ30 HMGB1 formed complexes with PGN, a known TLR2 ligand, and synergistically potentiated the inflammatory response in PBMCs.

Conclusions: We have demonstrated that TLR2 is a receptor for HMGB1 and this binding is negatively regulated by the C-terminal tail. HMGB1 did not induce functional activation of TLR2 while both full length HMGB1 and Δ30 HMGB1 potentiated the inflammatory activities of the TLR2 ligand PGN. We hypothesize that Δ30 HMGB1 generated in vivo by enzymatic cleavage could act as an enhancer of TLR2-mediated inflammatory activities.

Keywords: HMGB1, TLR2, Alarmin, Receptor, Protein-protein interactions, Inflammation

Background

High mobility group box 1 (HMGB1), originally described as a nuclear DNA-binding protein, was rediscovered as an endogenous inflammatory mediator released from dying and activated cells in response to infectious and sterile stimuli in the late 90s (Wang et al. 1999). HMGB1 has since been identified as a pathogenic mediator during sepsis, arthritis, cancer, drug-induced liver injury and stroke, among other diseases, and

inhibition of HMGB1 is beneficial in several experimental models (Andersson and Tracey 2011).

Structurally, HMGB1 expresses 215 amino acids organized into two DNA binding domains (boxes A and B) and a 30 amino acid long unstructured C-terminal acidic tail comprised of repeating glutamic and aspartic acid residues. Boxes A and B have a low sequence similarity (29%) but share a conserved global fold, consisting of three α-helices arranged in an L-like shape (Hardman et al. 1995; Weir et al. 1993). Biophyscial studies have shown that the tail interacts with residues in both boxes and the linker regions (Stott et al. 2010; Watson et al. 2007; Knapp et al. 2004). The interactions are dynamic with the protein alternating between "tail-bound" and

* Correspondence: hannah.aucott@ki.se
[1]Department of Medicine, Rheumatology Unit, Karolinska Institutet, Stockholm, Sweden
[3]Department of Medicine, Rheumatology Unit, Centre for Molecular Medicine (CMM) L8:04, Karolinska Hospital, 17176 Solna, Sweden
Full list of author information is available at the end of the article

"tail-unbound" conformations (Stott et al. 2010). Using circular dichroism spectroscopy Knapp et al. found that binding of the tail to specific residues within boxes A and B results in overall HMGB1 stabilization (Knapp et al. 2004). Moreover, binding of the tail to the boxes has been reported to modulate the interaction with other molecules including DNA and to regulate post-translational modifications (Lee and Thomas 2000; Muller et al. 2001; Sheflin et al. 1993; Stros et al. 1994; Pasheva et al. 2004).

Extracellular HMGB1 acts as an alarmin that interacts with multiple unrelated receptors to recruit and activate immune cells to the site of tissue damage. The receptor for advanced glycation end-products (RAGE), the toll-like receptor (TLR) family, C-X-C chemokine receptor 4 (CXCR4), cluster of differentiation 24 (CD24)/Siglec 10, TIM3 and integrin/Mac1 have all been described as HMGB1 receptors (Hori et al. 1995; Schiraldi et al. 2012; Das et al. 2016; Park et al. 2006; Chen et al. 2009; Gao et al. 2011; Chiba et al. 2012). Several members of the TLR family have been reported to interact with HMGB1 including TLR2, 4, 5 and 9 (Das et al. 2016; Yang et al. 2010; Park et al. 2004). Recent studies have defined HMGB1 binding to TLR4 and the subsequent NF-κB mediated cytokine production to be strictly regulated by post-translational cysteine redox modifications. Disulfide HMGB1 (dsHMGB1), containing a disulfide bridge between the two cysteine residues at positions 23 and 45 in box A and a reduced cysteine residue at position 106, binds to the TLR4/MD2 complex leading to NF-κB activation and expression of pro-inflammatory cytokines, including TNF (Yang et al. 2012; Yang et al. 2015). Complete reduction or oxidation of the three cysteine residues, generating fully reduced (frHMGB1) and sulfonyl (oxHMGB1) HMGB1 respectively, abolishes HMGB1-TLR4 mediated cytokine production (Yang et al. 2012). Likewise, mutation of the three cysteine residues to serines similarly abrogates HMGB1-TLR4 interactions (Venereau et al. 2012).

TLR2 and TLR4 were both suggested to be receptors for HMGB1 in a study by Park et al. in 2004 (Park et al. 2004) and since, the TLR2-HMGB1 axis has been suggested to contribute to the pathogenesis of several conditions including myocardial ischemia/reperfusion injury, peripheral artery disease, deep venous thrombosis and lupus nephritis (Stark et al. 2016; Feng et al. 2016; Mersmann et al. 2013; Sachdev et al. 2012; Xu et al. 2015). However, as compared to TLR4, much less is known about the mechanisms regulating the TLR2-HMGB1 interaction. TLR2 is found as a homodimer or a heterodimer in complex with TLR1 or 6 on the surface of a wide variety of cells including monocytes, tissue resident macrophages, T cells, B cells, dendritic cells and epithelial cells. Ligation of TLR2 activates MyD88-

mediated signalling pathways increasing expression of pro-inflammatory genes. Interestingly, in vitro analysis of the interaction between HMGB1 and TLR2 has produced conflicting data. Early studies using fluorescence resonance energy transfer (FRET) and co-immunoprecipitation experiments suggested that HMGB1 binds directly to TLR2 on the surface of macrophages inducing NF-κB activation (Park et al. 2006). In two separate studies, TLR2 was reported to mediate HMGB1-induced cytokine production in human embryonic kidney (HEK) cells overexpressing TLR2 (Yu et al. 2006) and cancer stem cells (Conti et al. 2013). However, in 2010 Yang et al. concluded that TLR2 is not a major receptor mediating HMGB1-induced cytokine production (Yang et al. 2010). They showed that TLR2 or RAGE deficiency did not reduce HMGB1-induced secretion of TNF, MIP-2, IL-6, IL-8 and IL-10, in contrast to TLR4 deficiency which completely abrogated HMGB1-dependent cytokine expression (Yang et al. 2010).

To clarify conflicting data in the literature, the aim of this study was to investigate if highly purified HMGB1 interacts with TLR2 and if so, to determine the functional outcome of the interaction. Our results reveal that binding of HMGB1 to TLR2 is negatively regulated by the acidic C-terminal tail domain, with truncated HMGB1 lacking the tail domain displaying dose-dependent binding to TLR2-Fc in contrast to full length HMGB1 (flHMGB1). We could not detect any functional consequence of the direct binding interaction between Δ30 HMGB1 and TLR2 in vitro. However, we can demonstrate that Δ30 HMGB1 forms complexes with known TLR2 ligands that enhance downstream signaling and cytokine production.

Methods

Preparation of recombinant HMGB1 proteins

For the experiment depicted in Fig. 1, in-house HMGB1 with a CBP tag was expressed and purified as previously described (Yang et al. 2010). Briefly, HMGB1 DNA was sub-cloned into the pCAL/n vector with a calmodulin binding protein (CBP) tag. The plasmid was transformed into *E.coli* BL21 (DE3) cells and cultured in 2-YT media. Protein expression was induced with the addition of 1 mM IPTG. HMGB1 was purified using calmodulin sepharose 4B resin (GE Healthcare). DNase I was added to remove any contaminating DNA, confirmed by GelRed staining of an agarose gel. Protein purity was verified by SDS-PAGE gel analysis with Coomassie blue staining. For the removal of contaminating endotoxin, the protein was incubated with 1% Triton X114 at 4 °C for 30 min, incubated for a further 10 min at 37 °C and centrifuged at 18,300 g at 25 °C for 10 min. Endotoxin levels were measured using the limulus amoebocyte

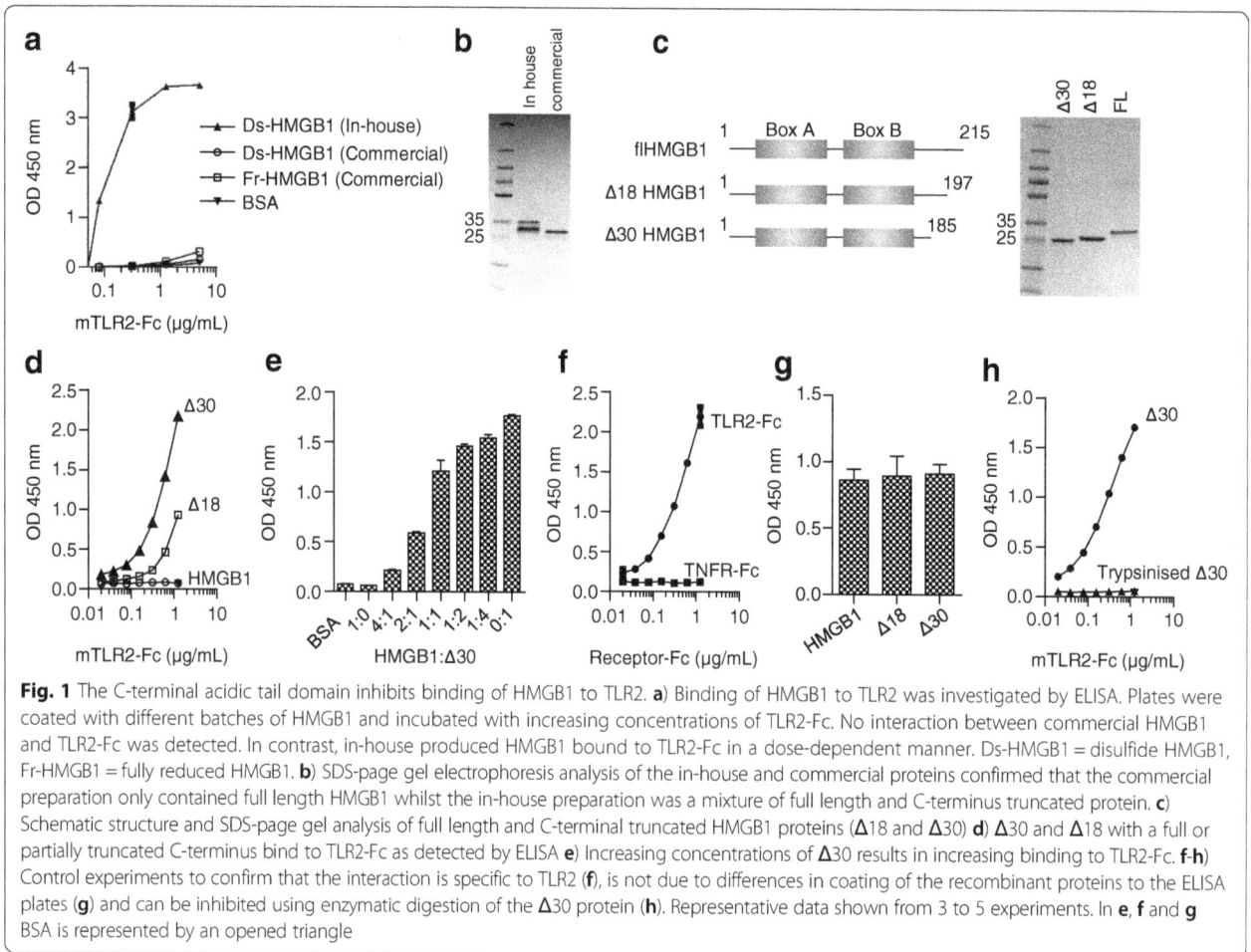

Fig. 1 The C-terminal acidic tail domain inhibits binding of HMGB1 to TLR2. **a**) Binding of HMGB1 to TLR2 was investigated by ELISA. Plates were coated with different batches of HMGB1 and incubated with increasing concentrations of TLR2-Fc. No interaction between commercial HMGB1 and TLR2-Fc was detected. In contrast, in-house produced HMGB1 bound to TLR2-Fc in a dose-dependent manner. Ds-HMGB1 = disulfide HMGB1, Fr-HMGB1 = fully reduced HMGB1. **b**) SDS-page gel electrophoresis analysis of the in-house and commercial proteins confirmed that the commercial preparation only contained full length HMGB1 whilst the in-house preparation was a mixture of full length and C-terminus truncated protein. **c**) Schematic structure and SDS-page gel analysis of full length and C-terminal truncated HMGB1 proteins (Δ18 and Δ30) **d**) Δ30 and Δ18 with a full or partially truncated C-terminus bind to TLR2-Fc as detected by ELISA **e**) Increasing concentrations of Δ30 results in increasing binding to TLR2-Fc. **f-h**) Control experiments to confirm that the interaction is specific to TLR2 (**f**), is not due to differences in coating of the recombinant proteins to the ELISA plates (**g**) and can be inhibited using enzymatic digestion of the Δ30 protein (**h**). Representative data shown from 3 to 5 experiments. In **e**, **f** and **g** BSA is represented by an opened triangle

lysate assay at the clinical laboratory, Karolinska University Hospital, Stockholm, Sweden.

Commercial ds- and fr-HMGB1 were purchased from HMG Biotech (Milan, Italy).

Tag free human flHMGB1 and Δ30 HMGB1 (lacking the C-terminal tail; residues 1–185) were cloned into the pETM-11 vector and expressed in *Escherichia coli* strain BL21 (DE3) cells. The proteins expressed a 6-residue N-terminal histidine tag (his-tag) with a tobacco etch virus (TEV) cleavable linker and were purified using Ni-sepharose affinity chromatography (HisTrap HP column, GE Healthcare, Uppsala, Sweden) on an ÄKTA explorer (GE Healthcare). A partially truncated HMGB1 (Δ18 HMGB1) was generated as a by-product during the production of the flHMGB1 protein and was co-purified during the affinity purification. Binding of the N-terminal his-tag to the column confirmed that the truncation was at the C-terminal tail domain. Truncated HMGB1 and flHMGB1 were separated using anion exchange chromatography on a HiTrap Q FF column (GE Healthcare) using an increasing salt concentration. The his-tag was cleaved using TEV protease (Protein science facility, Karolinska Institutet, Sweden) at a ratio of 1:20.

Endotoxin was removed using Triton-X114 two phase extraction (Aida and Pabst 1990); all proteins preparations had endotoxin levels below 0.03 EU/µg as measured using the limulus amebocyte lysate (LAL) assay (Department of Clinical Microbiology, Karolinska Universitetssjukhuset). Protein purity was confirmed using SDS-PAGE gel electrophoresis analysis.

TLR2 binding assay

96 well microtiter plates were coated with 40 nmol of protein (HMGB1, Δ18 HMGB1, Δ30 HMGB1) in PBS, pH 7.2 for 2 h at 37 °C. Plates were washed (0.05% Tween 20 in PBS, pH 7.2 was used as the buffer for all washing steps) and blocked with 1% bovine serum albumin (BSA) for 1 h. After washing, 0.2–1.25 µg/mL TLR2-Fc (R&D systems, UK) diluted in 1% BSA in PBS, pH 7.2 was added and plates were incubated for a further 2 h. For detection of bound TLR2-Fc, plates were first incubated with anti-human IgG HRP diluted in 1% BSA in PBS, pH 7.2 (1/1000; Dako, Agilent Technologies, Stockholm, Sweden) for 1 h and then 3, 3′, 5, 5′-Tetramethylbenzidine (TMB) substrate solution (Sigma Aldrich, Stockholm, Sweden). The reaction was stopped

by adding 2 N H_2SO_4. In control experiments, 0.2–1. 25 μg/mL Etanercept (TNFR-Fc; Pfizer, Sandwich, UK) or 80 ng/mL h2G7 antibody (humanized anti-HMGB1 (Lundback et al. 2016); the binding epitope for 2G7 is between residues 53 and 63 in HMGB1) was added in place of TLR2-Fc.

Enzymatic digestion of Δ30 HMGB1 was performed on column using immobilized trypsin according to the manufacturer's instructions (Promega, Madison, WI, USA). Briefly, the protein was denatured at 85 °C for 5 min, diluted in digestion buffer (50 mM ammonium bicarbonate, 40% ACN) and incubated on the column overnight at room temperature. Peptides were eluted in the recovery buffer (50 mM ammonium bicarbonate, 40% ACN, 0.02% TCA) by centrifugation and coated to ELISA plates as described previously.

HEK293 and alveolar macrophage (MH-S) cell culture conditions

HEK293 cells stably transfected with functional TLR2, TLR1/2 and TLR2/6 dimers (Invivogen, Toulouse, France) were cultured in DMEM (Sigma Aldrich) supplemented with heat inactivated fetal bovine serum (FBS) (10%; Sigma Aldrich), penicillin (100 U/mL)-streptomycin (100 μg/mL; Sigma Aldrich), L-glutamine (2 mM; Sigma Aldrich), nor-mocin (100 μg/mL; Invivogen) and blasticidin (10 μg/mL; Invivogen) at 37 °C with 5% CO_2.

The alveolar macrophage cell line, MH-S, (kindly provided by Fredrick Wermeling's laboratory, Karolinska Institutet, Stockholm, Sweden) was cultured in RPMI media (Sigma Aldrich) supplemented with heat inactivated FBS (10%; Sigma Aldrich), penicillin (100 U/mL)-streptomycin (100 μg/mL; Sigma Aldrich) and 2-mercaptoethanol (0.05 mM; Sigma Aldrich) at 37 °C with 5% CO_2.

For experiments, 0.05×10^4 cells were seeded in 96 well microtiter plates in serum free media and left to rest for 6 h. Recombinant proteins (flHMGB1 or Δ30 HMGB1) or positive controls (TLR4 control: LPS (Sigma Aldrich) and TLR2 controls: peptidoglycan (PGN, 2. 5 μg/mL) and Pam3CSK4 (2.5 μg/mL; Invivogen)) were diluted in PBS and added at indicated concentrations. Supernatants were collected 24 h after dosing and stored at -20 °C until analysis.

Whole blood assay

Blood was collected from adult healthy donors into sodium-heparin tubes and added to a 96 well microtiter plate (180 μL/well; 200 μL final volume). Recombinant proteins (flHMGB1 or Δ30 HMGB1) or controls (LPS (100 ng/mL), PGN (2.5 μg/mL) and Pam3CSK4 (2.5 μg/ mL)) were diluted in PBS and added at the concentrations indicated. Plates were incubated at 37 °C for 4 h. Samples were centrifuged at 2000 g for 10 min, the

serum was collected and stored at -20 °C until analysis. The study was approved by the North Ethical Committee in Stockholm, Sweden.

Peripheral blood mononuclear cells (PBMCs)

Blood was collected from adult healthy donors and PBMCs were purified using Ficoll centrifugation (Ficoll-Paque Plus, GE healthcare). Cells were seeded at 0.1×10^6 cells/well in a 96 well plate in Opti-MEM (Invitrogen) and cultured at 37 °C with 5% CO_2. Cells were treated with Δ30 HMGB1 or flHMGB1 (0–2000 ng/mL) alone or protein that had been pre-incubated with 20 ng/mL PGN for 16–18 h at 4 °C as 40 x stock solutions. The concentration of PGN was determined by performing a titration experiment and did not induce cytokine production alone. Supernatants were collected 24 h after protein addition. The study was approved by the Stockholm North Ethical Committee in Stockholm, Sweden.

Elisa

Cytokine levels were determined by ELISA according to the manufacturer's instructions (R&D systems, UK).

Statistical analysis

Statistical analysis was performed using graphpad Prism v6 software. Data was analyzed using a Kruskal-Wallis test with Dunn's multiple comparison correction. * $p \leq 0.05$, ** $p \leq 0.01$, *** $p \leq 0.001$.

Results

The C-terminal tail inhibits the interaction with TLR2

To investigate the binding of HMGB1 to TLR2, we coated ELISA plates with different batches of HMGB1 purified in-house (CBP-HMGB1) or purchased commercially (tag-free HMGB1) and incubated with increasing concentrations of TLR2-Fc. Since a number of recent studies have revealed that HMGB1 binding to TLR4 is strictly regulated by cysteine redox modifications, we tested the binding of both fr- and ds-HMGB1 isoforms. As shown in Fig. 1a, the in-house produced CBP-HMGB1 displayed dose-dependent binding to TLR2-Fc, in contrast to the commercial tag-free HMGB1 which did not interact with TLR2; either in the reduced or disulfide isoform. From our previous experience, we knew that recombinant HMGB1 produced in-house with an N-terminal tag often comprises of a mixture of full length and C-terminally truncated proteins, in contrast to commercial preparations, which only contain the flHMGB1 protein. We confirmed that this was the case using SDS-PAGE gel electrophoresis (Fig. 1b) and hypothesized that the difference in the ability to bind to TLR2 might be explained by the presence of the C-terminal truncated protein in the in-house produced HMGB1 batch.

To test this hypothesis, we purified a new batch of tag-free HMGB1 and separated the full length and truncated HMGB1 proteins using ion exchange chromatography (Additional file 1: Figure S1A & B). Protein purity was confirmed using SDS-PAGE gel electrophoresis (Fig. 1c) and accurate molecular weight (MW) was determined for the partially truncated proteins using mass spectrometric analysis. The results confirmed that the molecular weight was between 22.5 and 23.2 kDa, consistent with the loss of 13 to 18 residues from the C-terminal tail domain (referred to as Δ18; Additional file 1: Figure S1C). In addition, we also expressed and purified a protein with a full deletion of the C-terminal tail domain (Δ30; Fig. 1c).

The ability of the different HMGB1 proteins to bind to TLR2-Fc was investigated using the binding assay. Δ30 HMGB1 dose-dependently bound to TLR2-Fc as did Δ18 HMGB1 although to a much lower extent (Fig. 1d). In contrast to Δ18 HMGB1 and Δ30 HMGB1, full length tag-free HMGB1 did not interact with TLR2-Fc confirming that the binding interaction is inhibited in the presence of the C-tail domain. Moreover, protein mixtures with increasing concentrations of truncated HMGB1 compared to the FL protein displayed higher binding to TLR2-Fc (Fig. 1e and Additional file 1: Figure S2).

To confirm that the binding was specific to TLR2 and not caused by non-specific interactions with the Fc domain, plates were coated with Δ30 HMGB1 and incubated with increasing concentrations of TLR2 or TNFR-Fc. As shown in Fig. 1f, Δ30 HMGB1 did not interact with TNFR-Fc confirming the specificity to TLR2. Additionally, Δ30 HMGB1 did not bind to an irrelevant human IgG1 isotype control antibody (data not shown). Furthermore, all three HMGB1 proteins displayed equivalent binding to h2G7, a partly humanized anti-HMGB1 monoclonal antibody (Lundback et al. 2016) thus confirming that the results observed were not caused by differences in the coating of the proteins to the ELISA plates (Fig. 1g). Finally, to demonstrate that binding to TLR2-Fc was specific to Δ30 HMGB1 and not due to any potential protein contaminates, the protein was enzymatically digested using trypsin prior to the ELISA experiment. Enzymatically digested Δ30 HMGB1 did not bind to TLR2-Fc (Fig. 1h).

Pure Δ30 HMGB1 does not mediate TLR2-mediated cytokine production in vitro

In vivo TLR2 has been reported to signal as a homodimer or as a heterodimer complexed with TLR1 or TLR6. To elucidate the functional relevance of the interaction discovered between Δ30 and TLR2 in the binding studies, HEK293 cells expressing functional TLR2, 1/2 or 2/6 dimers were incubated with Δ30 HMGB1 or flHMGB1 for 24 h and the supernatants were analyzed for cytokine

production. Pam3CSK4 and PGN, known TLR2 ligands, were included as positive controls and induced IL-8 production in all of the cell lines. Δ30 HMGB1 and flHMGB1 did not induce cytokine production in the cells transfected with TLR2 or TLR2/6 (Fig. 2a). Moreover, Δ30 HMGB1 did not increase cytokine levels in the TLR1/2 transfected cells, compared to the PBS control. However, addition of flHMGB1 resulted in a non-significant dose-dependent increase in IL-8 production in the TLR1/2 cells.

To confirm that the absence of cytokine production in the TLR-transfected HEK293 cells was not due to the lack of additional co-factors that may be required for receptor binding and downstream signaling pathways, we isolated whole blood from healthy volunteers and incubated the cells with the recombinant HMGB1 proteins previously tested in the ELISA experiments. No cytokine production was detected in the PBS control or in the cells treated with Δ30 HMGB1 (Fig. 2b). flHMGB1, which did not interact with TLR2-Fc in the binding experiments (Fig. 1e), significantly increased IL-8 levels at 10 μg/mL but not at lower concentrations possibly by interacting with other receptors present on the cells including TLR4. Moreover, Δ30 HMGB1 did not induce cytokine production in the alveolar macrophage cell line expressing high levels of CD36, a co-receptor for TLR2 heterodimer signaling (Hoebe et al. 2005) (Fig. 2c).

HMGB1 acts in synergy with other molecules to enhance TLR2-mediated cytokine production

In addition to acting directly as a potent inflammatory mediator, it has previously been demonstrated that HMGB1 synergistically enhances the response to several endogenous and exogenous molecules including LPS, CXCL12 and IL-1β (Hreggvidsdottir et al. 2012; Hreggvidsdottir et al. 2009; Wahamaa et al. 2011; Schiraldi et al. 2012). Since we did not record any direct consequences of Δ30 HMGB1 binding to TLR2 we hypothesized that Δ30 HMGB1 may enhance TLR2-mediated responses. To test this, isolated PBMCs from healthy controls were incubated with Δ30 HMGB1 or flHMGB1 in complex with PGN. Addition of PBS, Δ30 HMGB1, flHMGB1 or PGN alone did not result in any detectable cytokine production (Fig. 3a). However, Δ30 HMGB1 and flHMGB1 in complex with PGN significantly enhanced IL-6 cytokine production by 7- and 6-fold respectively (Fig. 3a & b).

Discussion

A detailed understanding of HMGB1 signaling pathways is required to fully elucidate how HMGB1 contributes to disease pathogenesis and to identify novel therapeutic targets. It is becoming increasingly clear that post-translational modifications generate several different and functional HMGB1 isoforms that have the ability to

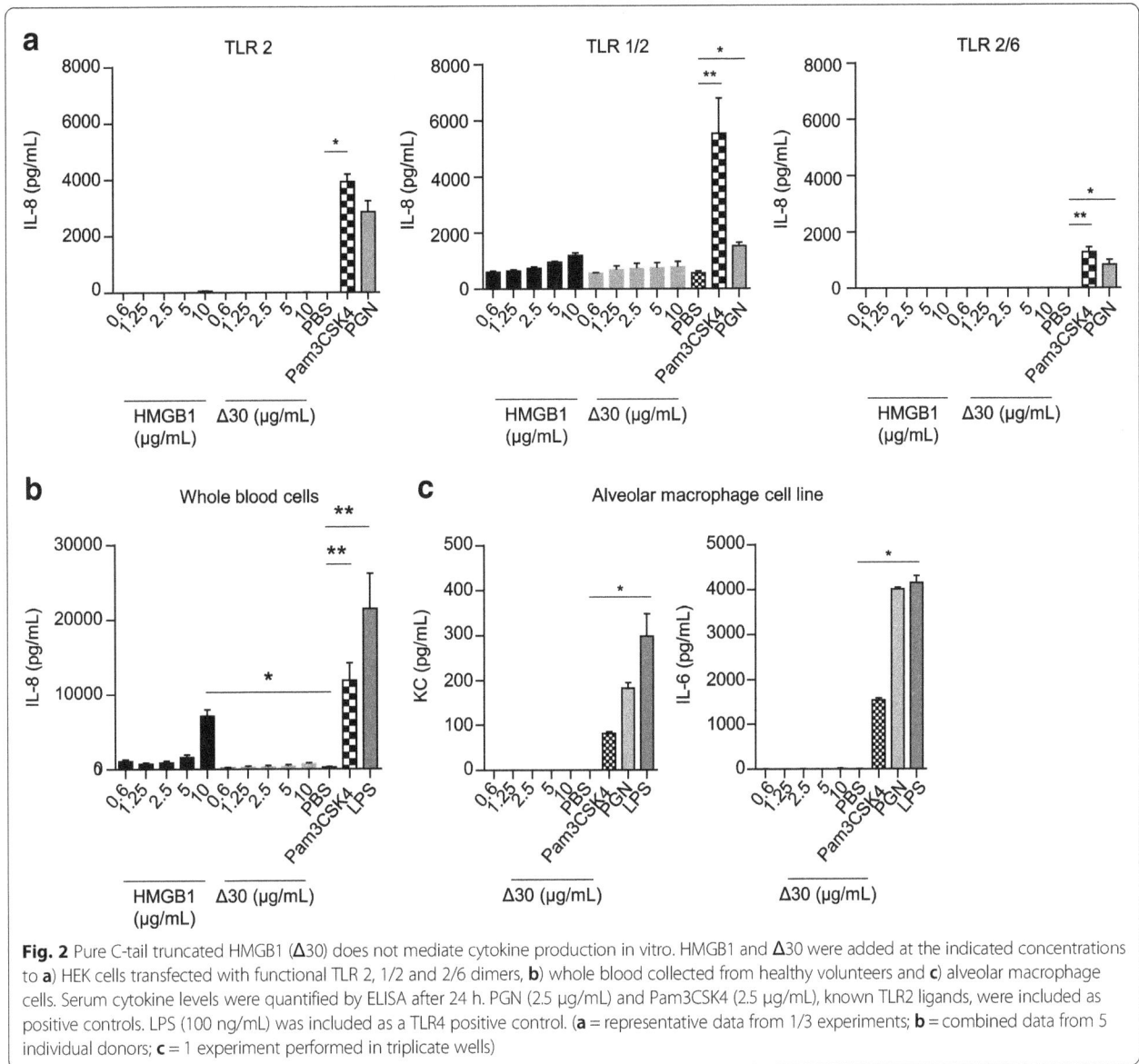

Fig. 2 Pure C-tail truncated HMGB1 (Δ30) does not mediate cytokine production in vitro. HMGB1 and Δ30 were added at the indicated concentrations to **a)** HEK cells transfected with functional TLR 2, 1/2 and 2/6 dimers, **b)** whole blood collected from healthy volunteers and **c)** alveolar macrophage cells. Serum cytokine levels were quantified by ELISA after 24 h. PGN (2.5 μg/mL) and Pam3CSK4 (2.5 μg/mL), known TLR2 ligands, were included as positive controls. LPS (100 ng/mL) was included as a TLR4 positive control. (**a** = representative data from 1/3 experiments; **b** = combined data from 5 individual donors; **c** = 1 experiment performed in triplicate wells)

interact with multiple unrelated receptors. While recent studies have defined HMGB1 binding to TLR4, little is known about the molecular requirements for HMGB1 interactions with TLR2. Consequently, the aim of this study was to investigate if TLR2 is a functional receptor for HMGB1 and if so, to identify the molecular requirements for binding. The results confirm that HMGB1 directly interacts with TLR2, but this interaction is inhibited by the presence of the C-terminal tail domain (Fig. 1d). Although it is able to directly bind to TLR2, highly purified Δ30 HMGB1 per se does not induce cytokine production via this receptor (Fig. 2), however it does act synergistically with known TLR2 ligands to potentiate their effects (Fig. 3).

In the current study, we are able to show that the conflicting findings previously reported on the HMGB1-TLR2 interaction are likely explained by the use of different sources of recombinant HMGB1. In our, and others, experience the expression of recombinant HMGB1 containing an N-terminal tag for purification purposes often results in the production of both flHMGB1 and a C-terminal truncated protein (Fig. 1c & Additional file 1: Figure S1) (Li et al. 2004). The generation of C-terminal truncated HMGB1 is most likely caused 1) by rapid degradation of the newly synthesized protein due to toxic effects of the acidic tail (Bianchi 1991; Lee et al. 1998) or 2) an inability of the bacteria to effectively transcribe the repetitive C-tail domain. As shown here, only truncated HMGB1 can interact with TLR2 (Fig. 1d). However, even a partial depletion of the tail (13–18 residues) is sufficient for TLR2 binding to occur (Fig. 1d). Further studies are needed to identify

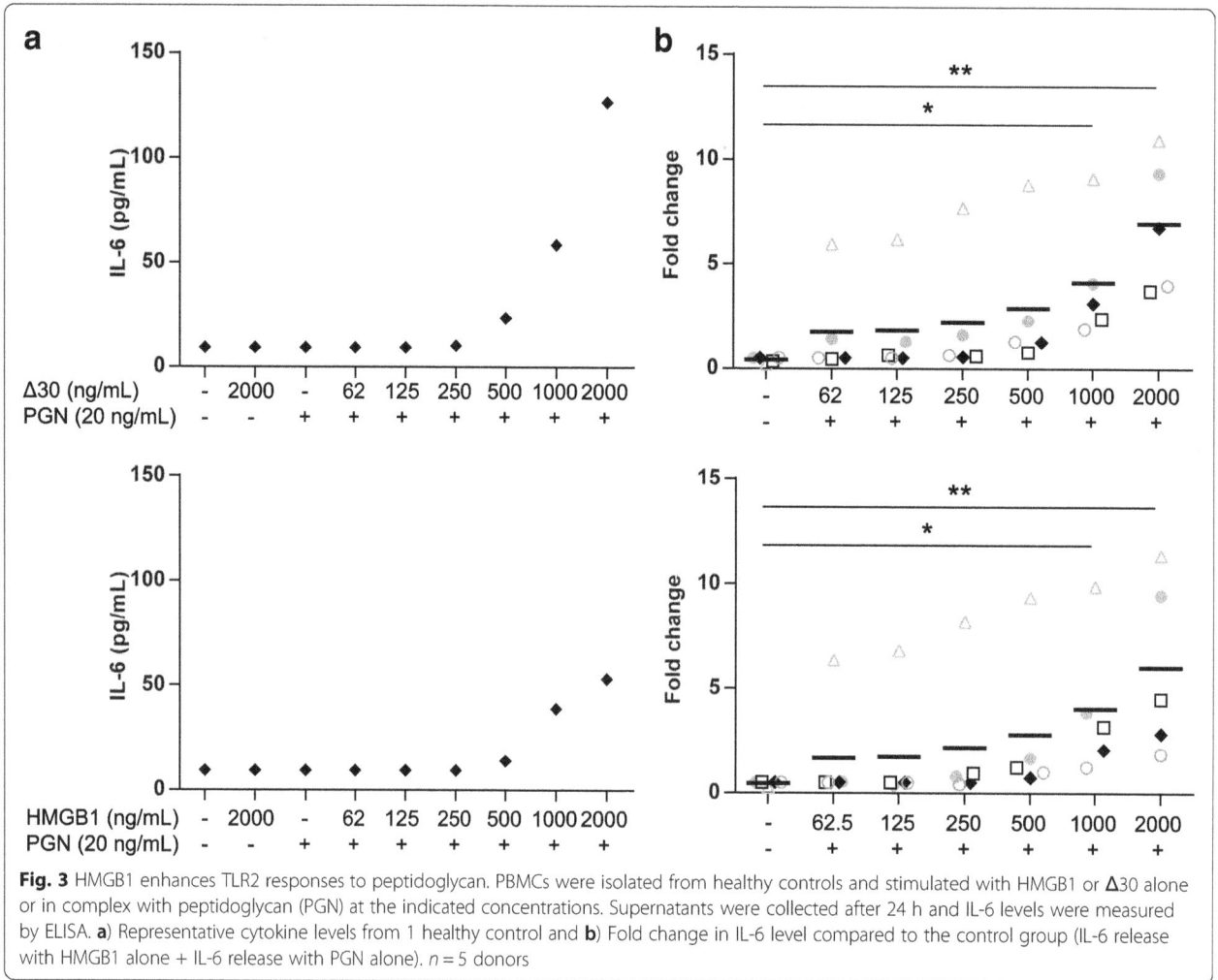

Fig. 3 HMGB1 enhances TLR2 responses to peptidoglycan. PBMCs were isolated from healthy controls and stimulated with HMGB1 or Δ30 alone or in complex with peptidoglycan (PGN) at the indicated concentrations. Supernatants were collected after 24 h and IL-6 levels were measured by ELISA. **a**) Representative cytokine levels from 1 healthy control and **b**) Fold change in IL-6 level compared to the control group (IL-6 release with HMGB1 alone + IL-6 release with PGN alone). n = 5 donors

whether the binding events are steered by electrostatic or hydrophobic forces and the critical residues required for the interaction.

The acidic tail regulates binding of HMGB1 to other molecules by interacting with the A and B boxes (Stott et al. 2010; Knapp et al. 2004). Interactions with box A are favoured and involve specific residues outside of the basic lysine-rich domains. Generally, depletion of the tail increases the affinity for molecules that bind to the boxes or linker residues. Removal of the tail increases the affinity for both linear and distored DNA structures and increases the DNA bending ability (Lee and Thomas 2000; Sheflin et al. 1993; Stros et al. 1994; Pasheva et al. 1998). In addition, acetylation of lysine 81 by CREB-binding protein (CBP) is inhibited when the C-terminus tail is present (Pasheva et al. 2004). The tail is required for binding to the H1 and H3 histones (Cato et al. 2008; Watson et al. 2013) and metformin (Horiuchi et al. 2017). Moreover, here we show that the tail inhibits binding of HMGB1 to TLR2 however, a recent study found that the tail is required for the interaction with

TLR5 (Das et al. 2016) suggesting that the tail regulates HMGB1 ligation to different TLRs.

Redox modification of the three cysteine residues present in HMGB1 regulates the inflammatory function and binding to TLR4 (Yang et al. 2010; Yang et al. 2012; Venereau et al. 2012). From these experiments it is difficult to define how the redox status impacts on the interaction of HMGB1 with TLR2. However, we observed that whilst the addition of H_2O_2 did not alter binding of Δ30 to TLR2-Fc, exposure to DTT reduced the interaction (Additional file 1: Figure S3A), indicating that redox modification may affect the binding. Treatment with H_2O_2 or DTT had no impact on the interaction between flHMGB1 and TLR2; in all cases flHMGB1 did not bind to TLR2 (Additional file 1: Figure S3B). This would suggest that although redox modification may contribute to the binding of HMGB1 to TLR2, it is the presence of the C-tail domain that is the major regulator of the interaction.

In additional to post-translational redox modifications, HMGB1 has been found to be a target for acetylation, phosphorylation, and methylation events (Tang et al. 2016). Acetylation of key lysine residues within the two nuclear localization signal (NLS) domains is required for cytoplasmic accumulation and active secretion of HMGB1 from monocytes and macrophages (Bonaldi et al. 2003). HMGB1 released from monocytes stimulated with LPS is also acetylated at several lysine residues found outside of the NLS sites (Lu et al. 2014). We speculate that acetylation of HMGB1 may alter the electrostatic potential and disrupt the interaction between the tail and the boxes possibly revealing the TLR2 binding sites in vivo, although this requires further investigation.

The interactions between the boxes and the tail may also be disrupted through the binding of a partner molecule to HMGB1. Previous studies have demonstrated that HMGB1 is able to interact with a wide variety of endogenous and exogenous molecules including Pam3CSK4, a synthetic TLR2 ligand (Hreggvidsdottir et al. 2009). HMGB1 complexes have enhanced pro-inflammatory activity and signal via the partner molecule receptor (Hreggvidsdottir et al. 2012). Here, we demonstrate that HMGB1 enhances PGN induced cytokine production via TLR2. HMGB1 also enhances PGN induced iNOS expression and nitric oxide release in macrophages (Chakraborty et al. 2013). Full length HMGB1 and Δ30 HMGB1 complexes with PGN induced comparable cytokine production (Fig. 3b), suggesting that the binding site(s) for PGN is located in the A box, B box or the linker residues. Binding of PGN to flHMGB1 may displace the interaction between the acidic tail and the boxes thereby exposing TLR2 binding epitopes.

HMGB1 complexes with LPS and CXCL12 mediate inflammation by enhancing cytokine production and inflammatory cell recruitment, respectively (Schiraldi et al. 2012; Hreggvidsdottir et al. 2009). We speculate that Δ30 HMGB1 may also bind to LPS and CXCL12 since the binding sites for both molecules have been mapped to boxes A and B, which are present in Δ30 HMGB1 and are likely to be exposed in the absence of the tail domain (Schiraldi et al. 2012; Youn et al. 2011). Δ30 HMGB1 also interacts with IL-1ß to enhance cytokine production in synovial fibroblasts isolated from arthritic patients (unpublished data from our lab).

Previous in vivo data suggests that the HMGB1-TLR2 axis may contribute to the pathogenesis of several inflammatory diseases, and that inhibition of this pathway may improve clinical outcome (Stark et al. 2016; Feng et al. 2016; Mersmann et al. 2013; Curtin et al. 2009). However, the results from the current study indicate that C-terminal truncated HMGB1 alone, containing no post-translational modification or binding partner, cannot signal via TLR2 to induce cytokine production (Fig. 2). Rather, our data suggests that HMGB1-TLR2 pro-inflammatory responses could be mediated by HMGB1-complexes (Fig. 3).

In the current study we have focused on investigating if HMGB1 induces TLR2-dependent cytokine production. However, recent studies also suggest a role for TLR2 in mediating protective and regenerative effects in models of skeletal muscle ischemia (Sachdev et al. 2012). Sachdev et al. found that TLR2 signalling reduces necrosis and promotes monocyte regeneration by attentuating HMGB1/TLR4 pathways (Xu et al. 2015). Moreover, TLR2 signalling is required for HMGB1-induced angiogenesis (Xu et al. 2015).

Conclusions

In summary, we have demonstrated that the C-terminal tail of HMGB1 negatively regulates the interaction with TLR2. The results from this study together with other reports thus indicate that binding of HMGB1 to different TLRs is differentially regulated. Disulfide full length HMGB1 interacts with TLR4 but cannot bind to TLR2 (Fig. 1a), which requires partial or full loss of the C-terminal tail (Fig. 1d). Binding of truncated HMGB1 to TLR2 does not appear to induce cytokine production alone, rather it acts in synergy with other TLR2 ligands. Further studies are needed to determine if a truncated HMGB1 protein similar to Δ18 or Δ30 exists in vivo and can be isolated from biological fluids. A study by Sterner and colleagues found that a C-terminal truncated HMGB1 protein may be present in calf thymus chromatin (Sterner et al. 1979). We hypothesize that such a protein may be generated by proteolytic cleavage of HMGB1 and that this molecule could act as an enhancer of TLR2-mediated inflammatory activities.

Abbreviations

BSA: Bovine serum albumin; CBP: Calmodulin-binding peptide; CD24: Cluster of differentiation 24; CXCR4: C-X-C chemokine receptor 4; dsHMGB1: Disulfide HMGB1; DTT: Dithiothreitol; flHMGB1: Full length HMGB1; frHMGB1: Fully reduced HMGB1; H_2O_2: Hydrogen peroxide; HEK: Human embryonic kidney; HMGB1: High mobility group box 1; LPS: Lipopolysaccharide; NLS: Nuclear localization signal; oxHMGB1: Sulfonyl HMGB1; PBMC: Peripheral blood mononuclear cell; PGN: Peptidoglycan; RAGE: Receptor for advanced glycation end-products; TEV: Tobacco etch virus; TLR: Toll-like receptor

Acknowledgements

Protein analysis was performed by the Proteomics Karolinska (PK/KI) core facility at Karolinska Institute, Stockholm.

Funding

The study was supported by grants from The Swedish Science Council, The Ceric center of Excellence, The Swedish Heart-Lung foundation and the Swedish Cancer foundation.

Authors' contributions

All authors were involved in the study design, data analysis and preparation of the manuscript. HA, AS and PL performed the experiments. All authors read and approved the final manuscript.

Competing interests

The authors declare that they have no competing interests.

Author details

[1]Department of Medicine, Rheumatology Unit, Karolinska Institutet, Stockholm, Sweden. [2]GE Healthcare Life Sciences, Uppsala, Sweden. [3]Department of Medicine, Rheumatology Unit, Centre for Molecular Medicine (CMM) L8:04, Karolinska Hospital, 17176 Solna, Sweden.

References

Aida Y, Pabst MJ. Removal of endotoxin from protein solutions by phase separation using triton X-114. J Immunol Methods. 1990;132(2):191–5.

Andersson U, Tracey KJ. HMGB1 is a therapeutic target for sterile inflammation and infection. Annu Rev Immunol. 2011;29:139–62.

Bianchi ME. Production of functional rat HMG1 protein in Escherichia coli. Gene. 1991;104(2):271–5.

Bonaldi T, et al. Monocytic cells hyperacetylate chromatin protein HMGB1 to redirect it towards secretion. EMBO J. 2003;22(20):5551–60.

Cato L, et al. The interaction of HMGB1 and linker histones occurs through their acidic and basic tails. J Mol Biol. 2008;384(5):1262–72.

Chakraborty R, Bhatt KH, Sodhi A. High mobility group box 1 protein synergizes with lipopolysaccharide and peptidoglycan for nitric oxide production in mouse peritoneal macrophages in vitro. Mol Immunol. 2013;54(1):48–57.

Chen GY, et al. CD24 and Siglec-10 selectively repress tissue damage-induced immune responses. Science. 2009;323(5922):1722–5.

Chiba S, et al. Tumor-infiltrating DCs suppress nucleic acid-mediated innate immune responses through interactions between the receptor TIM-3 and the alarmin HMGB1. Nat Immunol. 2012;13(9):832–42.

Conti L, et al. The noninflammatory role of high mobility group box 1/toll-like receptor 2 axis in the self-renewal of mammary cancer stem cells. FASEB J. 2013;27(12):4731–44.

Curtin JF, et al. HMGB1 mediates endogenous TLR2 activation and brain tumor regression. PLoS Med. 2009;6(1):e10.

Das N, et al. HMGB1 activates Proinflammatory signaling via TLR5 leading to allodynia. Cell Rep. 2016;17(4):1128–40.

Feng XJ, et al. TLR2 plays a critical role in HMGB1-induced glomeruli cell proliferation through the FoxO1 signaling pathway in lupus nephritis. J Interf Cytokine Res. 2016;36(4):258–66.

Gao HM, et al. HMGB1 acts on microglia Mac1 to mediate chronic neuroinflammation that drives progressive neurodegeneration. J Neurosci. 2011;31(3):1081–92.

Hardman CH, et al. Structure of the A-domain of HMG1 and its interaction with DNA as studied by heteronuclear three- and four-dimensional NMR spectroscopy. Biochemistry. 1995;34(51):16596–607.

Hoebe K, et al. CD36 is a sensor of diacylglycerides. Nature. 2005;433(7025):523–7.

Hori O, et al. The receptor for advanced glycation end products (RAGE) is a cellular binding site for amphoterin. Mediation of neurite outgrowth and co-expression of rage and amphoterin in the developing nervous system. J Biol Chem. 1995;270(43):25752–61.

Horiuchi T, et al. Metformin directly binds the alarmin HMGB1 and inhibits its proinflammatory activity. J Biol Chem. 2017;292(20):8436–46.

Hreggvidsdottir HS, et al. The alarmin HMGB1 acts in synergy with endogenous and exogenous danger signals to promote inflammation. J Leukoc Biol. 2009; 86(3):655–62.

Hreggvidsdottir HS, et al. High mobility group box protein 1 (HMGB1)-partner molecule complexes enhance cytokine production by signaling through the partner molecule receptor. Mol Med. 2012;18:224–30.

Knapp S, et al. The long acidic tail of high mobility group box 1 (HMGB1) protein forms an extended and flexible structure that interacts with specific residues within and between the HMG boxes. Biochemistry. 2004;43(38):11992–7.

Lee KB, Brooks DJ, Thomas JO. Selection of a cDNA clone for chicken high-mobility-group 1 (HMG1) protein through its unusually conserved 3'-untranslated region, and improved expression of recombinant HMG1 in Escherichia coli. Gene. 1998;225(1–2):97–105.

Lee KB, Thomas JO. The effect of the acidic tail on the DNA-binding properties of the HMG1,2 class of proteins: insights from tail switching and tail removal. J Mol Biol. 2000;304(2):135–49.

Li J, et al. Recombinant HMGB1 with cytokine-stimulating activity. J Immunol Methods. 2004;289(1–2):211–23.

Lu B, et al. JAK/STAT1 signaling promotes HMGB1 hyperacetylation and nuclear translocation. Proc Natl Acad Sci U S A. 2014;111(8):3068–73.

Lundback P, et al. A novel high mobility group box 1 neutralizing chimeric antibody attenuates drug-induced liver injury and postinjury inflammation in mice. Hepatology. 2016;64(5):1699–710.

Mersmann J, et al. Attenuation of myocardial injury by HMGB1 blockade during ischemia/reperfusion is toll-like receptor 2-dependent. Mediat Inflamm. 2013; 2013:174168.

Muller S, Bianchi ME, Knapp S. Thermodynamics of HMGB1 interaction with duplex DNA. Biochemistry. 2001;40(34):10254–61.

Park JS, et al. Involvement of toll-like receptors 2 and 4 in cellular activation by high mobility group box 1 protein. J Biol Chem. 2004;279(9):7370–7.

Park JS, et al. High mobility group box 1 protein interacts with multiple toll-like receptors. Am J Physiol Cell Physiol. 2006;290(3):C917–24.

Pasheva E, et al. In vitro acetylation of HMGB-1 and -2 proteins by CBP: the role of the acidic tail. Biochemistry. 2004;43(10):2935–40.

Pasheva EA, Pashev IG, Favre A. Preferential binding of high mobility group 1 protein to UV-damaged DNA. Role of the COOH-terminal domain. J Biol Chem. 1998;273(38):24730–6.

Sachdev U, et al. TLR2 and TLR4 mediate differential responses to limb ischemia through MyD88-dependent and independent pathways. PLoS One. 2012; 7(11):e50654.

Schiraldi M, et al. HMGB1 promotes recruitment of inflammatory cells to damaged tissues by forming a complex with CXCL12 and signaling via CXCR4. J Exp Med. 2012;209(3):551–63.

Sheflin LG, Fucile NW, Spaulding SW. The specific interactions of HMG 1 and 2 with negatively supercoiled DNA are modulated by their acidic C-terminal domains and involve cysteine residues in their HMG 1/2 boxes. Biochemistry. 1993;32(13):3238–48.

Stark K, et al. Disulfide HMGB1 derived from platelets coordinates venous thrombosis in mice. Blood. 2016;128(20):2435–49.

Sterner R, Vidali G, Allfrey VG. Discrete proteolytic cleavage of high mobility group proteins. Biochem Biophys Res Commun. 1979;89(1):129–33.

Stott K, et al. Tail-mediated collapse of HMGB1 is dynamic and occurs via differential binding of the acidic tail to the a and B domains. J Mol Biol. 2010; 403(5):706–22.

Stros M, Stokrova J, Thomas JO. DNA looping by the HMG-box domains of HMG1 and modulation of DNA binding by the acidic C-terminal domain. Nucleic Acids Res. 1994;22(6):1044–51.

Tang Y, et al. Regulation of posttranslational modifications of HMGB1 during immune responses. Antioxid Redox Signal. 2016;24(12):620–34.

Venereau E, et al. Mutually exclusive redox forms of HMGB1 promote cell recruitment or proinflammatory cytokine release. J Exp Med. 2012;209(9): 1519–28.

Wahamaa H, et al. High mobility group box protein 1 in complex with lipopolysaccharide or IL-1 promotes an increased inflammatory phenotype in synovial fibroblasts. Arthritis Res Ther. 2011;13(4):R136.

Wang H, et al. HMG-1 as a late mediator of endotoxin lethality in mice. Science. 1999;285(5425):248–51.

Watson M, Stott K, Thomas JO. Mapping intramolecular interactions between domains in HMGB1 using a tail-truncation approach. J Mol Biol. 2007;374(5): 1286–97.

Watson M, et al. Characterization of the interaction between HMGB1 and H3–a possible means of positioning HMGB1 in chromatin. Nucleic Acids Res. 2013;

Weir HM, et al. Structure of the HMG box motif in the B-domain of HMG1. EMBO J. 1993;12(4):1311–9.

Xu J, et al. TLR4 deters perfusion recovery and upregulates toll-like receptor 2 (TLR2) in ischemic skeletal muscle and endothelial cells. Mol Med. 2015;21: 605–15.

Yang H, et al. A critical cysteine is required for HMGB1 binding to toll-like receptor 4 and activation of macrophage cytokine release. Proc Natl Acad Sci U S A. 2010;107(26):11942–7.

Yang H, et al. Redox modification of cysteine residues regulates the cytokine activity of high mobility group box-1 (HMGB1). Mol Med. 2012;18:250–9.

Yang H, et al. MD-2 is required for disulfide HMGB1-dependent TLR4 signaling. J Exp Med. 2015;212(1):5–14.

Youn JH, et al. Identification of lipopolysaccharide-binding peptide regions within HMGB1 and their effects on subclinical endotoxemia in a mouse model. Eur J Immunol. 2011;41(9):2753–62.

Yu M, et al. HMGB1 signals through toll-like receptor (TLR) 4 and TLR2. Shock. 2006;26(2):174–9.

7

Over-expressed microRNA-181a reduces glomerular sclerosis and renal tubular epithelial injury in rats with chronic kidney disease via down-regulation of the TLR/NF-κB pathway by binding to CRY1

Lei Liu, Xin-Lu Pang, Wen-Jun Shang, Hong-Chang Xie, Jun-Xiang Wang and Gui-Wen Feng[*]

Abstract

Background: MicroRNAs (miRNAs) contribute to the progression of chronic kidney disease (CKD) by regulating renal homeostasis. This study explored the effects of miR-181a on CKD through the Toll-like receptor (TLR)/nuclear factor-kappa B (NF-κB) pathway by binding to CRY1.

Methods: Seventy male rats were selected and assigned into specific groups: miR-181a mimic, miR-181a inhibitor, and siRNA against CRY1, with each group undergoing different treatments to investigate many different outcomes. First, 24-h urinary protein was measured. ELISA was used to determine the serum levels of SOD, ROS, MDA, IL-1β, IL-6, and TNF-α. Biochemical tests for renal function were performed to measure albumin, uric acid, and urea in urine and urea nitrogen and creatinine in serum. The glomerulosclerosis index (GSI) and renal tubular epithelial (RTE) cell apoptosis were detected using PASM staining and TUNEL staining, respectively. Finally, RT-qPCR and western blot were done to determine miR-181a, CRY1, TLR2, TLR4, and NF-κB expression.

Results: CRY1 is the target gene of miR-181a, according to a target prediction program and luciferase assay. Rats diagnosed with CKD presented increases in 24-h urinary protein; GSI; RTE cell apoptosis rate; serum ROS, MDA, IL-1β, IL-6, and TNF-α; and CRY1, TLR2, TLR4, and NF-κB expression, as well as decreases in SOD level and miR-181a expression. Following transfection with either the miR-181a mimic or si-CRY1, 24-h urinary protein, renal damage, GSI, and cell apoptosis rate were all decreased. In addition, the overexpression of miR-181a or inhibition of CRY1 alleviated the degree of kidney injury through suppression of the TLR/NF-κB pathway.

Conclusion: miR-181a alleviates both GS and RTE injury in CKD via the down-regulation of the CRY1 gene and the TLR/NF-κB pathway.

Keywords: MicroRNA-181a, CRY1 gene, The TLR/NF-κB pathway, Chronic kidney disease, Glomerular sclerosis, Renal tubular epithelial injury

* Correspondence: drfengguiwen@163.com
Department of Kidney Transplantation, The First Affiliated Hospital of
Zhengzhou University, No. 1, Jianshe Road, Erqi District, Zhengzhou 450052,
Henan Province, People's Republic of China

Background

Chronic kidney disease (CKD) is a highly prevalent public health problem, and its incidence is rapidly increasing worldwide. Approximately 500 million people worldwide suffer from CKD, and the progression of the disease is much faster in the male population when compared with females (Gandolfo et al. 2004; Sampaio-Maia et al. 2016). CKD is characterized by certain adverse outcomes, including cardiovascular disease (CVD), kidney function failure, and premature death (Levey et al. 2005). The major histological findings in CKD patients are often glomerulosclerosis and tubulointerstitial fibrosis (Munoz-Felix et al. 2014). CKD can be classified based on the stages of disease severity, which are evaluated by measuring the body's glomerular filtration rate and albuminuria, as well as making a clinical diagnosis (Levey and Coresh 2012). Although the occurrence of CKD is age-independent, individuals over the age of 75 years are more susceptible to CKD (O'Hare et al. 2007). Significant advances have been made in controlling the progression of CVD, but the incidence and prevalence of CKD are still alarmingly high rates (Gaddam et al. 2016). Therefore, better studies and observations are necessary to provide a better understanding, diagnosis, and prognosis of CKD. A recent breakthrough has been the discovery that microRNAs (miRNAs), small non-coding RNA molecules, are involved in cancer (Lorenzen et al. 2011).

A member of the miR-181 family, miR-181a, functions as a mitochondrial miRNA in human kidneys (Marques et al. 2015; Su et al. 2015). Overexpression of miR-181a could very well enhance cell proliferation as well as reduce apoptosis of clear cell renal cell carcinoma via the down-regulation of KLF6 expression (Lei et al. 2017). Furthermore, Na et al. revealed that miR-181d could potentially target circadian rhythm genes, including cryptochrome1 (CRY1) and others (Na et al. 2009). CRY1, a circadian clock gene, is able to maintain its rhythmicity by inhibiting BMAL1/Clock transcriptional activity, thereby exerting pro-inflammation functions (Lee et al. 2013; Yang et al. 2015). For instance, down-regulating CRY activates pro-inflammatory cytokines via the nuclear factor-kappa B (NF-κB) pathway (Narasimamurthy et al. 2012). Up-regulated CRY1 could also potentially reduce the development of atherosclerosis by regulating the Toll-like receptor (TLR)/NF-κB pathway (Yang et al. 2015). The activation of the TLR2-MyD88-NF-κB pathway has been associated with the tubulointerstitial inflammation in CKD, further suggesting that the TLR/NF-κB pathway could be used as a potential target treatment for CKD (Ding et al. 2015).

Based on the aforementioned findings, we hypothesized that miR-181a, CRY1, and the TLR/NF-κB pathway are involved in the progression, incidence, and treatment of CKD. Few researchers have investigated the underlying mechanism of miR-181a in CKD via the TLR/NF-κB pathway. Therefore, we established a rat model to explore whether miR-181a influenced CKD by way of the TLR/NF-κB pathway via regulation of the CRY1 gene.

Materials

Ethics statement

All animal experiments in this study were conducted in accordance with guidelines for the use and care of laboratory animals.

Model establishment and transfection

A total of 70 male Sprague-Dawley (SD) rats aged 7 weeks and weighing approximately 210 ± 20 g were purchased from the Experimental Animal Centre of Southern Medical University. The rats were then randomly divided into two groups, with ten rats for the normal group and the remaining 60 rats for the CKD group, which were then used for the establishment of the CKD rat models through an intravenous injection of adriamycin into the tail vein (3 mg/kg) (Ding et al. 2014). Following 1 week of administration of adriamycin, the rats in the CKD group were classified into the following subcategories: blank (transfected without any sequences), negative control (NC) (transfected with fluorescence-labeled NC plasmids), miR-181a mimic (transfected with fluorescence-labeled miR-181a mimic plasmids), miR-181a inhibitor (transfected with fluorescence-labeled miR-181a inhibitor plasmids), si-CRY1 (transfected with fluorescence-labeled si-CRY1 plasmids), and miR-181a inhibitor + si-CRY1 (transfected with fluorescence-labeled miR-181a inhibitor + si-CRY1 plasmids). All transfected plasmids were designed and purchased by the Sangon Biotech Co., Ltd. (Shanghai, China). The rats in all CKD groups were injected with 0.002 μg plasmids via the tail vein, while the rats in the normal group were injected with an equal volume of normal saline via their tail vein. We collected 24-h urine samples from rats in each group at the end of the 4th week, along with their peripheral blood, which was extracted from the tail of rats to prepare the serum. The serum prepared from the peripheral blood was finally stored at − 20 °C for later use. The rats were then sacrificed following successful collection of the serum, and the kidneys were collected soon after and preserved. The renal capsule was then peeled off the kidney tissues, with some of the kidney tissues being preserved in 4% paraformaldehyde for cryostat sectioning, fluorescence microscopy detection, and terminal deoxyribonucleotidyl transferase (TDT)-mediated dUTP-digoxigenin nick end labelling (TUNEL) staining. Some of the cortex renis that remained was then placed in a 10% formaldehyde for pathological examination. The remaining kidney tissues were all preserved in liquid nitrogen to be used in later experiments.

Transfection of plasmids

Kidney tissues preserved with 4% paraformaldehyde overnight were then removed from their preservative and dehydrated using a sucrose solution until the kidney tissue settlement was noticeable at the bottom of the container. The tissues were then sliced into 45 μm sections at − 22 °C using a pre-cooled freezing microtome (HM525, SeaWorld Equipment Co., Ltd., Beijing, China), followed by dicing an appropriate amount of kidney tissue and soaking the pieces in a 6-well plate in ice-cold phosphate-buffered saline (PBS). The pathological slides were then treated with pre-gelatin to prevent tissue from falling off, sealed with anti-fluorescence quenching agents, and observed under a fluorescence microscope. Each field of vision was then photographed in both the bright field (natural light) and dark field (without natural light). The experiment was repeated 3 times.

Detection of 24-h urinary protein

Following the 4th week of observation, the 24-h urine was collected and its volume was recorded after all of the rats had been placed in a metal metabolic cage. Next, 5 mL of the collected 24-h urine was centrifuged at 3000 r/min to remove the sediment, stored in a freezer at 4 °C, and finally sent away to the laboratory for the quantitative determination of urinary protein. This experiment was repeated three times.

Enzyme-linked immunosorbent assay (ELISA)

Following the urinalysis, serum samples were centrifuged at 3000 r/min and the supernatant was taken. According to the instructions provided by the ELISA kit (YQ, Imun Bio-Tech Co., Ltd., Beijing, China), the contents of superoxide dismutase (SOD, E-33106), malondialdehyde (MDA, 10417R), reactive oxygen species (ROS, 10256R) (all from Shanghai Yuanye Bio-Technology Co., Ltd., Shanghai, China), interleukin-1β (IL-1β, E-30418), interleukin-6 (IL-6, E-30644), and tumor necrosis factor (TNF-α, E-30633) (all from Xiamen Huijia Biotechnology Co., Ltd., Xiamen, China) were all determined. All kits were purchased from Abcam (Cambridge, MA, USA). The optical density (OD) value of each well was evaluated at 450 nm in a microplate reader (BS-1101, Detie Laboratory Equipment Co., Ltd., Nanjing, China) after blank-control wells were set at zero. The experiments for each group were repeated three times.

Detection of renal functions

Urine samples were collected from each group to measure urea, uric acid, and albumin. After the urine had been collected, the rats were sacrificed via neck dislocation, allowing for the blood to be collected, and centrifuged at 2000 r/min at 4 °C for 10 min. The serum was then extracted, and serum creatinine and urea nitrogen were measured.

Hematoxylin-eosin (HE) staining

The kidney tissues were placed in a 10% neutral formaldehyde solution for over 24 h, after which they were rinsed under running tap water, conventionally dehydrated for 1 min, cleaned in xylene twice for 5 min, soaked in and embedded with paraffin, placed in the paraffin model, and finally left to cool on a cold bench. The paraffin sections were then stained using a hematoxylin (PT001, Shanghai Bogoo Science & Technology Co., Ltd., Shanghai, China) staining method at room temperature for a total of 10 min, followed by washing under running water for 30–60 s. The sections were then placed in eosin (0001-H, Beijing XinHuaLvYuan Science and Technology Co., Ltd., Beijing, China) at room temperature for 1 min, followed by dehydration in a gradient of ethanol and clearing in xylene I and xylene II (GD-RY1215–12, Shanghai Guduo Science and Technology Co., Ltd., Shanghai, China) twice for 1 min. After being sealed with neutral balsam, we observed the pathological changes of kidney tissues under a Caikon fluorescence microscope (PrimoStar iLED, Bioresearch & Technology Co., Ltd., Beijing, China). Glomerular hypertrophy was confirmed by measuring the mean glomerular perimeter of the 20 largest glomeruli (Uil et al. 2018). The experiment was repeated three times.

Periodic acid of Schiff-methenamine (PASM) staining

Paraffin sections of each group were dewaxed in water, oxidized with a 0.5% periodic acid for 30 min, and washed under both tap water and distilled water. After oxidizing with a 10% chromic acid for 20 min, the sections were then rinsed with distilled water, fixed in a 1% sodium sulfite solution for 30 s, washed with distilled water, and immersed under a hexamine-silver solution (JR00477, Shanghai Junrui Biotechnology Co., Ltd., Shanghai, China) for 30 min. The sections were then left to stand at a temperature of 65 °C for a total of 4 min for a water bath, after which they were removed and washed with distilled water and measured under a microscope until the black precipitate appeared in the glomerular capillary basement membrane. Following the appearance of the black precipitate, the sections were colored using a 0.1% auric chloride solution (G810493-5 g, Shanghai Chaoyan Biotechnology Co., Ltd., Shanghai, China) for 30 s, washed under running water for 10 min, and stained with hematoxylin and 0.5% eosin for a total of 3 min. After completing a conventional dehydration cycle, the sections were cleared, sealed, and observed (Other reagents were all prepared by our laboratory). Pathological changes of glomeruli were observed under a microscope, including the collapse or dissolution of the glomerular capillary network, formation of micro-thrombi in the renal capillary lumen, fracture in the renal capsule, and fibrin exuded and sclerotized in glomeruli. The sections were then further observed under the microscope (400 ×) in 20 random fields per slice. Glomerular basement membrane, reticular fibers, and type IV collagen were all discovered to be black, the nucleus was both blue and black, and the background was pink. The degree of the glomerular lesion was evaluated according to the glomerulosclerosis index (GSI). According to the proportion of GS accounting for the glomeruli, GSI was divided into 0–4 levels: grade 0, normal; grade 1, GSI of < 25%; grade 2, GSI of 25–50%; grade 3, GSI of 50–75%; grade 4, GSI of 75–100%. With the grade scoring determined, the GSI was then calculated using the following formula: GSI = [(1 × N1) + (2 × N2) + (3 × N3) + (4 × N4) / NT] × 100%, where N1-N4 indicate the numbers of glomeruli in grades 1–4 of glomerulosclerosis, respectively. Each experiment was conducted a total of 3 times.

Masson staining
Following the determination of the glomerulosclerosis index, the sections were dewaxed, dehydrated, stained with hematoxylin (PT001, Shanghai Bogoo Science & Technology Co., Ltd., Shanghai, China) for 8 min, and rinsed using tap water. After being placed in a mixture of 1% Ponceau (HL12202, Shanghai Haling Biotechnology Co., Ltd., Shanghai, China) and 1% fuchsin solution (HPBIO-SJ820, Shanghai Hepeng Biotechnology Co., Ltd., Shanghai, China) for 40 min, the reaction was terminated by addition of 1% glacial acetic acid and 1% molybdic acid solution, followed by addition of a mixture of 1% brilliant green and 1% phosphomolybdic acid in tap water. The sections were then conventionally dehydrated and mounted along with a neutral balata. The degree of the tubulointerstitial lesions was determined by observing both the normal and atrophic states of the renal tubules, as well as the degree of the inflammatory cell infiltration (other reagents were prepared by our laboratory). As a result, 20 fields of vision in each section were randomly selected to be observed under the microscope (400 ×). The basement membrane and the collagen fibers were stained either blue or green, the immune complex was stained red, and the nuclei were stained blue-brown. According to the ratios between the positive area of inflammatory cell infiltration, interstitial fibrosis, and the areas of glomeruli and renal tubules, the degree of the tubulointerstitial lesions was graded on a scale ranging between 0 and 4 points (0 points = negative area; 1 point = positive area < 10%; 2 points = 10–25% involvement of positive area; 3 points = 25–50% involvement of positive area; 4 points = positive area > 50%). Each experiment was conducted 3 times.

TUNEL staining
For the TUNEL staining process, kidney tissues were embedded in paraffin, sectioned, and stained according to the instructions provided by the TUNEL kit (40302ES20, Yeasen, USA). The nuclei of the apoptotic cells that were stained presented a brownish-yellow color, while the nuclei of normal cells were stained blue. The number of apoptotic cells in each renal field of vision was calculated using a digital pathologic slice scanner (6,504,523,001, Roche Diagnostics Ltd., Shanghai, China) from fields observed under a microscope (200 ×). Following the random selection of five fields of vision of each kidney section, the percentage of positive cells in each field was calculated, as was the average of all fields. The average proportion was the apoptotic index (AI). Each experiment was conducted a total of three times.

Dual luciferase reporter gene assay
The targeting regulatory relationship between miR-181a and the CRY1 gene was predicted with the bioinformatics prediction website http://www.microRNA.org, and a dual luciferase reporter gene assay was carried out to verify whether CRY1 was indeed a target gene of miR-181a. According to the binding sequence of the 3'UTR region of the combination of CRY1 mRNA and miR-181a, the target sequences as well as the mutation sequences were designed, and the target sequences were chemically synthesized; simultaneously, Xho I and Not I were added at the respective ends of the sequences. The fragments were cloned into the PUC57 vector. After identifying the positive clones, the recombinant plasmids were identified via DNA sequencing, after which they were further sub-cloned into the psiCHECK-2 vector and transformed into *Escherichia coli* DH5α cells to amplify the plasmids. The plasmids were then extracted following amplification according to the instructions provided by the Omega kit (D1100-50 T, Beijing Solarbio Science & Technology Co., Ltd., Beijing, China). Next, the cells were inoculated into a 6-well plate at a density rate of 2×10^5 cells per well. Following the adherence of the cells, they were transfected using the aforementioned inoculation method, cultured for a total of 48 h, and collected. The effect of miR-181a on the luciferase activity of the CRY1 3'-UTR in cells was examined according to the method provided by the dual luciferase gene assay kit (D0010, Beijing Solarbio Science & Technology Co., Ltd., Beijing, China). The fluorescence intensity was measured using a Glomax 20/20 luminometer fluorescence detector (E5311, Shaanxi Zhongmei Biotechnology Co., Ltd., Shaanxi, China). The aforementioned procedures were conducted in triplicate.

Reverse transcription quantitative polymerase chain reaction (RT-qPCR)
The total RNA was extracted from kidney tissues by using the miRNeasy Mini Kit (217,004, QIAGEN, Germany), and the primers for miR-181a, CRY1, TLR2,

TLR4, NF-κB, U6, and β-actin were all designed and simultaneously synthesized by TaKaRa Biotechnology Co. Ltd. (Liaoning, China) (Table 1). The sample RNA was reverse-transcribed into cDNA in a reaction system of 10 μL according to the instructions provided by PrimeScript TM RT reagent kit (RR036A, TaKaRa Biotechnology Co. Ltd., Liaoning, China). The conditions for the reaction system were reverse transcription at 37 °C 3 times (15 min each) and inactivation of reverse transcriptase at 85 °C for 5 s. Subsequently, we performed RT-qPCR according to the instructions provided by the SYBR® Premix Ex TaqTM II Kit (RR820A, TaKaRa Biotechnology Co. Ltd., Liaoning, China) using an ABI 7500 PCR machine (7500, ABI, USA). The PCR mix was 25 μL of SYBR® Premix Ex Taq™ II (2 ×), 2 μL of forward primer, 2 μL of reverse primer, 1 μL of ROX Reference Dye (50 ×), 4 μL of DNA template, and 16 μL of ddH$_2$O. The reaction conditions consisted of pre-denaturation at 95 °C for 30 s, 40 cycles of denaturation at 95 °C for 5 s, annealing at 60 °C for 30 s, and extension at 60 °C for 30 s. Afterwards, with 2 μg of total RNA as the template, U6 as the internal reference for miR-181a expression, and β-actin as the internal reference for the expression of CRY1, TLR2, TLR4, and NF-κB, the relative expression of miR-181a, CRY1, TLR2, TLR4, and NF-κB was analyzed by the $2^{-\triangle\triangle Ct}$ method, where $\triangle\triangle Ct = Ct_{\text{target gene}} - Ct_{\text{internal reference}}$. Each experiment was conducted in triplicate.

Western blot assay
The RIPA Kit (R0010, Beijing Solarbio Science & Technology Co., Ltd., Beijing, China) was used to extract total protein from fresh tissues, and the bicinchoninic acid (BCA) kit (G3522–1, Guangzhou JBCBIO Technologies Inc., Guangzhou, China) was used to determine the protein concentration. After protein separation with polyacrylamide gel electrophoresis (PAGE), the protein was transferred onto nitrocellulose (NC) membranes. The membranes were blocked using 5% bovine serum albumin (BSA) at room temperature for 1 h and incubated at 4 °C overnight with rabbit anti-rat primary antibodies (CRY1, ab3518, 1:2000; TLR2, ab213676, 1:800; TLR4, ab83444, 1 μg/ml; NF-κB, ab31432, 1:800). All of the antibodies were purchased from Abcam Inc., Cambridge, MA, USA. After washing with a PBS solution 5 times (5 min per wash), the membrane was incubated with a horseradish peroxidase (HRP)-labeled goat anti-IgG (1:5000, Beijing Zhongshan Biotechnology Co., Ltd., Beijing, China) and developed using an electrochemiluminescence (ECL) solution (WBKLS0500, Pierce, Rockford, IL, USA) for 1 min. Following the removal of the liquid, the membrane was covered with plastic wrap and exposed to an X-ray film (36209ES01, Qiancheng Biology Co., Ltd., Shanghai, China) for further observation. A quantitative protein analysis was conducted based on the ratio between the gray value of each protein and the gray value of β-actin using ImageJ software 1.48 μ (National Institutes of Health). Lastly, the membrane was developed in a darkroom and photographed. Each experiment was conducted in triplicate.

Statistical analysis
The statistical analysis was performed using the Statistical Package for the Social Sciences (SPSS) 21.0 software (IBM Corp. Armonk, NY, USA). The measurement data are expressed as the mean ± standard deviation. Differences between the two groups were compared using the t-test, while differences among multiple groups were compared using one-way analysis of variance (ANOVA). $p < 0.05$ was considered to be statistically significant.

Results
The plasmid in each group was successfully transfected
Green fluorescence was observed in each group under a standard microscope. The results (Fig. 1) revealed no obvious fluorescence in the normal and blank groups, while there was obvious green fluorescence in the NC, miR-181a mimic, miR-181a inhibitor, si-CRY1, and miR-181a mimic + si-CRY1 groups, indicating that the plasmid was successfully transfected in all seven groups.

Up-regulated miR-181a or down-regulated CRY1 reduces urinary protein levels of CKD
As seen in Fig. 2, the 24-h urinary protein at the end of the 4th week following transfection had significantly increased among the 6 CKD groups compared with the normal group ($p < 0.05$). No significant differences were

Table 1 Primer sequences for RT-qPCR

Genes	Primer sequences
miR-181a	F: 5'-GGGCAGCCTTAAGAGGA-3'
	R: 5'-CAGTGCGTGTCGTGGA-3'
CRY1	F: 5'-TCAGTTGGGAAGAAGGGATG-3'
	R: 5'-CATTGGGGTCTGTCCTCCTA-3'
TLR2	F: 5'-CGCTTCCTGAACTTGTCC-3'
	R: 5'-GGTTGTCACCTGCTTCCA-3'
TLR4	F: 5'-CTATCATCAGTGTATCGGTG-3'
	R: 5'-CAGTCCTCATTCTGGCTC-3'
NF-κB	F: 5'-ATTCAACAGATATACCACTGTCAAC-3'
	R: 5'-TGTTCTTCTCACTGGAGGCA-3'
U6	F: 5'-GCTTCGGCAGCATATACTAAAAT-3'
	R: 5'-CGCTTCACGAATTGTCATTGCGT-3'
β-actin	F: 5'-AGCCATGTACGTAGCCATCC-3'
	R: 5'-CTCTCAGCTGTGGTGGTGAA-3'

Notes: *RT-qPCR* reverse transcription quantitative polymerase chain reaction, *miR-181a* microRNA-181a, *CRY1* cryptochrome 1, *TLR2* toll-like receptor 2, *TLR4* toll-like receptor 4, *NF-κB* nuclear factor-kappa B, *F* forward, *R* reverse

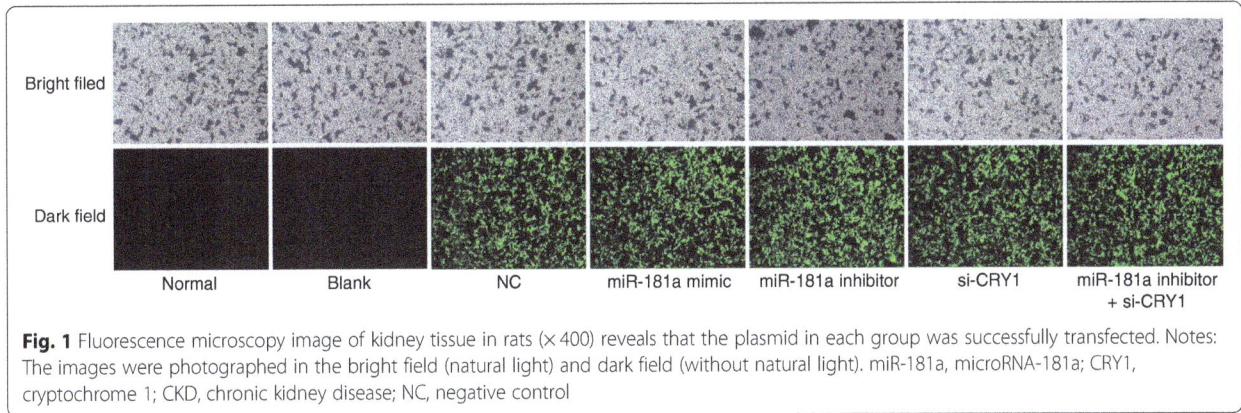

Fig. 1 Fluorescence microscopy image of kidney tissue in rats (× 400) reveals that the plasmid in each group was successfully transfected. Notes: The images were photographed in the bright field (natural light) and dark field (without natural light). miR-181a, microRNA-181a; CRY1, cryptochrome 1; CKD, chronic kidney disease; NC, negative control

observed in the 24-h urinary protein at the end of the 4th week following transfection between the blank and NC groups ($p > 0.05$). In comparison with the blank and NC groups, the 24-h urinary protein at the end of the 4th week following transfection had significantly declined in the miR-181a mimic and si-CRY1 groups, while it was elevated in the miR-181a inhibitor group ($p < 0.05$). However, 24-h urinary protein was not significantly different in the miR-181a inhibitor + si-CRY1 group ($p > 0.05$). These results indicate that up-regulation of miR-181a or down-regulation of CRY1 expression reduces urinary protein in CKD.

Up-regulated miR-181a or down-regulated CRY1 ameliorates renal damage in CKD

The biochemical tests of renal function (Tables 2 and 3) revealed significant increases in urine albumin, urine uric acid, urine urea, serum urea nitrogen, and serum creatinine at the end of the 4th week in the 6 CKD groups in comparison with the normal group (all $p < 0.05$). Again, no significant differences in the aforementioned indicators between the blank and NC groups were detected (all $p > 0.05$). When comparing the blank and NC groups, the contents of urine albumin, urine uric acid, urine urea, serum urea nitrogen, and serum creatinine in the miR-181a mimic group and si-CRY1 group all showed a significant decrease at the end of the 4th week following transfection, whereas they were all significantly increased in the miR-181a inhibitor group at the end of the 4th week after transfection ($p < 0.05$). There was no significant difference in the content of albumin, uric acid, urea, serum urea nitrogen, or serum creatinine in the miR-181a inhibitor + si-CRY1 group at the end of the 4th week following transfection (all $p > 0.05$) (Tables 2 and 3). The aforementioned findings suggest that the up-regulation of miR-181a or down-regulation of CRY1 reduces the degree of renal damage in CDK.

Up-regulated miR-181a or down-regulated CRY1 inhibits inflammatory infiltration and oxidation

The effects of miR-181a on inflammatory and oxidative conditions were assessed using an ELISA test. As illustrated in Fig. 3, the results showed that, compared with the normal group, ROS, MDA, IL-1β, IL-6, and TNF-α were up-regulated and SOD was down-regulated in the 6 CKD groups ($p < 0.05$). There were no significant differences in the previous parameters between the blank and NC groups ($p > 0.05$). In comparison with both the blank and NC groups, the miR-181a mimic and si-CRY1 groups had decreased ROS, MDA, IL-1β, IL-6, and

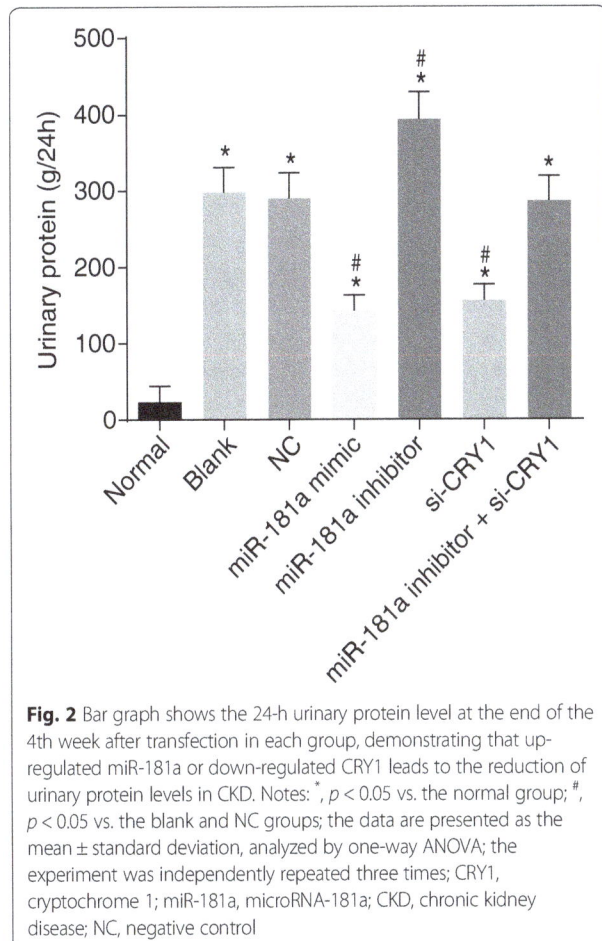

Fig. 2 Bar graph shows the 24-h urinary protein level at the end of the 4th week after transfection in each group, demonstrating that up-regulated miR-181a or down-regulated CRY1 leads to the reduction of urinary protein levels in CKD. Notes: *, $p < 0.05$ vs. the normal group; #, $p < 0.05$ vs. the blank and NC groups; the data are presented as the mean ± standard deviation, analyzed by one-way ANOVA; the experiment was independently repeated three times; CRY1, cryptochrome 1; miR-181a, microRNA-181a; CKD, chronic kidney disease; NC, negative control

Table 2 Upregulation of miR-181a or downregulation of CRY1 decreases the contents of urine albumin, uric acid, urea of CKD rats ($n = 10$)

Group	Urea (mmol/L)	Uric acid (μmol/L)	Albumin (g/L)
Normal	4.53 ± 0.75	152.32 ± 23.11	34.24 ± 5.12
Blank	48.16 ± 7.54[*]	256.71 ± 33.28[*]	20.97 ± 3.24[*]
NC	47.28 ± 7.23[*]	251.37 ± 32.14[*]	20.07 ± 3.13[*]
MiR-181a mimic	14.76 ± 2.31[*#]	193.48 ± 27.12[*#]	26.14 ± 4.12[*#]
MiR-181a inhibitor	67.82 ± 10.09[*#]	303.45 ± 33.23[*#]	13.92 ± 2.34[*#]
si-CRY1	14.24 ± 2.13[*#]	201.64 ± 25.96[*#]	28.18 ± 4.31[*#]
MiR-181a inhibitor + si-CRY1	46.82 ± 7.22[*]	248.39 ± 31.42[*]	23.26 ± 3.56[*]

Note: [*], $p < 0.05$ vs. the normal group; [#], $p < 0.05$ vs. the blank and NC groups; the data are presented as mean ± standard deviation and analyzed by one-way ANOVA.; the experiment was independently repeated three times
NC negative control, miR-181a microRNA-181a, CRY1 cryptochrome 1, CKD chronic kidney disease

TNF-α and increased SOD, while the miR-181a inhibitor group showed great elevation in the former values but a decline in SOD (all $p < 0.05$). There was no significant difference in ROS, MDA, IL-1β, IL-6, TNF-α, or SOD in the miR-181a inhibitor + si-CRY1 group compared with the blank and NC groups ($p > 0.05$). These results suggest that up-regulating miR-181a or down-regulating CRY1 expression suppresses both the inflammatory infiltration and oxidation.

Up-regulated miR-181a or down-regulated CRY1 reduces the degree of CKD

The transfection of the plasmids was observed using the HE staining method. As seen in Fig. 4, in comparison with the normal group, the other 6 groups had increased glomerular mesangial matrix, narrowed or damaged capillary lumen, adhesion of capillary plexus and cyst wall, and crescent formation in some glomeruli. There were

Table 3 Upregulation of miR-181a or downregulation of CRY1 decreases the contents of serum urea nitrogen and serum creatinine of CKD rats ($n = 10$)

Group	Serum urea nitrogen (mmol/L)	Serum creatinine (mmol/L)
Normal	3.47 ± 0.45	54.28 ± 8.34
Blank	8.39 ± 1.34[*]	94.39 ± 11.32[*]
NC	8.25 ± 1.24[*]	96.24 ± 11.34[*]
MiR-181a mimic	6.14 ± 0.83[*#]	70.73 ± 6.78[*#]
MiR-181a inhibitor	12.31 ± 2.12[*#]	113.65 ± 12.89[*#]
si-CRY1	6.06 ± 0.83[*#]	71.07 ± 6.75[*#]
MiR-181a inhibitor + si-CRY1	8.17 ± 1.23[*]	90.21 ± 11.31[*]

Note: [*], $p < 0.05$ vs. the normal group; [#], $p < 0.05$ vs. the blank and NC groups; the data are presented as mean ± standard deviation and analyzed by one-way ANOVA.; the experiment was independently repeated three times
NC negative control, miR-181a microRNA-181a, CRY1 cryptochrome 1, CKD chronic kidney disease

no significant differences in the pathological changes between the blank and NC groups. Compared with the blank and NC groups, the miR-181a mimic and si-CRY1 groups both showed a distinct glomus and renal balloon structure, evenly distributed endothelial cells and mesangial cells, as well as significantly reduced degrees of pathological changes. The miR-181a inhibitor group also presented with a severely deformed glomerular balloon, shrunken capillaries, and occlusion in parts of the vascular lumen, along with swelling, disorientation, and partial loss of RTE cells. There was no significant difference in the extent of the lesion in the miR-181a inhibitor + si-CRY1 group, indicating that up-regulation of miR-181a or down-regulation of CRY1 plays a significant part in reducing the degree of CKD.

Up-regulated miR-181a or down-regulated CRY1 reduces GSI

PASM staining was used to detect the GSI (Fig. 5). No obvious lesions were found in the glomeruli of the normal rats. In comparison with the normal group, an obvious collapse and dissolution of the glomerular capillary network, expansion in certain capillaries, micro-thrombosis in the renal capillary lumen, fractures in the renal capsule, a large number of inflammatory cells infiltrating the glomerulus, and a significant increase in GSI in the 6 CKD groups were all noticeable (all $p < 0.05$). There were no obvious differences in the pathological changes between the blank and NC groups ($p > 0.05$). In comparison with both the blank and NC groups, the pathological changes found among the miR-181a mimic group and the si-CRY1 group were significantly reduced, with the GSI showing a significant decline ($p < 0.05$). The pathological changes were significantly induced and the GSI increased in the miR-181a inhibitor group (all $p < 0.05$). The pathological changes in the miR-181a inhibitor + si-CRY1 group were not significantly different ($p > 0.05$). These findings indicate that the up-regulation of miR-181a or down-regulation of CRY1 expression can reduce the GSI.

Up-regulated miR-181a or down-regulated CRY1 reduces the degree of tubulointerstitial lesions

Next, we employed Masson staining to detect the degree of the tubulointerstitial lesions. As shown in Fig. 6, compared with the normal group, the remaining 6 groups showed signs of focal atrophy in the renal tubulus, renal interstitial lymphocyte infiltration, focal fibrosis, podocyte swelling, and higher levels of renal tubulointerstitial lesions (all $p < 0.05$). There was no significant difference in the degree of tubulointerstitial lesions between the blank and NC groups ($p > 0.05$). In comparison with both the blank and NC groups, the pathological changes and the degree of tubulointerstitial lesions were significantly less in both the miR-181a mimic and si-CRY1

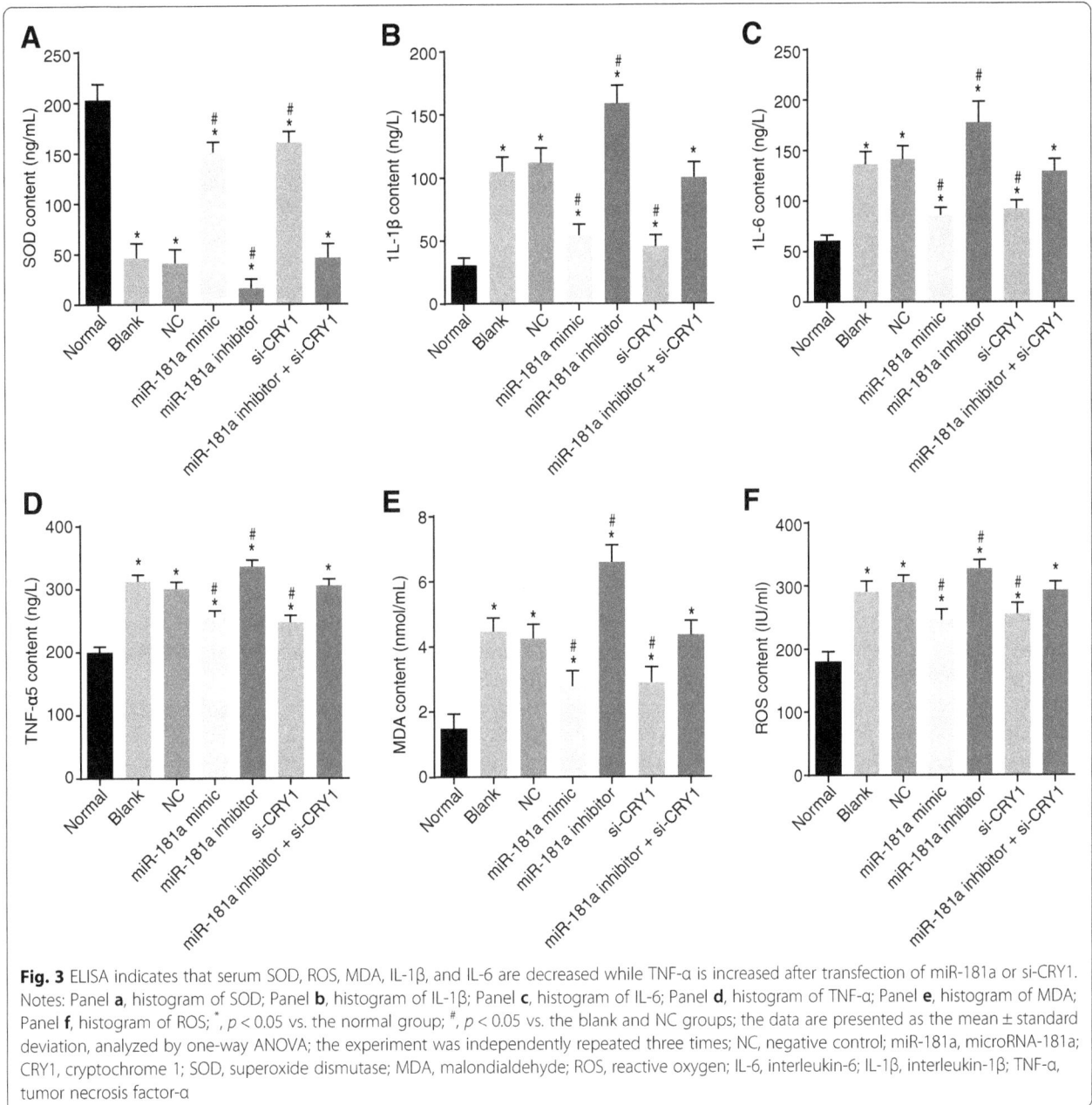

Fig. 3 ELISA indicates that serum SOD, ROS, MDA, IL-1β, and IL-6 are decreased while TNF-α is increased after transfection of miR-181a or si-CRY1. Notes: Panel **a**, histogram of SOD; Panel **b**, histogram of IL-1β; Panel **c**, histogram of IL-6; Panel **d**, histogram of TNF-α; Panel **e**, histogram of MDA; Panel **f**, histogram of ROS; *, $p < 0.05$ vs. the normal group; $^{#}$, $p < 0.05$ vs. the blank and NC groups; the data are presented as the mean ± standard deviation, analyzed by one-way ANOVA; the experiment was independently repeated three times; NC, negative control; miR-181a, microRNA-181a; CRY1, cryptochrome 1; SOD, superoxide dismutase; MDA, malondialdehyde; ROS, reactive oxygen; IL-6, interleukin-6; IL-1β, interleukin-1β; TNF-α, tumor necrosis factor-α

groups, while the pathological changes were greater and the degree of tubulointerstitial lesions higher in the miR-181a inhibitor group (all $p < 0.05$). No significant differences in the pathological changes in the miR-181a inhibitor + si-CRY group were detected ($p > 0.05$). The aforementioned results indicated that the up-regulation of miR-181a or down-regulation of CRY1 expression can immensely reduce the degree of the tubulointerstitial lesions.

Up-regulated miR-181a or down-regulated CRY1 inhibits apoptosis of RTE cell

RTE cell apoptosis was detected using the TUNEL staining method (Fig. 7). In comparison with the normal group, the apoptotic rate of the aforementioned apoptotic RTE cells was significantly higher in the remaining 6 groups ($p < 0.05$). No differences were found in the apoptotic rate between the blank and NC groups ($p > 0.05$). In comparison with both the blank and NC groups, the apoptotic rate of the RTE cells was considerably lower in the miR-181a mimic group and the si-CRY1 group, while it was elevated in the miR-181a inhibitor group (all $p < 0.05$). No significant differences were found in the apoptotic rate in the miR-181a inhibitor + si-CRY1 group ($p > 0.05$), indicating that either the up-regulation of miR-181a or down-regulation of CRY1 can directly inhibit the apoptosis process of RTE cells.

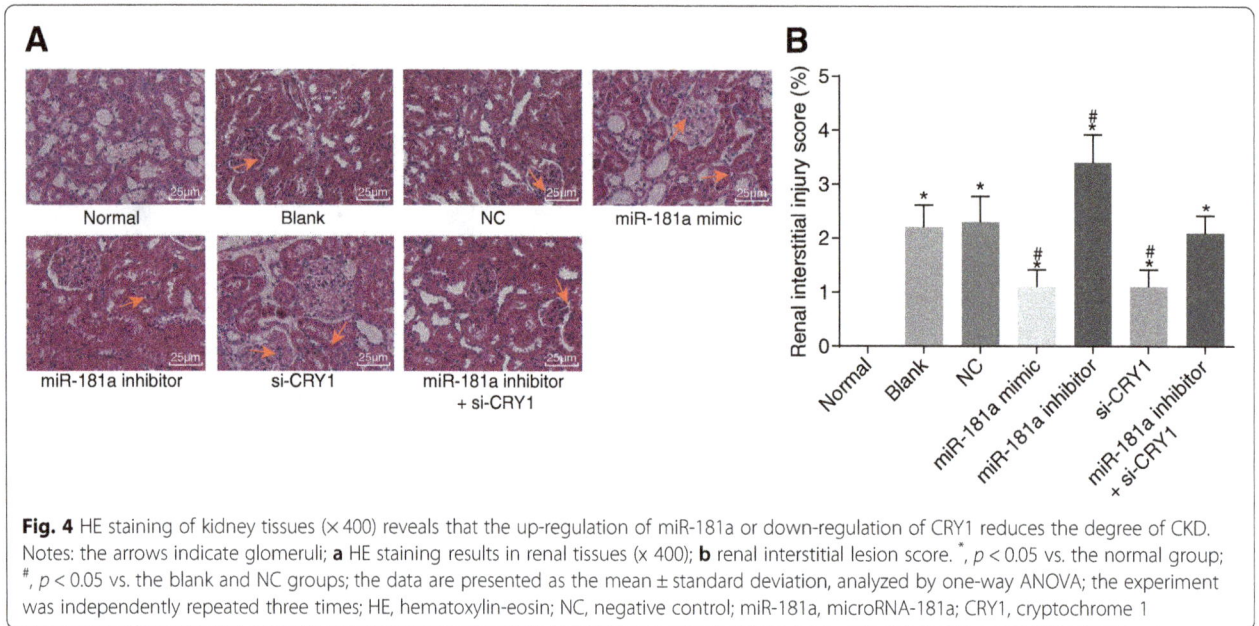

Fig. 4 HE staining of kidney tissues (× 400) reveals that the up-regulation of miR-181a or down-regulation of CRY1 reduces the degree of CKD. Notes: the arrows indicate glomeruli; **a** HE staining results in renal tissues (x 400); **b** renal interstitial lesion score. *, $p < 0.05$ vs. the normal group; #, $p < 0.05$ vs. the blank and NC groups; the data are presented as the mean ± standard deviation, analyzed by one-way ANOVA; the experiment was independently repeated three times; HE, hematoxylin-eosin; NC, negative control; miR-181a, microRNA-181a; CRY1, cryptochrome 1

CRY1 is a target gene of miR-181a

According to the analysis provided by online analysis software, there was a specific binding site between the CRY1 gene and miR-181a sequence, suggesting that CRY1 is a direct target gene of miR-181a (Fig. 8a). A dual luciferase reporter gene assay was used to verify this prediction. As depicted in Fig. 8b, the luciferase activity of the cells transfected with wild-type (Wt)-miR-181a/CRY1 in the miR-181a mimic group was significantly lower in comparison to the NC group ($p < 0.05$). No significant differences were observed, however, in the luciferase activity of the mutant (Mut) 3'UTR ($p > 0.05$). These results indicate that miR-181a can specifically bind to CRY1 and down-regulate the gene expression.

Up-regulated miR-181a or down-regulated CRY1 suppresses the activation of the TLR/NF-κB pathway by decreasing the mRNA expression of TLR/NF-κB pathway-related genes

The effect of miR-181a on the TLR/NF-κB pathway was analyzed using RT-qPCR. The results of the RT-qPCR are illustrated in Fig. 9. A notable increase in CRY1, TLR2, TLR4, and NF-κB mRNAs and a significant decrease in miR-181a expression in the 6 CKD groups were seen compared with the normal group (all $p < 0.05$). No significant difference was observed in miR-181a, CRY1, TLR2, TLR4, or NF-κB expression between the blank and NC groups ($p > 0.05$). The miR-181a mimic and si-CRY1 groups had reduced mRNA expression of CRY1, TLR2, TLR4, and

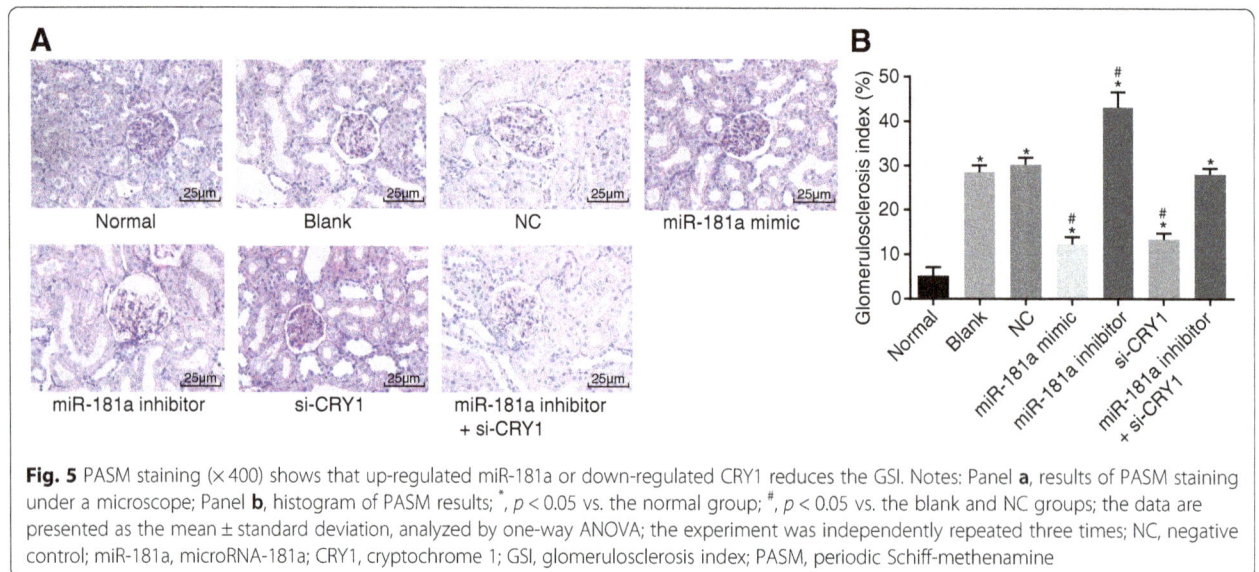

Fig. 5 PASM staining (× 400) shows that up-regulated miR-181a or down-regulated CRY1 reduces the GSI. Notes: Panel **a**, results of PASM staining under a microscope; Panel **b**, histogram of PASM results; *, $p < 0.05$ vs. the normal group; #, $p < 0.05$ vs. the blank and NC groups; the data are presented as the mean ± standard deviation, analyzed by one-way ANOVA; the experiment was independently repeated three times; NC, negative control; miR-181a, microRNA-181a; CRY1, cryptochrome 1; GSI, glomerulosclerosis index; PASM, periodic Schiff-methenamine

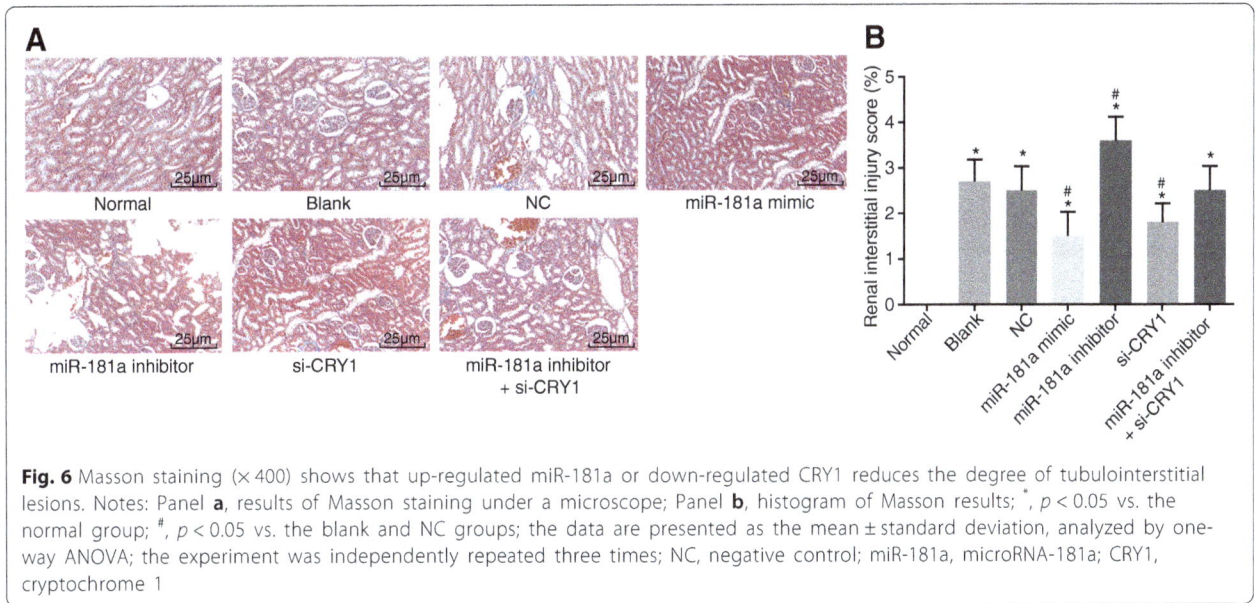

Fig. 6 Masson staining (× 400) shows that up-regulated miR-181a or down-regulated CRY1 reduces the degree of tubulointerstitial lesions. Notes: Panel **a**, results of Masson staining under a microscope; Panel **b**, histogram of Masson results; *, $p < 0.05$ vs. the normal group; #, $p < 0.05$ vs. the blank and NC groups; the data are presented as the mean ± standard deviation, analyzed by one-way ANOVA; the experiment was independently repeated three times; NC, negative control; miR-181a, microRNA-181a; CRY1, cryptochrome 1

NF-κB compared to the blank and NC groups ($p < 0.05$). miR-181a was up-regulated in the miR-181a mimic group ($p < 0.05$) while exhibiting no significant differences in the si-CRY1 group ($p > 0.05$). The mRNA changes in the miR-181a inhibitor group were opposite to those of the miR-181a mimic group. In the miR-181a inhibitor + si-CRY1 group, the expression of miR-181a was decreased ($p < 0.05$), with no significant differences in other indexes, compared to both the blank and NC groups ($p > 0.05$). These results show that the overexpression of miR-181a along with the silencing of CRY1 expression can suppress the activation of the TLR/NF-κB pathway.

Up-regulated miR-181a or down-regulated CRY1 inhibits the activation of the TLR/NF-κB pathway by decreasing the protein expression of TLR/NF-κB pathway-related genes

To further investigate whether miR-181a or CRY1 could affect the TLR/NF-κB pathway, CRY1, TLR2, TLR4, and NF-κB were detected using the western blot assay (Fig. 10). In comparison with the normal group, the CRY1, TLR2, TLR4, and NF-κB proteins were significantly elevated in the other 6 groups (all $p < 0.05$). All four proteins were similar between the blank and NC groups ($p > 0.05$). Compared with the blank and NC groups, all of those proteins were significantly decreased

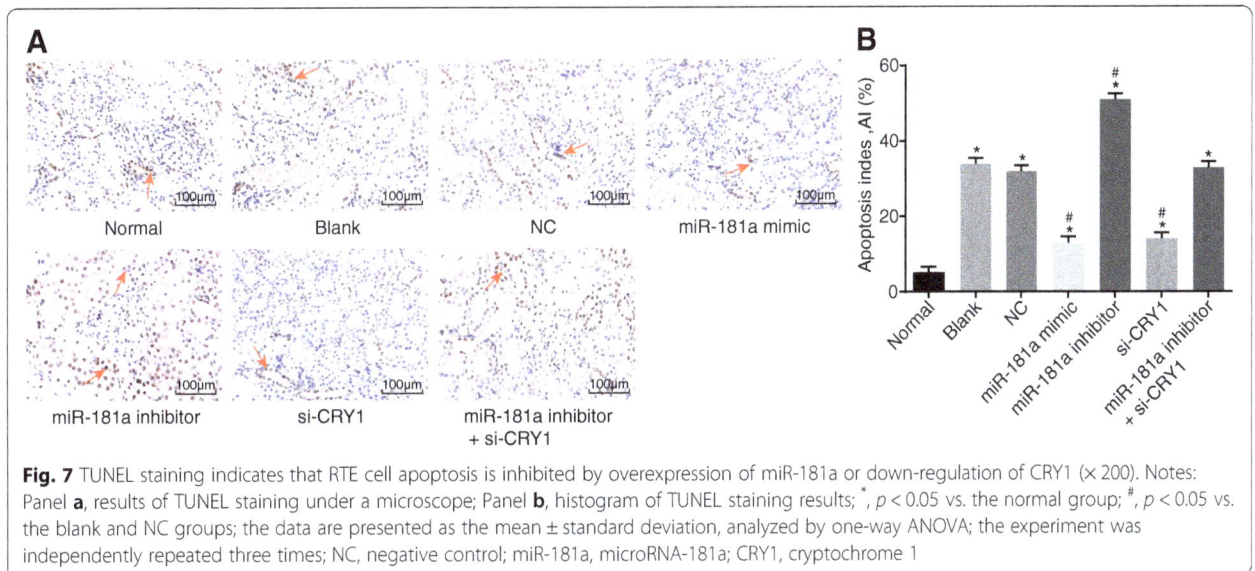

Fig. 7 TUNEL staining indicates that RTE cell apoptosis is inhibited by overexpression of miR-181a or down-regulation of CRY1 (× 200). Notes: Panel **a**, results of TUNEL staining under a microscope; Panel **b**, histogram of TUNEL staining results; *, $p < 0.05$ vs. the normal group; #, $p < 0.05$ vs. the blank and NC groups; the data are presented as the mean ± standard deviation, analyzed by one-way ANOVA; the experiment was independently repeated three times; NC, negative control; miR-181a, microRNA-181a; CRY1, cryptochrome 1

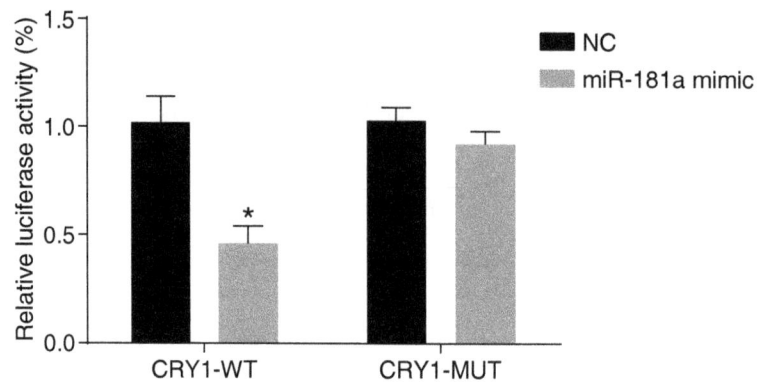

Fig. 8 A targeting/regulatory relationship between miR-181a and CRY1 is identified by the target prediction program and determination of luciferase activity. Notes: Panel **a**, predicted binding sites for miR-181a in the CRY1 3'UTR; Panel **b**, luciferase activity of cells transfected with CRY1-3'UTR-WT and CRY1-3'UTR-MUT; *, $p < 0.05$ vs. the NC group; the data are presented as the mean ± standard deviation, analyzed by t-test; the experiment was independently repeated three times; miR-181a, microRNA-181a; CRY1, cryptochrome 1; NC, negative control; UTR, untranslated region; WT, wild-type; MUT, mutant

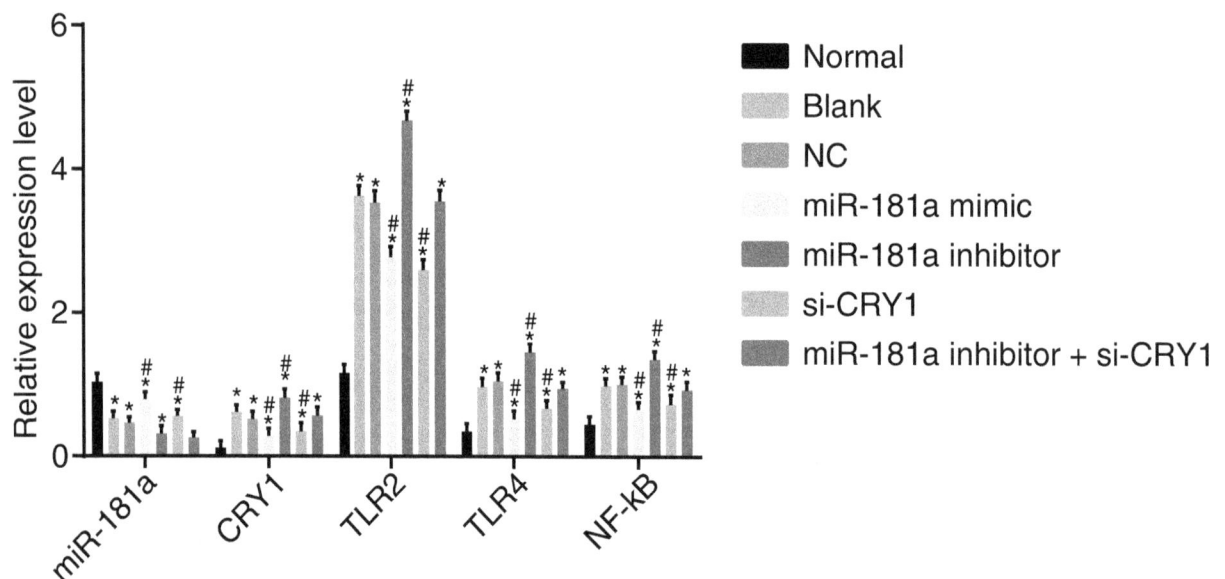

Fig. 9 RT-qPCR results demonstrate that up-regulated miR-181a or down-regulated CRY1 suppresses the activation of the TLR/NF-κB pathway by decreasing the mRNA expression of TLR/NF-κB pathway-related genes. Notes: *, $p < 0.05$ vs. the normal group; #, $p < 0.05$ vs. the blank and NC groups; the data are presented as the mean ± standard deviation, analyzed by one-way ANOVA; the experiment was independently repeated three times; NC, negative control; miR-181a, microRNA-181a; CRY1, cryptochrome 1; TLR2, Toll-like receptor 2; TLR4, Toll-like receptor 4; NF-κB, nuclear factor-kappa B; CKD, chronic kidney disease

in both the miR-181a mimic and si-CRY1 groups, while they were significantly increased in the miR-181a inhibitor group (all $p < 0.05$). No significant differences were detected in the miR-181a inhibitor + si-CRY1 group ($p > 0.05$). These results indicate that the overexpression of miR-181a or silencing of CRY1 expression can inhibit the activation of the TLR/NF-κB pathway.

Discussion

The inflammatory responses occurring during the progression of the damage of renal tissue as well as any tissue-related injury caused by CKD might develop into end-stage renal disease (Liu et al. 2013). miRNAs are important biomarkers in the diagnosis, prognosis, and prediction of renal development and disease (Neal et al. 2011; Xu et al. 2012). Based on these findings, the present study was conducted to investigate the effects of miR-181a and CRY1 on GS and RTE injury in CKD. Our results provide evidence that up-regulating miR-181a potentially suppresses the expression of CRY1 along with the activation of the TLR/NF-κB, thereby making a significant contribution to the alleviation of both GS and RTE injury of CKD.

Initially, our study revealed that miR-181a decreased the 24-h urinary protein levels of CKD and ameliorated its renal damage, which was reflected in the decreased contents of albumin, uric acid, urea, serum urea nitrogen, and serum creatinine after transfection. Serum albumin, uric acid, serum urea nitrogen and serum creatinine

can be used as parameters to evaluate CKD progression (Li et al. 2014). Up-regulating miR-181c also protects kidneys from CsA-induced renal injury and fibrosis through the suppression of the epithelial-mesenchymal transition (EMT) (Sun et al. 2017). Consistent with those findings, our study found that miR-181a inhibited both the GS and RTE injury in CKD, which was supported by an apparent decrease in the cell apoptosis rate and the levels of ROS, MDA, IL-1β, IL-6, and TNF-α in the miR-181a mimic group. In addition, the overexpression of miR-181a plays important roles in renal disease by inhibiting the cisplatin-induced apoptosis of tubular epithelial cells (Zhu et al. 2012). Another study reported that miR-181c suppresses the downstream production of pro-inflammatory mediators, such as TNF-α, IL-1β, and iNOS (Zhang et al. 2015). Moreover, the up-regulation of miR-181a further inhibits IL-6 and TNF-α in dendritic cells by targeting c-Fos (Wu et al. 2012). Although the aforementioned findings suggest that miR-181a could be a potentially important target in the treatment of CKD, further studies on its underlying mechanism were needed.

miRNAs affect the behaviors of malignant cells by silencing a variety of target genes, and regulating the downstream signaling pathways (Zhao et al. 2016). Our study provided evidence that CRY1 is indeed a target gene of miR-181a and that the elevation of miR-181a could lead to the direct down-regulation of CRY1.

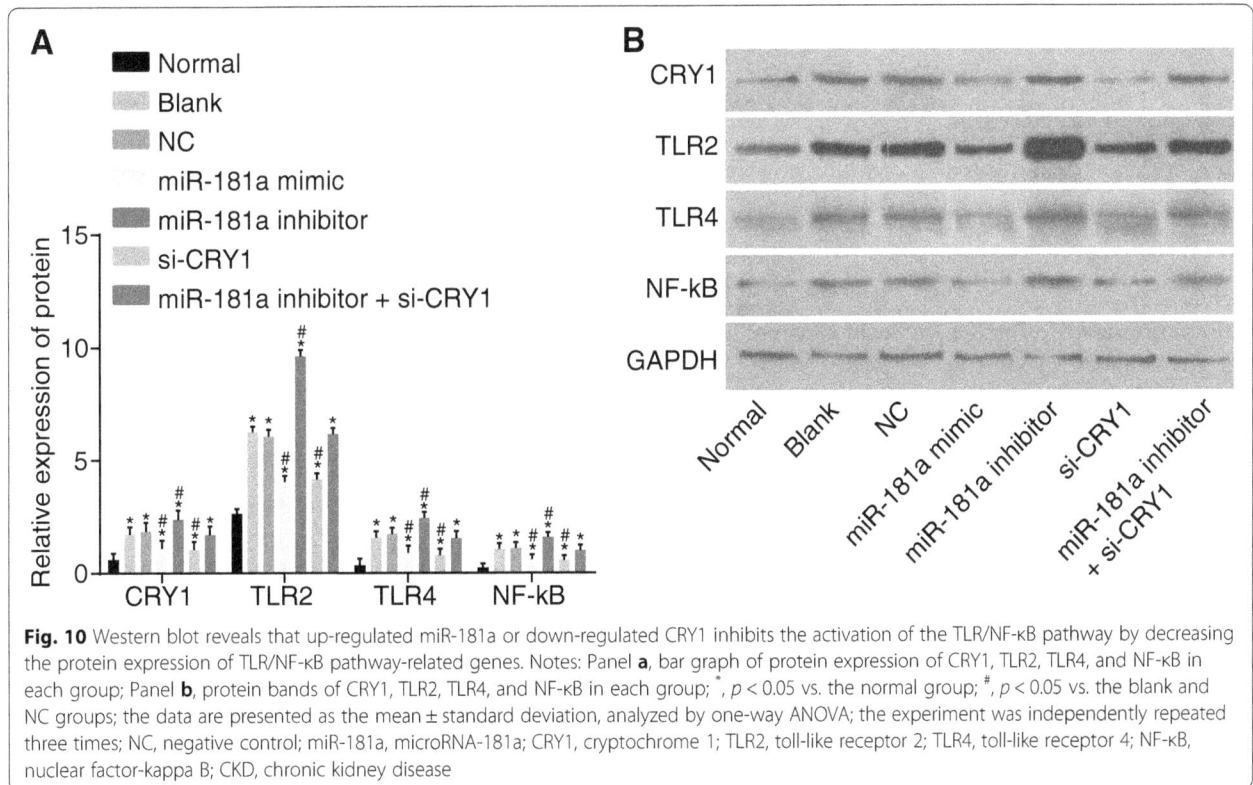

Fig. 10 Western blot reveals that up-regulated miR-181a or down-regulated CRY1 inhibits the activation of the TLR/NF-κB pathway by decreasing the protein expression of TLR/NF-κB pathway-related genes. Notes: Panel **a**, bar graph of protein expression of CRY1, TLR2, TLR4, and NF-κB in each group; Panel **b**, protein bands of CRY1, TLR2, TLR4, and NF-κB in each group; *, $p < 0.05$ vs. the normal group; #, $p < 0.05$ vs. the blank and NC groups; the data are presented as the mean ± standard deviation, analyzed by one-way ANOVA; the experiment was independently repeated three times; NC, negative control; miR-181a, microRNA-181a; CRY1, cryptochrome 1; TLR2, toll-like receptor 2; TLR4, toll-like receptor 4; NF-κB, nuclear factor-kappa B; CKD, chronic kidney disease

Moreover, miR-181d expression can also directly target the 3'-UTRs of CRY2 and FBXL3, providing information on its association with colorectal cancer (Guo et al. 2017). Our results and others' lead to the conclusion that an increased expression of miR-181a results in the down-regulation of CRY1, in turn promoting the GS and RTE injury in CKD.

NF-κB, a general nuclear transcription factor consisting of two glutenin subunits (p65 and p50), acts at the center of the inflammatory response and controls the gene expression of numerous inflammation-associated substances, including inflammatory cytokines (IL-1β, IL-6, IL-8, and TNF-α), as well as genes involved in ROS production (Jiang et al. 2014). Inhibiting the activation of the TLR4/NF-κB pathway reduces uric acid-induced EMT and inflammatory cytokine expression in the HK-2 cells of hyperuricemia nephropathy (Liu et al. 2017). Our findings show that TLR/NF-κB pathway-related proteins and inflammatory cytokines (IL-1β, IL-6 and TNF-α) were significantly reduced in both the miR-181a mimic and si-CRY1 groups, and over-expression of miR-181a seemed to reduce the GS and RTE injury by inhibiting the TLR/NF-κB pathway. Additionally, the inhibition of the TLR/NF-κB pathway by miR-181a could reduce inflammation in coronary artery disease (Hulsmans et al. 2012). Narasimamurthy et al. ascertained that the down-regulation of CRY, a core clock gene component, activates pro-inflammatory cytokines via the NF-κB pathway in chronic inflammatory disease (Narasimamurthy et al. 2012). There have also been various experimental and clinical data reports indicating TLRs are directly involved in the pathogenesis of urinary tract infections, acute kidney injury, and lupus nephritis (Chen et al. 2011; Ding et al. 2015; Moreth et al. 2014). We conclude that the up-regulation of miR-181a or down-regulation of CRY1 is directly associated with the inhibition of the TLR/NF-κB pathway, which reduces both the GS and RTE injury in CKD.

Conclusion

The overexpression of miR-181a could suppress both GS and RTE injury in patients diagnosed with CKD by down-regulating the expression of CRY1 via inhibition of the TLR/NF-κB pathway. Although the exact underlying mechanism of the regulation of the CKD metabolic pathway remains largely unknown, we believe that our findings improve our understanding of the specific mechanism by which the miR-181a-targeted CRY1 has an unfavorable effect on RTE cells in CKD via the TLR/NF-κB pathway.

Abbreviations

ANOVA: Analysis of variance; BCA: Bicinchoninic acid; BSA: Bovine serum albumin; CKD: Chronic kidney disease; CRY1: Cryptochrome 1; CVD: Cardiovascular disease; ECL: Electrochemiluminescence; ELISA: Enzyme-linked immunosorbent assay; EMT: Epithelial-mesenchymal transition; GSI: Glomerulosclerosis index; HE: Hematoxylin-eosin; HRP: Horseradish peroxidase; miRNA: microRNA; Mut: Mutant; NC: Negative control;

NC: Nitrocellulose; OD: Optical density; PAGE: Polyacrylamide gel electrophoresis; PASM: Periodic acid of Schiff-methenamine; PBS: Phosphate-buffered saline; RTE: Renal tubular epithelial; RT-qPCR: Reverse transcription–quantitative polymerase chain reaction; SD: Sprague-Dawley; SPSS: Statistical Package for the Social Sciences; TDT: Terminal deoxyribonucleotidyl transferase; Wt: Wild-type

Acknowledgments
We would like to give our sincere appreciation to the reviewers for their helpful comments on this article.

Authors' contributions
LL, X-LP, and G-WF designed the study. LL and G-WF collated the data, designed and developed the database, carried out data analyses and produced the initial draft of the manuscript. W-JS, H-CX, and J-XW contributed to drafting the manuscript. All authors have read and approved the final submitted manuscript.

Competing interests
The authors declare that they have no competing interests.

References
Chen J, John R, Richardson JA, Shelton JM, Zhou XJ, Wang Y, et al. Toll-like receptor 4 regulates early endothelial activation during ischemic acute kidney injury. Kidney Int. 2011;79:288–99.

Ding LH, Liu D, Xu M, Wu M, Liu H, Tang RN, et al. TLR2-MyD88-NF-kappaB pathway is involved in tubulointerstitial inflammation caused by proteinuria. Int J Biochem Cell Biol. 2015;69:114–20.

Ding ZH, Xu LM, Wang SZ, Kou JQ, Xu YL, Chen CX, et al. Ameliorating Adriamycin-induced chronic kidney disease in rats by orally administrated Cardiotoxin from Naja naja atra venom. Evid Based Complement Alternat Med. 2014;2014:621756.

Gaddam S, Gunukula SK, Lohr JW, Arora P. Prevalence of chronic kidney disease in patients with chronic obstructive pulmonary disease: a systematic review and meta-analysis. BMC Pulm Med. 2016;16:158.

Gandolfo MT, Verzola D, Salvatore F, Gianiorio G, Procopio V, Romagnoli A, et al. Gender and the progression of chronic renal diseases: does apoptosis make the difference? Minerva Urol Nefrol. 2004;56:1–14.

Guo X, Zhu Y, Hong X, Zhang M, Qiu X, Wang Z, et al. miR-181d and c-myc-mediated inhibition of CRY2 and FBXL3 reprograms metabolism in colorectal cancer. Cell Death Dis. 2017;8:e2958.

Hulsmans M, Sinnaeve P, Van der Schueren B, Mathieu C, Janssens S, Holvoet P. Decreased miR-181a expression in monocytes of obese patients is associated with the occurrence of metabolic syndrome and coronary artery disease. J Clin Endocrinol Metab. 2012;97:E1213–8.

Jiang GT, Chen X, Li D, An HX, Jiao JD. Ulinastatin attenuates renal interstitial inflammation and inhibits fibrosis progression in rats under unilateral ureteral obstruction. Mol Med Rep. 2014;10:1501–8.

Lee KH, Kim SH, Lee HR, Kim W, Kim DY, Shin JC, et al. MicroRNA-185 oscillation controls circadian amplitude of mouse Cryptochrome 1 via translational regulation. Mol Biol Cell. 2013;24:2248–55.

Lei Z, Ma X, Li H, Zhang Y, Gao Y, Fan Y, et al. Up-regulation of miR-181a in clear cell renal cell carcinoma is associated with lower KLF6 expression, enhanced cell proliferation, accelerated cell cycle transition, and diminished apoptosis. Urol Oncol. 2017;

Levey AS, Coresh J. Chronic kidney disease. Lancet. 2012;379:165–80.

Levey AS, Eckardt KU, Tsukamoto Y, Levin A, Coresh J, Rossert J, et al. Definition and classification of chronic kidney disease: a position statement from kidney disease: improving global outcomes (KDIGO). Kidney Int. 2005;67:2089–100.

Li L, Chang A, Rostand SG, Hebert L, Appel LJ, Astor BC, et al. A within-patient analysis for time-varying risk factors of CKD progression. J Am Soc Nephrol. 2014;25:606–13.

Liu H, Sun W, Wan YG, Tu Y, Yu BY, Hu H. Regulatory mechanism of NF-kappaB signaling pathway on renal tissue inflammation in chronic kidney disease and interventional effect of traditional Chinese medicine. Zhongguo Zhong Yao Za Zhi. 2013;38:4246–51.

Liu H, Xiong J, He T, Xiao T, Li Y, Yu Y, et al. High uric acid-induced epithelial-mesenchymal transition of renal tubular epithelial cells via the TLR4/NF-kB signaling pathway. Am J Nephrol. 2017;46:333–42.

Lorenzen JM, Haller H, Thum T. MicroRNAs as mediators and therapeutic targets in chronic kidney disease. Nat Rev Nephrol. 2011;7:286–94.

Marques FZ, Romaine SP, Denniff M, Eales J, Dormer J, Garrelds IM, et al. Signatures of miR-181a on renal transcriptome and blood pressure. Mol Med. 2015;

Moreth K, Frey H, Hubo M, Zeng-Brouwers J, Nastase MV, Hsieh LT, et al. Biglycan-triggered TLR-2- and TLR-4-signaling exacerbates the pathophysiology of ischemic acute kidney injury. Matrix Biol. 2014;35:143–51.

Munoz-Felix JM, Oujo B, Lopez-Novoa JM. The role of endoglin in kidney fibrosis. Expert Rev Mol Med. 2014;16:e18.

Na YJ, Sung JH, Lee SC, Lee YJ, Choi YJ, Park WY, et al. Comprehensive analysis of microRNA-mRNA co-expression in circadian rhythm. Exp Mol Med. 2009;41:638–47.

Narasimamurthy R, Hatori M, Nayak SK, Liu F, Panda S, Verma IM. Circadian clock protein cryptochrome regulates the expression of proinflammatory cytokines. Proc Natl Acad Sci U S A. 2012;109:12662–7.

Neal CS, Michael MZ, Pimlott LK, Yong TY, Li JY, Gleadle JM. Circulating microRNA expression is reduced in chronic kidney disease. Nephrol Dial Transplant. 2011;26:3794–802.

O'Hare AM, Choi AI, Bertenthal D, Bacchetti P, Garg AX, Kaufman JS, et al. Age affects outcomes in chronic kidney disease. J Am Soc Nephrol. 2007;18:2758–65.

Sampaio-Maia B, Simoes-Silva L, Pestana M, Araujo R, Soares-Silva IJ. The role of the gut microbiome on chronic kidney disease. Adv Appl Microbiol. 2016;96:65–94.

Su R, Lin HS, Zhang XH, Yin XL, Ning HM, Liu B, et al. MiR-181 family: regulators of myeloid differentiation and acute myeloid leukemia as well as potential therapeutic targets. Oncogene. 2015;34:3226–39.

Sun W, Min B, Du D, Yang F, Meng J, Wang W, et al. miR-181c protects CsA-induced renal damage and fibrosis through inhibiting EMT. FEBS Lett. 2017; 591:3588–99.

Uil M, Scantlebery AML, Butter LM, Larsen PWB, de Boer OJ, Leemans JC, et al. Combining streptozotocin and unilateral nephrectomy is an effective method for inducing experimental diabetic nephropathy in the 'resistant' C57Bl/6J mouse strain. Sci Rep. 2018;8:5542.

Wu C, Gong Y, Yuan J, Zhang W, Zhao G, Li H, et al. microRNA-181a represses ox-LDL-stimulated inflammatory response in dendritic cell by targeting c-Fos. J Lipid Res. 2012;53:2355–63.

Xu J, Li R, Workeneh B, Dong Y, Wang X, Hu Z. Transcription factor FoxO1, the dominant mediator of muscle wasting in chronic kidney disease, is inhibited by microRNA-486. Kidney Int. 2012;82:401–11.

Yang L, Chu Y, Wang L, Wang Y, Zhao X, He W, et al. Overexpression of CRY1 protects against the development of atherosclerosis via the TLR/NF-kappaB pathway. Int Immunopharmacol. 2015;28:525–30.

Zhang L, Li YJ, Wu XY, Hong Z, Wei WS. MicroRNA-181c negatively regulates the inflammatory response in oxygen-glucose-deprived microglia by targeting toll-like receptor 4. J Neurochem. 2015;132:713–23.

Zhao X, Zhou Y, Chen YU, Yu F. miR-494 inhibits ovarian cancer cell proliferation and promotes apoptosis by targeting FGFR2. Oncol Lett. 2016;11:4245–51.

Zhu HY, Liu MY, Hong Q, Zhang D, Geng WJ, Xie YS, et al. Role of microRNA-181a in the apoptosis of tubular epithelial cell induced by cisplatin. Chin Med J (Engl). 2012;125:523–6.

8

Myocyte-specific overexpressing HDAC4 promotes myocardial ischemia/reperfusion injury

Ling Zhang[2], Hao Wang[1], Yu Zhao[1], Jianguo Wang[1], Patrycja M. Dubielecka[2], Shougang Zhuang[2], Gangjian Qin[3], Y Eugene Chin[4], Race L. Kao[5] and Ting C. Zhao[1*]

Abstract

Background: Histone deacetylases (HDACs) play a critical role in modulating myocardial protection and cardiomyocyte survivals. However, Specific HDAC isoforms in mediating myocardial ischemia/reperfusion injury remain currently unknown.

We used cardiomyocyte-specific overexpression of active HDAC4 to determine the functional role of activated HDAC4 in regulating myocardial ischemia and reperfusion in isovolumetric perfused hearts.

Methods: In this study, we created myocyte-specific active HDAC4 transgenic mice to examine the functional role of active HDAC4 in mediating myocardial I/R injury. Ventricular function was determined in the isovolumetric heart, and infarct size was determined using tetrazolium chloride staining.

Results: Myocyte-specific overexpressing activated HDAC4 in mice promoted myocardial I/R injury, as indicated by the increases in infarct size and reduction of ventricular functional recovery following I/R injury. Notably, active HDAC4 overexpression led to an increase in LC-3 and active caspase 3 and decrease in SOD-1 in myocardium. Delivery of chemical HDAC inhibitor attenuated the detrimental effects of active HDAC4 on I/R injury, revealing the pivotal role of active HDAC4 in response to myocardial I/R injury.

Conclusions: Taken together, these findings are the first to define that activated HDAC4 as a crucial regulator for myocardial ischemia and reperfusion injury.

Keywords: Histone deacetylase4 (HDAC4) , Ischemia/reperfusion, Myocardial function

Background

Histone deacetylases (HDACs) are a group of enzymes that regulate gene expression by the modulation of their interactions with chromatin through the deacetylation of histones. The acetylation and deacetylation of chromatin histones are considered to be critical in the regulation of transcription in in the biological responses. Acetylation of histone is caused by histone acetyl transferase, which leads to nucleosomal relaxation and altered transcriptional activation. In contrast, histone deacetylase result in deacetylation and transcriptional repression (Turner 2000; McKinsey 2012).

Since the identification of HDAC 1 (Hassig et al. 1998), 18 HDACs have been identified and were classified into three distinct groups (Verdin et al. 2003). Class I HDACs consist of HDACs 1, 2, 3, and 8. Class II HDACs are further divided into the following: IIa (HDACs 4, 5, 7 and 9) and IIb (HDACs 6 and 10). It is notable that both HDAC 4 and HDAC 5 are highly expressed in the myocardium, brain and skeletal muscles, which indicates that both HDACs are important in modulating the biological function of these organs. (Fischle 1999; Grozinger et al. 1999; Wang et al. 1999). Class III HDACs were identified on the basis of sequence similarity with Sir, which includes SIRT1–7 and Sir2.

Recent studies have demonstrated that HDACs play an important role in the development of myocardial hypertrophy and ischemic injury (Antos et al. 2003; Kee et al.

---

* Correspondence: tzhao@bu.edu
[1]Department of Surgery, Boston University Medical School, Roger Williams Medical Center, 50 Maude Street, Providence, RI 02908, USA
Full list of author information is available at the end of the article

2006; Kong et al. 2006; Haberland et al. 2009; Granger et al. 2008). Inhibition of HDAC with chemical inhibitor trichostatin A attenuated cardiomyocyte hypertrophy. Likewise, pharmacological inhibition of HDACs suppressed myocardial hypertrophy and improved cardiac performance in vivo (Kong et al. 2006; Haberland et al. 2009). Furthermore, HDAC inhibition was found to be closely associated with the attenuation of myocardial ischemia and reperfusion injury in mice (Granger et al. 2008). More importantly, our extensive studies in animal models suggest that pharmacological inhibition of HDAC is considered to be one of the most important signals to reduce myocardial ischemia and reperfusion injury and improve cardiac performance (Zhao et al. 2007; Zhang et al. 2012a; Zhang et al. 2012b; Zhang et al. 2010). Additionally, we also demonstrated that HDAC inhibition or genetic inhibition of specific HDAC4 promoted myocardial repair through stimulating cardiac progenitor cells (Zhang et al. 2012a; Zhang et al. 2012b). Notably, we have found that HDAC inhibition increased the survival of embryonic stem cells through the reduction and degradation of HDAC4 isoform (Chen et al. 2011).

It is generally recognized that class II HDACs are critical to modulate cardiac injury, hypertrophy and development, but HDAC4 demonstrates very little activity. Most of the studies only focused on defining the function of the magnitude of HDAC expression rather than the activation of HDAC4, especially *activated* HDAC4, in modulating myocardial function. It is critical to identify the function of activated HDAC4 in the heart. These evidences indicate that HDAC4 is one of the most important class II HDACs in the heart and muscle and plays a critical role in modulating cardiac development, ischemic injury, and hypertrophy. In the present study, we created cardiac HDAC4 transgenic mice in which HDAC4 was activated to determine how active HDAC4 modulates myocardial injury. This will provide new insight into understanding the functional role of activated HDAC4 in heart disease.

Materials and methods
Generation of cardiac specific active HDAC4 mice
Creation of the mice carried out in Boston University transgenic core facility. A cDNA encoding an activated HDAC4 was cloned into an expression vector encoding alpha-myosine heavy chain (the α-MHC promoter, 5.4 kb), a cardiomyocyte-specific promoter at the multiple cloning site. After ligation, the construct was purified and verified by restriction enzyme digestion and sequencing. Transgenic mice were generated by microinjection of the α-MHC-HDAC4 DNA construct into fertilized FVB/n mouse eggs F_1 eggs. Founder mice and transgenic expression of HDAC4 were identified by

analysis of genomic DNA with primer A (5-CCTC GTTCCAGCTGTGGT-3); a sense primer specific to MHC promoter exon 2) and antisense primer B (5-AGCGCCAGGAGCTCCTGCTGC-3); specific to HDAC4 cDNA. The protocol for the animal experiments in this study was approved by IACUC, which is fully in agreement with the guidance for the Care and Use of Laboratory Animals published by the US National Institutes of Health.

Reagents and antibodies
Trichostatin A, 3-[4,5-dimethylthiazol-2-yl]-2,5- diphenyl-tetrazolium bromide (MTT) and 4,6-Diamidino-2-phenylindole (DAPI) were obtained from Life Technologies (Grand Island, NY). Primary antibodies including HDAC4 rabbit polyclonal and β-actin antibodies (Cell Signaling [Tm] (Beverly, MA), and primary active caspase 3 were purchased from Abcam (Cambridge, MA). SOD-1 and LC3 poly clonal primary antibodies was purchased from Santa Cruz biotechnology (Dallas, Texas). All chemicals for perfused hearts were purchased from Aldrich-Sigma (St. Louis, Missouri).

Langendorff isolated heart perfusion and functional measurement
The methodologies of Langendorff perfused system, ventricular function detection, and infarct size measurement has been described previously (Zhao et al. 2007). Briefly, adult male mice were anesthetized with a lethal intraperitoneal injection (i.p.) of sodium pentobarbital (120 mg/kg). The hearts were rapidly isolated and kept in ice-cold Krebs-Henseleit buffer. The isolated hearts were then cannulated through the ascending aorta in the isovolumetrically perfused system (Langendorff method) for retrograde perfusion using oxygenated Krebs-Henseleit buffer. They were then cannulated via the ascending aorta for retrograde perfusion by the Langendorff method using Krebs-Henseleit buffer containing 2.5 mmol/L of $CaCl_2 2H_2O$. During the course of the retrograde perfusion, Krebs-Henseleit buffer was continuously aerated with $95\%O_2{:}5\%CO_2$ to maintain the value of pH of Krebs-Henseleit buffer at 7.4. The Langendorff system was maintained at 37 °C, and the perfusion pressure was adjusted at a constant pressure of 55 mmHg. A water-filled latex balloon, attached to the tip of polyethylene tubing, was then inflated sufficiently to provide a left ventricular end-diastolic pressure (LVEDP) of about 10 mmHg. Left ventricular function was assessed by inserting a water-filled latex balloon into the left ventricle, which was connected to a pressure transducer and recorded through Power Lab recording system (ADInstruments, Bella Vista, AUSTRALIA). Ventricular functional parameters were measured, which include left ventricular end-diastolic pressure (LVEDP), left

ventricular systolic pressure (LVSP), left ventricular developed pressure (LVDP), rate pressure product (RPP), heart rate (HR), and coronary flow (CF).

Experimental protocol for myocardial I/R injury

Mice about 2 month old were randomized into four experimental groups that underwent the following treatments, as shown in the experimental protocol. *Control wild-type* and *α-MHC-HDAC4* mice were subjected to 30 min of stabilization and 30 min of ischemia followed by 30 min of reperfusion. To examine the contribution of HDAC4 to cardioprotection elicited by HDAC inhibition, we treated animals with HDAC inhibitor to determine whether HDAC inhibitor was able to attenuate the detrimental effects of HDAC4 over-expression in the heart. We utilized an established preconditioning protocol. Control wild-type and α-MHC-HDAC4 mice were treated (i.p. injection) with TSA 24 h before ischemia. Animals were divided into two additional groups: *TSA + Wild* type mice ($n = 5$), Wild type mice were injected with TSA (0.1 mg/kg ip); *TSA + α-MHC-HDAC4* mice (n = 5), α-MHC-HDAC4 mice were injected with TSA (0.1 mg/kg ip). Twenty-four hours later, the hearts were subjected to 30 min of ischemia followed by 30 min of reperfusion.

Measurement of myocardial infarction

Tetrazolium chloride (TTC) staining was employed to detect infarct size. After Langendorff perfusion, the hearts were then frozen in the refrigerator for a short period. Then, the frozen hearts were cut from apex to base into 1 mm thick slices. These slices were then placed in 10% TTC for 20 min. The cardiac sections were fixed in paraformaldehyde (4%) for photography. NIH ImageJ software was utilized to measure the area of viable and dead portion of tissues. The infarct size of each heart was determined and shown as the percentage of risk area, defined as the sum of total ventricular area minus cavities (Zhao et al. 2007).

Echocardiographic measurement of cardiac function

Cardiac functions of wild type and α-MHC-HDAC4 transgenic mice were assessed using echocardiographic measurements. Ventricular parameters include left ventricular internal dimension in end and systole (LVID;d and LVID;s); fractional shortening (FS) and ejection fraction (EF), which were described previously (Zhang et al. 2017).

Electrophoresis and western blot analysis

Protein extraction and western blot for analysis of protein expression were conducted as described as before (Zhao et al. 2007). In brief, myocardial tissues were isolated and then homogenized in cold lysis buffer containing protease inhibitor cocktails (Calbiochem, Billerica, MA). The protein lysates were subjected to centrifugation at 12,000 g at 4 °C for 15 min. The supernatant of these samples were then collected, and the protein concentration of the samples were determined using a Micro BCA Assay Kit (Thermo Scientific, Rockford, IL). The samples (50 μg/per lane) were loaded and run on SDS polyacrylamide gels at a constant voltage 100 V and transferred to polyvinylidene difluoride membrane at 24 V (PVDF). The PVDF was blocked in non-fat dry milk (5%) at room temperature for 1 h followed by incubation with individual primary antibodies, their respective polyclonal antibodies. Protein signals were then visualized by incubation with anti-rabbit horseradish peroxidase-conjugated secondary antibody and developed with ECL Chemiluminescence detection reagent (Amersham Pharmacia Biotech).

Immunohistochemistry

The cardiac tissues were fixed with buffered paraffin and then embedded samples were cut into 10 μm-thick sections. Tissue sections were de-paraffinized in xylene and then rehydrated at decreasing concentrations of ethanol, which was described in our previous protocol (Zhang et al. 2012a). Active caspase 3 was used to assess for apoptotic signals in the heart. LC-3 was used to determine the signal of autophagy in myocardium. Positive signals in term of active caspase 3 and LC-3 from cardiac sections were counted from 3 to 5 randomized fields. A detailed methodology of immunostaining for detection of active caspase-3 and LC3 was carried out as described in our previous protocol (Zhang et al. 2012a).

Measurement of HDAC activity

Measurement of cardiac HDAC activity was carried out by using by using a colorimetric HDAC activity assay kit (BioVision, Mountain View, CA).

Statistical analysis

All data, including ventricular function, infarct size, protein density, and immunostaining signals are expressed as mean ± SE. Differences among the groups were analyzed by one-way analysis of variance (ANOVA) followed by Bonferroni correction. Student's unpaired t test was conducted to compare the difference between groups. $p < 0.05$ was considered to be a significant difference between groups.

Results

Characterization of cardiac-specific HDAC4 mice

The HDAC4 proteins in the heart from MHC-HDAC4 levels were significantly higher than that of control wild type. In adult 2-month old mice, there was no differences in HDAC4 on other organs (Fig. 1a). The HDAC4 protein was increased in MHC-HDAC4 mice as compared to wild type (Fig. 1b). There is no difference in

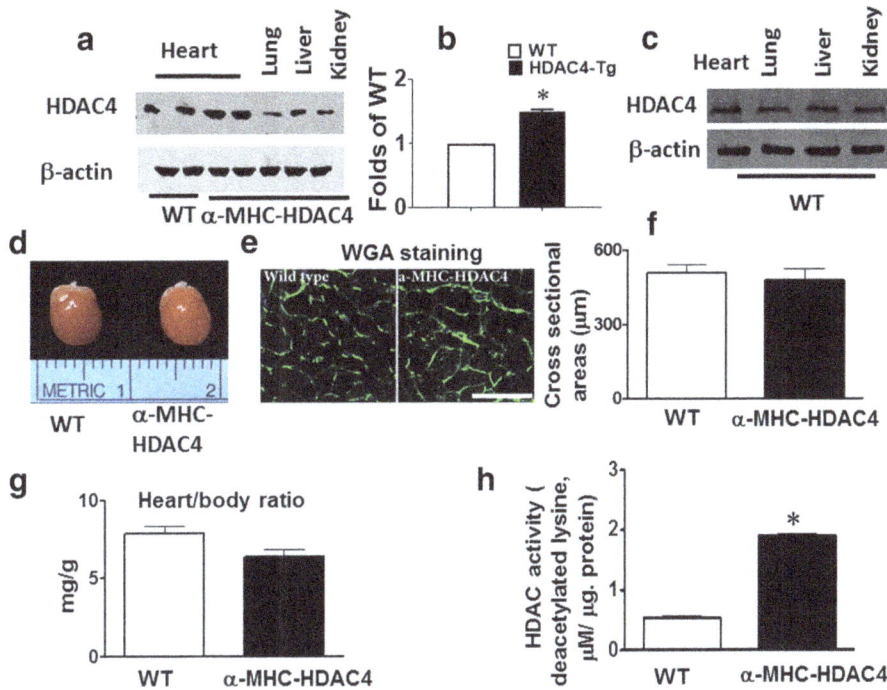

Fig. 1 Generation and characterization of cardiac myocyte-specific HDAC4 transgenic mice. **a** HDAC4 over-expression in α-MHC-HDAC4 mice and wild type mice; **b** Densitometric analysis of HDAC4 proteins from the heart; **c** HDAC4 proteins in heart and other organs in wild type mice (scale bar = 50 μm); **d** Isolated hearts from α-MHC-HDAC4 mice and wild type mice; **e** WGA staining of cardiomyocytes of α-MHC-HDAC4 mice and wild type mice; **f** Cardiomyocyte sizes in α-MHC-HDAC4 mice and wild type mice; **g** Heart/body weight ratio from α-MHC-HDAC4 mice and wild type mice; **h** HDAC activity measured from α-MHC-HDAC4 mice and wild type mice; values are present as Mean Values representing mean ± SE (n = 3–5/per group)

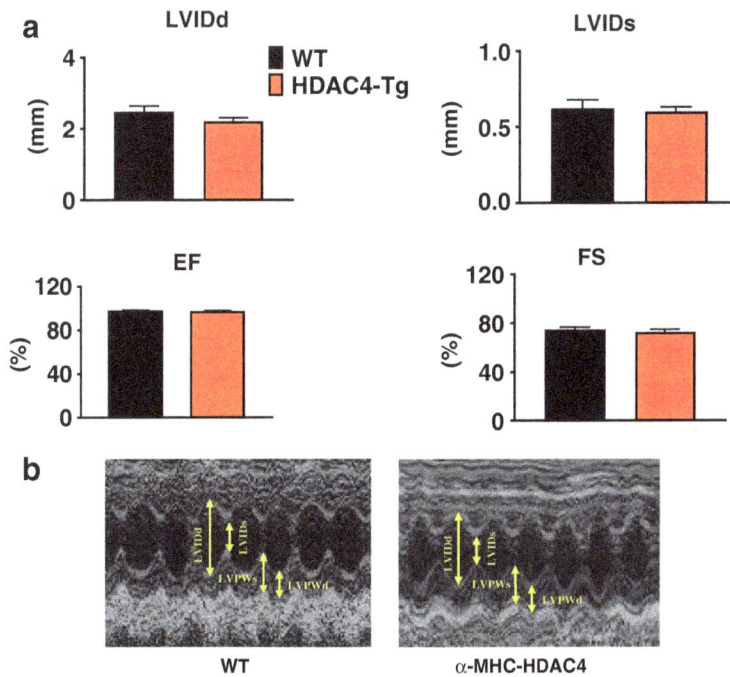

Fig. 2 Myocardial function of α-MHC-HDAC4 mice and wild type littermates. **a** Echocardiographic measurements of cardiac function from α-MHC-HDAC4 mice and wild type mice. Values represent mean ± SE (n = 5/per group). EF: Ejection fraction; FS: Fractional shortening; LVID: left ventricle internal diameter; **b** Representative image of M-Mode of echocardiographic measurements

HDAC4 proteins in the other organs wild type mice (Fig. 1c). There is no obvious abnormality except for heart size at whole organ level (Fig. 1d). There were no significant difference cardiomyocytes and the heart weight-body weight ratio between MHC-HDAC and wild-type mice at two-month-old age, which is consistent with the myocyte sizes detected by WGA (Fig. 1e–g). HDAC4 activity was also increased in MHC-HDAC4-Tg mice as compared to wild type mice (Fig. 1h). Echocardiographic measurements show no differences in cardiac function as indicated by LVIDs, LVIDd, EF, and FS at two-month of age between wild type and MHC-HDAC4 mice (Fig. 2).

Baseline ventricular functions prior to I/R
Baseline functional parameters, including left ventricular developed pressure (LVDP), LV-dP/dt max LV-dP/dt min, heart rate, and coronary effluent were recorded among control wild type and HDAC4 transgenic mice before subjection to I/R. The experimental protocol for I/R was shown in Fig. 3. As shown in Table 1, there were no significant differences among the groups before ischemia.

Infarct size
Myocardial infarct size, an index of irreversible myocardial injury, was measured. As shown in Fig. 4a, the infarct size following I/R in α-MHC-HDAC4 transgenic mice was ($43.6 \pm 0.6\%$) as compared with the wild type mice ($28.6 \pm 3.1\%$); the representative images are shown as Fig. 4b. This suggests that activation of HDAC4 increased infarct size in response to ischemia and reperfusion injury. However, following TSA treatment, the infarct size in α-MHC-HDAC4 transgenic mice group was reduced as compared to α-MHC-HDAC4 transgenic mice in absence of TSA treatment. The magnitude of infarct size in TSA-treated α-MHC-HDAC4 transgenic

mice is still larger than that of TSA-treated wild type mice. The data suggest that HDAC4 overexpression in the heart increased myocardial infarct size. It also indicates that the increase in the infarct size in α-MHC-HDAC4 transgenic mice was blocked by inhibition of HDAC4 activity.

Ventricular function recoveries following I/R
As shown in Fig. 5, left ventricular functional recovery declined dramatically as compared with baseline. However, as compared with the wild-type control, the post-ischemic LVEDP demonstrated a remarked elevation in MHC-HDAC4 mice ($p < 0.05$ vs Wild type), which was also accompanied with the reduction of RPP recovery MHC-HDAC4 at both 15 min (Fig. 5a) and 30 min (Fig. 5b) of reperfusion. The coronary effluent and heart rate demonstrated a slight decline as compared to pre-ischemic stage, but showed no difference following I/R between wild type and MHC-HDAC4 mice (Table 1).

We investigated whether, TSA, an HDAC inhibitor, could target HDAC4 to attenuate the depression of ventricular functional recoveries following I/R in MHC-HDAC4 mice. We delivered trichostatin A at a dose of 0.1 mg/kg, which has been shown to be protective in I/R injury, to both wild-type and MHC-HDAC4 mice. TSA treatment blocked the depression of the recovery of left ventricular functional recovery in MHC-HDAC4 mice (Fig. 5a and b). Thus, HDAC4 overexpression exacerbates myocardial I/R injury, and this process is attenuated by therapeutic delivery of chemical HDAC4 inhibitor.

Signaling mechanism of HDAC4 overexpression increased I/R injury
It was noticed that the HDAC inhibition-induced reduction in cell death was correlated with the suppression in autophagy (Cao et al. 2011). Autophagy was evaluated by western blot detection of the autophagosome associated lipidated

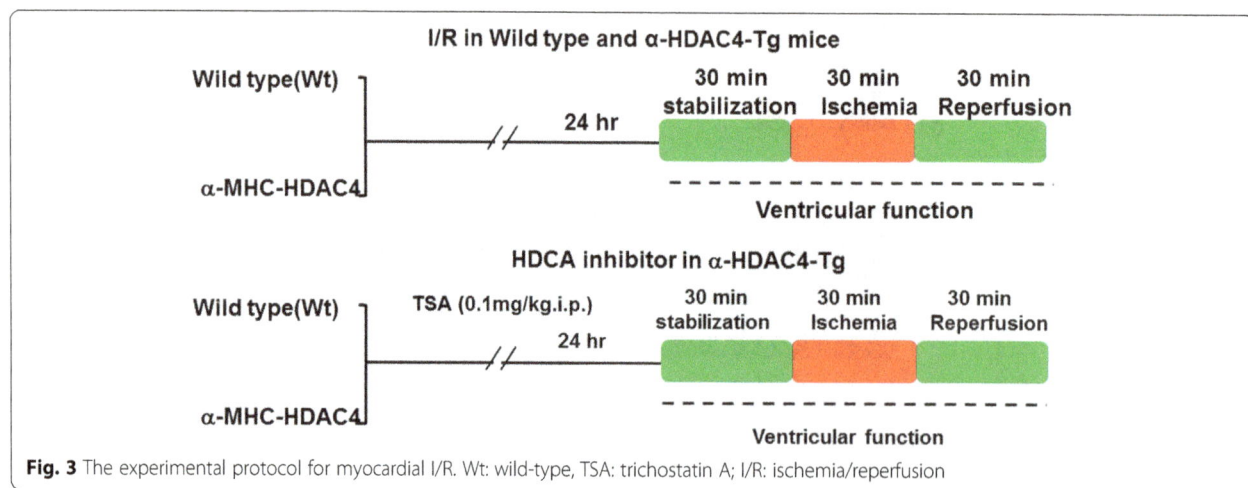

Fig. 3 The experimental protocol for myocardial I/R. Wt: wild-type, TSA: trichostatin A; I/R: ischemia/reperfusion

Table 1 Baseline ventricular function in Langendorff hearts

Groups	LVDP mmHg	LV-dP/dt max mmHg/s	LV-dP/dt min mmHg/s	CF ml/min	Heart rate bmp
WT	80 ± 10	2563 ± 337	2773 ± 437	3.6 ± 0.3	392 ± 38
MHC-HDAC4	106 ± 15	2757 ± 417	2843 ± 2521	2.8 ± 0.4	368 ± 28
TSA + WT	115 ± 6	3126 ± 168	3066 ± 82	3.8 ± 0.5	349 ± 29
TSA+ α-MHC-HDAC4	94 ± 8	3394 ± 258	3237 ± 180	3.6 ± 0.3	380 ± 34

LVDP Left ventricular develped pressure, *CF* coronary effluent, *TSA* trichostatin A
No significant differences were found between the experimental groups for any of the functional parameters (*n* = 4–5/per group)

isoform LC3 (LC3-II). The LC3-II level, relative to autophagy abundance, was detected in the ischemic heart of wild type mice, but overexpression of HDAC4 resulted in a significant increase in LC3-II in the heart (Fig. 6a and b), but this increased LC3-II was attenuated by treatment of TSA. Furthermore, activation of HDAC4 also increased active-caspase 3 and decreased SOD-1 signals (Fig. 6a and b). TSA treatment attenuated the effect of HDAC4 on active caspase 3 and SOD-1 levels in the heart. The immunostaining was also confirmed by an increase in caspase-3 positive nuclei in the HDAC4-Tg heart (Fig. 7a and b).

HDAC inhibition attenuated myocardial infarction in pig I/R model

As shown in Additional file 1: Figure S1a, there was no significant difference in the ratio of risk area/left

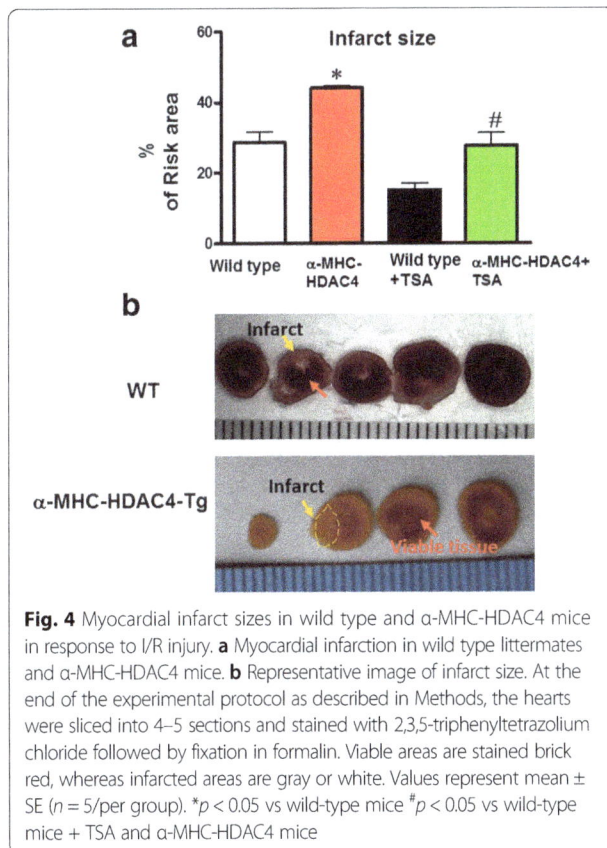

Fig. 4 Myocardial infarct sizes in wild type and α-MHC-HDAC4 mice in response to I/R injury. **a** Myocardial infarction in wild type littermates and α-MHC-HDAC4 mice. **b** Representative image of infarct size. At the end of the experimental protocol as described in Methods, the hearts were sliced into 4–5 sections and stained with 2,3,5-triphenyltetrazolium chloride followed by fixation in formalin. Viable areas are stained brick red, whereas infarcted areas are gray or white. Values represent mean ± SE (*n* = 5/per group). **p* < 0.05 vs wild-type mice *#p* < 0.05 vs wild-type mice + TSA and α-MHC-HDAC4 mice

ventricular area between control and TSA-treated groups. In contrast, as compared to the control group, TSA-treated group demonstrated a marked reduction in the ratio of infarct/risk area. Likewise, TSA treatment also manifested a significant reduction in infarct/left ventricular area. The representative histologic images are presented in Additional file 1: Figure S1b. The α-MHC-HDAC4 mice and wild type mice e results indicate that HDAC inhibition reduced myocardial infarction in the hearts exposed to I/R injury.

Discussion
Salient findings

In this study, we demonstrated that: 1) This is the first study to identify that overexpression of activated HDAC4, a major class II HDAC isoform in the heart exacerbates myocardial I/R injury, as indicated by the increase in infarct size and the reduction of myocardial function; 2) Over-expression of HDAC4-induced I/R injury was attenuated by delivery of HDAC inhibitor, TSA; 3) Furthermore, activated HDAC4 promoted I/R injury was associated with increased in autophagy, apoptosis and decreased SOD-1. These findings indicate that cardiac-specific activated HDAC4 reduces myocardial function and increases cardiac injury following I/R, which is associated with increased autophagy and apoptosis.

The roles of class II HDACs in cardiac development and hypertrophy were assessed in previous observations (Antos et al. 2003; Kee et al. 2006; Kong et al. 2006; Haberland et al. 2009; Granger et al. 2008). Class II HDAC4 only demonstrated a minimal enzymatic activity or lacked the activation in physiological condition. Importantly, cardiac injury or pathological stress resulted in enzymatic activation of HDAC4, suggesting that activated HDAC4 is more important for developing injury and serves as an effective target for potential therapy. In the present study, we created a cardiac-specific HDAC4 mouse model to provide the genetic and physiological evidence of HDAC4 in myocardial I/R. Our results indicated that specific activation of HDAC4 promotes myocardial injuries in the heart exposed to I/R, revealing that activated HDAC4 is crucial to modulate I/R injury. Previous reports indicated that the deletion of regular HDAC4 displayed premature ossification of developing

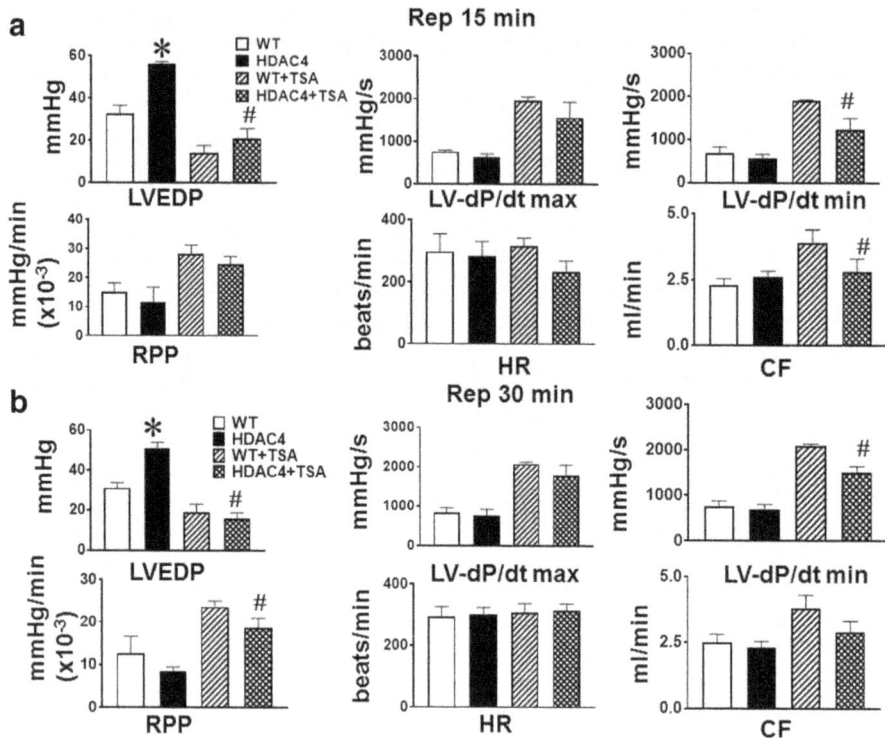

Fig. 5 Post-ischemic ventricular functional recovery following ischemia and reperfusion at the different times. **a** At 15 min of reperfusion; **b** At 30 min of reperfusion. Left ventricular (LV) function was assessed in isovolumetric hearts. The measured parameters include LV systolic pressure developed pressure (LVDP), LV-dP/dt max, LV-dP/dt min, heart rate (HR) and coronary effluents (CF). Values represent mean ± SE ($n = 4$–5/per group), $*p < 0.05$ vs wild type mice; $\#p < 0.05$ vs. α-MHC-HDAC4 mice

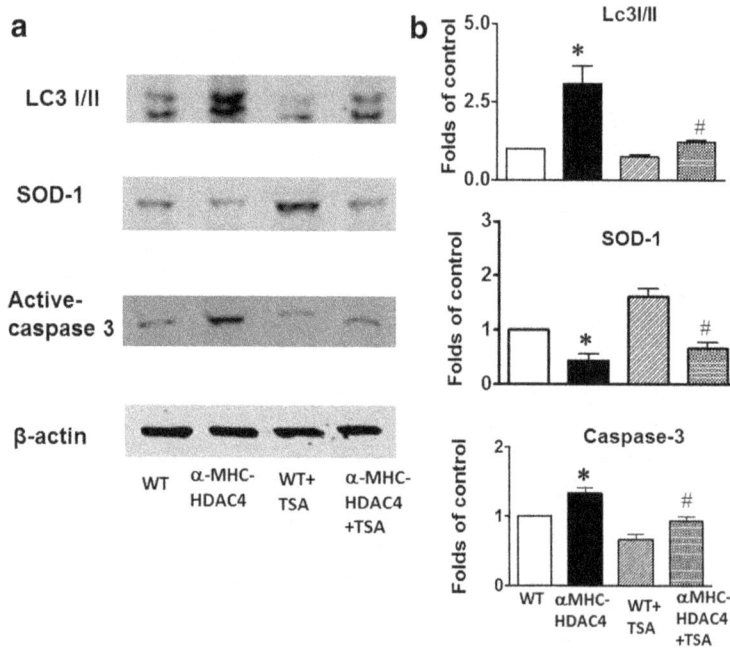

Fig. 6 Active HDAC4 increased active caspase 3 and autophagy and decreased SOD1. **a** Western blot showing increased active caspase-3, decreased SOD-1, and increased LC-3I/II in the heart from HDAC4 transgenic mice; **b** Densitometric analysis of each protein level relative to wild type ($n = 3$ per group); Values represent mean ± SE, $*p < 0.05$ vs WT; $\#p < 0.05$ vs WT + TSA. SOD: Superoxide dismutase; LC3: autophagosome associated lipidated isoform LC3

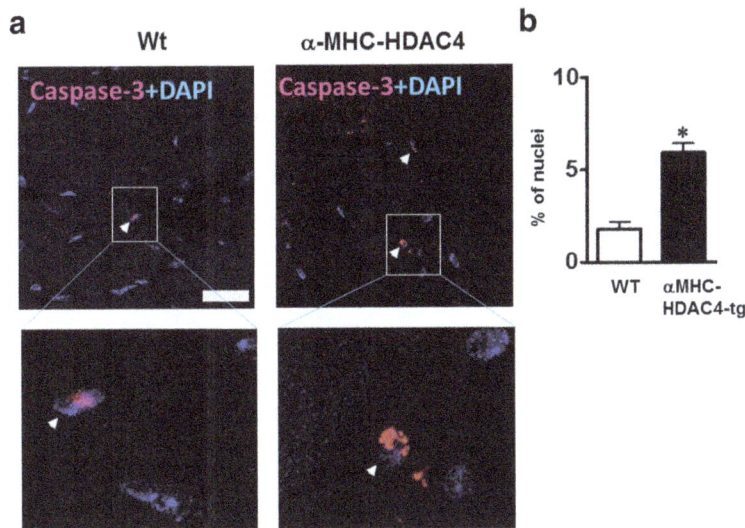

Fig. 7 Immunostaining detecting active caspase-3 in myocardium. **a** Immunostaining showing the increase of active caspase-3 positive signals in HDAC4-Tg mice vs wild type littermates. **b** Percentage of active caspase-3 positive nuclei in the myocardium following I/R. Values represent mean ± SE (n = 3 per group); Scale bar = 10μm

premature bone and early onset chondrocyte hypertrophy (Zhang et al. 2012c). In addition, over-expression of HDAC2 had augmented hypertrophy, but HDAC2 deficiency prevented attenuated cardiac hypertrophy (Trivedi et al. 2007). Likewise, transgenic mice with mutant HDAC4 displayed greater left ventricular hypertrophy and a larger cross-sectional area of LV myocytes (Ago et al. 2008). Even though all of these studies points out the importance of HDACs in contribution to cardiac failure and development. There is no information to define the role of activated HDAC4 in in mediating cardiac ischemia and reperfusion injury.

HDAC inhibitors were tested in many disease models to achieve their therapeutic effects by antagonize enzymatic activity of various HDACs. Our previous works and other observations have demonstrated that HDAC inhibitors elicited cardioprotective effects against myocardial ischemic injury (Zhao et al. 2007; Zhang et al. 2012a; Zhang et al. 2012b; Zhang et al. 2010; Chen et al. 2011). Although HDAC inhibitors were largely included to investigate the function of HDAC4 in various pathological models, however, non-specific effects of HDAC inhibitor demonstrated the limitation of assessing the role of specific HDAC isoforms. In our previous study, HDAC inhibitor (TSA) caused the degradation of HDAC4 in addition to the inhibition of HDAC activity. It is likely that the magnitude of HDAC4 content in HDAC4-Tg mice could be reduced due to the degradation of HDAC4. Therefore, we sought to include trichostatin A to see whether the physiological function of cardiac HDAC4 would be affected in response to ischemia and reperfusion injury. We also used the same dose

of TSA in wild type mice, which is consistent with our previous report showing that HDAC inhibitor demonstrated protective effects in wild type mice (Zhao et al. 2007). In this observation, delivery of HDAC inhibitor effectively blocked the deleterious effect of HDAC4 in I/R injury, revealing the importance of activated HDAC4 in contributing to I/R injury. This is supported by our previous studies in which cultured cardiomyocyte infected with HDAC4 increased hypoxic-induced cell damage, and trichostatin A antagonized the detrimental effect of HDAC4 in association with the reduction of HDAC4 (Du et al. 2015). Furthermore, HDAC4 was up-regulated in response to oxidant stress, and suppression of HDAC4 promoted embryonic stem cell-derived myogenesis and survival (Chen et al. 2011), implying that HDAC4 inhibition may function as a critical HDAC isoform attributable for the cardiac protective effect. More interestingly, we proceeded to define whether trichostatin A treatment could induce myocardial protection using a large animal model. Our results suggested that inhibition of HDAC protects the heart against ischemia/reperfusion injury in pig, as indicated by the reduction of myocardial infarct size. The finding provides a strong evidence demonstrating that HDAC inhibitor holds promise in developing a potential therapeutic strategy holding clinical implications in the future.

Signaling pathway involving activated HDAC4-induced I/R injury

It was noticed that the HDAC inhibition-induced reduction in cell death was correlated with the suppression in autophagy (Cao et al. 2011). This change in autophagic activity was thought to be linked with a variety of pathological conditions and recognized to be involved in ischemia and reperfusion injury. Interestingly, a previous report indicated that HDAC inhibition attenuated cardiac hypertrophy in association with the suppression of autophagy, establishing a correlation between HDAC and induction of autophagy in response to cardiac hypertrophy (Cao et al. 2011). In agreement with this observation, our finding indicates that overexpression of HDAC4 resulted in an increase in autophagy, which was also attenuated by TSA treatment. In addition, myocardial ischemia and reperfusion injury demonstrates an over-expression of HDAC4 in the heart caused by the reduction in anti-oxidant enzymes (SOD) and increase in apoptosis (Wang et al. 2017), which were prevented by TSA treatment. Our results indicate that the specific activation of HDAC4 promotes myocardial injuries in the heart exposed to I/R, which is associated with reduction of SOD-1 and increased apoptosis. It is also interesting to see the effects of TSA on other class II HDACs in HDAC4 overexpression mice in response to I/R injury in the future.

Conclusion

Our study provides direct evidence that active HDAC4 in the heart is crucial to promote myocardial I/R injury, and HDAC4-induced I/R injury can be attenuated by delivery of HDAC inhibitor. Furthermore, activated HDAC4-elicited cardiac injury was associated the increased autophagy, apoptosis and decreased SOD-1. Importantly, the studies provide new insight into understanding the molecular mechanism of active HDAC4 in I/R injury and hold promise in developing new therapeutic strategies to target active HDAC4.

Abbreviations
CF: Coronary effluents; EF: Ejection fraction; FS: Fractional shortening; HDAC4: Histone deacetylase 4; HR: Heart rate; I/R: Ischemia and reperfusion injury; LC3: Microtubule-associated protein light chain 3; LC3-II: Lapidated isoform of LC3, autophagy marker; LV: Left ventricular; LVDP: Left ventricular developed pressure; LVID: Left ventricle internal diameter; Rep: Reperfusion; SOD-1: Superoxide dismutase-1; TTC: Tetrazolium chloride; WGA: Wheat germ agglutinin

Acknowledgements
We thank the NIH for supporting the current study. We appreciate the editorial teams and reviewers for their constructive comments on this manuscript.

Funding
The work is supported by the National Heart, Lung, and Blood Institute Grants (R01 HL089405 and R01 HL115265).

Authors' contributions
LZ, JW, HW, RLK participated in data collection and image analysis; TCZ participated in manuscript preparation; YZ participated in preparation of Langendorff model; SZ, GQ, PMD participated in the experimental designs and helped to finalize the study. YEC and TCZ participated in interpretation of data. All authors read and approved the final manuscript.

Competing interests
The authors declare that they have no competing interests.

Author details
[1]Department of Surgery, Boston University Medical School, Roger Williams Medical Center, 50 Maude Street, Providence, RI 02908, USA. [2]Department of Emergency Medicine, Department of Medicine, Rhode Island Hospital, Brown University, Providence, RI, USA. [3]Feinberg Cardiovascular Research Institute, Northwestern University Feinberg School of Medicine, Chicago, USA. [4]Key Laboratory of Stem Cell Biology, Institutes of Health Sciences, Shanghai Institutes for Biological Sciences, Chinese Academy of Sciences, Shanghai, China. [5]Department of Surgery, East Tennessee State University, Johnson City, TN, USA.

References
Ago T, Liu T, Zhai P, Chen W, Li H, Molkentin JD, Vatner SF, Sadoshima J. A redox-dependent pathway for regulating class II HDACs and cardiac hypertrophy. Cell. 2008;133(6):978–93.

Antos CL, McKinsey TA, Dreitz M, Hollingsworth LM, Zhang CL, Schreiber K, Rindt H, Gorczynski RJ, Olson EN. Dose-dependent blockade to cardiomyocyte hypertrophy by histone deacetylase inhibitors. J Biol Chem. 2003;278:28930–7.

Cao DJ, Wang ZV, Battiprolu PK, Jiang N, Morales CR, Kong Y, Rothermel BA, Gillette TG, Hill JA. Histone deacetylase (HDAC) inhibitors attenuate cardiac hypertrophy by suppressing autophagy. Proc Natl Acad Sci U S A. 2011; 108(10):4123–8.

Chen HP, Denicola M, Qin X, Zhao Y, Zhang L, Long XL, Zhuang S, Liu PY, Zhao TC. HDAC inhibition promotes cardiogenesis and the survival of embryonic stem cells through proteasome-dependent pathway. J Cell Biochem. 2011; 112:3246–55.

Du J, Zhang L, Zhuang S, Qin GJ, Zhao TC. HDAC4 degradation mediates HDAC inhibition-induced protective effects against hypoxia/reoxygenation injury. J Cell Physiol. 2015;230(6):1321–31.

Fischle W. A new family of human histone deacetylases related to Saccharomyces cerevisiae HDA1p. J Biol Chem. 1999;274:11713–20.

Granger A, Abdullah I, Huebner F, Stout A, Wang T, Huebner T, Epstein JA, Gruber PJ. Histone deacetylase inhibition reduces myocardial ischemia-reperfusion injury in mice. FASEB J. 2008;22:3549–60.

Grozinger CM, Hassig CA, Schreiber SL. Three proteins define a class of human histone deacetylases related to yeast Hda1p. Proc Natl Acad Sci U S A. 1999; 96:4868–73.

Haberland M, Montgomery RL, Olson EN. The many roles of histone deacetylases in development and physiology: implications for disease and therapy. Nat Rev Genet. 2009;10:32–42.

Hassig CA, Tong JK, Fleischer TC, Owa T, Grable PG, Ayer DE, Schreiber SL. A role for histone deacetylase activity in HDAC1-mediated transcriptional repression. Proc Natl Acad Sci U S A. 1998;95:3519–24.

Kee HJ, Sohn IS, Kll N, Park JE, Qian YR, Yin Z, Ahn Y, Jeong MH, Bang YJ, Kim N, Kim JK, Kim KK, Epstein JA, Kook H. Inhibition of histone deacetylation blocks cardiac hypertrophy induced by angiotensin II infusion and aortic banding. Circulation. 2006;113:51–9.

Kong Y, Tannous P, Lu G, Berenji K, Rothermel BA, Olson EN, Hill JA. Suppression of class I and II histone deacetylases blunts pressure-overload cardiac hypertrophy. Circulation. 2006;113:2579–88.

McKinsey TA. Therapeutic potential for HDAC inhibitors in the heart. Annu Rev Pharmacol Toxicol. 2012;52:303–19.

Trivedi CM, Luo Y, Yin Z, Zhang M, Zhu W, Wang T, Floss T, Goettlicher M, Noppinger PR, Wurst W, Ferrari VA, Abrams CS, Gruber PJ, Epstein JA. Hdac2 regulates the cardiac hypertrophic response by modulating Gsk3 beta activity. Nat Med. 2007;13(3):324–31.

Turner BM. Histone acetylation and an epigenetic code. BioEssays. 2000;22:836–45.

Verdin E, Dequiedt F, Kasler HG. Class II histone deacetylases: versatile regulators. Trends Genet. 2003;19:286–93.

Wang AH, Bertos NR, Vezmar M, Pelletier N, Crosato M, Heng HH, Th'ng J, Han J, Yang XJ. HDAC4, a human histone deacetylase related to yeast HDA1, is a transcriptional corepressor. Mol Cell Biol. 1999;19:7816–27.

Wang H, Zhao YT, Zhang S, Dubielecka PM, Du J, Yano N, Chin YE, Zhuang S, Qin G, Zhao TC. Irisin plays a pivotal role to protect the heart against ischemia and reperfusion injury. J Cell Physiol. 2017;232(12):3775–85.

Zhang CL, McKinsey TA, Chang S, Antos CL, Hill JA, Olson EN. Class II histone deacetylases act as signal-responsive repressors of cardiac hypertrophy. Cell. 2012c;110(4):479–88.

Zhang L, Chen B, Zhao Y, Dubielecka PM, Wei L, Qin GJ, Chin YE, Wang Y, Zhao TC. Inhibition of histone deacetylase-induced myocardial repair is mediated by c-kit in infarcted hearts. J Biol Chem. 2012a;287:39338–48.

Zhang L, Du J, Yano N, Wang H, Zhao YT, Dubielecka PM, Zhuang S, Chin YE, Qin G, Zhao TC. Sodium butyrate protects -against high fat diet-induced cardiac dysfunction and metabolic disorders in type II diabetic mice. J Cell Biochem. 2017;118(8):2395–408.

Zhang L, Xin Q, Zhao Y, Fast L, Zhuang S, Liu P, Cheng G, Zhao TC. Inhibition of histone deacetylases preserves myocardial performance and prevents cardiac remodeling through stimulation of endogenous angiomyogenesis. J Pharmacol Exp Ther. 2012b;341:285–93.

Zhang LX, Zhao Y, Cheng G, Guo TL, Chin YE, Liu PY, Zhao TC. Targeted deletion of NF-kappaB p50 diminishes the cardioprotection of histone deacetylase inhibition. Am J Physiol Heart Circ Physiol. 2010;298:H2154–63.

Zhao TC, ChengG ZLX, Tseng YT, Padbury JF. Inhibition of histone deacetylases triggers pharmacologic preconditioning effects against myocardial ischemic injury. Cardiovasc Res. 2007;76:473–81.

9

Loss of Transient Receptor Potential Melastatin 3 ion channel function in natural killer cells from Chronic Fatigue Syndrome/ Myalgic Encephalomyelitis patients

Hélène Cabanas[1,2*] [iD], Katsuhiko Muraki[3], Natalie Eaton[1,2], Cassandra Balinas[1,2], Donald Staines[1,2] and Sonya Marshall-Gradisnik[1,2]

Abstract

Background: Chronic Fatigue Syndrome (CFS)/ Myalgic Encephalomyelitis (ME) is a debilitating disorder that is accompanied by reduced cytotoxic activity in natural killer (NK) cells. NK cells are an essential innate immune cell, responsible for recognising and inducing apoptosis of tumour and virus infected cells. Calcium is an essential component in mediating this cellular function. Transient Receptor Potential Melastatin 3 (TRPM3) cation channels have an important regulatory role in mediating calcium influx to help maintain cellular homeostasis. Several single nucleotide polymorphisms have been reported in *TRPM3* genes from isolated peripheral blood mononuclear cells, NK and B cells in patients with CFS/ME and have been proposed to correlate with illness presentation. Moreover, a significant reduction in both TRPM3 surface expression and intracellular calcium mobilisation in NK cells has been found in CFS/ME patients compared with healthy controls. Despite the functional importance of TRPM3, little is known about the ion channel function in NK cells and the epiphenomenon of CFS/ME. The objective of the present study was to characterise the TRPM3 ion channel function in NK cells from CFS/ME patients in comparison with healthy controls using whole cell patch-clamp techniques.

Methods: NK cells were isolated from 12 age- and sex-matched healthy controls and CFS patients. Whole cell electrophysiology recording has been used to assess TRPM3 ion channel activity after modulation with pregnenolone sulfate and ononetin.

Results: We report a significant reduction in amplitude of TRPM3 current after pregnenolone sulfate stimulation in isolated NK cells from CFS/ME patients compared with healthy controls. In addition, we found pregnenolone sulfate-evoked ionic currents through TRPM3 channels were significantly modulated by ononetin in isolated NK cells from healthy controls compared with CFS/ME patients.

Conclusions: TRPM3 activity is impaired in CFS/ME patients suggesting changes in intracellular Ca^{2+} concentration, which may impact NK cellular functions. This investigation further helps to understand the intracellular-mediated roles in NK cells and confirm the potential role of TRPM3 ion channels in the aetiology and pathomechanism of CFS/ME.

Keywords: Transient receptor potential Melastatin 3, Calcium, Chronic fatigue syndrome/Myalgic encephalomyelitis, Natural killer cells, Flow cytometry, Patch-clamp

* Correspondence: h.cabanas@griffith.edu.au
[1]School of Medical Science, Griffith University, Gold Coast, QLD, Australia
[2]The National Centre for Neuroimmunology and Emerging Diseases, Menzies Health Institute Queensland, Griffith University, Gold Coast, QLD, Australia
Full list of author information is available at the end of the article

Background

Chronic Fatigue Syndrome/ Myalgic Encephalomyelitis (CFS/ME) is a complex and debilitating disorder hallmarked by persistent or relapsing chronic fatigue that is inadequately alleviated by rest (Fukuda et al., 1994). At least four concurrent symptoms related to multiple systems including the immune, neurological, musculoskeletal, gastrointestinal, and cardiovascular systems accompany this unexplained fatigue (Carruthers et al., 2011). Without a pathology test, diagnosis is complex and relies on different case definitions that address the characteristics of CFS/ME (Carruthers et al., 2011; Jason et al., 2015). Although the Centers for Disease Control and Prevention (CDC) criteria are widely employed, this definition has been considered too broad in its symptom requirements (Johnston et al., 2013). Thus, the definition of CFS/ME was revised producing the Canadian Consensus Criteria (CCC) and finally in 2011 a more specific definition was established known as the International Consensus Criteria (ICC) to assist diagnosis (Carruthers et al., 2011). The underlying aetiology of CFS/ME remains unknown. However, a consistent feature of CFS/ME in the literature is immune dysfunction, and more precisely a significant reduction in Natural Killer (NK) cell cytotoxicity, a hallmark of NK cell function (Brenu et al., 2012; Brenu et al., 2011; Curriu et al., 2013; Hardcastle et al., 2015; Huth et al., 2016a; Klimas et al., 1990; Maher et al., 2005; Natelson et al., 2002; Nijs & Frémont, 2008; Sharpe et al., 1991; Siegel et al., 2006; Stanietsky & Mandelboim, 2010).

NK cells are effector lymphocytes of the innate immune system that eliminate pathogens and tumour cells, in addition to immune cell activation and cytokine production (Vivier et al., 2008). NK cells can be divided into five different phenotypes determined by their expression of cell-surface molecules including CD56 and CD16. The two main mature NK cell subtypes are CD56^{bright}CD16^{dim} and CD56^{dim}CD16^{bright}. CD56^{bright}CD16^{dim} NK cells exist as the minority in peripheral blood as efficient cytokine producers (Cooper et al., 2001). The CD56^{dim}CD16^{bright} subset constitutes 90% of human peripheral NK cells with significantly higher cytotoxic activity than CD56^{bright} NK cells as they contain an abundance of cytolytic proteins. Additionally, the presence of the low-affinity Fc-γ receptor CD16 facilitates the activation of antibody-dependent cellular cytotoxicity (ADCC) (Moretta, 2010; Stabile et al., 2015). Differences in NK cell phenotypes and significantly reduced peripheral NK cell numbers resulting in significant reduction in NK cell cytotoxicity, have been reported in CFS/ME and implicated in disease severity (Brenu et al., 2013; Hardcastle et al., 2015; Lanier, 2003; Maher et al., 2005; Nijs & Frémont, 2008). Importantly, NK cells require calcium (Ca^{2+}) to regulate cellular functions including NK cell cytotoxicity. Indeed, numerous steps including adhesion to the target cell, activation of surface receptors, microtubule reorganisation, polarisation of secretory granules and release of lytic proteins, including granzyme A and granzyme B, creation of the immune synapse, formation of perforin pores, and finally granzyme-induced target cell apoptosis require tight regulation of Ca^{2+} signalling (Anasetti et al., 1987; Henkart, 1985; Kass & Orrenius, 1999; Schwarz et al., 2013).

Transient Receptor Potential (TRP) ion channels can trigger specific Ca^{2+}-dependent signal transduction pathways regulating many biological processes in both excitable and nonexcitable cells (Gees et al., 2010). TRP channels represent a large and diverse family of nonselective cation channels that are widely expressed and respond to a wide range of chemical and physical stimuli (Voets et al., 2005). Moreover, genetic variations in TRP genes and noxious stimuli have been implicated in several pain-related pathological conditions/modalities, including inflammatory, neuropathic, visceral and dental pain, as well as pain associated with cancer (Mickle et al., 2016; Nilius, 2007). The mammalian TRP channels are divided into subgroups according to amino acid sequence similarities: TRPC (canonical), TRPM (melastatin), TRPV (vanilloid), TRPA (ankyrin), TRPML (mucolipin), and TRPP (polycystin) (Clapham et al., 2001). TRP cation channel subfamily M member 3 (TRPM3) is a Ca^{2+}-permeable nonselective cation channel, expressing a calmodulin binding region on the N-terminus which plays a role in activation of Ca^{2+} dependent signalling pathways (Holakovska et al., 2012; Lee et al., 2003; Oberwinkler & Philipp, 2014). The human *TRPM3* gene encodes for many different TRPM3 isoforms due to alternative splicing and exon usage, leading to channels with divergent pore and gating properties (Frühwald et al., 2012; Oberwinkler et al., 2005; Thiel et al., 2013). In particular, the TRPM3α2 isoform has been characterized as being highly permeable for Ca^{2+} and other divalent cations (Frühwald et al., 2012). TRPM3 ion channels are highly expressed in neurons of dorsal root ganglia, where they serve as thermosensitive channels implicated in the detection of noxious heat (Vriens et al., 2011). Furthermore, TRPM3 has been identified in a number of tissues and cell types, including pancreatic beta cells, brain, pituitary gland, eye, kidney, and adipose tissue, that serve many different functions (Hoffmann et al., 2010; Oberwinkler & Philipp, 2014; Wagner et al., 2008). While expressed ubiquitously in mammalian cells, the roles and functions of TRPM3 have yet to be determined in immune cells and more particularly in NK cells, where TRPM3 has been previously identified without electrophysiological evaluation (Nguyen et al., 2017; Nguyen et al., 2016).

TRPM3 ion channels are quickly (< 100 ms) and reversibly activated by a neuronal steroid, Pregnenolone sulfate (PregS) (Wagner et al., 2008). The precursor, pregnenolone is derived from cholesterol and sulphated in vivo for biological actions in the immune and central nervous systems. It is associated with memory and cognition, neuronal myelination, activation of neurotransmitter-gated channels, modulation of glutamate–nitric oxide–guanosine $3',5'$-(cyclic) phosphate pathways, maintenance of glucose and insulin homeostasis and the management of noxious stimuli (Harteneck, 2013; Nilius & Voets, 2008). Stimulation of TRPM3 with PregS in pancreatic beta-cells induces an intracellular signalling cascade, involving a rise in intracellular Ca^{2+} concentration ($[Ca^{2+}]_i$), activation of the protein kinases Raf and extracellular signal-regulated kinases (ERK), resulting in the regulation of different cellular processes and a change in gene expression pattern (Thiel et al., 2013). However, it is notable that concentrations of PregS were sometimes high (30–100 μM), causing non-specific effects without TRPM3. On the other hand, a natural compound, deoxybezoin ononetin, has been identified as a selective and potent blocker of PregS-induced TRPM3 currents in TRPM3-expressing dorsal root ganglia neurones and TRPM3 transfected HEK293 cells (Straub et al., 2013). Therefore, both use of TRPM3 agonist and blocker are critical to identify the activity of TRPM3 currents in native cells.

Regulation and importance of TRPM3 channels in NK cells and the epiphenomenon of CFS/ME is relatively unknown. Five single nucleotide polymorphisms (SNPs) (rs6560200, rs1106948, rs12350232, rs11142822, rs1891301) have been identified in *TRPM3* genes in CFS/ME patients (Marshall-Gradisnik et al., 2016). A recent investigation characterising TRPM3 related responses in NK cells and B lymphocytes found a significant reduction in expression of TRPM3 on the NK cell surface in CFS/ME patients compared with healthy controls (HC) (Nguyen et al., 2016). Moreover, isolated NK cells from CFS/ME patients have impaired TRPM3 activity following PregS stimulation, resulting in impaired Ca^{2+} mobilisation and reduced NK cell cytotoxicity (Nguyen et al., 2017). These results strongly suggest the importance of TRPM3 in the pathophysiology of CFS/ME. However, as the electrophysiological characterisation of endogenous TRPM3 channels on isolated NK cells is lacking, we aimed to characterise TRPM3 channel currents using whole cell patch-clamp measurements in HC and CFS/ME patients after modulation with PregS and ononetin. This novel approach may help to understand the clinical importance of TRPM3 in the pathomechanism of CFS/ME.

Methods

Participant recruitment
Six CFS/ME patients and six age- and sex-matched HC were recruited using the National Centre for Neuroimmunology and Emerging Diseases (NCNED) research database.

Participants were screened using a comprehensive questionnaire corresponding with the CDC, CCC and ICC case definitions. All six CFS/ME patients were defined by the CCC. HC reported no incidence of fatigue and were in good health without evidence of illness. Participants were excluded from this study if they reported history of smoking, autoimmune diseases, cardiac disease, diabetes or other co-morbidities.

Two of the six CFS/ME patients reported regular administration of non-steroidal anti-inflammatory for pain relief. No participants reported use of pharmacological agents that directly or indirectly influence TRPM3 or Ca^{2+} signalling.

This investigation was approved by the Griffith University Human Research Ethics Committee (HREC/15/QGC/63).

Peripheral blood mononuclear cell isolation and natural killer cell isolation
A total of 85 ml of whole blood was collected in ethylenediaminetetraacetic acid (EDTA) tubes between 8:00 am and 12:00 am. Routine full blood analysis was performed within 4h of collection for red blood cell count, white blood cell count and granulocyte cell count.

Peripheral blood mononuclear cells (PBMCs) were isolated from 80 ml of whole blood by centrifugation over a density gradient medium (Ficoll-Paque Premium; GE Healthcare, Uppsala, Sweden) as previously described (Brenu et al., 2011; Munoz & Leff, 2006). PBMCs were stained with trypan blue (Invitrogen, Carlsband, CA, USA) to determine cell count and cell viability. PBMCs were adjusted to a final concentration of 5×10^7 cells/ml for NK cell isolation.

NK cells were isolated by immunomagnetic selection using an EasySep Negative Human NK Cell Isolation Kit (Stem Cell Technologies, Vancouver, BC, Canada). NK Cell purification was determined using flow cytometry. NK cells were incubated for 20 min at room temperature in the presence of CD56 FITC (0.25 μg/5 μl) and CD3 PE Cy7 (0.25 μg/20 μl) monoclonal antibodies (BD Bioscience, San Jose, CA, USA) as previously described (Nguyen et al., 2017).

Whole cell electrophysiology recording
Borosilicate glass capillaries with an outside diameter of 1.5 mm and inside diameter of 0.86 mm (Harvard Apparatus, Holliston, MA, USA) were used as patch pipettes. Pipette resistance when filled with pipette solution was 8–12 MΩ. The pipettes were mounted on a CV203BU head-stage (Molecular Devices, Sunnyvale, CA, USA) connected to a 3-way coarse manipulator and a micro-manipulator (Narishige, Tokyo, Japan). Electrical signals were amplified and recorded using an Axopatch 200B amplifier and PClamp 10.7 software (Molecular Devices, Sunnyvale, CA, USA). Data were filtered at 5 kHz and

sampled digitally at 10 kHz via a Digidata 1440A analogue to digital converter (Molecular Devices, Sunnyvale, CA, USA). The voltage-ramp protocol was a step from a holding potential of + 10 mV to – 90 mV, followed by a 0.1 s ramp to + 110 mV, before returning to + 10 mV (repeated every 10 s). The liquid junction potential between the pipette and bath solutions (– 10 mV) was corrected. A leak current component was not subtracted from the recorded currents. Electrode was filled with the intracellular pipette solution containing 30 mM CsCl, 2 mM MgCl$_2$, 110 mM L-Aspartic acid, 1 mM EGTA, 10 mM HEPES, 4 mM ATP, 0.1 mM GTP, adjusted pH to 7.2 with CsOH and osmolality of 290 mOsm/L with D-mannitol. The pipette solution was filtered using a 0.22 μm membrane filter (Sigma-Aldrich, St. Louise, MO, USA), divided into aliquots and stored at – 20 °C. Bath solution contained: 130 mM NaCl, 10 mM CsCl, 1 mM MgCl$_2$, 1.5 mM CaCl$_2$2H$_2$O, 10 mM HEPES, adjusted pH to 7.4 with NaOH and osmolality 300 mOsm/L with D-glucose. All reagents were purchased from Sigma-Aldrich, except for ATP and GTP that were purchased from Sapphire Bioscience. TRPM3 currents were stimulated by adding 100 μM PregS (Tocris Bioscience, Bristol, UK) to the bath solution, whereas PregS-induced TRPM3 currents were blocked by adding 10 μM ononetin (Tocris Bioscience, Bristol, UK). All measurements were performed at room temperature. The authors removed the possibility of chloride current involvement in TRPM3 assessment by using L-Aspartic acid in the intracellular pipette solution. Unstable currents were also removed from the analysis. This ensured only TRPM3 function was assessed.

Statistical analysis

Cytometry data was exported from FacsDiva v8.1 and analysed using SPSS v24 (IBM Corp, Version 24, Armonk, NY, USA) and GraphPad Prism v7 (GraphPad Software Inc., Version 7, La Jolla, CA, USA). Electrophysiological data were analysed using pCLAMP 10.7 software (Molecular Devices, Sunnyvale, CA, USA). Origin 2018 (OriginLab Corporation, Northampton, MA, USA) and GraphPad Prism v7 (GraphPad Software Inc., Version 7, La Jolla, CA, USA) were used for statistical analysis and data presentation. The Shapiro-Wilk test was used to determine population normality. Statistical comparison was performed using the Mann-Whitney U test (Table 1, Fig. 1 and Fig. 3e), and Fishers exact test (Fig. 3g), to determine any significant differences. Significance was set at $p < 0.05$ and the data are presented as mean ± SEM unless otherwise stated.

Results

Participant characteristics and blood parameters

A total of twelve age- and sex-matched participants were included for this investigation. Demographic and clinical

Table 1 Blood parameters and patient demographic

	CFS/ME	HC	P Value
Age (years)	42.5 ± 6.05	42.8 ± 5.47	0.872
Gender n(%)			
Male	2 (20%)	2 (20%)	1.000
Female	4 (80%)	4 (80%)	
BMI (kg/m^2)	23.54 ± 0.54	23.35 ± 1.37	0.240
SF-36			
Fatigue (%)	30.42 ± 8.91	77.92 ± 6.25	*0.009*
General Health (%)	31.25 ± 5.97	74.31 ± 4.50	*0.004*
Physical Functioning (%)	70.83 ± 6.64	93.33 ± 4.77	*0.015*
Role Physical (%)	20.83 ± 9.64	87.50 ± 12.5	*0.009*
Role Emotional (%)	59.38 ± 9.24	96.88 ± 3.13	*0.004*
Social Functioning (%)	37.5 ± 5.59	95.83 ± 4.17	*0.002*
Body Pain (%)	49.17 ± 5.27	84.17 ± 8.41	*0.015*
Pathology			
White Cell Count (×10^9/L)	5.58 ± 0.30	7.13 ± 0.49	*0.03*
Lymphocytes (×10^9/L)	1.99 ± 0.2	1.75 ± 0.22	0.423
Neutrophils (× 10^9/L)	3.03 ± 0.23	4.78 ± 0.42	*0.01*
Monocytes (× 10^9/L)	0.41 ± 0.05	0.39 ± 0.06	0.748
Eosinophils (×10^9/L)	0.12 ± 0.02	0.18 ± 0.06	0.936
Basophils (× 10^9/L)	0.04 ± 0.01	0.04 ± 0.002	0.799
Platelet (× 10^9/L)	265.0 ± 23.36	266.17 ± 15.70	1.00
Red Cell Count (× 10^{12}/L)	4.63 ± 0.09	4.69 ± 0.13	0.63
Haematocrit	0.41 ± 0.01	0.42 ± 0.01	0.624
Haemoglobin (g/L)	135.0 ± 3.52	139.67 ± 5.21	0.687

SF-36 scores were analysed using participant questionnaire responses. Results from routine full blood analysis in CFS/ME patients and HC. Data presented as mean ± SD. *Abbreviations: CFS/ME, chronic fatigue syndrome/myalgic encephalomyelitis; HC, healthy controls; BMI, body mass index*

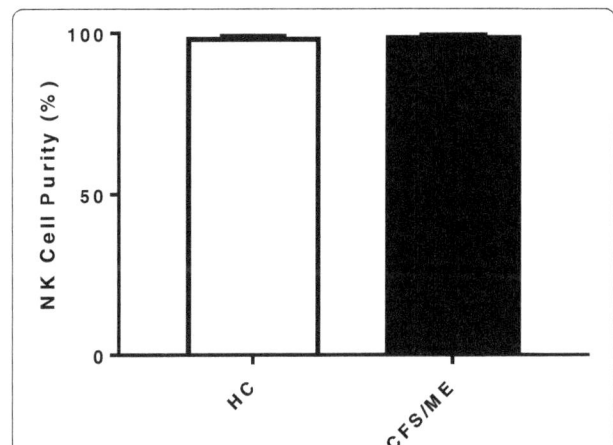

Fig. 1 Natural Killer cell purity. Bar graphs representing isolated NK cell purity for HC and CFS/ME patients. Data presented as mean ± SEM. HC = 98.07% ± 0.80 and CFS/ME = 98.28% ± 0.58. Abbreviations: CFS/ME, chronic fatigue syndrome/myalgic encephalomyelitis; HC, healthy controls; NK cell, natural killer cell

data for patients are summarised in Table 1. There was no significant difference in age or gender between patients and HC. The 36-Item Short Form Survey (SF-36) was used to determine participant health-related-quality of life. As expected, there was a significant difference in SF-36 scores between CFS/ME patients and HC. Moreover, while there was a significant difference in white cell count and neutrophils, all results remained within normal range for age and sex as provided by the Gold Coast University Hospital Pathology Unit, NATA accredited laboratory.

Natural killer cell purity

NK cell purity ($CD3^-/CD56^+$) was 98.07% ± 0.80 for HC and 98.28% ± 0.58 for CFS/ME patients (Fig. 1) as determined by flow cytometry. There was no significant difference in NK cell purity in CFS/ME patients compared with HC.

TRPM3 activity after Pregnenolone sulfate stimulation

A whole-cell patch-clamp technique was used to measure endogenous TRPM3 activity, enabling a small size of current recordings under voltage-clamp conditions and observation of the typical shape of the TRPM3 current–voltage relationship ($I–V$) (Fig. 2). We used 100 μM PregS to stimulate the channels as TRPM3 is minimally expressed in NK cells (Nguyen et al., 2017; Nguyen et al., 2016). As expected, the ionic current evoked by PregS was relatively small (Fig. 2a and e) in NK cells isolated from HC and we report a typical $I–V$ of TRPM3, which had a clear outward rectification (Fig. 2b). In contrast, the amplitude of ionic current after PregS stimulation was significantly smaller (Fig. 2c, d) in NK cells from CFS/ME patients than that from HC (Fig. 2e, $p < 0.0001$), suggesting impaired TRPM3 channel activity after PregS stimulation in CFS/ME patients.

TRPM3 activity after ononetin modulation

Ononetin effectively inhibits PregS-evoked Ca^{2+}-influx and ionic currents through TRPM3 channels (Straub et al., 2013). Therefore, to confirm that TRPM3 activity is involved in ionic currents evoked by PregS in NK cells, we next used 10 μM ononetin to modulate the channels (Fig. 3). As shown in Fig. 3a, the ionic currents evoked by PregS were effectively inhibited by simultaneous application of ononetin in isolated NK cells from HC. Moreover, the $I–V$ of ononetin sensitive currents was outwardly-rectified and typical for TRPM3 (Fig. 3b). In contrast, ionic currents in the presence of PregS were mostly resistant to ononetin in isolated NK cells from CFS/ME patients (Fig. 3c, d), in comparison with HC (Fig. 3e, f, g ($p = 0.0005$)), showing significant loss of the TRPM3 channel activity in CFS/ME patients.

Discussion

Our previous investigations have proposed that NK cells from CFS/ME patients have significantly reduced expression of TRPM3 and subsequent reduction in intracellular Ca^{2+} mobilisation compared with HC (Nguyen et al., 2017; Nguyen et al., 2016). This present study used electrophysiological methods to characterise endogenous TRPM3 activity in peripheral NK cells from HC and CFS/ME patients. We provide evidence suggesting PregS-dependent channel activity for TRPM3 is significantly lower in CFS/ME patients compared with HC. Moreover, ionic currents in CFS/ME patients were resistant to ononetin in the presence of PregS.

The patch clamp technique is regarded as a gold standard for ion channel research and offers direct insight into ion channel properties through the characterization of ion channel activity. In this study, we characterised, for the first time, the TRPM3 ion channel current in isolated human NK cells. We report a significant reduction amplitude of TRPM3 current after PregS stimulation in isolated NK cells from CFS/ME patients compared with HC. This is consistent with our previous findings showing significantly reduced TRPM3 expression as well as significantly reduced intracellular Ca^{2+} mobilisation in isolated NK cells from CFS/ME patients compared with HC (Nguyen et al., 2017; Nguyen et al., 2016). In addition, we found PregS-evoked ionic currents through TRPM3 channels were significantly modulated by ononetin in isolated NK cells from HC compared with CFS/ME patients. Indeed, isolated NK cells from CFS/ME were resistant to ononetin suggesting that PregS may activate non-TRPM3 cationic currents in CFS/ME patients. Alternatively, CFS/ME patients may express different spliced isoforms of TRPM3 that are non-sensitive to ononetin. Although we demonstrate TRPM3 channel activity dysfunction in CFS/ME patients, further investigations are required to elucidate the mechanisms involved in the impaired TRPM3 channel activity as well as the different TRPM3 isoform types that are expressed in NK cells.

Previous electrophysiological investigations have shown that TRPM3 forms an ion channel permeable to Ca^{2+}, sodium (Na^+), magnesium (Mg^{2+}), and manganese (Mn^{2+}) (Grimm et al., 2005; Oberwinkler et al., 2005). Ca^{2+} plays an important role in intracellular signalling pathways, cell differentiation and division, apoptosis, and transcriptional events. In non-excitable cells, such as immune cells, a main Ca^{2+} entry pathway is known as store-operated Ca^{2+} entry (SOCE) and some TRP ion channels are associated with this pathway. While the sub-family TRPC have been traditionally associated with this important cellular mechanism (Cheng et al., 2013; Ong et al., 2016; Salido et al., 2009), recent research has also identified TRPM3 as a component for SOCE in

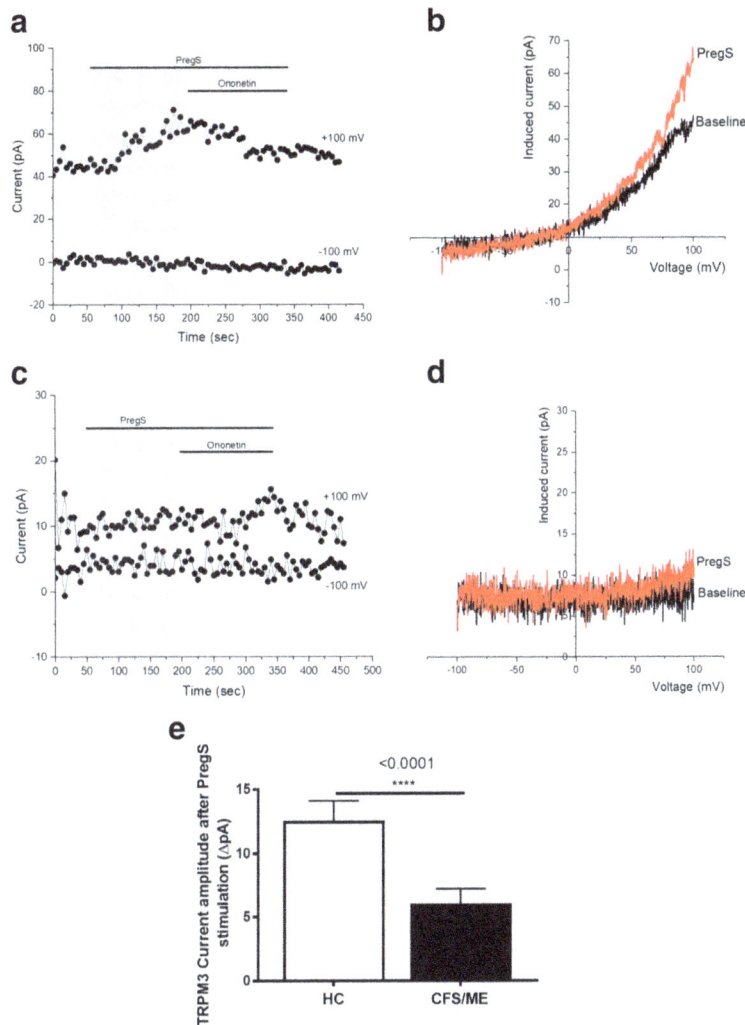

Fig. 2 TRPM3 activity after PregS stimulation. Data were obtained under whole-cell patch clamp conditions. **a** A representative time-series of current amplitude at + 100 mV and − 100 mV showing the effect of 100 μM PregS on ionic currents in isolated NK cells from HC. **b** I–V before and after PregS stimulation in a cell corresponding with (**a**). **c** A representative time-series of current amplitude at + 100 mV and − 100 mV showing the effect of 100 μM PregS on ionic currents in isolated NK cells from CFS/ME patients. **d.** I–V before and after PregS stimulation in a cell as shown in (**c**). **e** Bar graphs representing TRPM3 current amplitude at + 100 mV after stimulation with 100 μM PregS in CFS/ME patients ($N = 6$; $n = 33$) compared with HC (N = 6; $n = 29$). Data are represented as mean ± SEM. Abbreviations: CFS/ME, chronic fatigue syndrome/myalgic encephalomyelitis; HC, healthy control; NK, natural killer

white matter of the central nervous system (CNS) (Papanikolaou et al., 2017). Upon TRPM3 channel activation, changes in $[Ca^{2+}]_i$ occur, resulting in the regulation of many biological processes that correspond to an array of cells expressing this channel. TRPM3 is located and linked to vascular smooth muscle contraction, modulation of glucose-induced insulin release from pancreatic islets, detection of noxious heat in dorsal root ganglia and development of epithelial cells of the choroid plexus, as well as function of oligodendrocytes and neurons (Hoffmann et al., 2010; Oberwinkler et al., 2005; Vriens et al., 2011; Wagner et al., 2008). Therefore, dysregulation of TRPM3 family, affecting SOCE and more generally, Ca^{2+} signalling has significant implications for cell regulatory machinery.

Significant reduction in NK cell cytotoxicity is a consistent feature reported in CFS/ME patients (Brenu et al., 2012; Brenu et al., 2011; Curriu et al., 2013; Hardcastle et al., 2015; Huth et al., 2016a; Klimas et al., 1990; Maher et al., 2005; Natelson et al., 2002; Nijs & Frémont, 2008; Sharpe et al., 1991; Siegel et al., 2006; Stanietsky & Mandelboim, 2010). NK cell cytotoxic activity is a Ca^{2+} dependent process, which drives the intracellular microtubule reorganisation, polarisation of cytoplasmic granules, release of lytic proteins and the creation of the immune synapse (Anasetti et al., 1987; Henkart, 1985). Moreover, Ca^{2+}-dependent cytotoxic processes allow for the production and recruitment of lytic proteins (Voskoboinik et al., 2015). Following cytotoxic granule

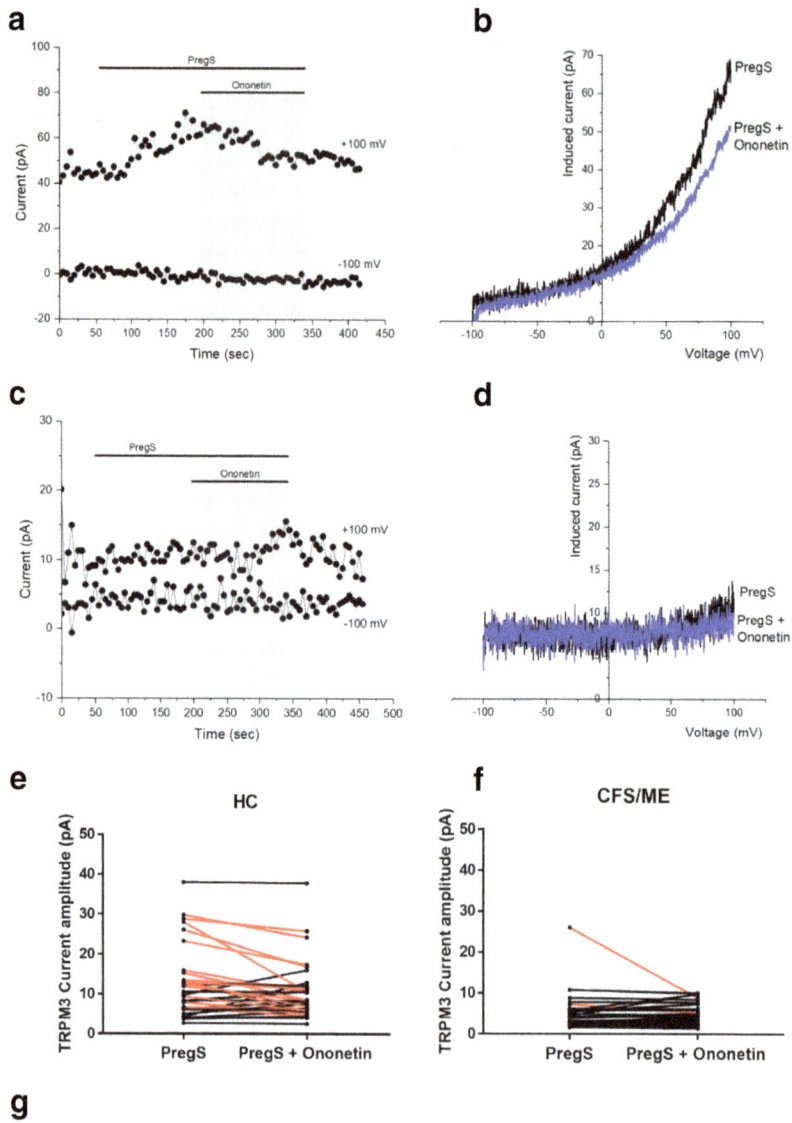

a

b

c

d

e HC

f CFS/ME

g

Data analysed	Sensitive	Insensitive	Total	P Value
HC	16	17	33	
CFS/ME	2	26	28	
Total	18	43	61	0.0005

Percentage of row total	Sensitive	Insensitive
HC	48.48%	51.52%
CFS/ME	7.14%	92.86%

Fig. 3 (See legend on next page.)

Fig. 3 TRPM3 activity after ononetin modulation. Data were obtained under whole-cell patch clamp conditions. **a.** A representative time-series of current amplitude at + 100 mV and − 100 mV showing the effect of 10 μM ononetin on ionic currents in the presence of PregS in isolated NK cells from HC. **b** *I–V* before and after application of ononetin in a cell as shown in (**a.**). **c** A representative time-series of current amplitude at + 100 mV and − 100 mV showing the effect of 10 μM ononetin on ionic currents in the presence of PregS in isolated NK cells CFS/ME patients. **d.** *I–V* before and after application of ononetin in a cell as shown in (**c.**). **e. f** Scatter plots representing change of each current amplitude before and after ononetin application in all NK cells from HC and CFS/ME patients. Each cell represented as red lines had reduction in currents by ononetin. **g** Table summarizing data for sensitive and insensitive cells to 10 μM ononetin in HC (N = 6; n = 33) compared to CFS/ME patients (N = 6; *n* = 28). Data are analysed with Fisher's exact test. Abbreviations: CFS/ME, chronic fatigue syndrome/myalgic encephalomyelitis; HC, healthy controls

delivery to the immune synapse, the formation of perforin pores and granzyme-induced cell apoptosis are highly dependent on Ca^{2+} (Orrenius et al., 2003; Voskoboinik et al., 2005). Previous studies have reported impaired Ca^{2+} signalling in NK cells from CFS/ME patients demonstrated through changes to ERK1/2 and mitogen-activated protein kinase (MAPK) pathways (Chacko et al., 2016; Huth et al., 2016b). CFS/ME patients have significantly decreased ERK1/2 following incubation with K562 cells (Huth et al., 2016b). ERK1/2 is activated in a Phosphatidylinositol-4,5-bisphosphate 3-kinase ($P1_3K$)-dependent manner that may also be associated with cytoplasmic Ca^{2+} ion levels through activation of TRPM3 (Lee et al., 2003). In the absence of phosphatidylinositol 4,5-biphosphate (PIP_2), TRPM3 is not activated, resulting in reduced cytosolic Ca^{2+} (Tóth et al., 2015). Previous research completed by Nguyen and colleagues reported that the expression of TRPM3 ion channel and $[Ca^{2+}]_i$ were significantly reduced in NK cells from CFS/ME patients (Nguyen et al., 2017). In addition, ERK1/2 requires Ca^{2+} as the final activator to initiate NK cell lysis (Huth et al., 2016b). Changes in Ca^{2+} signalling may impair cytokine production, including Interferon (IFN)-γ and Tumor Necrosis Factor (TNF), therefore interfering with systemic inflammation and anti-tumour responses (Romee et al., 2013). Previous investigations have reported both an increased and decreased inflammatory profile of CFS/ME patients along with reduced IFN-γ (Klimas et al., 1990; Lorusso et al., 2009). TRPM3-related Ca^{2+} dysfunction may then result in a reduction of $[Ca^{2+}]_i$, which may lower the function and cytotoxic capacity of the NK cells in CFS/ME patients.

Importantly, TRPM3 ion channels have a role in the detection of heat and in pain transmission in the CNS (Held et al., 2015). TRPM3 has been previously identified as a nociceptor channel involved in acute heat sensing and inflammatory heat hyperalgesia, and thus as a potential target for analgesic treatments (Vriens et al., 2011). Dysregulation of thermoregulatory responses has been reported in CFS/ME patients (Wyller et al., 2007). Generalised pain is a characteristic of CFS/ME and occurs in the absence of overt tissue damage, and this is suggestive of potential CNS impairments (Barnden et al., 2015; Barnden et al., 2016; Shan et al., 2016; Shan et al.,

2017). Our present findings suggest TRPM3 ion channels may be involved in the pathomechansim of CFS/ME and hence have a possible role in nociception and thermoregulation.

While this study provides evidence of TRPM3 channel activity dysfunction in CFS/ME patients, this study is not without limitations with the low sample numbers. Indeed, these findings need to be validated in a larger cohort of patients. Additionally, the use of high and single doses of PregS and Ononetin may reduce the drugs specificity and selectivity and consequently modulate other non-TRPM3 cationic currents. Further investigations are also required to assess the impact of PregS and Ononetin on the different TRPM3 isoforms. This could explain the differences observed between HC and CFS/ME patients as well as within groups. Finally, TRPM4, TRPM5, TRPM2 and TRPM7 surface expression has been reported on B cells, bone marrow cells, splenic cells, lymph node B cells and T and mast cells (Zierler et al., 2017), suggesting our recent findings may also be pertinent to other TRPM channel functions and Ca^{2+} – mediated roles, such as SOCE.

Conclusions
We have demonstrated impaired TRPM3 activity in CFS/ME patients through electrophysiological investigations in NK cells after modulation with PregS and ononetin. As TRPM3 is widely distributed in the body, particularly brain, eye, cardiovascular system, gastrointestinal system and pancreas, we assert that widespread changes in TRPM3 function in key body systems may contribute to CFS/ME. We suggest changes to Ca^{2+} ion concentration in the cytosol and intracellular stores result from changes in TRPM3 function, which may impact NK cellular functions. Therefore, Ca^{2+} signalling pathways could be an alternative therapeutic target in CFS/ME because of their importance in various cellular processes. This investigation confirms the potential role of TRPM3 ion channels in the aetiology and pathomechanism of CFS/ME, and could suggest potential therapeutic targets and/or prognostic markers.

Abbreviations

$[Ca^{2+}]_i$: Intracellular Ca^{2+} concentration; ADCC: Antibody-dependent cellular cytotoxicity; BMI: Body Mass Index; Ca^{2+}: Calcium; CCC: Canadian Consensus Criteria; CDC: Centers for Disease Control and Prevention; CFS/ME: Chronic Fatigue Syndrome/Myalgic Encephalomyelitis; CNS: Central nervous system; EDTA: Ethylendiaminetetraacetic acid; ERK: Extracellular signal-regulated kinases; HC: Healthy controls; ICC: International Consensus Criteria; IFN: Interferon; MAPK: Mitogen-activated protein kinase; Mg^{2+}: Magnesium; Mn^{2+}: Manganese; Na^+: Sodium; NCNED: National Centre for Neuroimmunology and Emerging Diseases; NK: Natural killer; PBMCs: Peripheral blood mononuclear cells; PI_3K: Phosphatidylinositol-4, 5-bisphosphate 3-kinase; PIP_2: Phosphatidylinositol 4,5-bisphosphate; PregS: Pregnenolone sulfate; SF-36: 36-Item Short Form Survey; SNPs: Single nucleotide polymorphisms; SOCE: Store-operated Ca^{2+} entry; TNF: Tumour necrosis factor; TRP: Transient Receptor Potential; TRPA: Transient Receptor Potential Ankyrin; TRPC: Transient Receptor Potential Canonical; TRPM: Transient Receptor Potential Melastatin; TRPML: Transient Receptor Potential Mucolipin; TRPP: Transient Receptor Potential POlycystin; TRPV: Transient Receptor Potential Vanilloid

Funding

This study was supported by the Mason Foundation, McCusker Charitable Foundation, Stafford Fox Medical Research Foundation, Mr. Douglas Stutt, Alison Hunter Memorial Foundation, Buxton Foundation, Blake Beckett Trust, Henty Donation, and the Change for ME Charity.

Authors' contributions

HC, KM, SM-G and DS designed the study and wrote the manuscript with contributions from other authors. HC, NE and CB performed experiments. HC and KM performed data analysis. All authors read and approved the final manuscript.

Competing interests

The authors declare that they have no competing interest.

Author details

[1]School of Medical Science, Griffith University, Gold Coast, QLD, Australia.
[2]The National Centre for Neuroimmunology and Emerging Diseases, Menzies Health Institute Queensland, Griffith University, Gold Coast, QLD, Australia.
[3]Laboratory of Cellular Pharmacology, School of Pharmacy, Aichi-Gakuin University, Chikusa, Nagoya, Japan.

References

Anasetti C, Martin PJ, June CH, Hellstrom KE, Ledbetter JA, Rabinovitch PS, et al. Induction of calcium flux and enhancement of cytolytic activity in natural killer cells by cross-linking of the sheep erythrocyte binding protein (CD2) and the fc-receptor (CD16). J Immunol. 1987;139:1772–9.

Barnden LR, Crouch B, Kwiatek R, Burnet R, Del Fante P. Evidence in chronic fatigue syndrome for severity-dependent upregulation of prefrontal myelination that is independent of anxiety and depression. NMR Biomed. 2015;28:404–13.

Barnden LR, Kwiatek R, Crouch B, Burnet R, Del Fante P. Autonomic correlations with MRI are abnormal in the brainstem vasomotor Centre in chronic fatigue syndrome. Neuroimage Clin. 2016;11:530–7.

Brenu EW, Hardcastle SL, Atkinson GM, van Driel ML, Kreijkamp-Kaspers S, Ashton KJ, et al. Natural killer cells in patients with severe chronic fatigue syndrome. Auto Immun Highlights. 2013;4:69–80.

Brenu EW, van Driel ML, Staines DR, Ashton KJ, Hardcastle SL, Keane J, et al. Longitudinal investigation of natural killer cells and cytokines in chronic fatigue syndrome/myalgic encephalomyelitis. J Transl Med. 2012;10:88.

Brenu EW, van Driel ML, Staines DR, Ashton KJ, Ramos SB, Keane J, et al. Immunological abnormalities as potential biomarkers in chronic fatigue syndrome/Myalgic encephalomyelitis. J Transl Med. 2011;9;81.

Carruthers BM, van de Sande MI, De Meirleir KL, Klimas NG, Broderick G, Mitchell T, et al. Myalgic encephalomyelitis: international consensus criteria. J Intern Med. 2011;270:327–38.

Chacko A, Staines DR, Johnston SC, Marshall-Gradisnik SM. Dysregulation of protein kinase gene expression in NK cells from chronic fatigue syndrome/ Myalgic encephalomyelitis patients. Gene Regul Syst Bio. 2016;10:85–93.

Cheng KT, Ong HL, Liu X, Ambudkar IS. Contribution and regulation of TRPC channels in store-operated Ca2+ entry. Curr Top Membr. 2013;71:149–79.

Clapham DE, Runnels LW, Strübing C. The TRP ion channel family. Nat Rev Neurosci. 2001;2:387–96.

Cooper MA, Fehniger TA, Caligiuri MA. The biology of human natural killer-cell subsets. Trends Immunol. 2001;22:633–40.

Curriu M, Carrillo J, Massanella M, Rigau J, Alegre J, Puig J, et al. Screening NK-, B- and T-cell phenotype and function in patients suffering from Chronic Fatigue Syndrome. J Transl Med. 2013;11:68.

Frühwald J, Camacho Londoño J, Dembla S, Mannebach S, Lis A, Drews A, et al. Alternative splicing of a protein domain indispensable for function of transient receptor potential melastatin 3 (TRPM3) ion channels. J Biol Chem. 2012;287:36663–72.

Fukuda K, Straus SE, Hickie I, Sharpe MC, Dobbins JG, Komaroff A. The chronic fatigue syndrome: a comprehensive approach to its definition and study. International chronic fatigue syndrome study group. Ann Intern Med. 1994;121:953–9.

Gees M, Colsoul B, Nilius B. The Role of Transient Receptor Potential Cation Channels in Ca2+ Signaling. Cold Spring Harb Perspect Biol. 2010 [cited 2018 May 3];2. Available from: https://www.ncbi.nlm.nih.gov/pmc/articles/ PMC2944357/

Grimm C, Kraft R, Schultz G, Harteneck C. Activation of the melastatin-related cation channel TRPM3 by D-erythro-sphingosine [corrected]. Mol Pharmacol. 2005;67:798–805.

Hardcastle SL, Brenu EW, Johnston S, Nguyen T, Huth T, Wong N, et al. Characterisation of cell functions and receptors in Chronic Fatigue Syndrome/ Myalgic Encephalomyelitis (CFS/ME). BMC Immunol. 2015 [cited 2018 May 3];16. Available from: https://www.ncbi.nlm.nih.gov/pmc/articles/PMC4450981/

Harteneck C. Pregnenolone sulfate: from steroid metabolite to TRP channel ligand. Molecules. 2013;18:12012–28.

Held K, Voets T, Vriens J. TRPM3 in temperature sensing and beyond. Temperature (Austin). 2015;2:201–13.

Henkart PA. Mechanism of lymphocyte-mediated cytotoxicity. Annu Rev Immunol. 1985;3:31–58.

Hoffmann A, Grimm C, Kraft R, Goldbaum O, Wrede A, Nolte C, et al. TRPM3 is expressed in sphingosine-responsive myelinating oligodendrocytes. J Neurochem. 2010;114:654–65.

Holakovska B, Grycova L, Jirku M, Sulc M, Bumba L, Teisinger J. Calmodulin and S100A1 protein interact with N terminus of TRPM3 channel. J Biol Chem. 2012;287:16645–55.

Huth TK, Brenu EW, Ramos S, Nguyen T, Broadley S, Staines D, et al. Pilot study of natural killer cells in chronic fatigue syndrome/Myalgic encephalomyelitis and multiple sclerosis. Scand J Immunol. 2016a;83:44–51.

Huth TK, Staines D, Marshall-Gradisnik S. ERK1/2, MEK1/2 and p38 downstream signalling molecules impaired in CD56dimCD16+ and CD56brightCD16dim/ − natural killer cells in Chronic Fatigue Syndrome/Myalgic Encephalomyelitis patients. J Transl Med. 2016b [cited 2018 May 10];14. Available from: https:// www.ncbi.nlm.nih.gov/pmc/articles/PMC4839077/

Jason LA, Kot B, Sunnquist M, Brown A, Evans M, Jantke R, et al. Chronic fatigue syndrome and Myalgic encephalomyelitis: toward an empirical case definition. Health Psychol Behav Med. 2015;3:82–93.

Johnston S, Brenu EW, Staines D, Marshall-Gradisnik S. The prevalence of chronic fatigue syndrome/ myalgic encephalomyelitis: a meta-analysis. Clin Epidemiol. 2013;5:105–10.

Kass GE, Orrenius S. Calcium signaling and cytotoxicity. Environ Health Perspect. 1999;107:25–35.

Klimas NG, Salvato FR, Morgan R, Fletcher MA. Immunologic abnormalities in chronic fatigue syndrome. J Clin Microbiol. 1990;28:1403–10.

Lanier LL. Natural killer cell receptor signaling. Curr Opin Immunol. 2003;15:308–14.

Lee N, Chen J, Sun L, Wu S, Gray KR, Rich A, et al. Expression and characterization of human transient receptor potential melastatin 3 (hTRPM3). J Biol Chem. 2003;278:20890–7.

Lorusso L, Mikhaylova SV, Capelli E, Ferrari D, Ngonga GK, Ricevuti G. Immunological aspects of chronic fatigue syndrome. Autoimmun Rev. 2009; 8:287–91.

Maher KJ, Klimas NG, Fletcher MA. Chronic fatigue syndrome is associated with diminished intracellular perforin. Clin Exp Immunol. 2005;142:505–11.

Marshall-Gradisnik S, Huth T, Chacko A, Johnston S, Smith P, Staines D. Natural killer cells and single nucleotide polymorphisms of specific ion channels and receptor genes in myalgic encephalomyelitis/chronic fatigue syndrome. Appl Clin Genet. 2016;9:39–47.

Mickle AD, Shepherd AJ, Mohapatra DP. Nociceptive TRP Channels: Sensory Detectors and Transducers in Multiple Pain Pathologies. Pharmaceuticals (Basel). 2016 [cited 2018 May 16];9. Available from: https://www.ncbi.nlm.nih.gov/pmc/articles/PMC5198047/

Moretta L. Dissecting CD56dim human NK cells. Blood. 2010;116:3689–91.

Munoz NM, Leff AR. Highly purified selective isolation of eosinophils from human peripheral blood by negative immunomagnetic selection. Nat Protoc. 2006;1: 2613–20.

Natelson BH, Haghighi MH, Ponzio NM. Evidence for the presence of immune dysfunction in chronic fatigue syndrome. Clin Diagn Lab Immunol. 2002;9:747–52.

Nguyen T, Johnston S, Clarke L, Smith P, Staines D, Marshall-Gradisnik S. Impaired calcium mobilization in natural killer cells from chronic fatigue syndrome/ myalgic encephalomyelitis patients is associated with transient receptor potential melastatin 3 ion channels. Clin Exp Immunol. 2017;187:284–93.

Nguyen T, Staines D, Nilius B, Smith P, Marshall-Gradisnik S. Novel identification and characterisation of transient receptor potential melastatin 3 ion channels on natural killer cells and B lymphocytes: effects on cell signalling in chronic fatigue syndrome/Myalgic encephalomyelitis patients. Biol Res. 2016;49:27.

Nijs J, Frémont M. Intracellular immune dysfunction in myalgic encephalomyelitis/chronic fatigue syndrome: state of the art and therapeutic implications. Expert Opin Ther Targets. 2008;12:281–9.

Nilius B. TRP channels in disease. Biochim Biophys Acta. 2007;1772:805–12.

Nilius B, Voets T. A TRP channel-steroid marriage. Nat Cell Biol. 2008;10:1383–4.

Oberwinkler J, Lis A, Giehl KM, Flockerzi V, Philipp SE. Alternative splicing switches the divalent cation selectivity of TRPM3 channels. J Biol Chem. 2005;280: 22540–8.

Oberwinkler J, Philipp SE. TRPM3. Handb Exp Pharmacol. 2014;222:427–59.

Ong HL, de Souza LB, Ambudkar IS. Role of TRPC channels in store-operated calcium entry. Adv Exp Med Biol. 2016;898:87–109.

Orrenius S, Zhivotovsky B, Nicotera P. Regulation of cell death: the calcium-apoptosis link. Nat Rev Mol Cell Biol. 2003;4:552–65.

Papanikolaou M, Lewis A, Butt AM. Store-operated calcium entry is essential for glial calcium signalling in CNS white matter. Brain Struct Funct. 2017;222: 2993–3005.

Romee R, Foley B, Lenvik T, Wang Y, Zhang B, Ankarlo D, et al. NK cell CD16 surface expression and function is regulated by a disintegrin and metalloprotease-17 (ADAM17). Blood. 2013;121:3599–608.

Salido GM, Sage SO, Rosado JA. TRPC channels and store-operated ca(2+) entry. Biochim Biophys Acta. 2009;1793:223–30.

Schwarz EC, Qu B, Hoth M. Calcium, cancer and killing: the role of calcium in killing cancer cells by cytotoxic T lymphocytes and natural killer cells. Biochim Biophys Acta. 2013;1833:1603–11.

Shan ZY, Kwiatek R, Burnet R, Del Fante P, Staines DR, Marshall-Gradisnik SM, et al. Progressive brain changes in patients with chronic fatigue syndrome: a longitudinal MRI study. J Magn Reson Imaging. 2016;44:1301–11.

Shan ZY, Kwiatek R, Burnet R, Del Fante P, Staines DR, Marshall-Gradisnik SM, et al. Medial prefrontal cortex deficits correlate with unrefreshing sleep in patients with chronic fatigue syndrome. NMR Biomed. 2017;30

Sharpe MC, Archard LC, Banatvala JE, Borysiewicz LK, Clare AW, David A, et al. A report--chronic fatigue syndrome: guidelines for research. J R Soc Med. 1991; 84:118–21.

Siegel SD, Antoni MH, Fletcher MA, Maher K, Segota MC, Klimas N. Impaired natural immunity, cognitive dysfunction, and physical symptoms in patients with chronic fatigue syndrome: preliminary evidence for a subgroup? J Psychosom Res. 2006;60:559–66.

Stabile H, Nisti P, Morrone S, Pagliara D, Bertaina A, Locatelli F, et al. Multifunctional human CD56 low CD16 low natural killer cells are the prominent subset in bone marrow of both healthy pediatric donors and leukemic patients. Haematologica. 2015;100:489–98.

Stanietsky N, Mandelboim O. Paired NK cell receptors controlling NK cytotoxicity. FEBS Lett. 2010;584:4895–900.

Straub I, Mohr F, Stab J, Konrad M, Philipp S, Oberwinkler J, et al. Citrus fruit and fabacea secondary metabolites potently and selectively block TRPM3. Br J Pharmacol. 2013;168:1835–50.

Thiel G, Müller I, Rössler OG. Signal transduction via TRPM3 channels in pancreatic β-cells. J Mol Endocrinol. 2013;50:R75–83.

Tóth BI, Oberwinkler J, Voets T. Phosphoinositide regulation of TRPM channels – TRPM3 joins the club! Channels (Austin). 2015;10:83–5.

Vivier E, Tomasello E, Baratin M, Walzer T, Ugolini S. Functions of natural killer cells. Nat Immunol. 2008;9:503–10.

Voets T, Talavera K, Owsianik G, Nilius B. Sensing with TRP channels. Nat Chem Biol. 2005;1:85–92.

Voskoboinik I, Thia M-C, Fletcher J, Ciccone A, Browne K, Smyth MJ, et al. Calcium-dependent plasma membrane binding and cell lysis by perforin are mediated through its C2 domain: a critical role for aspartate residues 429, 435, 483, and 485 but not 491. J Biol Chem. 2005;280:8426–34.

Voskoboinik I, Whisstock JC, Trapani JA. Perforin and granzymes: function, dysfunction and human pathology. Nat Rev Immunol. 2015;15:388–400.

Vriens J, Owsianik G, Hofmann T, Philipp SE, Stab J, Chen X, et al. TRPM3 is a nociceptor channel involved in the detection of noxious heat. Neuron. 2011; 70:482–94.

Wagner TFJ, Loch S, Lambert S, Straub I, Mannebach S, Mathar I, et al. Transient receptor potential M3 channels are ionotropic steroid receptors in pancreatic beta cells. Nat Cell Biol. 2008;10:1421–30.

Wyller VB, Godang K, Mørkrid L, Saul JP, Thaulow E, Walløe L. Abnormal thermoregulatory responses in adolescents with chronic fatigue syndrome: relation to clinical symptoms. Pediatrics. 2007;120:e129–37.

Zierler S, Hampe S, Nadolni W. TRPM channels as potential therapeutic targets against pro-inflammatory diseases. Cell Calcium. 2017;67:105–15.

10

B-1a cells protect mice from sepsis-induced acute lung injury

Monowar Aziz[1][*] [iD], Yasumasa Ode[1], Mian Zhou[1], Mahendar Ochani[1], Nichol E. Holodick[2,4], Thomas L. Rothstein[2,4] and Ping Wang[1,3]

Abstract

Background: Sepsis morbidity and mortality are aggravated by acute lung injury (ALI) or acute respiratory distress syndrome (ARDS). Mouse B-1a cells are a phenotypically and functionally unique sub-population of B cells, providing immediate protection against infection by releasing natural antibodies and immunomodulatory molecules. We hypothesize that B-1a cells ameliorate sepsis-induced ALI.

Methods: Sepsis was induced in C57BL/6 mice by cecal ligation and puncture (CLP). PBS or B-1a cells were adoptively transferred into the septic mice intraperitoneally. After 20 h of CLP, lungs were harvested and assessed by PCR and ELISA for pro-inflammatory cytokines (IL-6, IL-1β) and chemokine (MIP-2) expression, by histology for injury, by TUNEL and cleaved caspase-3 for apoptosis, and by myeloperoxidase (MPO) assay for neutrophil infiltration.

Results: We found that septic mice adoptively transferred with B-1a cells significantly decreased the mRNA and protein levels of IL-6, IL-1β and MIP-2 in the lungs compared to PBS-treated mice. Mice treated with B-1a cells showed dramatic improvement in lung injury compared to PBS-treated mice after sepsis. We found apoptosis in the lungs was significantly inhibited in B-1a cell injected mice compared to PBS-treated mice after sepsis. B-1a cell treatment significantly down-regulated MPO levels in the lungs compared to PBS-treated mice in sepsis. The protective outcomes of B-1a cells in ALI was further confirmed by using B-1a cell deficient CD19$^{-/-}$ mice, which showed significant increase in the lung injury scores following sepsis as compared to WT mice.

Conclusions: Our results demonstrate a novel therapeutic potential of B-1a cells to treat sepsis-induced ALI.

Keywords: B-1a cells, Sepsis, Acute lung injury, Inflammation, Neutrophils, IL-10

Background

Based on the Third International Consensus Definitions for Sepsis and Septic Shock (Sepsis-3), sepsis is defined as "life-threatening organ dysfunction caused by a dys-regulated host response to infection" (Singer et al. 2016). In the United States, there are approximately 1 million cases of sepsis annually, with a mortality rate up to 40% (Vincent et al. 2014; Martin et al. 2006; Aziz et al. 2013). The lungs are particularly susceptible to injury during sepsis, and more than 50% of patients with sepsis develop acute lung injury (ALI) or acute respiratory distress syndrome (ARDS) (Sevransky et al. 2009; Gu et al.

2014). The pathophysiology of sepsis-induced ALI is less well understood. Antibiotics and supportive measures are the only treatments available for patients with sepsis and ALI, and these measures have limited impact on the high mortality rates of sepsis.

Immune cells recognize pathogen-associated molecular patterns (PAMPs) via their toll-like receptors (TLRs) to exaggerate "cytokine storm", which trigger inflammation and impair tissue function during sepsis (Aziz et al. 2013; Barton and Medzhitov 2003; Foster and Medzhitov 2009). Neutrophil infiltration in lungs is a major pathophysiological hallmark of ALI. Uncontrolled migration of neutrophils into lungs leads to exaggerated production of cytokines, chemokines, myeloperoxidase (MPO), reactive oxygen species (ROS), nitric oxide (NO), and neutrophil extracellular traps (NETs) causing

* Correspondence: maziz1@northwell.edu
[1]Center for Immunology and Inflammation, The Feinstein Institute for Medical Research, 350 Community Dr, Manhasset, NY 11030, USA
Full list of author information is available at the end of the article

unrestrained inflammation, lung dysfunction and death (Aziz et al. 2013; Grommes and Soehnlein 2011; Abraham 2003; Lee and Downey 2001; Brinkmann et al. 2004; Kaplan and Radic 2012; Delgado-Rizo et al. 2017). Thus, regulating the exaggerated function of neutrophils and their uncontrolled infiltration into lungs serves as an effective therapeutic tool in ALI. The early onset of pro-inflammatory cytokine storm, often contributing to the lung injury in sepsis, can be reversed by the actions of anti-inflammatory cytokines such as interleukin (IL)-10 (Cinel and Opal 2009; Kono et al. 2006). We recently demonstrated the beneficial role of IL-10 producing B-1a cells in sepsis by controlling the systemic levels of pro-inflammatory cytokines, chemokines and bacterial loads (Aziz et al. 2017), while their role in ALI remained unknown. Elucidation of the novel role of B-1a cells in lungs during sepsis will not only improve our understanding of ALI pathophysiology, but also help us to develop effective therapeutics against ALI.

In mouse, B cells consist of various subpopulations, which include follicular (FO), marginal zone (MZ) and B-1 B cells (Aziz et al. 2015). The role of FO and MZ B cells collectively known as B-2 cells in the early immune response and inflammatory cytokine production during sepsis has been demonstrated previously (Kelly-Scumpia et al. 2011; Honda et al. 2016). B-1 cells comprising a minor portion of the total B cells in mice display unique features in terms of their phenotype, localization, development, signaling and function (Aziz et al. 2015; Martin and Kearney 2001; Kantor et al. 1992). The surface phenotype of murine B-1 cells is $B220^{lo}$, IgM^{hi}, IgD^{lo}, $CD23^-$, $CD19^{hi}$ and $CD43^+$ (Aziz et al. 2017; Aziz et al. 2015; Kantor et al. 1992). B-1 cells can be further divided into B-1a and B-1b cells, depending on their surface expression of CD5 (Kantor et al. 1992; Berland and Wortis 2002). B-1a cells are predominantly localized in the peritoneal cavity; however, a small portion of B-1a cells can also be found in the respiratory tract, intestinal tissues, lymph nodes, spleen and bone marrow (Aziz et al. 2015; Yenson and Baumgarth 2014). B1a cells can secrete large amounts of natural IgM and IgA that are capable of recognition and clearance of invading pathogens (Aziz et al. 2015; Grönwall et al. 2012; Vas et al. 2012). Natural antibodies have antigen specificity for a number of microbial epitopes such as phospholipids and lipopolysaccharides (LPS) (Grönwall et al. 2012; Vas et al. 2012). Murine B-1a cells are known to produce ample amount of IL-10 and granulocyte macrophage colony stimulating factor (GM-CSF), which attenuate excessive inflammation during sepsis (Aziz et al. 2017; Aziz et al. 2015; Rauch et al. 2012).

Recent findings demonstrate an active role of B-1a cells for protection against lung infection caused by influenza virus (Baumgarth et al. 1999; Baumgarth et al. 2000; Choi and Baumgarth 2008). During influenza virus infection B-1a cells migrate from serosal cavities to the lungs, where they secrete natural Abs and other immunomodulatory molecules to protect rodents against influenza virus infection (Baumgarth et al. 2000; Choi and Baumgarth 2008). Consistently, in various animal models of ALI initiated by direct instillation of LPS, *E. coli* or *S. pneumoniae*, B-1a cells were shown to migrate from the pleural cavity to the lung parenchymal tissues, where they secrete GM-CSF and IgM to protect rodents against ALI (Weber et al. 2014). A recent study has demonstrated that due to the loss of function of natural IgM as secreted from the B-1a cells could be the cause of poor prognostic outcomes of lung infection in aged animals (Holodick et al. 2016). The beneficial role of B-1a cells in lungs was shown in virus and bacterial infections, as well as in young over old mice with *S. pneumoniae* infection, indicating that these cells play a pivotal role in lung diseases. Nonetheless, their role in sepsis-induced ALI remains unknown.

In the current study, we aimed to study the role of B-1a cells in ALI during sepsis. Our study for the first time revealed the protective role of B-1a cells against sepsis-induced ALI by controlling exaggerated inflammation and infiltration of neutrophils in lungs. Thus, B-1a cells could represent a promising therapeutic in sepsis-induced ALI.

Methods
Animals
Wild-type (WT) C57BL/6 mice obtained from Taconic (Albany, NY) and B6.129P2(C)CD19$^{tm1(cre)cgn}$/J (CD19$^{-/-}$) mice obtained from The Jackson Laboratory were housed in a temperature and light controlled room and fed a standard laboratory diet. For all experiments male 8- to 10-week-old 21–28 g of body weight (BW) mice were used. Animals were randomly assigned to sham, vehicle control and B-1a cell treatment groups. Number of animals estimated in each group was based on our previous study on an animal model of sepsis (Aziz et al. 2017). All animal protocols were approved by our Institutional Animal Care and Use Committee.

Murine model of polymicrobial sepsis
Mice were anesthetized with 2% isofluorane inhalation and underwent cecal ligation and puncture (CLP). A 2-cm incision was made to the abdominal wall, and the cecum was exposed and ligated 0.5 cm from the tip with 4–0 silk suture. A 22-gauge needle was used to make one puncture through and through to the distal cecum, extruding a small amount of fecal contents. The cecum was replaced into the abdominal cavity, and the exposed abdominal wall was closed in two layers with running 4–0 silk suture. In sham-operated mice only laparotomy

was performed, but their cecum was not ligated and punctured. Animals were resuscitated with 1 ml of normal saline subcutaneously. In another experiment, WT and CD19$^{-/-}$ mice were subjected to either sham or CLP operation following the above CLP protocol.

Adoptive transfer of murine B-1a cells

Murine B-1a cells in peritoneal washouts were stained with FITC-B220 (clone RA3-6B2), Pacific Blue-CD23 (clone B3B4), and PE-Cy5-CD5 (clone 53-7.3) obtained from BD Biosciences (San Diego, CA). B-1a cells with phenotype, CD23$^-$B220^{lo}CD5^{int} were sort-purified using a BD Biosciences Influx instrument. Post-sort analysis showed PerC B-1a cells to be ≥98% pure. Sort-purified B-1a cells were washed with PBS and then suspended in PBS for adoptive transfer into septic mice through intraperitoneal (i.p.) injection. At the time of CLP operation, 5×10^5 B-1a cells suspended in 150 μl of PBS were delivered into the peritoneal cavity and the abdominal wound was closed with running 4–0 silk suture. As vehicle negative control, 150 μl of PBS was injected into the abdomen of CLP-operated mice. The animals were allowed food and water ad libitum, and at 20 h after CLP operation and B-1a cell transfer the animals were euthanized and lungs were collected for various ex vivo analyses.

Quantitative real-time PCR assay

Total RNA was extracted from lung tissues using TRIzol reagent (Invitrogen; Carlsbad, CA) and reverse-transcribed into cDNA using reverse transcriptase enzyme (Applied Biosystems; Foster City, CA). The PCR reaction was performed in 20 μl of final volume containing 0.08 μM of forward and reverse primer, 2 μl of 10–20× diluted original cDNA, and 10 μl SYBR Green PCR Master Mix (Applied Biosystems) using Applied Biosystems 7300 real-time PCR machine. Mouse β-actin served as an internal control gene for normalization. Relative expression of mRNA was represented as fold change in comparison to the sham group. The sense and anti-sense primer sequences of mouse genes are, IL-6 (NM_031168): 5′-CCGGAGAGGAGACTTCACA G-3′ and 5′-GGAAATTGGGGTAGGAAGGA-3′; IL-1β (NM_008361): 5′-CAGGATGAGGACATGAGCACC-3′ and 5′-CTCTGCAGACTCAAACTCCAC-3′; tumor necrosis factor-α (TNF-α) (NM_013693.2): 5′-AGACCCTCA CACTCAGATCATCTTC-3′ and 5′-TTGCTACGA CGTGGGCTACA-3′; interferon γ (IFNγ) (NM_008337): 5′-GGCTTTGCAGCTCTTCCTC-3′ and 5′-CCAG TTCCTCCAGATATCCAA-3′; IL-10 (NM_010548): 5′-CAGCCGGGAAGACAATAA CT-3′ and 5′-GCAT TAAGGAGTCGGTTAGCA-3′; MIP-2 (NM_009140): 5′-CCCTGGTTC AGAAAATCATCCA-3′ and 5′-GCTC CTCCTTTCCAGGTCAGT-3′; β-actin (NM_007393): 5′-CGTGAAAAGATGACCCAGATCA-3′ and 5′-TGGT ACGACCAGAGGCATACAG-3′.

ELISA

The lung tissue was crushed in liquid nitrogen, and approximately 50 mg of powdered tissues were dissolved in 500 μl of lysis buffer (10 mM Hepes, pH 7.4, 5 mM MgCl$_2$, 1 mM DTT, 1% Triton X-100, and 2 mM each of EDTA and EGTA), and subjected to sonication on ice. Protein concentration was determined by the BioRad protein assay reagent (Hercules, CA). Equal amounts (50 μg) of proteins were loaded into respective enzyme-linked immunosorbent assay (ELISA) wells for assessment of IL-6, IL-1β, TNF-α, IFNγ, IL-10 and MIP-2 by using the kits obtained from BD Biosciences, and IgM by using the kit from Bethyl Laboratories, Inc., Montgomery, TX.

Lung tissue histology

Formalin fixed and paraffin embedded lung tissue blocks were sectioned at 5 μm thickness and placed on glass slides. Lung tissue sections were stained with hematoxylin & eosin (H&E) and observed under a light microscope. Morphological changes were scored as nil (0), mild (1), moderate (2), or severe (3) injury based on the presence of exudates, hyperemia or congestion, infiltration of neutrophils, alveolar hemorrhage, presence of debris, and cellular hyperplasia, in a blinded fashion (Aziz et al. 2012; Hirano et al. 2015). The sums of scores of different animals were averaged and plotted on a bar graph.

Myeloperoxidase assay

A total of 50–100 mg of liquid nitrogen-based powered lung tissues were homogenized in KPO$_4$ buffer containing 0.5% hexa-decyl-trimethyl-ammonium bromide (Sigma-Aldrich, St. Louis, MO) using a sonicator with the samples placed in ice. After centrifuging, the supernatant was diluted in reaction solution which contains O-Dianisidine dihydrochloride (Sigma-Aldrich) and H$_2$O$_2$ (ThermoFisher Scientific, Waltham, MA) as substrate. Rate of change in optical density (ΔOD) between 1 and 4 min was measured at 460 nm to calculate myeloperoxidase (MPO) activity (Aziz et al. 2012).

TUNEL assay

The presence of apoptotic cells in lung tissue sections was determined using a terminal deoxynucleotide transferase dUTP nick end labeling (TUNEL) assay kit (Roche Diagnostics, Indianapolis, IN). Briefly, lung tissues were fixed in 10% phosphate buffered formalin and were then embedded into paraffin and sectioned at 5 μm following standard histology procedures. Lung sections were dewaxed, rehydrated and equilibrated in Tris buffered saline (TBS). The sections were then digested with 20 μg/mL proteinase K$^+$ for 20 min at room temperature. The lung tissue sections were then washed and incubated with a cocktail containing terminal deoxynucleotidyl transferase enzyme and fluorescence labeled nucleotides and examined under a fluorescence micro-scope (Nikon Eclipse Ti-S, Melville, NY).

Caspase-3 enzyme activity assay

The caspase-3 enzyme activity in lung tissues was assessed by a fluorimetric assay system kit (Sigma, Saint Louis, MO). Lung tissues were homogenized in liquid nitrogen, and approximately 50 mg of powdered tissues were dissolved in 500 µl of lysis buffer, which contains a cocktail of 10 mM Hepes, pH 7.4, 5 mM $MgCl_2$, 1 mM DTT, 1% Triton X-100, and 2 mM each of EDTA and EGTA, and then subjected to sonication by placing the samples in ice. Protein concentration was measured by the Bio Rad protein assay reagent (Hercules). Equal amounts of proteins in a 5 µl volume were added to the 100 µl assay buffer (20 mM Hepes, pH 7.4, 5 mM DTT, 2 mM EDTA, and 0.1% CHAPS) containing 10 µM DEVD-AMC substrate molecule and the

rate of changes of fluorescence intensity at 37 °C were measured at 370 nm (excitation wavelength) and 450 nm (emission wavelength) in a fluorometer (Synergy H1, BioTek, Winooski, VT). The caspase-3 enzyme activity was expressed as mM AMC/min/g of protein (Aziz et al. 2012).

Statistical analysis

Figure preparation and data analyses were performed by using SigmaPlot 12.5 software (Systat Software Inc., San Jose, CA). Data represented in the figures are expressed as mean ± standard error (SE). One way analysis of variance (ANOVA) was used for comparison among multiple groups and the significance was determined by the Student-Newman-Keuls (SNK) test. Paired two-tailed Student's t-test was applied for two-group comparisons. Significance was determined as $p \leq 0.05$ between experimental groups.

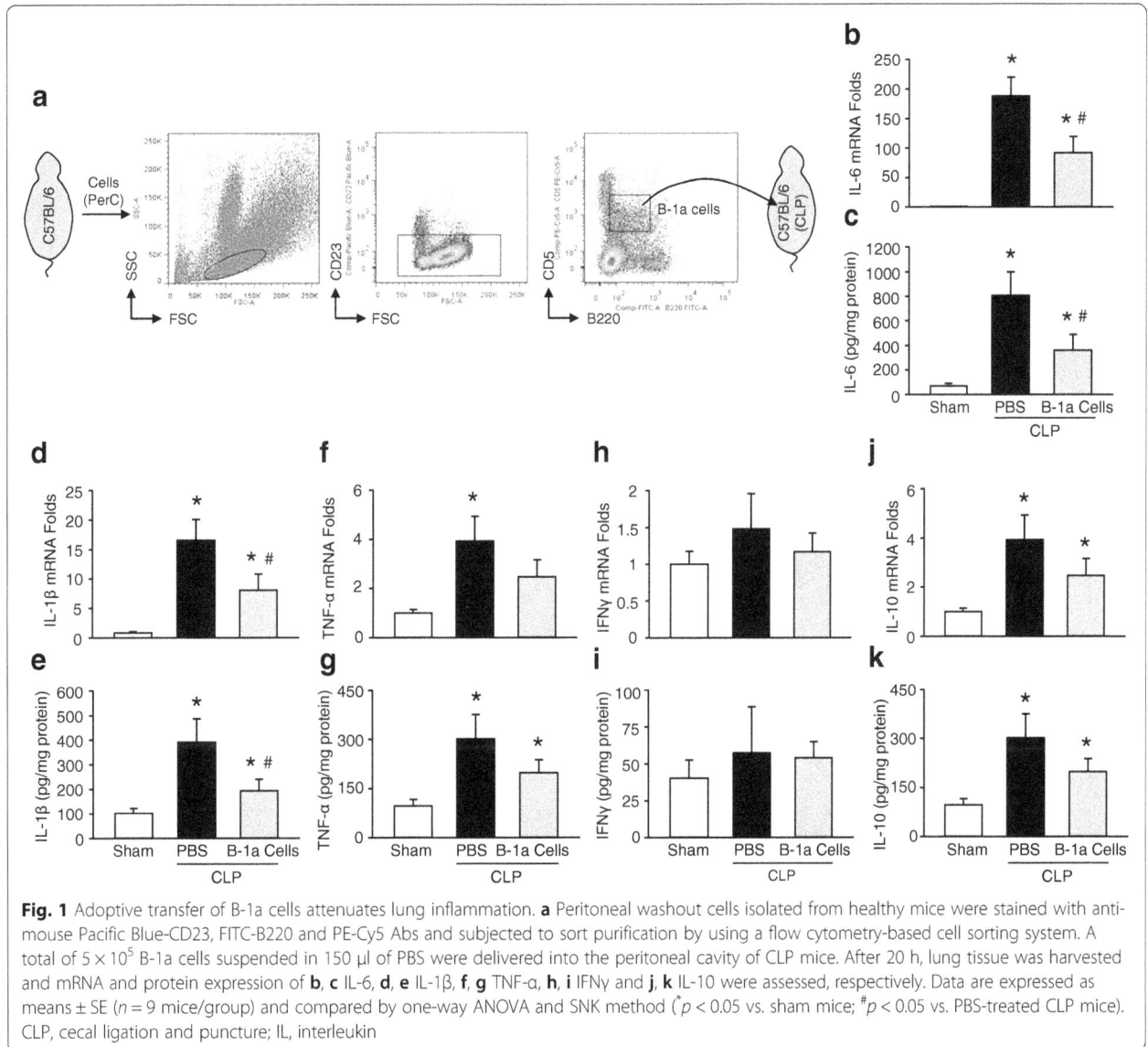

Fig. 1 Adoptive transfer of B-1a cells attenuates lung inflammation. a Peritoneal washout cells isolated from healthy mice were stained with anti-mouse Pacific Blue-CD23, FITC-B220 and PE-Cy5 Abs and subjected to sort purification by using a flow cytometry-based cell sorting system. A total of 5×10^5 B-1a cells suspended in 150 µl of PBS were delivered into the peritoneal cavity of CLP mice. After 20 h, lung tissue was harvested and mRNA and protein expression of b, c IL-6, d, e IL-1β, f, g TNF-α, h, i IFNγ and j, k IL-10 were assessed, respectively. Data are expressed as means ± SE ($n = 9$ mice/group) and compared by one-way ANOVA and SNK method ($^*p < 0.05$ vs. sham mice; $^#p < 0.05$ vs. PBS-treated CLP mice). CLP, cecal ligation and puncture; IL, interleukin

Results

B-1a cells attenuate the expression of pro-inflammatory cytokines in the lungs during sepsis

Peritoneal B-1a cells were sort-purified based on $CD23^-B220^{lo}CD5^{int}$ surface phenotype from healthy mice and then injected into mice immediately after CLP operation (Fig. 1a). At 20 h after CLP operation, lungs were harvested to assess the expression of pro- and anti-inflammatory cytokines. Expression of IL-6 and IL-1β in lung tissue from CLP mice was significantly up-regulated compared to sham-operated mice, while the adoptive transfer of B-1a cells significantly down-regulated expression of IL-6 and IL-1β by 51 and 54%, respectively at the mRNA and 55 and 51%, respectively at the protein level (Fig. 1b-e). We found significant up-regulation of the expression of TNF-α at mRNA and protein levels in the lung tissues of CLP mice, while there was a trend towards down-regulation of TNF-α expression in lungs of B-1a cell-treated CLP mice as compared to vehicle-treated CLP mice (Fig. 1f, g). We

could not find significant increase of the expression of IFNγ at both mRNA and protein levels in lungs at 20 h of CLP, which could be due to the fact that its up-regulation might occur at earlier time point after CLP operation, and therefore 20 h after CLP was too late to determine its up-regulation in lung tissues (Fig. 1h, i). Similar to the patterns of expression of pro-inflammatory cytokines, we found significant up-regulation of IL-10 expression at mRNA and protein levels in the lung tissues following CLP operation as compared to sham-operated mice (Fig. 1j, k). We noticed a trend towards decreasing the expression of IL-10 in lungs of B-1a cell-treated CLP mice as compared to vehicle-treated CLP mice, reflecting the remission of inflammation after B-1a cell treatment in septic mice (Fig. 1j, k).

Treatment of septic mice with B-1a cells attenuates lung injury scores

Histological images of lung tissue showed decreased levels of alveolar congestion, exudate, interstitial and

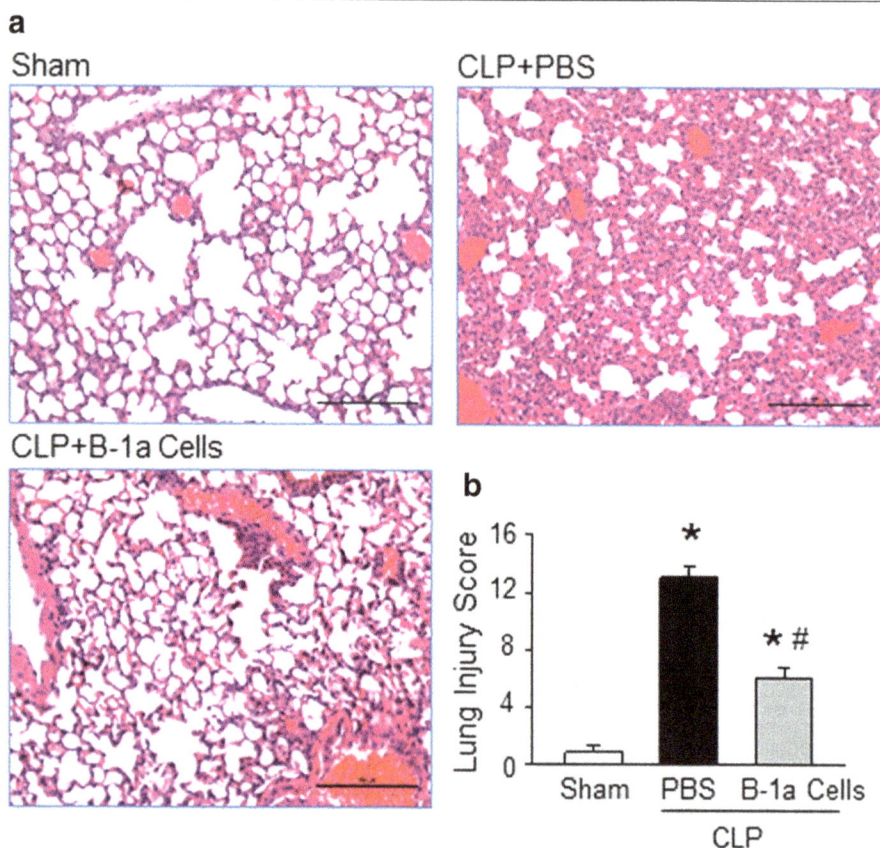

Fig. 2 Treatment with B-1a cells improves the histopathological *score* of lung tissue damage in sepsis. **a** Lung tissue was collected after 20 h from sham-operated, and either PBS- or B-1a cell-treated CLP mice and stained with H&E. Each slide was observed under light microscopy at × 100 original magnification in a blinded fashion. Representative images for each group are shown. Scale bar, 100 μm. **b** Histological injury scores of the lungs in different groups were quantified as described in Materials and Methods. Data from three independent experiments are expressed as means ± SE (*n* = 6 mice/group) and compared by one-way ANOVA and SNK method ($^*p < 0.05$ vs. shams; $^\#p < 0.05$ vs. PBS-treated CLP mice). CLP, cecal ligation and puncture; H&E, hematoxylin and eosin

alveolar cellular infiltrates, intra-alveolar capillary hemorrhages, and damage of epithelial architecture, in B-1a cell-treated CLP mice as compared to PBS-treated CLP mice (Fig. 2a). These histological changes were reflected in a significant decrease in lung tissue injury score, in B-1a cell-treated mice compared to PBS-treated CLP mice by a mean value of 54% (Fig. 2b). On the other hand, the sham-operated mouse lungs showed normal histological architecture.

B-1a cells attenuate chemokine and MPO levels in the lungs of septic mice

Chemokines such as MIP-2 play a pivotal role in the infiltration of neutrophils in lungs during sepsis (Aziz et al. 2013; Abraham 2003). In lung tissue following sepsis, we noticed significant up-regulation of MIP-2 expression compared to sham mice, while the mice treated with B-1a cells significantly reduced the expression of MIP-2 by 49 and 46%, respectively at the mRNA and protein levels compared to PBS-treated CLP mice (Fig. 3a, b). The neutrophil infiltration in lungs as measured by the amount of MPO showed significant inhibition in B-1a cell-treated mice by 41% as compared to PBS-treated mice during CLP (Fig. 3c).

Treatment with B-1a cells attenuates apoptosis in the lung during sepsis

Sepsis resulted in a significant increase in the number of apoptotic cells in lungs (Aziz et al. 2013; Aziz et al. 2012). Here, we noticed that the septic mice treated with B-1a cells experienced a significant decrease in the numbers of apoptotic cells by 56% compared to PBS-treated septic mice (Fig. 4a, b). Furthermore, following sepsis we noticed a significant increase of the activation of caspase-3, the rate-limiting enzyme for apoptosis in the lungs, compared to sham-operated mice. However, the treatment of septic mice with B-1a cells significantly reduced the level of active caspase-3 by mean values of 52%, compared to PBS-treated septic mice (Fig. 4c).

Treatment with B-1a cells restores IgM levels in lung tissues during sepsis

About 80% of the IgM present in the blood are natural IgM which comes from the B-1a cells and its levels are high at steady-state (Aziz et al. 2015). We previously showed that during sepsis the circulatory (blood) level of IgM were decreased during sepsis, while after adoptive transfer of B-1a cells in the septic mice increased the level of IgM in the blood (Aziz et al. 2017). In addition to this, within the peritoneal cavity (local infectious foci) the IgM levels were also increased following treatment of septic mice with B-1a cells (Aziz et al. 2017). To know whether or not IgM is present in the lungs and their levels are altered during sepsis, we assessed IgM levels

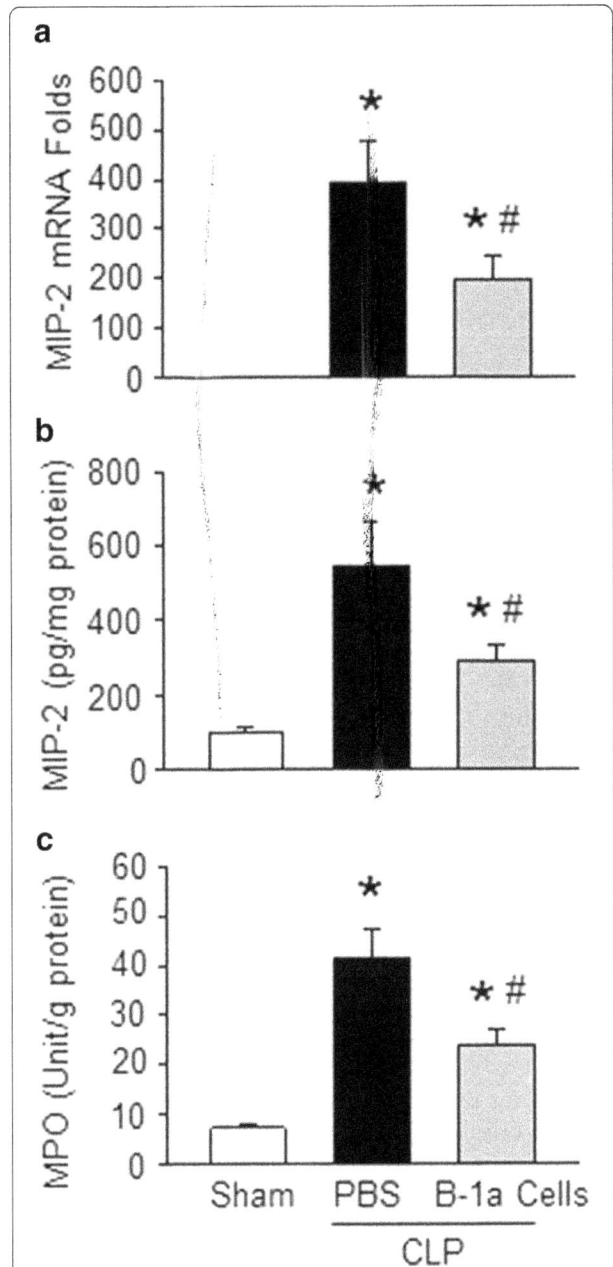

Fig. 3 B-1a cells attenuate MIP-2 and MPO levels in lungs after sepsis. a, b At the time of CLP, mice were treated with either PBS as vehicle or 5×10^5 PerC B-1a cells in 150 µl of PBS by i.p. injection. After 20 h, lung tissue was harvested and mRNA and protein expression of MIP-2 were assessed, respectively. c MPO activity in lungs of sham-operated, and PBS or B-1a cell-treated CLP mice was determined. Data are expressed as means ± SE ($n = 9$ mice/group from 3 independent experiments) and compared by one-way ANOVA and SNK method ($^*p < 0.05$ vs. shams; $^\#p < 0.05$ vs. PBS-treated CLP mice). CLP, cecal ligation and puncture; MIP-2, macrophage-inflammatory protein-2; MPO, myeloperoxidase

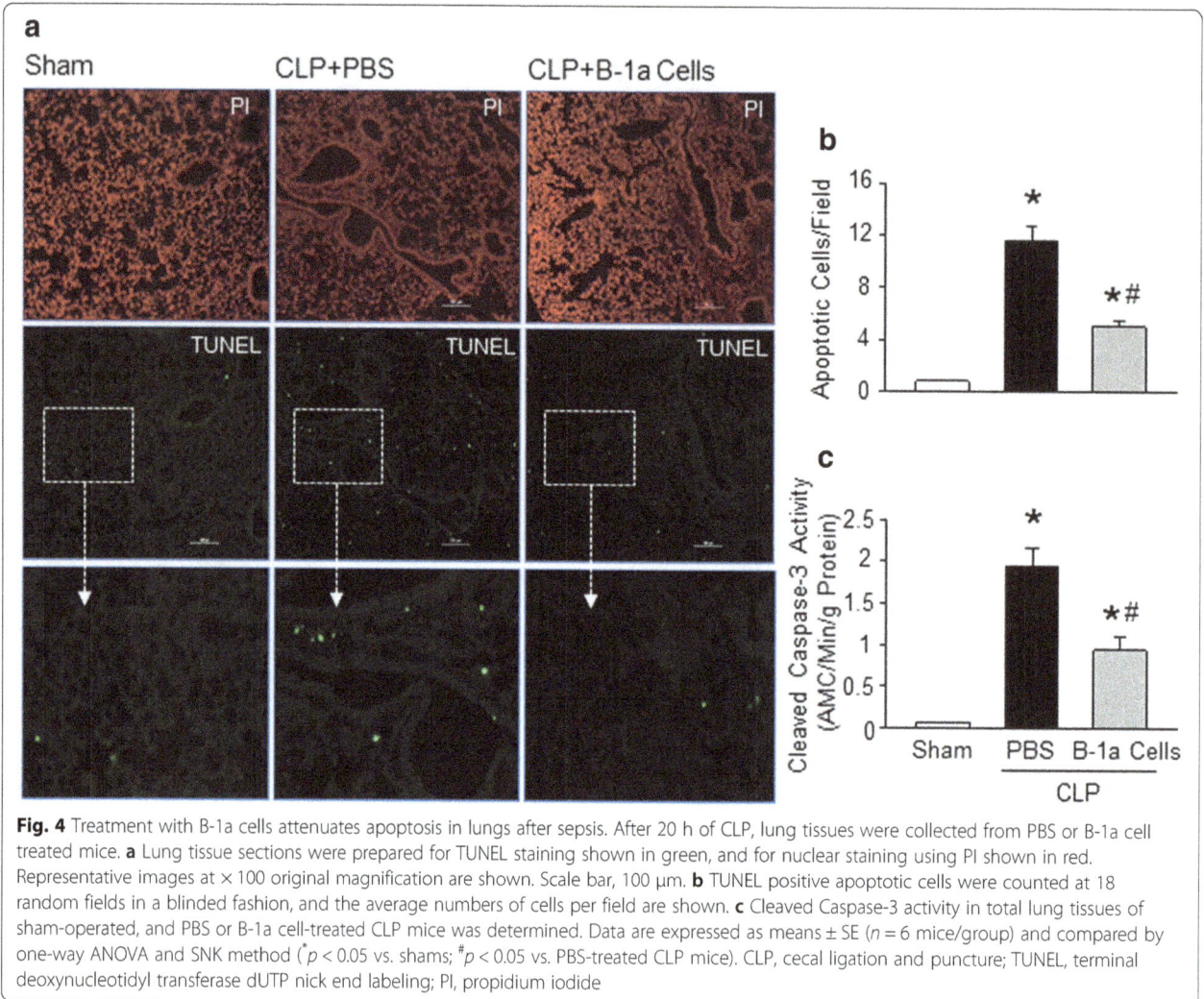

Fig. 4 Treatment with B-1a cells attenuates apoptosis in lungs after sepsis. After 20 h of CLP, lung tissues were collected from PBS or B-1a cell treated mice. **a** Lung tissue sections were prepared for TUNEL staining shown in green, and for nuclear staining using PI shown in red. Representative images at × 100 original magnification are shown. Scale bar, 100 μm. **b** TUNEL positive apoptotic cells were counted at 18 random fields in a blinded fashion, and the average numbers of cells per field are shown. **c** Cleaved Caspase-3 activity in total lung tissues of sham-operated, and PBS or B-1a cell-treated CLP mice was determined. Data are expressed as means ± SE ($n = 6$ mice/group) and compared by one-way ANOVA and SNK method ($^*p < 0.05$ vs. shams; $^\#p < 0.05$ vs. PBS-treated CLP mice). CLP, cecal ligation and puncture; TUNEL, terminal deoxynucleotidyl transferase dUTP nick end labeling; PI, propidium iodide

in the lung tissues in sham and CLP-operated vehicle- or B-1a cell-treated mice. We found that during sepsis IgM levels in the lungs were significantly decreased as compared to sham mice, while treatment of CLP mice with B-1a cells significantly increased the level of IgM in the lungs (Fig. 5). Therefore, the B-1a cell-mediated protection against sepsis-induced ALI could be mediated through both systemic and local increase of IgM.

Deficiency of B-1a cells in CD19$^{-/-}$ mice exacerbates lung injury

B cells express the co-receptor CD19, which serves as a positive regulator of B cell receptor (BCR) signaling and is critical for B cell development and activation (Aziz et al. 2017; Aziz et al. 2015; Haas et al. 2005). It has been shown that transgenic mice over expressing CD19 generate excess B-1a cells which provide protection against infection, while CD19-deficient mice lack B-1a cells and are susceptible to infection (Haas et al. 2005). We examined CD19$^{-/-}$ mice to determine whether or not the

deficiency of B-1a cells would exacerbate lung injury during sepsis. Following CLP, histological images of the lung tissues showed increased levels of alveolar congestion, exudate, interstitial and alveolar cellular infiltrates, intra-alveolar capillary hemorrhages, and extensive damage of epithelial architecture in CD19$^{-/-}$ mice as compared to WT mice (Fig. 6a). These histological changes were reflected in a significant increase in lung tissue injury score in CD19$^{-/-}$ mice compared to WT mice by a mean value of 54% after CLP (Fig. 6b).

Discussion

B-1a cells are part of innate immune system and exhibit unique phenotypic, developmental, localizations, signaling and functional characteristics that differ from the conventional B-2 cells (Aziz et al. 2015). B-1a cells are innate-like, while B-2 cells are adaptive-type immune-reactive lymphoid cells. B-1a cells spontaneously secrete germline-like, polyreactive natural antibody (IgM), which acts as a first line of defense by

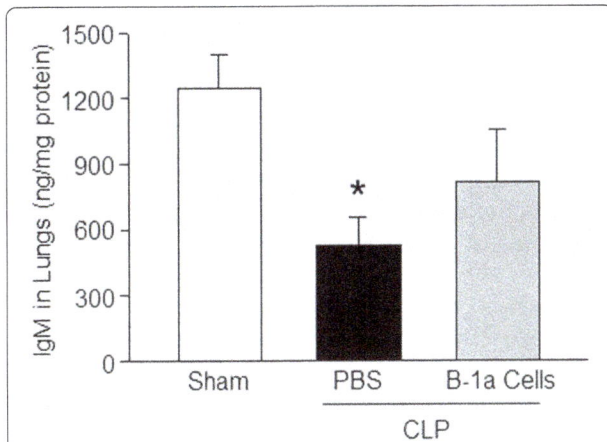

Fig. 5 Treatment with B-1a cells increases IgM levels in the lungs following sepsis. A total of 5×10^5 sorted B-1a cells were delivered into the peritoneal cavity of CLP mice. After 20 h, lung tissue was harvested from sham, PBS-, and B-1a cell-treated mice and assessed IgM levels in total extracted proteins by ELISA. Data are expressed as means ± SE (n = 9 mice/group) and compared by one-way ANOVA and SNK method (*p < 0.05 vs. sham mice). CLP, cecal ligation and puncture; ELISA, enzyme-linked immunosorbent assay

neutralizing a wide range of pathogens (Aziz et al. 2015; Grönwall et al. 2012). B-1a cells are known to produce several immunomodulatory molecules either spontaneously or in the presence of stimulation, which attenuate infectious and inflammatory diseases including influenza, pneumonia, atherosclerosis, inflammatory bowel disease, autoimmunity, obesity and diabetes mellitus [reviewed in (Aziz et al. 2015)]. Recently, the beneficial role of B-1a cells in sepsis has been reported (Aziz et al. 2017; Rauch et al. 2012), and this was shown to be mediated through the control of excessive systemic inflammation and bacterial burdens. Nonetheless, the role of B-1a cells in mitigating inflammation and injuries to the remote organs especially lungs, during sepsis was not known. In the current study, we primarily focused on the role of B-1a cells in attenuating ALI during sepsis.

Using a mouse model of sepsis, we previously showed that the numbers of B-1a cells in peritoneal cavity, spleen and bone-marrow were significantly decreased (Aziz et al. 2017). Adoptive transfer of syngeneic B-1a cells into septic mice significantly attenuated systemic inflammatory and injury parameters as well as bacterial burden in the blood and peritoneal cavity (Aziz et al.

a

WT-sham

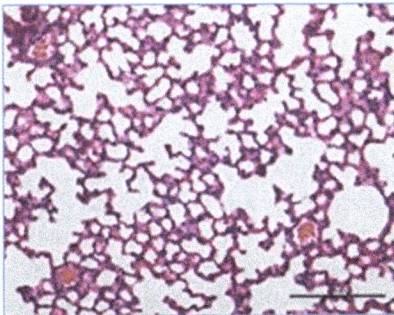

CD19⁻ᐟ⁻-Sham

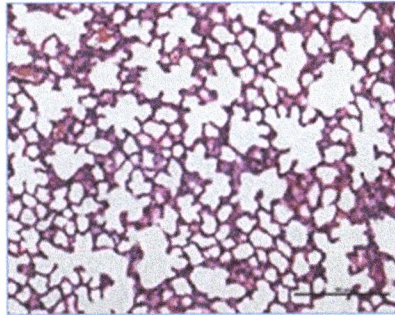

WT-CLP

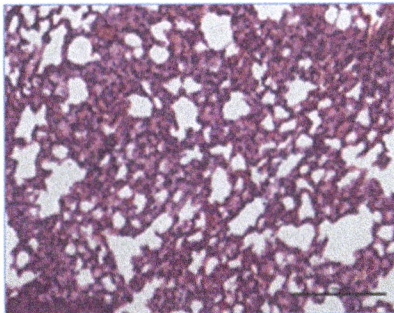

CD19⁻ᐟ⁻-CLP

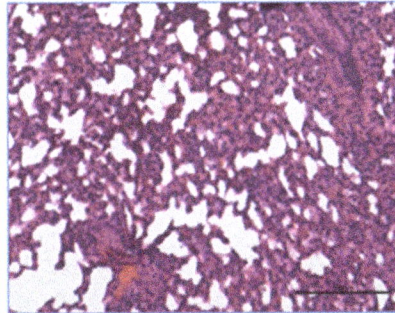

b

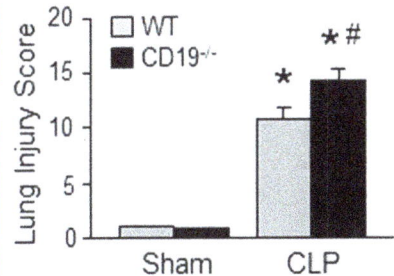

Fig. 6 Deficiency of B-1a cells exaggerates lung injury during sepsis. **a** After 20 h of CLP induced in WT and CD19$^{-/-}$ mice, lung tissues were harvested and stained with H&E. The slides were observed under light microscopy at × 100 original magnification in a blinded fashion. Representative images for each group are shown. Scale bar, 100 μm. **b** Histological injury scores of the lungs in WT and CD19$^{-/-}$ mice were quantified as described in Materials and Methods. Data obtained from three independent experiments are expressed as means ± SE (n = 6 mice/group) and compared by one-way ANOVA and SNK method (*p < 0.05 vs. shams; #p < 0.05 vs. WT CLP mice). CLP, cecal ligation and puncture; H&E, hematoxylin and eosin

2017). In the current study, we found that the adoptive transfer of murine B-1a cells into septic mice significantly attenuated the expression of pro-inflammatory cytokines IL-6 and IL-1β in the lungs. We also found overall improvement of lung injury scores in B-1a cell-treated mice during sepsis. The attenuation of sepsis-induced lung injury was correlated with reduced levels of chemokine expression, neutrophil infiltration as assessed by MPO, and cellular apoptosis through the down-regulation of caspase-3 activity. We previously demonstrated B-1a cell–deficient CD19$^{-/-}$ mice were more susceptible to infectious inflammation, thereby causing an increased mortality rate in sepsis (Aziz et al. 2017). Here, we also found that the CD19$^{-/-}$ mice showed significantly increased levels of lung injury scores as compared to WT mice after sepsis, thus suggesting the pivotal beneficial role of B-1a cells to protect mice from ALI during sepsis. The improvement of systemic inflammation and lung injury and inflammation after administration of B-1a cells in septic animals can be better reflected in their survival outcomes. In our previous study, we demonstrated significant improvement of the survival outcome in B-1a cell-treated mice over that of PBS-treated mice with sepsis (Aziz et al. 2017). By contrast, the B-1a cell deficient CD19$^{-/-}$ mice had significantly reduced rate of survival as compared to the WT mice during sepsis (Aziz et al. 2017).

The crosstalk effect between B-1a cells and macrophages has been demonstrated in previous reports (Thies et al. 2013; Barbeiro et al. 2011). B-1a cells produce IL-10 in response to LPS stimulation (Aziz et al. 2017; Barbeiro et al. 2011). In B-1a cells and macrophages co-cultures, production of pro-inflammatory cytokines was lower and the production of anti-inflammatory cytokine IL-10 was higher than in macrophage monocultures (Barbeiro et al. 2011). Interestingly, co-culture of IL-10$^{-/-}$ B-1a cells and WT macrophages did not reduce the levels of the pro-inflammatory cytokines (Aziz et al. 2017), indicating the pivotal regulatory role of B-1a cells in controlling inflammation. Beside these in vitro findings, we demonstrated the beneficial role of B-1a cells during sepsis through the production of anti-inflammatory cytokine IL-10 (Aziz et al. 2017). Lungs contain resident alveolar macrophages which during sepsis become activated to produce excessive amounts of pro-inflammatory cytokines and chemokines (Aziz et al. 2012; Moldoveanu et al. 2009). However, we noticed significant decreases in the expression of pro-inflammatory cytokines IL-6 and IL-1β and chemokine MIP-2 in the lungs of B-1a cell-treated mice during sepsis. Since B-1a cells are known to produce excessive amounts of anti-inflammatory cytokine IL-10, it is therefore understandable that the B-1a cells could temper the pro-inflammatory responses of alveolar macrophages and thus protect mice from ALI during sepsis.

B-1a cells can serve as antigen presenting cells, providing effective signaling to T-cells via CD80 and CD86 molecules, which are expressed on B-1a cells (Aziz et al. 2015). Therefore, in parallel to study the crosstalk effect between B-1a cells and macrophages, it would be of interest for future studies to elucidate the novel role of B-1a cells on T cells in the lungs during sepsis.

GM-CSF is mainly produced by the innate response activator (IRA) B cells (Rauch et al. 2012). Our current study focused on the effect of IL-10- and IgM-producing B-1a cells in sepsis-induced ALI. In our previous study, we demonstrated that the septic mice treated with IL-10$^{-/-}$ B-1a cells did not show protection against sepsis (Aziz et al. 2017), thus pointing to the role of B-1a cell-secreted IL-10 to exert beneficial role in sepsis. We also demonstrated that the levels of GM-CSF in B-1a cells between WT and IL-10$^{-/-}$ mice strains following sepsis were remained same (Aziz et al. 2017), indicating that the lack of IL-10 in B-1a cells could be detrimental in sepsis without affecting the levels of GM-CSF. Future studies focusing on the role of GM-CSF producing IRA B cells will help reveal the importance of IRA B cells in sepsis-induced ALI.

In sepsis, irresistible migration of neutrophils into the lungs leads to endothelial cell injury and sustained inflammation (Aziz et al. 2013; Aziz et al. 2012; Hirano et al. 2015; Hirano et al. 2016). The patients with ARDS represent huge infiltration of neutrophils in the lung tissues which correlates with the severity of lung injury as a result of releasing ample amounts of proteolytic enzymes and pro-inflammatory mediators from the infiltrated neutrophils into the lung tissue beds (Abraham 2003; Williams and Chambers 2014). Thus, it is suggested that the regulation of neutrophil infiltration into the lungs could be an effective therapeutic approach in septic-induced ALI. Here, in the current study, we noticed dramatic reduction of neutrophil infiltration in the lungs as measured by MPO and chemokine MIP-2 levels which ultimately led to diminished lung tissue injury in the B-1a cell-treated mice. Although the direct roles of B-1a cells on macrophages and T cells had been delineated previously, the effect of B-1a cells on neutrophils is largely unknown. Elucidation of the direct role of B-1a cells on neutrophils will provide additional insights into the pathophysiology of ALI in sepsis.

In the context of lung injury and inflammation caused by viral and bacterial infections, several reports have already demonstrated the beneficial role of B-1a cells in protecting mice from lung injury, mainly mediated through the release of natural IgM (Baumgarth et al. 1999; Baumgarth et al. 2000; Weber et al. 2014). Natural IgM secreted from B-1a cells eliminates invading pathogens and also scavenges dying cells, which in turn can attenuate inflammation and tissue injury (Grönwall et al.

2012; Vas et al. 2012). On the other hand, mice lacking natural IgM are prone to develop autoimmune diseases because of the failure to neutralize/remove antigens and apoptotic cells to maintain homeostasis (Aziz et al. 2015; Boes et al. 2000). In the current study, we noticed significant reduction in the number of apoptotic cells in the lungs following B-1a cell treatment in septic mice. Although here we did not assess the phagocytic clearance of apoptotic cells by professional phagocytes, we found that the septic mice treated with B-1a cells showed reduced levels of caspase-3 activity, indicating inhibition of cellular apoptosis by B-1a cell treatment. It has been demonstrated that endothelial cell pyroptosis, a form of cell death, may result in sepsis-induced ALI through the activation of caspases (Cheng et al. 2017; Aziz et al. 2014). Since the pyroptotic cells also undergo DNA fragmentation and, like apoptotic cells show positive TUNEL staining (Mariathasan et al. 2005), our TUNEL assay data in lung tissues pointed to the possibility of decreased pyroptosis of lung cells following treatment of septic mice with B-1a cells. Further studies by staining the lung tissue sections with endothelial cell marker CD31 Ab, TUNEL and caspase-1 Ab will help confirm the status of endothelial cell pyroptosis in lungs during sepsis, and also demonstrate the inhibitory effect of B-1a cells for endothelial cell pyroptosis during sepsis.

During influenza virus infection, the therapeutic potential of murine B-1a cells was mainly generated by their enrichment at the lungs as a result of their translocation from serosal cavities where they are generally localized at the steady-state condition (30). Following their translocation into lungs, B-1a cells autonomously secrete natural Abs and other immunomodulatory molecules to protect hosts against influenza virus infection (Aziz et al. 2015; Baumgarth et al. 1999; Baumgarth et al. 2000). In line with this fact, Weber, et al. showed B-1a cells migrate from the pleural cavity to the interstitial lung tissues, where they produce ample amount of GM-CSF and natural Abs to protect the host from endotoxin or *S. pneumoniae*-induced ALI in mice (Weber et al. 2014). In the current study utilizing murine model of sepsis, B-1a cells could be enriched into the lungs as a result of their translocation from the site of origin to protect mice against lung inflammation.

In the current study, we injected septic mice with B-1a cells at the time of CLP operation, the post-treatment of septic mice with B-1a cells would help advance our current therapeutic strategy towards more clinically relevant circumstances. We basically chose to treat mice with B-1a cells immediately after CLP rather than post-surgery because most of the pro-inflammatory cytokines and chemokines are expressed early/hyperdynamic phase in sepsis, reaching maximum levels around 10–12 h after CLP and then returns to normal levels (Aziz

et al. 2013; Bosmann and Ward 2013; Rittirsch et al. 2008). Therefore, in order to obtain optimal inhibition of pro-inflammatory cytokines and chemokines by the treatment of B-1a cells, we chose time of treatment at CLP induction instead of a later time point. We delivered the B-1a cells into the septic mice through the intraperitoneal route; however, administration of B-1a cells intravenously would help shift this laboratory strategy to bedside approaches.

In the present study, we used C57BL/6 WT mice, also known as B6 mice obtained from the Taconic to compare the outcomes of sepsis-induced ALI with B6 background B-1a cell deficient CD19$^{-/-}$ mice obtained from the Jackson lab. Our previous studies on B6 background of mice of Taconic and Jackson lab showed similar outcomes in their survival in CLP-induced sepsis (Giangola et al. 2013; Qiang et al. 2013). However, since the immune responses of mice may vary among various strains and vendors (Otto et al. 2016), we consider this as one of our limitations in experimental designing. Further studies using control WT mice and CD19$^{-/-}$ mice from the same vendor will strengthen our present finding of the beneficial effect of B-1a cells on ALI during sepsis.

Conclusions

We identified the beneficial role of murine B-1a cells in sepsis-induced ALI through the mitigation of inflammation and injury to the lungs. Recently, a B cell population in human has been identified which represents functional characteristics that match with murine B-1a cells, including autonomous production of natural IgM, constitutive basal expression of intracellular signal transduction molecules, and effective stimulation of T lymphocytes (Aziz et al. 2015; Griffin et al. 2011; Rothstein et al. 2013). Our current study demonstrating the role of mouse B-1a cells in sepsis-induced ALI further focuses on identifying valuable lessons that may be applicable to human B-1a cells.

Abbreviations

ALI: Acute lung injury; ARDS: Acute respiratory distress syndrome; BCR: B-cell receptor; CLP: Cecal ligation and puncture; ELISA: Enzyme-linked immunosorbent assay; FO: Follicular; GM-CSF: Granulocyte-macrophage colony-stimulating factor; LPS: Lipopolysaccharides; MIP-2: Macrophage-inflammatory protein-2; MPO: Myeloperoxidase; MZ: Marginal zone; NETs: Neutrophil extracellular traps; NO: Nitric oxide; PAMP: Pathogen-associated molecular pattern; PBS: Phosphate-buffered saline; ROS: Reactive oxygen species; TLR: Toll-like receptor; TUNEL: Terminal deoxynucleotide transferase dUTP nick end labeling

Acknowledgements

We thank the NIH for supporting the study.

Funding
This study was supported by the National Institutes of Health (NIH) grants R35GM118337, R01GM053008 and R01GM057468 to PW and R01AI029690 to TLR.

Authors' contributions
PW conceived the idea of the project. MA, TLR and PW designed the experiments. MA, NEH, YO, MZ and MO performed the experiments. MA, MO and YO performed CLP and measured lung parameters. MZ performed lung IHC. NEH sorted murine PerC B-1a cells and maintained CD19$^{-/-}$ mice breeders. MA analyzed the data and wrote the manuscript. TLR and PW reviewed and edited the manuscript. All authors read and approved the final manuscript.

Competing interests
The authors declare that they have no competing interests.

Author details
[1]Center for Immunology and Inflammation, The Feinstein Institute for Medical Research, 350 Community Dr, Manhasset, NY 11030, USA. [2]Center for Oncology and Cell Biology, The Feinstein Institute for Medical Research, Manhasset, New York 11030, USA. [3]Department of Surgery and Molecular Medicine, Donald and Barbara Zucker School of Medicine at Hofstra/Northwell, Manhasset, New York 11030, USA. [4]Present Address: Western Michigan University Homer Stryker M.D. School of Medicine, 1000 Oakland Drive, Kalamazoo, MI 49008, USA.

References
Abraham E. Neutrophils and acute lung injury. Crit Care Med. 2003;31:S195–9.

Aziz M, Holodick NE, Rothstein TL, Wang P. The role of B-1 cells in inflammation. Immunol Res. 2015;63:153–66.

Aziz M, Holodick NE, Rothstein TL, Wang P. B-1a cells protect mice from sepsis: critical role of CREB. J Immunol. 2017;199:750–60.

Aziz M, Jacob A, Wang P. Revisiting caspases in sepsis. Cell Death Dis. 2014; 5:e1526.

Aziz M, Jacob A, Yang WL, Matsuda A, Wang P. Current trends in inflammatory and immunomodulatory mediators in sepsis. J Leukoc Biol. 2013;93:329–42.

Aziz M, Matsuda A, Yang WL, Jacob A, Wang P. Milk fat globule-epidermal growth factor-factor 8 attenuates neutrophil infiltration in acute lung injury via modulation of CXCR2. J Immunol. 2012;189:393–402.

Barbeiro DF, et al. B-1 cells temper endotoxemic inflammatory responses. Immunobiology. 2011;216:302–8.

Barton GM, Medzhitov R. Toll-like receptor signaling pathways. Science. 2003;300: 1524–5.

Baumgarth N, Herman OC, Jager GC, Brown L, Herzenberg LA. Innate and acquired humoral immunities to influenza virus are mediated by distinct arms of the immune system. Proc Natl Acad Sci U S A. 1999;96:2250–5.

Baumgarth N, et al. B-1 and B-2 cell-derived immunoglobulin M antibodies are nonredundant components of the protective response to influenza virus infection. J Exp Med. 2000;192:271–80.

Berland R, Wortis HH. Origins and functions of B-1 cells with notes on the role of CD5. Annu Rev Immunol. 2002;20:253–300.

Boes M, et al. Accelerated development of IgG autoantibodies and autoimmune disease in the absence of secreted IgM. Proc Natl Acad Sci U S A. 2000;97: 1184–9.

Bosmann M, Ward PA. The inflammatory response in sepsis. Trends Immunol. 2013;34:129–36.

Brinkmann V, et al. Neutrophil extracellular traps kill bacteria. Science. 2004;303: 1532–5.

Cheng KT, et al. Caspase-11-mediated endothelial pyroptosis underlies endotoxemia-induced lung injury. J Clin Invest. 2017;127:4124–35.

Choi YS, Baumgarth N. Dual role for B-1a cells in immunity to influenza virus infection. J Exp Med. 2008;205:3053–64.

Cinel I, Opal SM. Molecular biology of inflammation and sepsis: a primer. Crit Care Med. 2009;37:291–304.

Delgado-Rizo V, et al. Neutrophil extracellular traps and its implications in inflammation: an overview. Front Immunol. 2017;8:81.

Foster SL, Medzhitov R. Gene-specific control of the TLR-induced inflammatory response. Clin Immunol. 2009;130:7–15.

Giangola MD, et al. Growth arrest-specific protein 6 attenuates neutrophil migration and acute lung injury in sepsis. Shock. 2013;40:485–91.

Griffin DO, Holodick NE, Rothstein TL. Human B1 cells in umbilical cord and adult peripheral blood express the novel phenotype CD20+ CD27+ CD43+ CD70. J Exp Med. 2011;208:67–80.

Grommes J, Soehnlein O. Contribution of neutrophils to acute lung injury. Mol Med. 2011;17:293–307.

Grönwall C, Vas J, Silverman GJ. Protective roles of natural IgM antibodies. Front Immunol. 2012;3:66.

Gu WJ, Wan YD, Tie HT, Kan QC, Sun TW. Risk of acute lung injury/acute respiratory distress syndrome in critically ill adult patients with pre-existing diabetes: a meta-analysis. PLoS One. 2014;9:e90426.

Haas KM, Poe JC, Steeber DA, Tedder TF. B-1a and B-1b cells exhibit distinct developmental requirements and have unique functional roles in innate and adaptive immunity to S. pneumoniae. Immunity. 2005;23:7–18.

Hirano Y, Aziz M, Wang P. Role of reverse transendothelial migration of neutrophils in inflammation. Biol Chem. 2016;397:497–506.

Hirano Y, et al. Neutralization of osteopontin attenuates neutrophil migration in sepsis-induced acute lung injury. Crit Care. 2015;19:53.

Holodick NE, Vizconde T, Hopkins TJ, Rothstein TL. Age-related decline in natural IgM function: diversification and selection of the B-1a cell pool with age. J Immunol. 2016;196:4348–57.

Honda S, et al. Marginal zone B cells exacerbate endotoxic shock via interleukin-6 secretion induced by Fcα/μR-coupled TLR4 signalling. Nat Commun. 2016;7: 11498.

Kantor AB, Stall AM, Adams S, Herzenberg LA. Differential development of progenitor activity for three B-cell lineages. Proc Natl Acad Sci U S A. 1992; 89:3320–4.

Kaplan MJ, Radic M. Neutrophil extracellular traps: double-edged swords of innate immunity. J Immunol. 2012;189:2689–95.

Kelly-Scumpia KM, et al. B cells enhance early innate immune responses during bacterial sepsis. J Exp Med. 2011;208:1673–82.

Kono H, et al. The Kupffer cell protects against acute lung injury in a rat peritonitis model: role of IL-10. J Leukoc Biol. 2006;79:809–17.

Lee WL, Downey GP. Neutrophil activation and acute lung injury. Curr Opin Crit Care. 2001;7:1–7.

Mariathasan S, Weiss DS, Dixit VM, Monack DM. Innate immunity against Francisella tularensis is dependent on the ASC/caspase-1 axis. J Exp Med. 2005;202:1043–9.

Martin F, Kearney JF. B1 cells: similarities and differences with other B cell subsets. Curr Opin Immunol. 2001;13:195–201.

Martin GS, Mannino DM, Moss M. The effect of age on the development and outcome of adult sepsis. Crit Care Med. 2006;34:15–21.

Moldoveanu B, et al. Inflammatory mechanisms in the lung. J Inflamm Res. 2009;2:1–11.

Otto GP, et al. Clinical chemistry reference intervals for C57BL/6J, C57BL/6N, and C3HeB/FeJ mice (Mus musculus). J Am Assoc Lab Anim Sci. 2016;55:375–86.

Qiang X, et al. Cold-inducible RNA-binding protein (CIRP) triggers inflammatory responses in hemorrhagic shock and sepsis. Nat Med. 2013;19:1489–95.

Rauch PJ, et al. Innate response activator B cells protect against microbial sepsis. Science. 2012;335:597–601.

Rittirsch D, Flierl MA, Ward PA. Harmful molecular mechanisms in sepsis. Nat Rev Immunol. 2008;8:776–87.

Rothstein TL, Griffin DO, Holodick NE, Quach TD, Kaku H. Human B-1 cells take the stage. Ann N Y Acad Sci. 2013;1285:97–114.

Sevransky JE, et al. Mortality in sepsis versus non-sepsis induced acute lung injury. Crit Care. 2009;13:R150.

Singer M, et al. The third international consensus definitions for sepsis and septic shock (Sepsis-3). JAMA. 2016;315:801–10.

Thies FG, et al. Cross talk between peritoneal macrophages and B-1 cells in vitro. PLoS One. 2013;8:e62805.

Vas J, Grönwall C, Marshak-Rothstein A, Silverman GJ. Natural antibody to apoptotic cell membranes inhibits the proinflammatory properties of lupus autoantibody immune complexes. Arthritis Rheum. 2012;64:3388–98.

Vincent JL, et al. Assessment of the worldwide burden of critical illness: the intensive care over nations (ICON) audit. Lancet Respir Med. 2014;2:380–6.

Weber GF, et al. Pleural innate response activator B cells protect against pneumonia via a GM-CSF-IgM axis. J Exp Med. 2014;211:1243–56.

Williams AE, Chambers RC. The mercurial nature of neutrophils: still an enigma in ARDS? Am J Physiol Lung Cell Mol Physiol. 2014;306:L217–30.

Yenson V, Baumgarth N. Purification and immune phenotyping of B-1 cells from body cavities of mice. Methods Mol Biol. 2014;1190:17–34.

11

Genome-wide meta-analysis identifies novel loci associated with parathyroid hormone level

Antonela Matana[1], Dubravka Brdar[2], Vesela Torlak[2], Thibaud Boutin[3], Marijana Popović[1], Ivana Gunjača[1], Ivana Kolčić[4], Vesna Boraska Perica[1], Ante Punda[2], Ozren Polašek[4], Maja Barbalić[1], Caroline Hayward[3] and Tatijana Zemunik[1*]

Abstract

Background: Parathyroid hormone (PTH) is one of the principal regulators of calcium homeostasis. Although serum PTH level is mostly accounted by genetic factors, genetic background underlying PTH level is insufficiently known. Therefore, the aim of this study was to identify novel genetic variants associated with PTH levels.

Methods: We performed GWAS meta-analysis within two genetically isolated Croatian populations followed by replication analysis in a Croatian mainland population and we also combined results across all three analyzed populations. The analyses included 2596 individuals. A total of 7,411,206 variants, imputed using the 1000 Genomes reference panel, were analysed for the association. In addition, a sex-specific GWAS meta-analyses were performed.

Results: Polymorphisms with the lowest P-values were located on chromosome 4 approximately 84 kb of the 5′ of *RASGEF1B* gene. The most significant SNP was rs11099476 ($P = 1.15 \times 10^{-8}$). Sex-specific analysis identified genome-wide significant association of the variant rs77178854, located within *DPP10* gene in females only ($P = 2.21 \times 10^{-9}$). There were no genome-wide significant findings in the meta-analysis of males.

Conclusions: We identified two biologically plausible novel loci associated with PTH levels, providing us with further insights into the genetics of this complex trait.

Keywords: Parathyroid hormone, Genome-wide association analysis, Meta-analysis

Background

Parathyroid hormone (PTH) plays a critical role in the regulation of bone mineral metabolism and calcium homeostasis (DeLuca, 1986). PTH regulates serum calcium levels by stimulating osteoclast activity within bone in order to release calcium. Circulating PTH enhances the reabsorption of calcium in distal nephrons and induces the synthesis of the vitamin D active metabolite 1,25-dihydroxyvitamin D $(1,25(OH)_2D_3)$ within the kidney (Kumar & Thompson, 2011; Kumar et al., 1991; Khundmiri et al., 2016). The $1,25(OH)_2D_3$ stimulates intestinal calcium absorption and moreover, has a syner-

gistic effect with PTH in bone resorption by stimulating proliferation of osteoclasts (Kumar & Thompson, 2011; Kumar et al., 1991; Khundmiri et al., 2016).

Variations in PTH synthesis and secretion are regulated by serum levels of calcium and phosphate, as well as by $1,25(OH)_2D_3$ (Kumar & Thompson, 2011; Gago et al., 2005). Decreases in serum levels of calcium and increases in serum levels of phosphate stimulate the secretion of PTH, while $1,25(OH)_2D_3$ decreases PTH secretion (Silver & Levi, 2005). Regulation of PTH secretion in response to variations in serum calcium is mediated by the calcium-sensing receptors on the membrane of parathyroid cells (Kumar & Thompson, 2011; Brent et al., 1988). $1,25(OH)_2D_3$ associates with the vitamin D receptor and thus represses the transcription of PTH. The secretion of PTH is also indirectly altered by

* Correspondence: tzemunik@mefst.hr
[1]Department of Medical Biology, University of Split, School of Medicine, Šoltanska 2, Split, Croatia
Full list of author information is available at the end of the article

$1,25(OH)_2D_3$ and its regulation of calcium-sensing receptor expression (Kumar & Thompson, 2011). Serum phosphate regulates PTH mRNA and serum PTH levels independently of changes in either serum calcium or $1,25(OH)_2D_3$ levels (Kilav et al., 1995).

The most common pathological condition of excessive secretion of parathyroid hormone is hyperparathyroidism. Primary hyperparathyroidism is due to hypersecretion of the parathyroid gland, while secondary hyperparathyroidism can result from conditions that lead to hypocalcemia, especially observed in patients with chronic kidney disease (Fraser, 2009). Hypoparathyroidism, parathyroid hormone deficiency, is an uncommon condition that occurs mostly due to surgical removal of the parathyroid gland (Abate & Clarke, 2017).

Both environmental and genetic factors influence serum PTH levels. It is estimated that 60% of the variation in PTH concentrations is genetically determined. (Hunter et al., 2001). However, the genetic background underlying PTH level is not yet well understood.

Only one high-density genome-wide association study (GWAS) of PTH concentration has been reported to date (Robinson-Cohen et al., 2017). Robinson-Cohen et al. identified five significantly associated loci, including the strongest associated SNP rs6127099 located upstream of *CYP24A1*, a gene that encodes the primary catabolic enzyme for 1.25 $(OH)_2D$ (Robinson-Cohen et al., 2017). The other significantly associated loci were intronic variant rs4074995 within *RGS14* (regulator of G-protein signaling 14), rs219779 adjacent to *CLDN14* (Claudin 14), rs4443100 located near *RTDR1* (RSPH14, radial spoke head 14 homolog) and rs73186030 located near *CASR* (calcium-sensing receptor) gene (Robinson-Cohen et al., 2017). However, only three of these five loci (rs6127099, rs4074995 and rs219779) were replicated within an independent sample. Altogether, the five reported loci explained only 4.2% of the variance in circulating PTH, suggesting that additional genetic variants remain undiscovered.

The aim of our study is identification of novel loci associated with the parathyroid function, by performing a GWAS meta-analysis of plasma PTH levels within two genetically isolated Croatian populations (Korcula and Vis) following by replication analysis in the urban population of Split. To maximize the power of the study, we additionally performed meta-analysis for PTH plasma levels in all three Croatian populations. We also conducted gender-specific GWAS meta-analyses.

Methods
Study cohorts

This study was performed on samples from three Croatian populations: from the Dalmatian islands of Korcula and Vis and the mainland city of Split, within the large-scale project of "10,001 Dalmatians" (Rudan et al., 2009). A detailed description of the cohorts is provided in Table 1. The Korcula population is genetically isolated from Croatian Mainland, while Vis population is genetically isolated from Croatian Mainland and surrounding islands (Vitart et al., 2008). For all study populations, we excluded participants who underwent parathyroid surgery, as well as individuals who had PTH level < 5 pg/ml, which is near the minimum PTH assay detection limit (4.3 pg/ml). After these exclusions, the number of individuals available with PTH level and genotype data was 806 in Korcula, 831 in Vis and 959 in Split. In all three cohorts there were no participants who reported serious renal disease that could affect PTH concentration. The study was approved by the Research Ethics Committees in Croatia and Scotland and all participants provided informed consent. All analyses were in accordance with the relevant guidelines and regulations.

Genotyping and imputation

Additional file 1: Table S1 shows cohort-summary information on genotyping, imputation and quality control procedures. The final numbers of single nucleotide polymorphisms (SNPs) included in analyses were 9,182,797 for the Korcula sample, 8,865,173 for the Vis sample and 8,777,560 for the Split sample. The number of overlapping SNPs present in all three cohorts was 7,411,206.

Table 1 Characteristics of study participants

Variables	Korcula	Vis	Split
N with PTH and GWAS data	863	834	960
N underwent parathyroid surgery	1	0	1
N with PTH level < 5 pg/ml	56	3	3
Sample size used in the analyses	806	831	959
Women, N (%)	524 (65%)	486 (58%)	586 (61%)
Median age, (q_L,q_U)	57 (47, 67)	57 (45,69)	52 (40, 61)
Median PTH, pg/ml (q_L,q_U)	19.9 (13.7, 29.1)	25.9 (18.4, 32.1)	21.6 (17.2, 26.5)

N: number of individuals; q_L: lower quartile, q_U: upper quartile

Measurement of PTH

Plasma PTH levels were determined by radio-immunoassay method (RIA) in the Laboratory of Bio-chemistry, Department of Nuclear Medicine, University Hospital Split. RIA ran on the Scintillation counter liquid samples, Capintec, and 125I served as a marker. The concentrations of PTH in the plasma were determined using commercial kits (DIAsource hPTH -120 min-IRMA Kit, DIAsource ImmunoAssays S.A, Belgium). The reference range of plasma PTH levels is 12.26–35.50 pg/ml.

Statistical analyses

We performed genome-wide association analysis within each data set and then conducted a meta-analysis of two genetically isolated cohorts (Korcula and Vis) followed by replication analysis in the cohort of the mainland city of Split. To maximize the study power, we also performed a further meta-analysis of all three cohorts.

Genome-wide association analyses

Association analysis for the Split sample was carried out using a combination of R-package GenABEL and SNPTEST software, while for the Korcula and Vis samples analyses were conducted using R-packages GenABEL and VariABEL (Aulchenko et al., 2007; Marchini et al., 2007; Struchalin et al., 2012).

PTH levels were adjusted for age and sex using linear regression analysis and the calculated residuals were inverse-Gaussian transformed to achieve a normal distribution. GWAS was performed on transformed residuals using linear mixed model which accounts for population structure and relatedness. Association statistics for each SNP, including effect size estimates (β-estimates), standard errors and p-values were calculated under an additive genetic model.

Prior to performing the meta-analysis we calculated genomic inflation factors (lambdas) in individual data sets. No adjustments were necessary ($\lambda_{Korcula} = 1.026$, $\lambda_{Vis} = 1.001$, $\lambda_{Split} = 0.99$).

Meta-analysis

Meta-analysis was carried out using the R-package MetABEL (R: A Language and Environment for Statistical Computing, 2018). Meta-analysis was conducted using the inverse-variance fixed-effects method on overlapping SNPs based on the β-estimates and standard errors from each study. Meta-analyses showed no significant evidence for inflated statistics (both $\lambda_{Korcula - Vis}$ and $\lambda_{Korcula - Vis - Split}$ were 1.01), thus no genomic correction was applied. To visualize results of the meta-analysis, Manhattan and quantile-quantile (QQ) plots were created using R-package qqman (Turner, 2014). Regional association plots for loci of interest

(±400 kb) were produced using Locus Zoom based on hg19 genome build and 1000 genomes EUR population as the linkage disequilibrium (LD) population (Pruim et al., 2010). Forest plots for the most associated SNP were created using R-package MetABEL. To confirm the genotyping quality for the most associated SNPs in the regions, cluster plots were visually inspected using the Illumina GenomeStudio software package. If the SNP of interest was not directly genotyped, but imputed, then cluster plots were examined for directly genotyped SNPs in high LD with the SNP of interest ($r^2 > 0.8$), located on the same chromosome and less than 400 kb apart. A genome-wide significance of association was defined as $p - value \leq 5 \times 10^{-8}$. Power calculations were performed using Quanto version 1.2.4 for quantitative traits (WJ MJ, 2006).

Sex-specific analyses

In order to identify sex-specific effects we performed GWAS analyzing males and females separately in each cohort. We used the same procedures as in the primary analyses with the exception of the gender covariate. Association results were meta-analyzed using the inverse-variance fixed-effects method. The total sample sizes were 1596 in women and 1000 in men.

Results
Meta-analyses

In each population, a separate genome-wide association study of PTH levels was conducted. We meta-analyzed two genetically isolated cohorts, Korcula and Vis (Additional file 1: Figure S1), and then replicated results in the Split population. A total of 1637 individuals were included in the meta-analysis and 959 in the replication analysis (Table 1). The most associated SNP was rs4616742 (reference allele C, $\beta = 0.18$, $SE = 0.04$, $P = 4.42 \times 10^{-7}$). The SNP is located near protein coding gene *RASGEF1B* (RASGEF Domain Family Member 1B). All top SNPs, located on the chromosome 4 near *RASGEF1B* gene with $P < 10^{-6}$ from meta-analysis of 'genetically isolated populations' reached $P < 0.05$ in the Split population.

To maximize the study power, we performed a meta-analysis of all three cohorts. In total, 2596 individuals were included in the meta-analysis (Table 1). The results are shown in Fig. 1a. As seen from the quantile-quantile plot there was no early deviation from expected P values (Fig. 1b). Four SNPs, representing one locus, reached genome-wide significance. As in the meta-analysis of two genetically isolated cohorts, SNPs with the lowest P-values were located on chromosome 4 near *RASGEF1B*. The most associated SNP was rs11099476 ($P = 1.15 \times 10^{-8}$), which explained 1.14% of the variance in PTH. We found the T allele of the rs11099476 to be associated

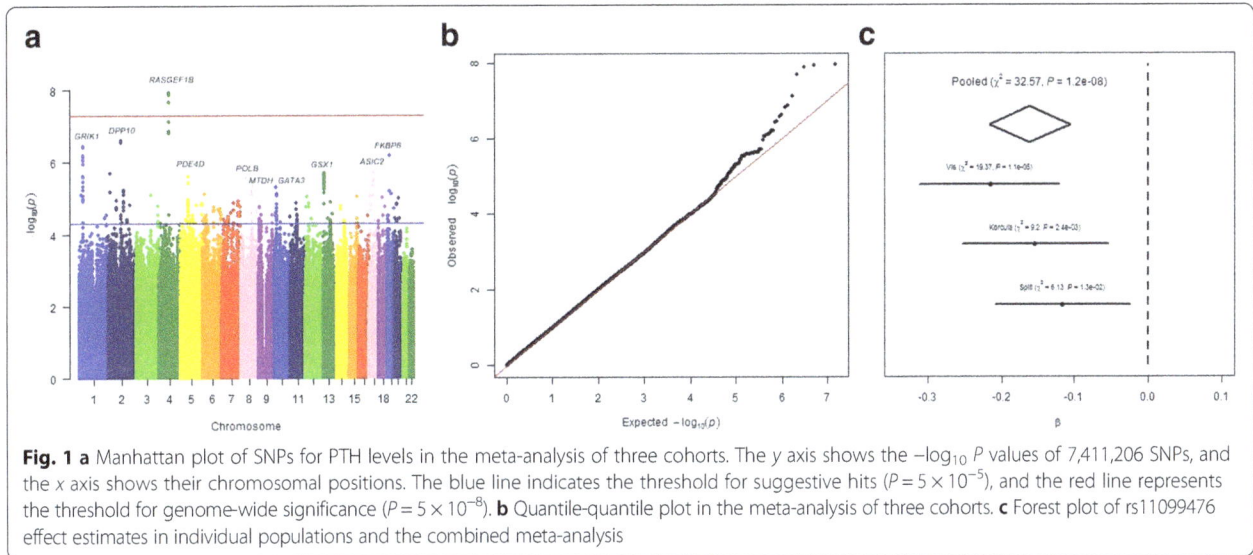

Fig. 1 a Manhattan plot of SNPs for PTH levels in the meta-analysis of three cohorts. The y axis shows the $-\log_{10} P$ values of 7,411,206 SNPs, and the x axis shows their chromosomal positions. The blue line indicates the threshold for suggestive hits ($P = 5 \times 10^{-5}$), and the red line represents the threshold for genome-wide significance ($P = 5 \times 10^{-8}$). **b** Quantile-quantile plot in the meta-analysis of three cohorts. **c** Forest plot of rs11099476 effect estimates in individual populations and the combined meta-analysis

with higher PTH level ($\beta = 0.16$, $SE = 0.03$). Effect sizes were in the same direction across all three cohorts (Fig. 1c). The regional association plot for rs11099476 is given in Fig. 2a. The identified SNP, rs11099476, is in high LD with the top SNP from meta-analysis of 'genetically isolated populations', rs4616742 ($r^2 = 0.9$). These results indicated that associated locus is becoming more significant as the sample size increases and confirmed the consistency of our top finding.

Analysis also revealed several suggestive loci ($P < 5 \times 10^{-6}$), including rs77178854 in the *DPP10* gene ($P = 2.46 \times 10^{-7}$), rs481121 near the *GRIK3* gene ($P = 3.58 \times 10^{-7}$), rs76615278 in the *FKBP8* gene ($P = 6.34 \times 10^{-7}$), rs1875872 near the *ASIC2* gene ($P = 1.94 \times 10^{-6}$), rs9512841 near the *GSX1* gene ($P = 2.01 \times 10^{-6}$), rs191686630 in the *PDE4D* gene, rs3136797 in the *POLB* gene ($P = 2.68 \times 10^{-6}$), rs499177 near the *MTDH* gene and rs58726672 near the *GATA3* gene ($P = 4.77 \times 10^{-6}$) (Table 2).

Sex-specific analyses

We searched for gender-specific loci by performing sex-specific GWAS meta-analysis, analyzing females and males separately in each cohort. The results for females are shown in Fig. 3. The top hit detected in the meta-analysis of all three cohorts, rs77178854, located within *DPP10* gene, reached genome-wide significance (reference allele C, $\beta = 0.82$, $SE = 0.14$, $P = 2.21 \times 10^{-9}$) in females (Table 3). Effect sizes were in the same direction across all three cohorts (Fig. 3c). Regional association plot of the identified SNP is shown in Fig. 2b. No single locus reaching genome wide significance was identified in males (Additional file 1: Table S2).

Discussion

In this GWAS meta-analysis of three Croatian populations we identified a novel genome-wide significant locus associated with plasma PTH level near gene *RASGEF1B* on chromosome 4. We also identified a sex-specific significant association in females in the *DPP10* gene.

The significance of the identified polymorphism rs11099476 was most influenced by the Vis population, which is isolated from the Croatian Mainland and surrounding islands, then by the Korcula population which is isolated from the Croatian Mainland and the least contributed by the mainland city of Split population (Fig. 2c). However, although the locus significance was most affected by the isolated populations, significance has been amplified in the meta-analysis of all three cohorts compared to meta-analysis of 'genetically isolated populations'.

The identified common variant rs11099476 accounts for 1.14% of population variance in plasma PTH. *RASGEF1B* is the guanine nucleotide exchange factor with specificity for Rap2A, a member of Rap subfamily of Ras-like G proteins (Yaman et al., 2009). Rap2 subfamily contains Rap2A and Rap2B, which share about 90% sequence homology (Paganini et al., 2006). Rap2A protein binds GDP to GTP and exhibits a low intrinsic GTPase activity in the presence of Mg^{2+} (Lerosey et al., 1991), while Rap2B increases intracellular calcium level and phosphorylation level of extracellular signal-related kinase (ERK) 1/2 (Di et al., 2015). Variations near *RASGEF1B* gene have been associated with height (He et al., 2015; Allen et al., 2010). Height is positively correlated with calcium absorption efficiency which is important determinant of calcium balance (Abrams et al., 2005). Some evidence of association was also found for variations in this gene and bone density, hip, and cystatin C

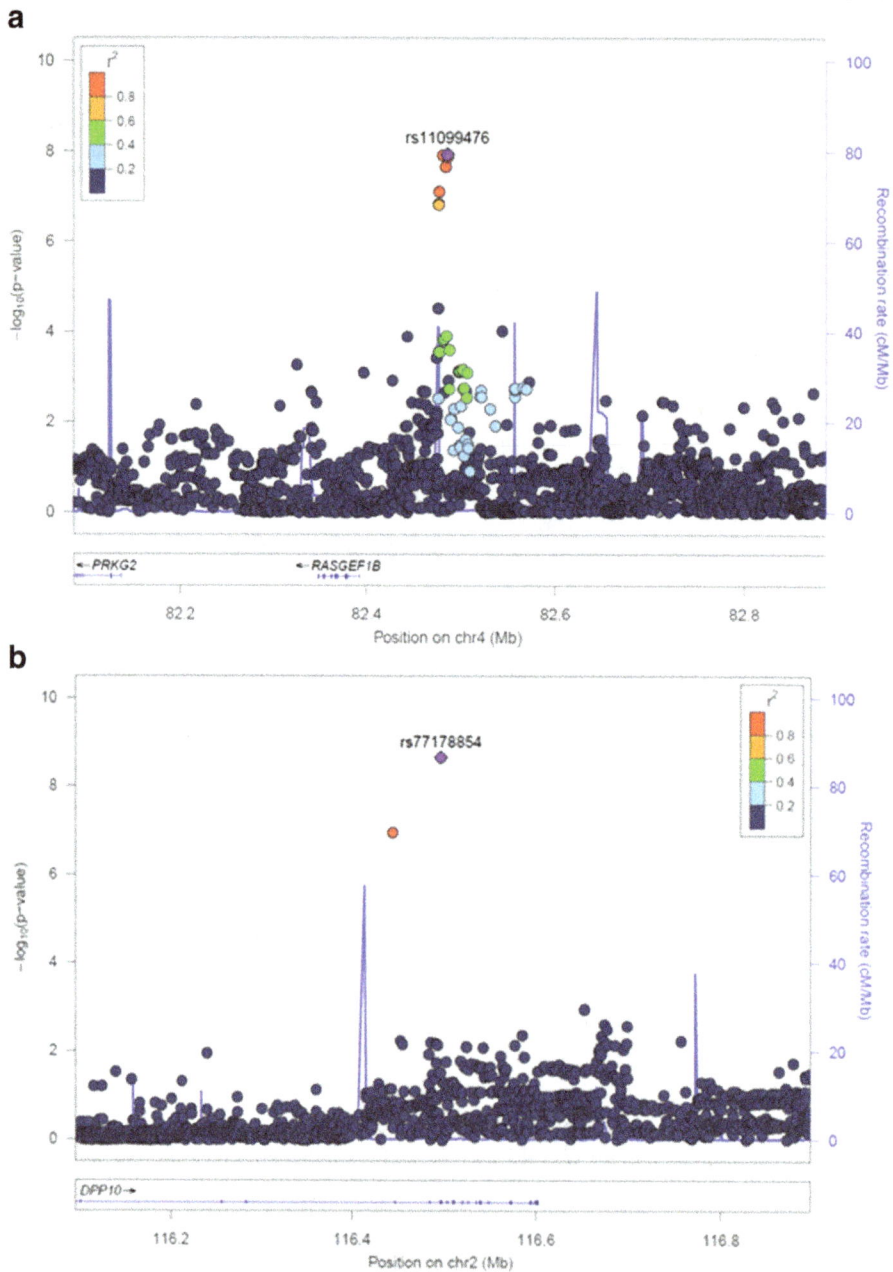

Fig. 2 a Regional association plot for the chromosome 4 locus rs11099476 in the meta-analysis of three cohorts. **b** Regional association plot for the chromosome 2 locus rs77178854 in the sex-stratified meta-analysis of three cohorts among females. SNPs are plotted by position against association with PTH (−log10 P values). The purple diamond highlights the most significant, whereas the colors of other variant represent LD with most significant SNP

in serum (Kiel et al., 2007; Kottgen et al., 2010). PTH is a significant negative predictor of bone mineral density at the hip (Sneve et al., 2008). Cystatin C in serum is a biomarker of kidney function, and chronic kidney disease (Kottgen et al., 2010). Disturbed kidney function can influence PTH stimulated calcium reabsorption and synthesis of 1,25(OH)$_2$D$_3$ (Kumar & Thompson, 2011; Kumar et al., 1991; Khundmiri et al., 2016). However, to understand the mechanism underlying the observed

association further functional studies of *RASGEF1B* will be needed.

Although no signals other than rs11099476 reached genome-wide significance, several candidate loci showed suggestive evidence of association. Particularly interesting is the variant near *GATA3* gene since mutations in this gene are the cause of hypoparathyroidism with sensorineural deafness and renal dysplasia (Van Esch et al., 2000). Of note, in a previous large GWA meta-analysis, variant

Table 2 Associations of top single nucleotide polymorphisms($P < 5 \times 10^{-6}$) with PTH concentrations

SNP	Chr	Position	Nearest Gene	Effect Allele	Other Allele	EAF Korcula	EAF Vis	EAF Split	GnomAD EAF	β	SE	P value
rs11099476	4	82,486,056	RASGEF1B	T	A	0.57	0.55	0.54	0.59	0.16	0.03	1.15×10^{-8}
rs77178854	2	116,496,539	DPP10	C	G	0.97	0.98	0.99	0.98	0.58	0.11	2.46×10^{-7}
rs481121	1	37,203,485	GRIK1	A	G	0.56	0.56	0.58	0.49	0.14	0.03	3.58×10^{-7}
rs76615278	19	18,654,588	FKBP8	G	A	0.84	0.83	0.82	*	0.20	0.04	6.34×10^{-7}
rs1875872	17	31,795,716	ASIC2	A	G	0.62	0.65	0.65	0.65	0.14	0.03	1.94×10^{-6}
rs9512841	13	28,309,646	GSX1	G	A	0.51	0.52	0.53	0.58	0.13	0.03	2.01×10^{-6}
rs191686630	5	58,477,398	PDE4D	A	T	0.11	0.16	0.21	*	0.19	0.04	2.36×10^{-6}
rs3136797	8	42,226,805	POLB	C	G	0.98	0.99	0.98	0.99	0.57	0.12	2.68×10^{-6}
rs499177	8	98,472,201	MTDH	T	C	0.46	0.57	0.45	0.44	0.13	0.03	4.66×10^{-6}
rs58726672	10	8,407,822	GATA3	C	T	0.98	0.98	0.98	0.98	0.57	0.13	4.77×10^{-6}

Top SNPs were defined as the SNP with lowest P value within a 500 kb window
Chr: chromosome; EAF: effect allele frequency; GnomAD EAF: effect allele frequency from Genome Aggregation Database; β: effect size; SE: standard error
*variants without frequency information in Genome Aggregation Database

near *GATA3* gene was found to be associated with serum calcium (O'Seaghdha et al., 2013).

Given the reported differences in PTH level between males and females, we performed sex-specific analyses (Wei et al., 2015; Serdar et al., 2017). Our study supports the sex-specificity underlying PTH level. Sex-stratified analysis in women identified a novel locus associated with PTH. The identified locus is the intron variant rs77178854, located within *DPP10* gene. *DPP10* encodes a membrane protein that is a member of the serine proteases family, which binds specific voltage-gated potassium channels and alters their expression and biophysical properties. It is highly expressed in brain, pancreas, spinal cord and adrenal gland (Allen et al., 2003), and may serve as a prognostic marker in colorectal cancer (Park et al., 2013). It is interesting to note that Aigner et al. showed that high serum PTH concentrations were associated with distal colorectal cancer in women but not in men (Aigner et al., 2015). The existence of *DPP10* in endocrine cells indicate that the protein might also have an additional role in the regulation of hormone secretion (Bezerra et al., 2015), which also supports our finding. Further studies of *DPP10* will be needed to clarify this result.

The only previously published high-density GWAS for PTH levels did not identify *RASGEF1B* or *DPP10* at a genome-wide significant level, despite having a sample size of over 29,155 participants (22, 653 in discovery stage and 6502 in replication analysis) (Robinson-Cohen et al., 2017). The possible explanation could be an increased relative effect of these loci in our populations due to the reduced genetic and environmental heterogeneity found in two out of three cohorts (i.e., Korcula and Vis) (Rudan et al., 2008) compared to the urban populations used in the

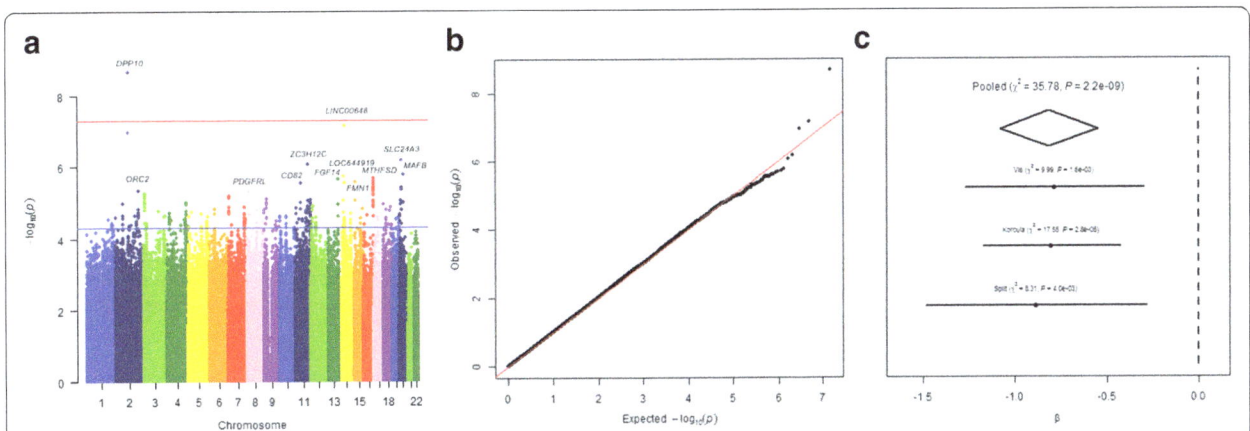

Fig. 3 a Manhattan plot of SNPs for PTH levels in the sex-stratified meta-analysis of three cohorts among females. The y axis shows the $-\log_{10} P$ values of 7,411,206 SNPs, and the x axis shows their chromosomal positions. The blue line indicates threshold for suggestive hits ($P = 5 \times 10^{-5}$), and red line represents the threshold for genome-wide significance ($P = 5 \times 10^{-8}$). **b** Quantile-quantile plot in the sex-stratified meta-analysis of three cohorts among females. **c** Forest plot of rs77178854 effect estimates in individual populations and the combined meta-analysis among females

Table 3 Associations of top single nucleotide polymorphisms($P < 5 \times 10^{-6}$) with PTH concentrations among females

SNP	Chr	Position	Nearest Gene	Effect Allele	Other Allele	EAF Korcula	EAF Vis	EAF Split	GnomAD EAF	β	SE	P value
rs77178854	2	116,496,539	DPP10	C	G	0.98	0.97	0.99	0.98	0.82	0.14	2.21×10^{-9}
rs1890709	14	49,101,833	LINC00648	A	G	0.38	0.30	0.33	0.31	0.20	0.04	7.12×10^{-8}
rs16981087	20	19,739,954	SLC24A3	G	C	0.80	0.78	0.77	0.81	0.22	0.04	6.99×10^{-7}
rs661171	11	110,016,519	ZC3H12C	G	T	0.74	0.70	0.71	0.70	0.20	0.04	8.94×10^{-7}
rs74629672	20	39,105,870	MAFB	T	A	0.95	0.94	0.94	0.96	0.43	0.09	1.68×10^{-6}
rs1349573	14	41,403,160	LOC644919	G	A	0.05	0.05	0.06	0.03	0.45	0.10	1.94×10^{-6}
rs3866634	16	86,567,929	MTHFSD	G	A	0.93	0.92	0.93	0.91	0.32	0.07	2.14×10^{-6}
rs7997888	13	102,759,325	FGF14	A	G	0.04	0.04	0.04	0.15	0.49	0.10	2.19×10^{-6}
rs5024438	15	33,077,401	FMN1	G	A	0.72	0.70	0.79	*	0.23	0.05	2.76×10^{-6}
rs77796218	11	44,580,581	CD82	C	T	0.97	0.96	0.97	0.98	0.49	0.10	2.84×10^{-6}
rs13406545	2	201,792,123	ORC2	T	A	0.15	0.19	0.18	0.23	0.21	0.05	4.54×10^{-6}
rs2588129	8	17,462,468	PDGFRL	A	G	0.04	0.02	0.02	0.11	0.54	0.12	4.57×10^{-6}

Top SNPs were defined as the SNP with lowest P value within a 500 kb window

Chr: chromosome; EAF: effect allele frequency; GnomAD EAF: effect allele frequency from Genome Aggregation Database; β: effect size; SE: standard error
*variants without frequency information in Genome Aggregation Database

analysis of Robinson-Cohen et al. *(Robinson-Cohen et al., 2017)*. Previously reported *CYP24A1*, *RGS14* and *CLDN14* variants associated with PTH level (Robinson-Cohen et al., 2017) had the same directions of effect in our study as originally reported but did not show significant associations, probably due to limited sample size of our study or specificity of isolated populations (Additional file 1: Table S3).

The greatest strengths of our study include a comprehensive set of genetic variants examined and ethnically homogeneous sample. We had sufficient data to confidently detect an association for the identified *RASGEF1B* locus, since our meta-analysis had 92% power to detect associated SNP with an effect size of 0.19 and minor allele frequency of 0.45 at the genome-wide level of significance. Furthermore, meta-analysis performed in females only had 86% power to detect *DPP10* locus with an effect size of 0.82 and minor allele frequency of 0.02 at the genome-wide level of significance. Meta-analysis performed in males only had 84% power to detect SNPs with an effect size of 0.35 and minor allele frequency of 0.3 at the genome-wide level of significance. The main limitation of our study is the modest sample size used in the analysis, reducing statistical power for detecting additional associations with smaller effect sizes or minor allele frequencies. Nevertheless, we have identified novel, previously unsuspected and biological plausible associations with PTH variation. Further replication analysis would be required to confirm our findings and to discover additional genetic variants underlying PTH levels in order to explain more of the variability in PTH variations.

Conclusions

In summary, in a GWA meta-analysis of PTH levels we identified a novel significant locus rs11099476 located near a guanine nucleotide exchange factor *RASGEF1B*. The finding appears to be consistent based on analyses of meta-GWAS across all three analyzed cohorts and meta-GWAS across two isolated populations followed by replication analysis in the mainland cohort. Our work also includes the first gender-specific GWAS performed to date and revealed significant association for an intron variant rs77178854 located within the *DPP10* gene in women, indicating the possibility that sex-specificity is underlying PTH level. To conclude, findings from this study improve the current knowledge of the genetic factors regulating PTH levels and their validation in independent populations would be beneficial.

Abbreviations
GWAS: genome-wide association study; PTH: Parathyroid hormone; RIA: radio-immunoassay method; SNP: single nucleotide polymorphism

Acknowledgments
We would like to thank all participants of this study and acknowledge invaluable support of the local teams in Zagreb and Split, especially that of the Institute for Anthropological Research, Zagreb, Croatia.

Funding
The Croatian Science Foundation funded this work under the project "Identification of new genetic loci implicated in regulation of thyroid and parathyroid function" (grant no. 1498).
The "10 001 Dalmatians" project was funded by grants from the Medical Research Council (UK), European Commission Framework 6 project

EUROSPAN (Contract No.LSHG-CT-2006-018947), the Republic of Croatia Ministry of Science, Education and Sports research grant (216–1080315-0302), the Croatian Science Foundation (grant 8875), CEKOM (Ministry of Economy, Entrepreneurship and Crafts) and the Research Centre of Excellence in Personalized Medicine (Ministry of Science and Education).

Authors' contributions

TZ conceived the study idea; OP, CH, TZ, VBP, IK and MB formed the biobank "10 001 Dalmatians"; VT, DB and AP performed the measurements of parathyroid hormones and verified the relevance of the results; TB performed imputation of the data; AM, MP, IG researched the data; AM performed the statistical analysis and drafted the manuscript; TZ, CH, MB, MP, IG, VBP and OP contributed to the discussion, review and editing of the manuscript; all authors approved the final version of the manuscript.

Competing interests

The authors declare that they have no competing interests.

Author details

[1]Department of Medical Biology, University of Split, School of Medicine, Šoltanska 2, Split, Croatia. [2]Department of Nuclear Medicine, University Hospital Split, Spinciceva 1, Split, Croatia. [3]MRC Human Genetics Unit, University of Edinburgh, Western General Hospital, Crewe Road, Edinburgh, UK. [4]Department of Public Health, University of Split, School of Medicine Split, Šoltanska 2, Split, Croatia.

References

Abate EG, Clarke BL. Review of hypoparathyroidism. Front Endocrinol. 2017;7

Abrams SA, Griffin IJ, Hawthorne KM, Liang LL. Height and height Z-score are related to calcium absorption in five- to fifteen-year-old girls. Journal of Clinical Endocrinology & Metabolism. 2005;90:5077–81.

Aigner E, Stadlmayr A, Huber-Schonauer U, Zwerina J, Husar-Memmer E, Niederseer D, Eder SK, Stickel F, Pirich C, Schett G, et al. Parathyroid hormone is related to dysplasia and a higher rate of distal colorectal adenoma in women but not men. Hormones & Cancer. 2015;6:153–60.

Allen HL, Estrada K, Lettre G, Berndt SI, Weedon MN, Rivadeneira F, Willer CJ, Jackson AU, Vedantam S, Raychaudhuri S, et al. Hundreds of variants clustered in genomic loci and biological pathways affect human height. Nature. 2010;467:832–8.

Allen M, Heinzmann A, Noguchi E, Abecasis G, Broxholme J, Ponting CP, Bhattacharyya S, Tinsley J, Zhang YM, Holt R, et al. Positional cloning of a novel gene influencing asthma from chromosome 2q14. Nat Genet. 2003;35: 258–63.

Aulchenko YS, Ripke S, Isaacs A, Van Duijn CM. GenABEL: an R library for genome-wide association analysis. Bioinformatics. 2007;23:1294–6.

Bezerra GA, Dobrovetsky E, Seitova A, Fedosyuk S, Dhe-Paganon S, Gruber K. Structure of human dipeptidyl peptidase 10 (DPPY): a modulator of neuronal Kv4 channels. Sci Rep. 2015;5

Brent GA, Leboff MS, Seely EW, Conlin PR, Brown EM. Relationship between the concentration and rate of change of calcium and serum intact parathyroid-hormone levels in normal humans. Journal of Clinical Endocrinology & Metabolism. 1988;67:944–50.

DeLuca HF. The metabolism and functions of vitamin D. Adv Exp Med Biol. 1986; 196:361–75.

Di JH, Huang H, Qu DB, Tang JJ, Cao WJ, Lu Z, Cheng Q, Yang J, Bai J, Zhang YP, Zheng JN. Rap2B promotes proliferation, migration, and invasion of human breast cancer through calcium-related ERK1/2 signaling pathway. Sci Rep. 2015;5

Fraser WD. Hyperparathyroidism. Lancet. 2009;374:145–58.

Gago EV, Cadarso-Suarez C, Perez-Fernandez R, Burgos RR, Mugica JD, Iglesias CS. Association between vitamin D receptor FokI polymorphism and serum parathyroid hormone level in patients with chronic renal failure. J Endocrinol Investig. 2005;28:117–21.

He MA, Xu M, Zhang B, Liang J, Chen P, Lee JY, Johnson TA, Li HX, Yang XB, Dai JC, et al. Meta-analysis of genome-wide association studies of adult height in east Asians identifies 17 novel loci. Hum Mol Genet. 2015;24:1791–800.

Hunter D, De Lange M, Snieder H, MacGregor AJ, Swaminathan R, Thakker RV, Spector TD. Genetic contribution to bone metabolism, calcium excretion, and vitamin D and parathyroid hormone regulation. J Bone Miner Res. 2001; 16:371–8.

Khundmiri SJ, Murray RD, Lederer E. PTH and vitamin D. Comprehensive Physiology. 2016;6:561–601.

Kiel DP, Demissie S, Dupuis J, Lunetta KL, Murabito JM, Karasik D. Genome-wide association with bone mass and geometry in the Framingham heart study. Bmc Medical Genetics. 2007;8

Kilav R, Silver J, Navehmany T. Parathyroid-hormone gene-expression in Hypophosphatemic rats. J Clin Investig. 1995;96:327–33.

Kottgen A, Pattaro C, Boger CA, Fuchsberger C, Olden M, Glazer NL, Parsa A, Gao XY, Yang Q, Smith AV, et al. New loci associated with kidney function and chronic kidney disease. Nat Genet. 2010;42:376–U334.

Kumar R, Cahan DH, Madias NE, Harrington JT, Kurtin P, Dawsonhughes BF. Vitamin-D and calcium-transport. Kidney Int. 1991;40:1177–89.

Kumar R, Thompson JR. The regulation of parathyroid hormone secretion and synthesis. J Am Soc Nephrol. 2011;22:216–24.

Lerosey I, Chardin P, Degunzburg J, Tavitian A. The product of the Rap2 gene, member of the Ras superfamily - biochemical-characterization and site-directed mutagenesis. J Biol Chem. 1991;266:4315–21.

Marchini J, Howie B, Myers S, McVean G, Donnelly P. A new multipoint method for genome-wide association studies by imputation of genotypes. Nat Genet. 2007;39:906–13.

O'Seaghdha CM, Wu HS, Yang Q, Kapur K, Guessous I, Zuber AM, Kottgen A, Stoudmann C, Teumer A, Kutalik Z, et al. Meta-analysis of genome-wide association studies identifies six new loci for serum calcium concentrations. PLoS Genet. 2013;9

Paganini S, Guidetti GF, Catricala S, Trionfini P, Panelli S, Balduini C, Torti M. Identification and biochemical characterization of Rap2C, a new member of the rap family of small GTP-binding proteins. Biochimie. 2006;88:285–95.

Park HS, Yeo HY, Chang HJ, Kim KH, Park JW, Kim BC, Baek JY, Kim SY, Kim DY. Dipeptidyl peptidase 10, a novel prognostic marker in colorectal Cancer. Yonsei Med J. 2013;54:1362–9.

Pruim RJ, Welch RP, Sanna S, Teslovich TM, Chines PS, Gliedt TP, Boehnke M, Abecasis GR, Willer CJ. LocusZoom: regional visualization of genome-wide association scan results. Bioinformatics. 2010;26:2336–7.

R: A Language and Environment for Statistical Computing 2018 [http://www.R-project.org/].

Robinson-Cohen C, Lutsey PL, Kleber ME, Nielson CM, Mitchell BD, Bis JC, Eny KM, Portas L, Eriksson J, Lorentzon M, et al. Genetic variants associated with circulating parathyroid hormone. J Am Soc Nephrol. 2017;28:1553–65.

Rudan I, Carothers AD, Polasek O, Hayward C, Vitart V, Biloglav Z, Kolcic I, Zgaga L, Ivankovic D, Vorko-Jovic A, et al. Quantifying the increase in average human heterozygosity due to urbanisation. Eur J Hum Genet. 2008;16:1097–102.

Rudan I, Marusic A, Jankovic S, Rotim K, Boban M, Lauc G, Grkovic I, Dogas Z, Zemunik T, Vatavuk Z, et al. "10 001 Dalmatians:" Croatia launches its National Biobank. Croatian Medical Journal. 2009;50:4–6.

Serdar MA, Can BB, Kilercik M, Durer ZA, Aksungar FB, Serteser M, Coskun A, Ozpinar A, Unsal I. Analysis of changes in parathyroid hormone and 25 (oh) vitamin D levels with respect to age, gender and season: a data mining study. Journal of Medical Biochemistry. 2017;36:73–83.

Silver J, Levi R. Regulation of PTH synthesis and secretion relevant to the management of secondary hyperparathyroidism in chronic kidney disease. Kidney Int. 2005;67:S8–S12.

Sneve M, Emaus N, Joakimsen RM, Jorde R. The association between serum parathyroid hormone and bone mineral density, and the impact of smoking: the Tromso study. Eur J Endocrinol. 2008;158:401–9.

Struchalin MV, Amin N, Eilers PHC, van Duijn CM, Aulchenko YS. An R package "VariABEL" for genome-wide searching of potentially interacting loci by testing genotypic variance heterogeneity. BMC Genet. 2012;13

Turner SD: qqman: an R package for visualizing GWAS results using Q-Q and manhattan plots. biorXiv DOI: 101101/005165 2014.

Van Esch H, Groenen P, Nesbit MA, Schuffenhauer S, Lichtner P, Vanderlinden G, Harding B, Beetz R, Bilous RW, Holdaway I, et al. GATA3 haplo-insufficiency causes human HDR syndrome. Nature. 2000;406:419–22.

Vitart V, Rudan I, Hayward C, Gray NK, Floyd J, Palmer CN, Knott SA, Kolcic I, Polasek O, Graessler J, et al. SLC2A9 is a newly identified urate transporter influencing serum urate concentration, urate excretion and gout. Nat Genet. 2008;40:437–42.

Wei QS, Chen ZQ, Tan X, Su HR, Chen XX, He W, Deng WM. Relation of age, sex and bone mineral density to serum 25-Hydroxyvitamin D levels in Chinese women and men. Orthop Surg. 2015;7:343–9.

Gauderman WJ MJ: QUANTO 1.1: a computer program for power and sample size calculations for genetic-epidemiology studies.: University of Southern California; 2006.

Yaman E, Gasper R, Koerner C, Wittinghofer A, Tazebay UH. RasGEF1A and RasGEF1B are guanine nucleotide exchange factors that discriminate between rap GTP-binding proteins and mediate Rap2-specific nucleotide exchange. FEBS J. 2009;276:4607–16.

12

Leukemia inhibitory factor inhibits erythropoietin-induced myelin gene expression in oligodendrocytes

Georgina Gyetvai, Cieron Roe, Lamia Heikal, Pietro Ghezzi[*] and Manuela Mengozzi

Abstract

Background: The pro-myelinating effects of leukemia inhibitory factor (LIF) and other cytokines of the gp130 family, including oncostatin M (OSM) and ciliary neurotrophic factor (CNTF), have long been known, but controversial results have also been reported. We recently overexpressed erythropoietin receptor (EPOR) in rat central glia-4 (CG4) oligodendrocyte progenitor cells (OPCs) to study the mechanisms mediating the pro-myelinating effects of erythropoietin (EPO). In this study, we investigated the effect of co-treatment with EPO and LIF.

Methods: Gene expression in undifferentiated and differentiating CG4 cells in response to EPO and LIF was analysed by DNA microarrays and by RT-qPCR. Experiments were performed in biological replicates of $N \geq 4$. Functional annotation and biological term enrichment was performed using DAVID (Database for Annotation, Visualization and Integrated Discovery). The gene-gene interaction network was visualised using STRING (Search Tool for the Retrieval of Interacting Genes).

Results: In CG4 cells treated with 10 ng/ml of EPO and 10 ng/ml of LIF, EPO-induced myelin oligodendrocyte glycoprotein (*MOG*) expression, measured at day 3 of differentiation, was inhibited ≥ 4-fold ($N = 5$, $P < 0.001$). Inhibition of EPO-induced *MOG* was also observed with OSM and CNTF. Analysis of the gene expression profile of CG4 differentiating cells treated for 20 h with EPO and LIF revealed LIF inhibition of EPO-induced genes involved in lipid transport and metabolism, previously identified as positive regulators of myelination in this system. In addition, among the genes induced by LIF, and not by differentiation or by EPO, the role of suppressor of cytokine signaling 3 (SOCS3) and toll like receptor 2 (TLR2) as negative regulators of myelination was further explored. LIF-induced *SOCS3* was associated with *MOG* inhibition; Pam3, an agonist of TLR2, inhibited EPO-induced *MOG* expression, suggesting that TLR2 is functional and its activation decreases myelination.

Conclusions: Cytokines of the gp130 family may have negative effects on myelination, depending on the cytokine environment.

Keywords: Central glia-4, Multiple sclerosis, Myelin oligodendrocyte glycoprotein, SOCS3, TLR2

Background

Oligodendrocytes (OLs), the myelinating cells of the central nervous system (CNS), produce the myelin sheath that provides physical protection and metabolic support to the axons and allows efficient conduction of action potential (Philips & Rothstein, 2017). In chronic inflammatory diseases, such as multiple sclerosis (MS), damage to OLs causes demyelination, impairs axonal function and leads to progressive degeneration of axons (Franklin & Gallo, 2014; Tauheed et al., 2016).

Remyelination, the process by which OL progenitor cells (OPCs) differentiate and mature to produce myelin that wraps demyelinated axons, can occur in the adult brain, where a wide-spread population of OPCs is present. Remyelination is usually highly efficient after injury and in the first stages of MS, but declines with aging and disease progression. Remyelination failure is a major determinant of progressive axonal degeneration and permanent neurological disability in chronic demyelinating

* Correspondence: P.Ghezzi@bsms.ac.uk
Department of Clinical and Experimental Medicine, Brighton & Sussex Medical School, Brighton BN1 9PS, UK

diseases. Since OPCs are present in adult aging brain and in MS lesions, a block in differentiation and not a lack of OPCs seems responsible for remyelination failure (Franklin & Gallo, 2014; Kremer et al., 2015; Chamberlain et al., 2016).

The main immunomodulating drugs approved for MS can delay disease progression but do not prevent progressive disability since do not repair existing damage. Remyelinating therapies are needed. In the last years, several remyelinating strategies have been attempted, and drugs that inhibit negative signals (e.g. antibodies to LINGO-1) or provide positive stimulation (e.g. clemastine fumarate) are in the translational pipeline, but no remyelinating drugs are currently available (Kremer et al., 2015; Cadavid et al., 2017; Green et al., 2017; Bove & Green, 2017).

The observations that remyelination can be achieved in aging brain when appropriate exogenous factors are provided (Ruckh et al., 2012) and transplantation of neuronal precursors increases remyelination mainly by immunomodulatory mechanisms (Martino & Pluchino, 2006) suggest that direct administration of neuroprotective factors, as opposed to transplantation of stem cells, might be a good remyelinating strategy.

In the last 20 years, erythropoietin (EPO) has emerged as a potential candidate for neuroprotective and neuroregenerative treatment in injury and disease of the nervous system (Sargin et al., 2010). Interestingly, EPO improves cognitive performance in healthy animals and humans and in disease, including in MS (Ehrenreich et al., 2007; Robinson et al., 2018; Li et al., 2018). Although the mechanism is still largely unknown, we and others showed that EPO acts directly on OLs to increase myelination in vitro and in vivo (Sugawa et al., 2002; Cervellini et al., 2013; Hassouna et al., 2016; Gyetvai et al., 2017).

In a recent study aimed at identifying cytokines exhibiting protective and regenerative functions similar to EPO by "functional clustering", leukemia inhibitory factor (LIF) emerged as one of the cytokines functionally similar to EPO (Mengozzi et al., 2014).

LIF is a member of the interleukin-6 (IL-6) cytokine family that signals through the LIF receptor (LIFR) and the cytokine receptor glycoprotein 130 (gp130), the latter shared with all the other cytokines of the IL-6 family, including ciliary neurotrophic factor (CNTF) and oncostatin M (OSM). LIF downstream signaling pathways include the JAK/STAT3, the PI3K/AKT and the MAPK/ERK pathways (Nicola & Babon, 2015; Davis & Pennypacker, 2018).

LIF is a pleiotropic cytokine that can have diverse and opposite effects on different cell types, resulting in stimulation or inhibition of cell proliferation, differentiation and inflammation (Nicola & Babon, 2015; Davis & Pennypacker, 2018; Slaets et al., 2010; Cao et al., 2011; Linker et al., 2008; Ulich et al., 1994). It is currently believed to play a crucial role in the response to injury, particularly in the CNS (Slaets et al., 2010). Its expression is increased in cerebral ischemia, spinal cord injury, Alzheimer's disease, Parkinson's disease, seizure and MS (Nicola & Babon, 2015; Slaets et al., 2010; Vanderlocht et al., 2006; Mashayekhi & Salehi, 2011).

In the CNS, LIF can act on immune, neuronal and glial cells (Davis & Pennypacker, 2018). Many studies point to a direct action on OLs. In particular, LIF is required in development for the correct maturation of OLs; in addition, in vivo and in vitro, both endogenous and exogenous LIF protect OLs from cell death and increase their proliferation, differentiation and maturation (Nicola & Babon, 2015; Davis & Pennypacker, 2018; Slaets et al., 2010; Stankoff et al., 2002; Ishibashi et al., 2006; Emery et al., 2006).

Studies in LIF knock-out mice and exogenous LIF administration have highlighted its protective action in many models of demyelination (Nicola & Babon, 2015; Davis & Pennypacker, 2018; Slaets et al., 2010; Emery et al., 2006; Marriott et al., 2008), suggesting the possible therapeutic use of LIF and LIF inducers in demyelinating diseases, including MS (Slaets et al., 2010; Vela et al., 2016; Metcalfe, 2018).

Coadministration of neuroprotective agents rather than a single agent may be more effective. In this regard, EPO was previously reported to synergise with insulin-like growth factor (IGF)-1 to protect against neuronal damage (Digicaylioglu et al., 2004; Kang et al., 2010).

We have previously used an in vitro model of myelination, CG4 OPC transduced to overexpress erythropoietin receptor (EPOR), to study the mechanisms by which EPO increases myelin gene expression (Gyetvai et al., 2017). Aim of this study was to investigate whether co-treatment with EPO and LIF was more effective than EPO alone and the mechanisms involved. Surprisingly, we found that LIF strongly inhibited EPO-induced myelination. By gene expression profiling, we investigated the mechanisms mediating LIF inhibitory effects at the early stage of the OL differentiation process.

Methods

Cell culture and generation of CG4 cells expressing EPOR

Rat CG4 OPC overexpressing the EPO receptor (CG4-EPOR) were generated and cultured as reported in our previous studies (Cervellini et al., 2013; Gyetvai et al., 2017). As previously shown, wild type CG4 do not express EPOR and do not respond to EPO (Cervellini et al., 2013). However, primary OLs express low levels of EPOR under physiological conditions (Sugawa et al., 2002), and EPOR is induced in the CNS in pathologies where EPO has protective functions (Siren et al., 2001); in particular, injury induces EPOR expression in OLs (Ott et al., 2015). By overexpressing EPOR in CG4 cells, we set up an in vitro system that allowed us to characterise the mechanisms mediating EPO differentiating and myelinating effects in

OLs, mimicking an in vivo situation of injury or disease, where EPOR would be up-regulated.

CG4-EPOR cells, for simplicity referred to as CG4, were used throughout this study. Briefly, CG4 cells were cultured in poly-L-ornithine-coated 6-well plates (320,000 cells in 4 ml of medium per well). They were maintained at the progenitor stage by culture in growth medium (GM), consisting of Dulbecco's modified Eagle medium (DMEM) (Sigma-Aldrich) supplemented with biotin (10 ng/ml), basic fibroblast growth factor (bFGF; 5 ng/ml), platelet-derived growth factor (PDGF; 1 ng/ml), N1 supplement (all from Sigma-Aldrich) and 30% B104-conditioned medium, obtained as previously reported (Cervellini et al., 2013; Gyetvai et al., 2017). After overnight culture, the cells were induced to differentiate into OLs by switching to differentiation-promoting medium (DM), consisting of DMEM-F12 (Invitrogen/ThermoFisher Scientific) supplemented with progesterone (3 ng/ml), putrescine (5 μg/ml), sodium selenite (4 ng/ml), insulin (12.5 μg/ml), transferrin (50 μg/ml), biotin (10 ng/ml), thyroxine (0.4 μg/ml) and glucose (3 g/l) (all from Sigma-Aldrich), as reported (Cervellini et al., 2013; Gyetvai et al., 2017). Undifferentiated cells are bipolar; after 2 days of differentiation the cells acquire about 90% of multipolar morphology. Differentiated CG4 cells express myelin proteins, including MOG, a marker of myelin deposition in these cells (Louis et al., 1992; Solly et al., 1996). After 3 h in DM, some of the cells were treated with recombinant human EPO (Creative Dynamics), recombinant mouse LIF (Sigma-Aldrich), recombinant rat OSM (Peprotech), recombinant rat CNTF (Peprotech), or Pam3CSK4 (Pam3; Invivo-Gen). Human EPO is approximately 80% homologous to rodent EPO, and it is biologically active on rat cells (Gyetvai et al., 2017). Mouse and rat LIF share 92% sequence homology (Willson et al., 1992), and mouse LIF is biologically active on rat cells (Takahashi et al., 1995).

RNA extraction

For the microarray experiment, total RNA was extracted and analysed as reported, using the miRNeasy system and protocol (QIAGEN) (Gyetvai et al., 2017). For all the other experiments, total RNA was extracted with QIAzol (QIAGEN), following the instructions of the manufacturer, and RNA purity and concentration were determined using a NanoDrop ND-1000 (NanoDrop Technologies/ThermoFisher Scientific).

RT-qPCR

Reverse transcription (RT) and real time qPCR were carried out as reported (Gyetvai et al., 2017; Mengozzi et al., 2012), using TaqMan® gene expression assays (Applied Biosystems/ThermoFisher Scientific) and Brilliant III qPCR master mix (Stratagene/Agilent Technologies).

Gene expression was quantified using the ΔΔCt method, according to Applied Biosystems' guidelines. Results were normalized to *HPRT1* expression (reference gene) and expressed as fold change (FC) or as $\log_2$ FC vs one of the control samples, chosen as the calibrator, as previously reported (Mengozzi et al., 2012).

Microarrays

All experimental conditions were performed in quadruplicate; undifferentiated cells were cultured in quadruplicate but only 3 random samples were used for microarray analysis and all of the 4 samples for qPCR validation. Results from 27 arrays are analysed and presented in this study: 3 undifferentiated (undif) and 4 differentiated (dif), 4 differentiated+EPO (EPO), 4 differentiated+EPO + LIF (EPO + LIF) at each time point (at 4 h and 23 h of differentiation; 1 h and 20 h after treatment with EPO and LIF respectively). RNA was amplified, labelled and hybridised onto Single Colour SurePrint G3 Rat GE 8x60K Microarrays (AMADID:028279; Agilent) at Oxford Gene Technology, Oxford, UK. Following hybridisation, the arrays were scanned to derive the array images. Feature extraction software v10.7.3.1 was used to generate the array data from the images.

Microarray data analysis

Raw data in standard format from the microarray experiment have been deposited in the Gene Expression Omnibus (GEO) database of the National Center for Biotechnology Information (NCBI) (Barrett et al., 2013) and are accessible through GEO Series accession number GSE84687 (http://www.ncbi.nlm.nih.gov/geo). Raw data were normalised and analysed using GeneSpring (Agilent) and Excel (Microsoft) softwares. Transcript expression levels ($\log_2$ of the gProcessed Signal) between the experimental groups were compared by Student's *t* test, obtaining uncorrected *P* values. Subsequent multiple comparison corrections were performed using the Benjamini-Hochberg (BH) False Discovery Rate (FDR) procedure, obtaining adjusted *P* values (BH adj. *P* values). Fold change in the expression was calculated as the ratio between the average of the gProcessed Signals of the various groups and expressed as $\log_2$. Differences in expression with a BH adj. *P* value < 0.05 and an absolute fold change ≥1.5 ($\log_2$ fold change ≥0.58) were considered statistically significant.

Functional annotation and biological term enrichment was performed using the DAVID v6.8 database (Database for Annotation, Visualization and Integrated Discovery) available online (https://david.ncifcrf.gov) (Huang da et al., 2009). Categories with *P* values < 0.05 were considered significantly enriched.

Gene-gene interaction networks were visualised using the STRING v10.5 database (Search Tool for the Retrieval of

Interacting Genes/Proteins) available online (http://string-db.org). STRING assigns to each reported functional association a confidence score, which is dependent on both the experimental method on which the functional association prediction is based, and on the reliability of computational approaches used for prediction. We used all active prediction methods, and a confidence score > 0.4.

Results

LIF induces *MOG* with a bell-shaped dose response curve

CG4 cells, a largely used in vitro model of myelination, can be differentiated to produce myelin proteins, including myelin basic protein (MBP), a marker of differentiation, and MOG, a marker of myelin deposition(Louis et al., 1992; Solly et al., 1996). In previous studies, we have validated this model and shown that expression of MOG mRNA correlated with production of the protein, measured by western blot (Cervellini et al., 2013). Therefore, in this study we measured MOG mRNA as a marker of myelination in differentiated CG4 cells.

CG4 cells were differentiated for 3 days in DM with or without increasing concentrations of LIF ranging from 0.004 to 10 ng/ml. LIF increased *MOG* expression with a peak at 0.2 ng/ml and had no effect at the higher dose of 10 ng/ml, showing a bell-shaped dose response curve (Fig. 1a). In contrast, our previous results had shown that in these cells EPO still increased *MOG* expression at high doses, up to 400 ng/ml, although the expression plateaus after 10 ng/ml (Cervellini et al., 2013).

LIF inhibits EPO-induced *MOG* expression

To investigate whether LIF synergised with EPO in increasing *MOG* expression, the cells were co-stimulated with EPO at 10 ng/ml and with LIF at 0.2 and 10 ng/ml. No synergistic or additive effect was observed; surprisingly, LIF markedly inhibited EPO-induced *MOG* expression at the high dose (10 ng/ml, Fig. 1b), and some inhibition was also observed at the low dose (0.2 ng/ml, Fig. 1c), which had a positive effect on *MOG* induction when added alone (Fig. 1a). Since EPO at high doses still increased MOG expression in these cells, as mentioned above and reported in a previous study (Cervellini et al., 2013), whereas LIF was less effective at high dose (10 ng/ml) than at low dose (0.2 ng/ml; Fig. 1a), these results suggest the LIF might induce a negative feedback that inhibits both its own and EPO's pro-myelinating effects.

Of note, LIF at 10 ng/ml inhibited also EPO-induced myelin basic protein (MBP) expression at the same time point (at day 3 of differentiation): *MBP* mRNA as FC vs control, mean ± SD, $N = 8$; EPO: 3.7 ± 1.3, $P < 0.001$ vs control; EPO + LIF: 1.5 ± 0.4, $P < 0.001$ vs EPO alone by two-tailed Student's t-test).

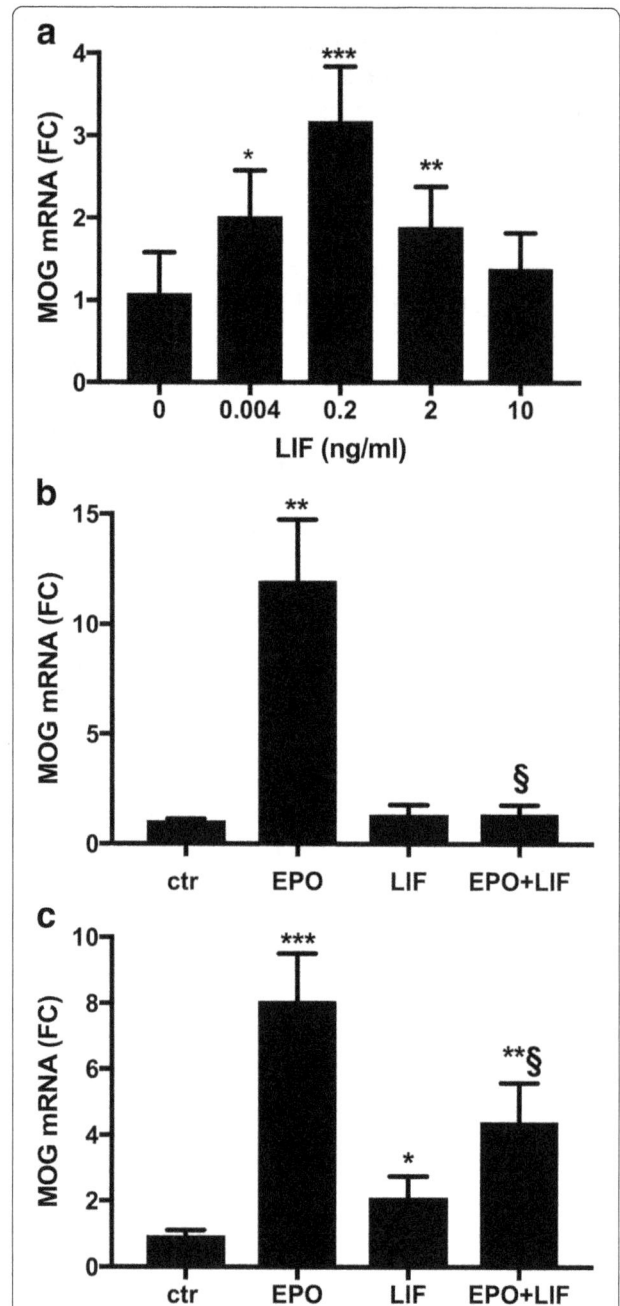

Fig. 1 LIF induces MOG mRNA with a bell-shaped dose-response curve and inhibits EPO-induced MOG expression. Cells cultured for 1 day in growth medium (GM) were switched to differentiation medium (DM). After 3 h in DM the cells were treated with the indicated concentrations of LIF (**a**) or with or without EPO (10 ng/ml) and LIF (10 ng/ml, panel **b**; 0.2 ng/ml, **c**). MOG gene expression was measured by RT-qPCR at day 3 of differentiation. Results are expressed as fold change (FC) vs one of the control samples (no LIF in panel **a** and ctr in **b** and **c**). Data are the mean ± SD of seven samples from two independent experiments assayed in duplicate (**a**) or of quadruplicate samples assayed in duplicate and representative or five (**b**) or two (**c**) independent experiments; * $P < 0.05$, **$P < 0.01$, ***$P < 0.001$ vs control; § $P < 0.01$ vs EPO alone by two-tailed Student's t-test

LIF-induced changes in gene expression

To investigate the mechanisms by which LIF inhibits EPO-induced myelin gene expression, we performed a gene expression microarray study to identify the genes regulated by LIF in cells co-cultured with EPO and LIF, in which EPO-induced myelin gene expression was inhibited. We reasoned that co-culture with LIF might inhibit the effect of EPO by two mechanisms: i) inhibiting the expression of "positive regulators" of myelination increased by EPO; ii) increasing the expression of "negative regulators" of myelination, which are likely to be unchanged or decreased by differentiation or by EPO.

Analysis of the transcripts regulated by differentiation and further regulated by addition of EPO at 1 h and 20 h has been reported elsewhere (Gyetvai et al., 2017). Here we focussed on the genes regulated by LIF, selected by comparing EPO + LIF vs EPO at 1 h and 20 h and setting a fold change (FC) cut-off of 1.5 ($\log_2$ FC 0.58) and P value < 0.05 after applying the BH correction for multiple tests.

Negative regulators of myelination induced by LIF at 1 h

The gene expression profile of EPO-treated CG4 cells at 1 h and the effect of differentiation alone, previously reported (Gyetvai et al., 2017), is summarised in Fig. 2a; differentiation affected 878 genes, of which 461 were upregulated and 417 downregulated; treatment of differentiating cells with EPO for 1 h affected only 5 genes, which were all upregulated. Only 3 of these were affected and further increased by LIF (Fig. 2a and Additional file 1).

Since at the early time point LIF did not inhibit any EPO-induced gene, we focussed on the idea that it might induce negative regulators of myelination, whose expression would likely be either unchanged or decreased by culture in DM with or without EPO. When comparing EPO + LIF vs EPO, 82 genes were increased (Fig. 2a). Of these, 7 genes were excluded because they were also increased by differentiation alone (4, Additional file 2) or by EPO (3, Additional file 1). Therefore 75 genes that were either downregulated or not changed by differentiation, not altered by EPO and finally upregulated by LIF remained.

Network analysis of the remaining 75 genes (28 + 47, Fig. 2a) using the STRING database highlighted hubs centered on *STAT3* and *SOCS3* which included *Myd88*, part of toll-like receptor (TLR) signaling (Fig. 2b). A list of all the 75 genes, their fold change in expression levels by LIF (EPO + LIF vs EPO) and by differentiation (differentiated vs undifferentiated) is reported in Additional file 3.

EPO-induced positive regulators of myelination inhibited by LIF at 20 h

The gene expression profile of EPO-treated CG4 cells and the effect of differentiation at 20 h have been previously reported (Gyetvai et al., 2017). In Fig. 3a, the genes affected by LIF have been included.

At this time point EPO increased the expression of a number of genes, potential positive regulators of myelination, including 43 genes upregulated also by differentiation alone and 113 unaffected by differentiation. Addition of LIF decreased 7 of the 43 genes increased by EPO and differentiation, and 9 of the 113 genes increased only by EPO, as summarized in the Venn diagram in Fig. 3b (left). We focussed on the 16 putative positive regulators of myelination inhibited by LIF (green arrows, Fig. 3b), listed in Table 1. Functional annotation analysis of this subset of genes using the DAVID software highlighted enriched gene ontology biological process (GO:BP) and KEGG pathways categories involved in fatty acid transport, storage and oxidation; genes belonging to these categories included *CD36*, *Pnlip*, *Plin2*, *Ppargc1a* (Table 2). Of note, LIF inhibited also *Ptpre*, a protein tyrosine phosphatase which, among other effects, inhibits MAPK/ERK activation and that we previously identified as one of the top EPO-induced genes (Gyetvai et al., 2017).

Negative regulators of myelination induced by LIF at 20 h

As at the 1 h time point, we then searched for potential LIF-induced negative regulators at 20 h. These were selected by comparing EPO + LIF and EPO and setting a cut-off of FC > 1.5 ($\log_2$ FC > 0.58) and BH adj. P value < 0.05. As shown in Fig. 3a and in the Venn diagram in Fig. 3b (right), among the transcripts unchanged by either EPO and/or differentiation alone, we identified 256 genes increased by addition of LIF; out of 1272 genes decreased by differentiation, 69 genes were increased by LIF; among the 37 genes downregulated by EPO, 2 were increased by LIF. In total, 327 genes unchanged or decreased by differentiation or EPO were increased by LIF (full list Additional file 4).

STRING interaction analysis of the 71 genes induced by LIF and also decreased by differentiation (69) or EPO (2) (right red arrows, Fig. 3b), and therefore more likely to be putative negative regulators of myelination, highlighted a network of highly connected genes focused around *STAT3*, *SOCS3* and *TLR2* (Fig. 3c).

High expression of LIF-induced *SOCS3* is associated with reduced *MOG* expression

Since *SOCS3*, downstream of STAT3, was highly induced by LIF at both time points, and its expression in OLs can inhibit LIF-induced myelination in vivo in mice (Emery et al., 2006), we explored further its involvement in LIF-mediated inhibition of myelination.

The mRNA expression of *SOCS3* from the microarray experiment was validated by RT-qPCR using the same RNA used for the microarray experiment; inhibition of *SOCS3* by differentiation and induction by LIF at 1 h, reported in Additional file 3, were confirmed (*SOCS3* mRNA as $\log_2$ FC, mean ± SD, $N = 4$;

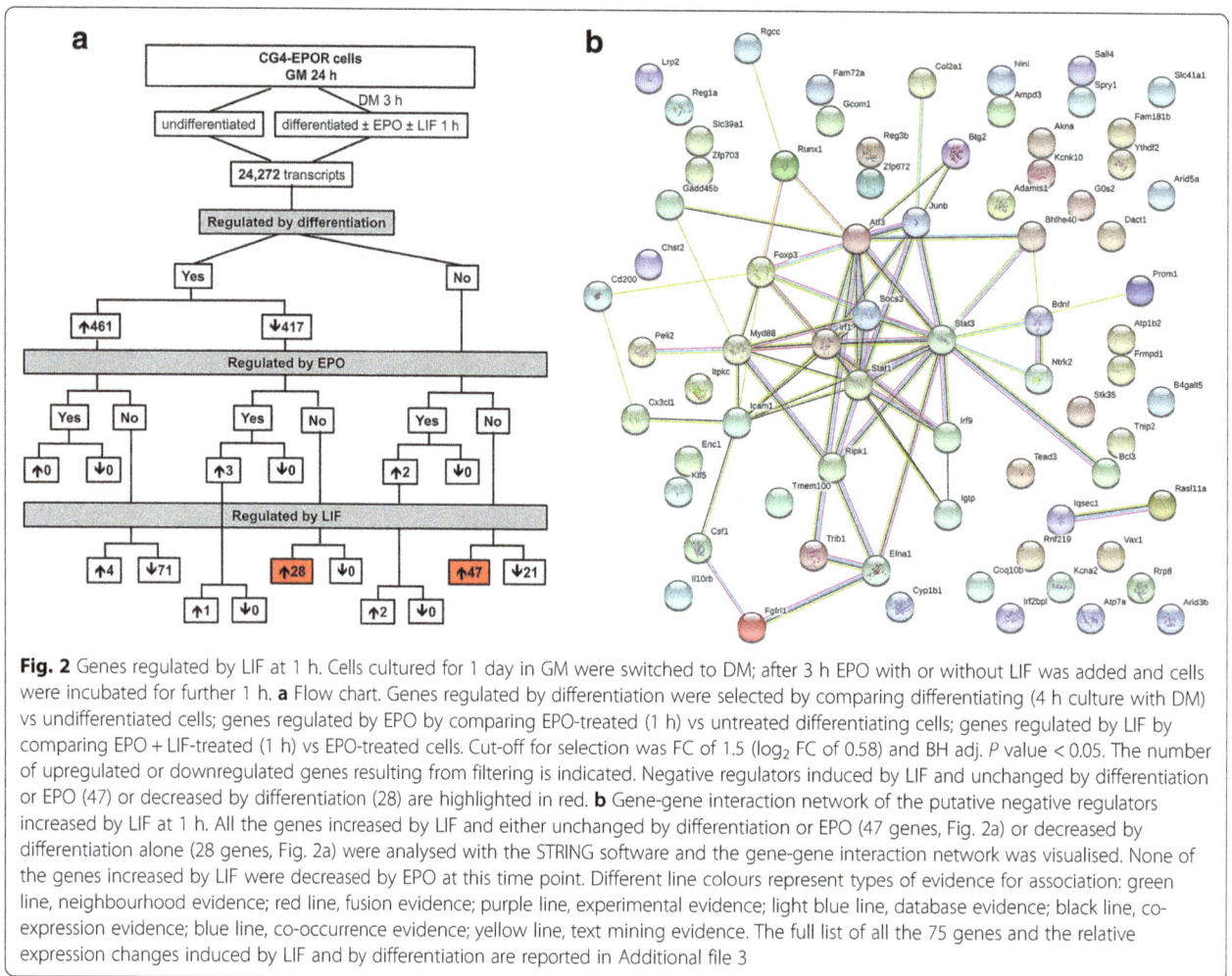

Fig. 2 Genes regulated by LIF at 1 h. Cells cultured for 1 day in GM were switched to DM; after 3 h EPO with or without LIF was added and cells were incubated for further 1 h. **a** Flow chart. Genes regulated by differentiation were selected by comparing differentiating (4 h culture with DM) vs undifferentiated cells; genes regulated by EPO by comparing EPO-treated (1 h) vs untreated differentiating cells; genes regulated by LIF by comparing EPO + LIF-treated (1 h) vs EPO-treated cells. Cut-off for selection was FC of 1.5 (log$_2$ FC of 0.58) and BH adj. P value < 0.05. The number of upregulated or downregulated genes resulting from filtering is indicated. Negative regulators induced by LIF and unchanged by differentiation or EPO (47) or decreased by differentiation (28) are highlighted in red. **b** Gene-gene interaction network of the putative negative regulators increased by LIF at 1 h. All the genes increased by LIF and either unchanged by differentiation or EPO (47 genes, Fig. 2a) or decreased by differentiation alone (28 genes, Fig. 2a) were analysed with the STRING software and the gene-gene interaction network was visualised. None of the genes increased by LIF were decreased by EPO at this time point. Different line colours represent types of evidence for association: green line, neighbourhood evidence; red line, fusion evidence; purple line, experimental evidence; light blue line, database evidence; black line, co-expression evidence; blue line, co-occurrence evidence; yellow line, text mining evidence. The full list of all the 75 genes and the relative expression changes induced by LIF and by differentiation are reported in Additional file 3

dif vs undif: − 2.8 ± 0.2, P < 0.001; EPO + LIF vs EPO: 1.9 ± 0.3, P < 0.001 by two-tailed Student's t-test).

In independent experiments, *SOCS3* expression was dose-dependently induced by LIF (Fig. 4a). Furthermore, co-stimulation of EPO-treated cells with LIF which, as shown in Fig. 1b, inhibits EPO-induced *MOG* expression, induced high levels of *SOCS3* at 1 h (Fig. 4b).

The association between MOG inhibition and induction of high levels of SOCS3 was confirmed with OSM or CNTF, cytokines also belonging to the IL-6 family. At concentrations equimolar to the high dose of LIF (10 ng/ml), also OSM and CNTF inhibited EPO-induced MOG (Fig. 4c), and induced high levels of *SOCS3* at 1 h (*SOCS3* mRNA as FC vs control, mean ± SD, N = 4; OSM: 8.1 ± 1.7, P < 0.001; CNTF: 5.2 ± 1.7, P < 0.01 by two-tailed Student's t-test). Of note, at a lower dose (0.13 ng/ml), equimolar to 0.2 ng/ml of LIF, OSM induced MOG expression, whereas CNTF had no effect (*SOCS3* mRNA as FC vs control, mean ± SD, N = 4; OSM: 3.2 ± 0.7, P < 0.001; CNTF: 1.4 ± 0.2, P = 0.19 by two-tailed Student's t-test).

TLR2 engagement inhibits EPO-induced MOG

Among the negative regulators induced by LIF, *TLR2* was also highlighted as a highly connected hub by STRING analysis at 20 h (Fig. 3c). Microarray expression of *TLR2* was validated by RT-qPCR using the same RNA used for the microarray experiment, confirming the inhibition of *TLR2* by differentiation and the very high induction by LIF at 20 h reported in Additional file 4 (*TLR2* mRNA as log$_2$ FC, mean ± SD, N = 4; dif vs undif: − 1.5 ± 0.5, P < 0.01; EPO + LIF vs EPO: 3.6 ± 0.3, P < 0.001 by two-tailed Student's t-test).

We therefore assessed the functional relevance of this finding using the TLR2 agonist Pam3. As shown in Fig. 4d, TLR2 activation inhibited EPO-induced *MOG* expression at the same extent as LIF and potentiated LIF inhibition.

Discussion

Although there is ample evidence in the literature that LIF and other cytokines of the IL-6 family, including CNTF, have pro-myelinating activities in vivo and in vitro (Nicola & Babon, 2015; Davis & Pennypacker, 2018; Slaets et al., 2010; Metcalfe, 2018), we report here

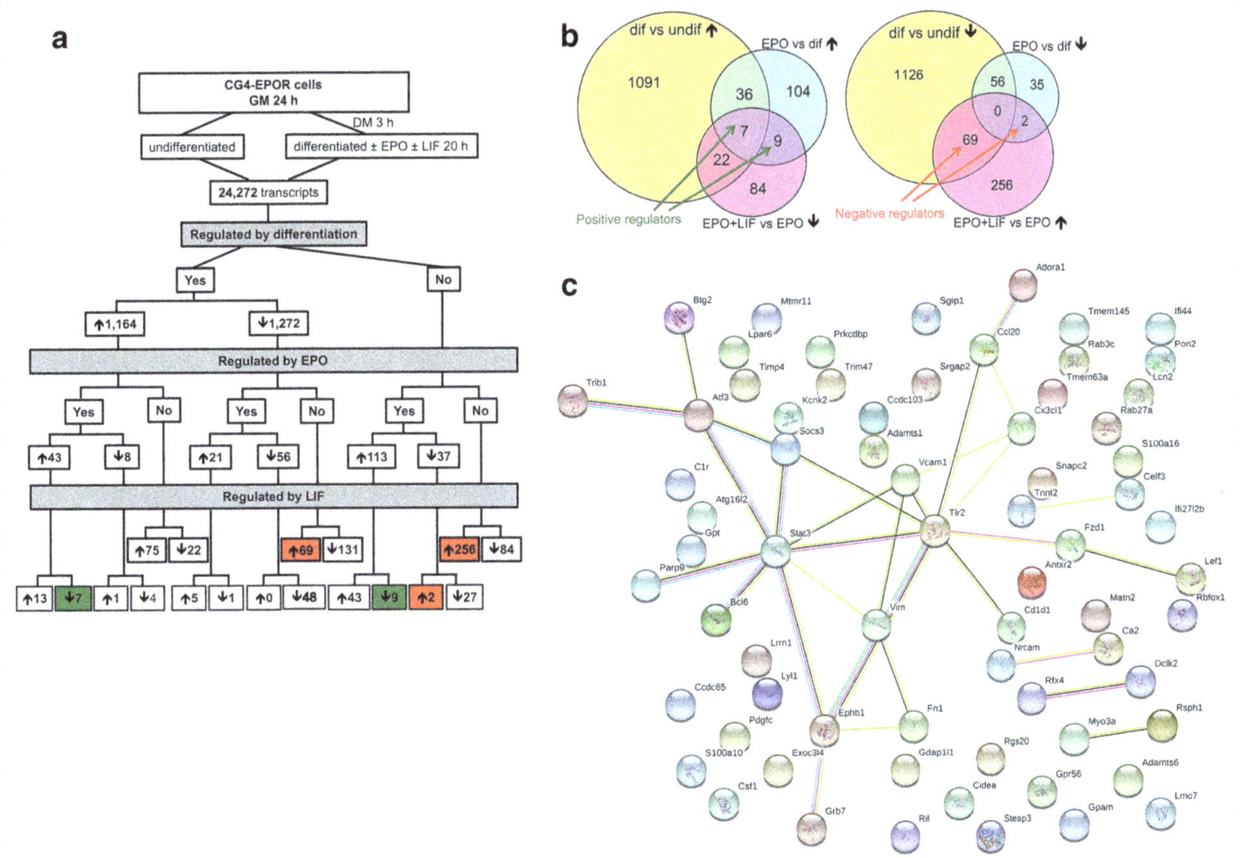

Fig. 3 Genes regulated by LIF at 20 h. Cells cultured for 1 day in GM were switched to DM; after 3 h EPO with or without LIF was added for 20 h. **a** Flow chart. Genes regulated by differentiation, EPO and LIF were selected as in the legend to Fig. 2. Positive regulators induced by EPO and inhibited by LIF are highlighted in green (16, of which 7 induced also by differentiation). Negative regulators induced by LIF and unchanged by differentiation or EPO (256) or decreased by differentiation (69) or by EPO (2) are highlighted in red. **b** Venn diagrams showing positive regulators inhibited by LIF (left; EPO-induced genes unchanged or induced by differentiation, 9 and 7 respectively, green arrows) and negative regulators induced by LIF (right; 256 unchanged by differentiation or EPO; 69 and 2 decreased by differentiation or EPO respectively, red arrows). The genes changed in opposite directions by EPO and differentiation are not included in **b**. These are: 8 genes increased by differentiation but decreased by EPO and 21 genes increased by EPO but decreased by differentiation (**a**). In addition, the left diagram (positive regulators) does not include the genes decreased by LIF but also decreased by differentiation or EPO (4 + 1 + 48 + 131 + 27 = 211; **a**). The right diagram (negative regulators) does not include the genes increased by LIF but also increased by EPO or differentiation (13 + 1 + 75 + 5 + 43 = 137; **a**). Dif, differentiated; undif, undifferentiated. **c** Gene-gene interaction network of the putative negative regulators increased by LIF at 20 h. All the genes increased by LIF and decreased by differentiation alone (69 genes, **a**) or by EPO alone (2 genes, **a**) were analysed with the STRING software as described in the legend to Fig. 2. The full list of all the 71 genes is reported in Additional file 4

that LIF can inhibit myelination in vitro. Specifically, in CG4 OPC induced to differentiate into OLs in the presence of EPO, co-treatment with LIF inhibited EPO-induced *MOG* expression. Of note, LIF inhibition was observed in CG4 cells transduced to overexpress EPOR, and therefore optimised to respond to EPO. We had previously used this in vitro system to study the mechanisms by which EPO increased myelin gene expression (Gyetvai et al., 2017), using *MOG* as a readout since its expression is associated with myelin deposition in these cells (Solly et al., 1996). Compared to cells incubated in DM alone, treatment with EPO consistently induced high levels of *MOG* expression, which were strongly inhibited by LIF. The effect was more marked

at high LIF concentrations (10 ng/ml), but inhibition was also noted at lower concentrations (0.2 ng/ml), which per se could slightly increase *MOG* expression. All together these observations highlight the strength of the inhibitory effect of LIF.

Our data may seem in contrast with many studies observing LIF pro-myelinating effects (Nicola & Babon, 2015; Davis & Pennypacker, 2018; Slaets et al., 2010; Metcalfe, 2018). However, no effect of LIF on OL differentiation had been previously described (Barres et al., 1993; Kahn & De Vellis, 1994; Park et al., 2001; interestingly, one study reported inhibitory effects of high LIF doses (more than 5 ng/ml) on OPC differentiation (Ishibashi et al., 2006). The ability of LIF to inhibit the

Table 1 Genes increased by EPO and inhibited by LIF at 20 h

ProbeName	Gene	EPO + LIF vs EPO		EPO vs differentiation	
		Log₂FC	BH adj.P	Log₂FC	BH adj.P
A44P792784	Htr2c	−1.98	6.0E-04	5.14	5.1E-05
A64P128810	RGD1565355	−1.79	7.2E-04	5.11	9.3E-05
A64P113795	LOC100365047	−1.58	1.2E-02	2.06	3.9E-03
A64P057188	**Shroom2**[a]	−1.52	5.5E-03	1.73	1.6E-02
A64P054808	CD36[a]	−1.47	1.1E-03	6.98	1.5E-04
A44P305482	Ppargc1a	−1.43	3.9E-03	1.48	1.6E-02
A44P335776	Chodl	−1.42	6.3E-03	1.89	5.9E-03
A44P158758	Calcr	−1.40	1.3E-02	1.78	1.9E-02
A64P15946	**Pmp2**[a]	−1.16	1.4E-02	5.24	1.5E-05
A64P025432	**LOC498829**	−1.04	6.0E-03	1.06	1.1E-02
A44P194803	**Baalc**	−1.03	3.1E-03	1.93	7.0E-04
A64P137130	Ptpre	−0.94	1.4E-02	4.01	3.5E-04
A44P254984	Pnlip	−0.89	4.8E-03	0.92	5.2E-03
A42P839964	Plin2	−0.79	8.7E-03	1.33	2.8E-03
A42P826938	**LRRTM1**	−0.63	3.9E-03	1.11	6.4E-04
A42P646991	**Mag**	−0.59	1.7E-02	1.34	7.9E-03

All the genes increased by EPO and inhibited by LIF at 20 h are listed. In bold the genes also increased by differentiation. The full list of the genes increased by EPO and differentiation at 20 h was previously reported (Gyetvai et al., 2017). [a]Genes represented by 2 probes consistently changed by EPO in the same direction, of which only the most significantly changed one is shown

pro-myelinating effects of other cytokines had not previously been reported.

LIF activates STAT3, which has a key role in myelination (Steelman et al., 2016). However, LIF signaling is tightly regulated. LIF-induced SOCS3, downstream of STAT3, inhibits STAT3 phosphorylation and excessive induction of inflammatory genes (Yasukawa et al., 2003),

and is one of the main mechanisms through which LIF inhibits IL-6-induced differentiation of T helper (Th)17 cells (Cao et al., 2011). In the present study, LIF-induced SOCS3 expression was associated with a reduction of EPO-induced MOG at high concentration of LIF. In addition, also OSM and CNTF, cytokines of the IL-6 family, used at equimolar LIF concentrations at which they induced similar levels of SOCS3 as compared to LIF (reported above in the Results section), inhibited EPO-induced MOG expression. These observations, together with previous results documenting increased myelination in SOCS3 knock-out mice (Emery et al., 2006), suggest that SOCS3 might play a role in LIF inhibition of MOG expression. SOCS3 induction might explain the lower levels of MOG observed at high doses of LIF compared to low dose, and inhibition of EPO-induced MOG. Of note, SOCS3 can inhibit EPO-induced STAT5 activation (Sasaki et al., 2000; Bachmann et al., 2011).

We investigated whether LIF might directly inhibit the expression of positive regulators of myelination induced by EPO. By gene expression profiling, we found that LIF downregulated genes involved in lipid transport and metabolism previously found to be increased by EPO, including CD36, Ppargc1a, Pnlip and Plin2 (Gyetvai et al., 2017). Preferential downregulation of these genes by LIF strengthens the hypothesis that they might have a role in mediating EPO myelinating effects.

LIF inhibitory effects reported here cannot exclusively be correlated with an action on differentiated cells; LIF might also act on undifferentiated cells.

In this regard, LIF inhibited PTPRE, a tyrosine phosphatase induced by EPO that, among other effects, inhibits MAPK/ERK phosphorylation. We had previously shown that inhibitors of ERK in this system potentiate

Table 2 Enriched KEGG pathways and GO:BP categories among the genes increased by EPO and inhibited by LIF at 20 h

Category	Term	Fold enrichment	Gene symbols	P value
KEGG	Fat digestion and absorption	87.7	Pnlip, CD36, RGD1565355	3.4E-04
KEGG	Adipocytokine signaling pathway	44.5	CD36, Ppargc1a, RGD1565355	1.3E-03
GO:BP	Intestinal cholesterol absorption	730.6	PnlipP, CD36	2.5E-03
KEGG	Insulin resistance	30.3	CD36, Ppargc1a, RGD1565355	2.9E-03
GO:BP	Response to drug	11.1	CD36, Plin2, Htr2c, PPARGC1A	3.7E-03
KEGG	AMPK signaling pathway	26.3	CD36, PPARGC1A, RGD1565355	3.8E-03
GO:BP	Cell surface receptor signaling pathway	22.8	Calcr, CD36, RGD1565355	6.1E-03
GO:BP	Long-chain fatty acid transport	243.5	CD36, Plin2	7.5E-03
GO:BP	Fatty acid oxidation	182.7	CD36, Ppargc1a	1.0E-02
GO:BP	Lipid storage	108.2	CD36, Plin2	1.7E-02
GO:BP	Response to lipid	97.4	Pnlip, CD36	1.9E-02
GO:BP	Receptor internalization	69.6	Calcr, CD36	2.6E-02
KEGG	Malaria	37.7	CD36, RGD1565355	4.5E-02

DAVID Functional Annotation Chart analysis showing the overrepresented GO:BP categories and KEGG pathways among the genes increased by EPO and decreased by LIF at 20 h. The fold enrichment and the significance of enrichment (P value) are reported

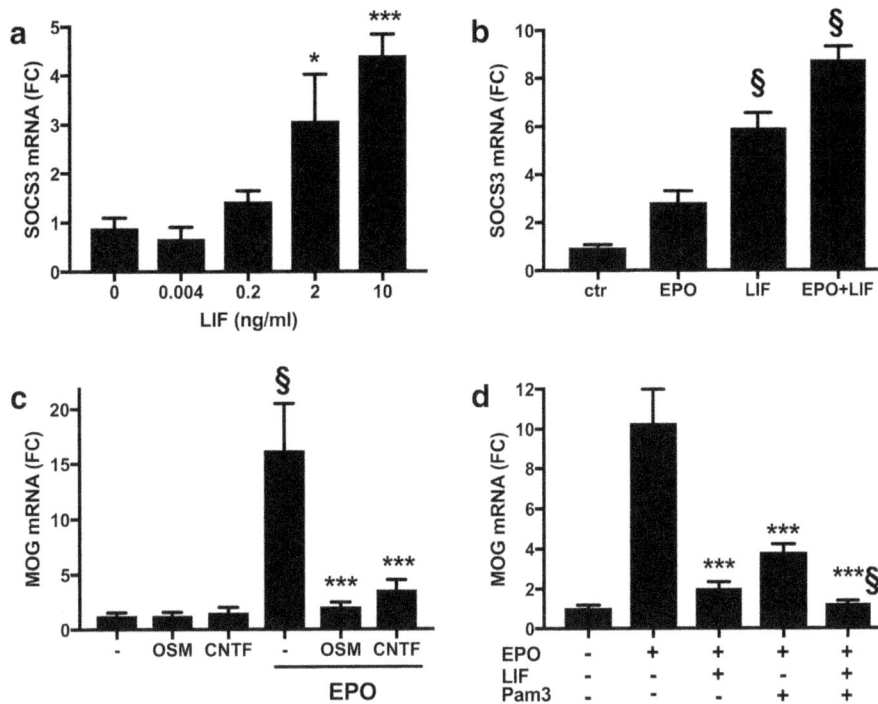

Fig. 4 Role of SOCS3 and TLR2 in mediating LIF inhibition. **a-b** LIF induction of SOCS3 is associated with a reduction in MOG expression (shown in Fig. 1). Cells cultured for 1 day in GM were switched to DM; after 3 h they were treated with the indicated concentrations of LIF (**a**), or with or without EPO (10 ng/ml) and LIF (10 ng/ml; **b**). After 1 h, SOCS3 mRNA was measured by RT-qPCR. Results, expressed as fold change (FC) vs one of the control (ctr) samples (no LIF in **a**) are the mean ± SD of quadruplicate samples assayed in duplicate and are representative of two independent experiments; $*$ $P < 0.05$, $***$ $P < 0.001$ vs control (no LIF); § $P < 0.001$ vs EPO by two-tailed Student's t-test. **c** OSM and CNTF inhibit EPO-induced MOG expression. Cells cultured as above were treated with or without EPO (10 ng/ml) and OSM or CNTF (both at 6.5 ng/ml, equimolar concentrations to LIF 10 ng/ml). MOG gene expression was measured by RT-qPCR at day 3. Results, expressed as above, are the mean ± SD of eight samples from two independent experiments assayed in duplicate; $***$ $P < 0.001$ vs EPO alone; § $P < 0.001$ vs untreated by two-tailed Student's t-test. **d** TLR2 engagement inhibits EPO-induced MOG expression. Cells were differentiated in the absence or in the presence of EPO (10 ng/ml), with or without LIF (10 ng/ml) or Pam3 (1 µg/ml), a TLR2/1 ligand. MOG expression was measured at day 3 by RT-qPCR. Results, expressed as above, are the mean ± SD of quadruplicate samples assayed in duplicate and are representative of two independent experiments; $***P < 0.001$ vs EPO alone; § $P < 0.01$ vs EPO + LIF by two-tailed Student's t-test

myelination, in support of the hypothesis that activation of ERK might sustain proliferation of OPCs and inhibit the start of differentiation (Gyetvai et al., 2017). Both EPO and LIF can induce ERK activation (Gyetvai et al., 2017; Nicola & Babon, 2015). However, EPO induces the feedback inhibitor *PTPRE*. Inhibition of *PTPRE* by LIF might prolong ERK activation in OPCs, inhibiting differentiation.

In addition, other than being pro-myelinating cytokines, LIF and other members of the IL-6 family, such as CNTF, are essential in development for inducing astrocyte differentiation. LIF can also increase astrocyte differentiation in vitro, although the presence of extracellular matrix factors may be required (Nicola & Babon, 2015). CG4 cells are bipotential OL type-2 astrocyte (O-2A) progenitors that can be induced to differentiate into type-2 astrocytes or into mature OLs (Louis et al., 1992; Solly et al., 1996). In primary OLs and CG4 cells LIF can induce the astrocyte marker GFAP (Kahn & De Vellis, 1994; Gresle et al., 2015), an observation that we have confirmed (Additional file 4). It is therefore possible that LIF, if present at the very early stages of the OL differentiation process, could interfere by inducing astrocyte differentiation. Although this is a very controversial issue, the presence of O-2A progenitors in vivo, and even in pathological conditions, has been suggested (Franklin & Blakemore, 1995; Virard et al., 2006).

Among the possible negative regulators induced by LIF, we noticed components of the TLR pathways, including TLR2 and Myd88, an adaptor protein used by almost all TLRs. Other than microbial products, the TLRs recognize endogenous danger-associated molecular patterns (DAMPs) released from injured tissues which regulate inflammatory responses (Lee et al., 2013). All cells of the CNS express the TLRs, including OLs which preferentially express TLR2 and TLR3 (Bsibsi et al., 2002; Sloane et al., 2010). TLR2 is upregulated in experimental models of MS and in MS demyelinating lesions, where it is also expressed by OLs (Sloane et al., 2010; Zekki et al., 2002; Esser et al., 2018); TLR2 activation inhibits OL maturation, an effect not shared by all TLRs (Sloane et al., 2010). We show here that TLR2 is functional in OLs, and its activation inhibits myelin gene expression.

Whether TLR2 has a role in mediating LIF inhibitory effects will of course depend on the presence of TLR2 ligands. TLR2, by forming homodimers and heterodimers with TLR1 or TLR6, can bind a broad range of ligands, including Gram-positive bacterial cell wall components, endogenous DAMPs such as heat shock proteins (HSPs) and high mobility group protein B1 (HMGB1), and fragments of extracellular matrix (ECM) molecules, such as hyaluronan (Piccinini & Midwood, 2010; Miranda-Hernandez & Baxter, 2013). Of note, TLR2 ligands, including hyaluronan, HMGB1 and peptidoglycan, a component of Gram-positive bacteria, have been detected in EAE and in MS lesions (Back et al., 2005; Visser et al., 2006; Andersson et al., 2008), suggesting that LIF-induction of TLR2 in OLs might actually lead to inhibition of remyelination.

Although LIF has an important role in promoting myelination (Slaets et al., 2010; Stankoff et al., 2002; Metcalfe, 2018), its pleiotropic nature, and its ability to induce proliferation inhibiting differentiation or vice versa, may result in negative myelinating effects at certain stages of the myelination process, likely when undifferentiated OL progenitors should stop proliferating and start differentiating. In pathological conditions, including MS, remyelination, especially at later disease stages, is insufficient to re-establish motor and cognitive performance. MS lesions may contain large numbers of poorly differentiated OPCs and immature OLs, suggesting that in many cases the main cause of remyelination failure is not a lack of OPCs, but rather an inability of these cells to differentiate into mature myelin producing cells (Franklin & Gallo, 2014; Kremer et al., 2015; Chamberlain et al., 2016). The presence of LIF in MS lesions (Vanderlocht et al., 2006) might contribute to inhibit OPC differentiation and remyelination.

Moreover, our findings show that, when considering the action of cytokines on myelination, one should consider that they act on a tightly regulated network, where each cytokine can affect the action of another. Identifying these regulatory networks may be important as different cytokines may be up- or down-regulated in disease conditions and this may have pharmacological relevance when cytokines are administered as neuroprotective or neuroreparative agents. Although the effectiveness of EPO in MS is unclear and recent clinical trials have not shown an efficacy (Schreiber et al., 2017), research is still active on EPO mimetics or derivatives with different biological properties (Culver et al., 2017; Bonnas et al., 2017); clinical trials with EPO in optic neuritis are ongoing after positive indications from phase 2 trials (Suhs et al., 2012; Diem et al., 2016) and its use to improve traumatic brain injury is still open (Counter et al., 1994). Likewise, there is interest in the potential use of LIF in the therapy of MS (Slaets et al., 2010; Metcalfe, 2018). The

tight regulation of LIF signaling pathways that might negatively affect remyelination, shown here, needs to be taken into account in designing combination therapies and dose-finding studies. Additionally, increased blood and cerebrospinal fluid levels of LIF (Mashayekhi & Salehi, 2011), IL-11 (Zhang et al., 2015), CNTF (Massaro et al., 1997) and IL-6 (Wullschleger et al., 2013) have been found in MS patients, thus raising the possibility of them affecting the response to EPO.

Of course we should bear in mind the limitations of our study. The use of a cell line, although largely used for basic studies on myelination, limits the external validity of our findings, and only in vivo experiments in models of demyelination could indicate the in vivo relevance of the pathways that we have identified.

Conclusion

This study reports that the IL-6 family cytokine LIF can inhibit EPO-induced myelin gene expression in OLs. LIF's promyelinating effects have long been known, but controversial results have also been reported. The pleiotropic activities of LIF, which can inhibit or stimulate proliferation or differentiation and exhibit inflammatory or anti-inflammatory action, together with the tight inhibitory feedback mechanisms that regulate its signaling pathways, and its ability to induce negative regulators, such as TLR2, can translate into inhibition of myelination, depending on the stage of OL differentiation and on the cytokine environment. Further studies on the mechanisms by which endogenous cytokines positively and negatively affect myelination may lead to the identification of therapeutic targets and new drugs essential to improve remyelination in demyelinating diseases.

Additional files

Additional file 1: Genes increased by EPO in differentiating cells at 1 h. Genes changed more than 1.5-fold (absolute $\log_2$ FC > 0.58), BH adj. *P* value < 0.05 in EPO-treated vs untreated differentiating cells are listed; ns = not significant. There were no genes decreased by EPO at this time point. The relative change in differentiating (dif) vs undifferentiated (undif) cells and in EPO + LIF vs EPO-treated cells are also reported. *Represented by 2 probes consistently increased by EPO of which only the most significantly changed one is shown (xlsx file). (XLSX 10 kb)

Additional file 2: Genes increased by LIF and by differentiation at 1 h. These genes have been identified by comparing EPO + LIF vs EPO and differentiating (dif) vs undifferentiated (undif) cells, setting a threshold of $\log_2$ FC ≥ 0.58 and BH adj. *P* value < 0.05. *Represented by 2 probes consistently increased by LIF of which only the most significantly changed one is shown (xlsx file). (XLSX 10 kb)

Additional file 3: Genes increased by LIF and unchanged or decreased by differentiation or EPO at 1 h. The genes increased more than 1.5-fold ($\log_2$ FC ≥ 0.58), BH adj. *P* value < 0.05 in EPO + LIF vs EPO-treated differentiating cells are listed; ns = not significant. For genes represented by 2 probes (*) consistently increased by LIF, only the one increased more significantly is shown (xlsx file). (XLSX 20 kb)

Additional file 4: Genes increased by LIF and unchanged or decreased by differentiation or EPO at 20 h. The genes increased more than 1.5-fold (log$_2$ FC ≥ 0.58), BH adj. P value < 0.05 in EPO + LIF vs EPO-treated differentiating cells are listed; ns = not significant. For genes represented by 2 probes (*) consistently increased by LIF, only the one increased more significantly is shown (xlsx file). (XLSX 63 kb)

Abbreviations
BH: Benjamini-Hochberg; CD36: Cluster of differentiation 36; CG4: Central glia-4; CNS: Central nervous system; CNTF: Ciliary neurotrophic factor; DAMP: Damage-associated molecular patterns; DAVID: Database for Annotation, Visualization and Integrated Discovery; DM: Differentiation medium; EPO: Erythropoietin; EPOR: Erythropoietin receptor; ERK: Extracellular signal-regulated kinases; GM: Growth medium; GO:BP: Gene ontology biological process; gp130: Glycoprotein 130; HPRT1: Hypoxanthine phosphoribosyltransferase 1; HSP: Heat shock protein; JAK: Janus kinase; LIF: Leukemia inhibitory factor; LIFR: Leukemia inhibitory factor receptor; MAPK: Mitogen-activated protein kinase; MOG: Myelin oligodendrocyte glycoprotein; MS: Multiple sclerosis; Myd88: Myeloid differentiation primary response 88; O-2A: Oligodendrocyte-type-2 astrocyte; OL: Oligodendrocyte; OPC: Oligodendrocyte progenitor cell; OSM: Oncostatin M; PI3K: Phosphatidylinositol-3-kinase; Plin2: Perilipin 2; Pnlip: Pancreatic lipase; Ppargc1a: Peroxisome proliferator-activated receptor gamma coactivator 1 alpha; Ptpre: Protein tyrosine phosphatase receptor type E; qPCR: Quantitative polymerase chain reaction; RT: Reverse transcription; SOCS3: Suppressor of cytokine signaling 3; STAT3: Signal transducer and activator of transcription 3; STRING: Search Tool for the Retrieval of Interacting Genes; TLR: Toll like receptor

Acknowledgments
The authors thank Alexander Annenkov for providing the CG4-EPOR cells used in this study.

Funding
Supported by the RM Philips Trust (PG), the Brighton Centre for Regenerative Medicine and Devices (CRMD), University of Brighton (GG) and the Brighton and Sussex Medical School as part of the Independent Research Project of CR.

Authors' contributions
GG, CR, LH, MM performed experiments, analyzed and interpreted results; GG, MM, PG designed experiments; GG, MM and PG wrote the manuscript; all authors critically revised and approved the final manuscript. All authors read and approved the final manuscript.

Competing interests
The authors declare they have no competing interests as defined by *Molecular Medicine*, or other interests that might be perceived to influence the results and discussion reported in this paper.

References
Andersson A, Covacu R, Sunnemark D, Danilov AI, Dal Bianco A, Khademi M, Wallstrom E, Lobell A, Brundin L, Lassmann H, et al. Pivotal advance: HMGB1 expression in active lesions of human and experimental multiple sclerosis. J Leukoc Biol. 2008;84(5):1248–55.

Bachmann J, Raue A, Schilling M, Bohm ME, Kreutz C, Kaschek D, Busch H, Gretz N, Lehmann WD, Timmer J, et al. Division of labor by dual feedback regulators controls JAK2/STAT5 signaling over broad ligand range. Mol Syst Biol. 2011;7:516.

Back SA, Tuohy TM, Chen H, Wallingford N, Craig A, Struve J, Luo NL, Banine F, Liu Y, Chang A, et al. Hyaluronan accumulates in demyelinated lesions and inhibits oligodendrocyte progenitor maturation. Nat Med. 2005;11(9):966–72.

Barres BA, Schmid R, Sendtner M, Raff MC. Multiple extracellular signals are required for long-term oligodendrocyte survival. Development. 1993;118(1):283–95.

Barrett T, Wilhite SE, Ledoux P, Evangelista C, Kim IF, Tomashevsky M, Marshall KA, Phillippy KH, Sherman PM, Holko M, et al. NCBI GEO: archive for functional genomics data sets--update. Nucleic Acids Res. 2013;41(Database issue):D991–5.

Bonnas C, Wustefeld L, Winkler D, Kronstein-Wiedemann R, Dere E, Specht K, Boxberg M, Tonn T, Ehrenreich H, Stadler H, et al. EV-3, an endogenous human erythropoietin isoform with distinct functional relevance. Sci Rep. 2017;7(1):3684.

Bove RM, Green AJ. Remyelinating pharmacotherapies in multiple sclerosis. Neurotherapeutics. 2017;14(4):894–904.

Bsibsi M, Ravid R, Gveric D, van Noort JM. Broad expression of toll-like receptors in the human central nervous system. J Neuropathol Exp Neurol. 2002;61(11):1013–21.

Cadavid D, Balcer L, Galetta S, Aktas O, Ziemssen T, Vanopdenbosch L, Frederiksen J, Skeen M, Jaffe GJ, Butzkueven H, et al. Safety and efficacy of opicinumab in acute optic neuritis (RENEW): a randomised, placebo-controlled, phase 2 trial. Lancet Neurol. 2017;16(3):189–99.

Cao W, Yang Y, Wang Z, Liu A, Fang L, Wu F, Hong J, Shi Y, Leung S, Dong C, et al. Leukemia inhibitory factor inhibits T helper 17 cell differentiation and confers treatment effects of neural progenitor cell therapy in autoimmune disease. Immunity. 2011;35(2):273–84.

Cervellini I, Annenkov A, Brenton T, Chernajovsky Y, Ghezzi P, Mengozzi M. Erythropoietin (EPO) increases myelin gene expression in CG4 oligodendrocyte cells through the classical EPO receptor. Mol Med. 2013;19:223–9.

Chamberlain KA, Nanescu SE, Psachoulia K, Huang JK. Oligodendrocyte regeneration: its significance in myelin replacement and neuroprotection in multiple sclerosis. Neuropharmacology. 2016;110(Pt B):633–43. https://doi.org/10.1016/j.neuropharm.2015.10.010.

Counter CM, Botelho FM, Wang P, Harley CB, Bacchetti S. Stabilization of short telomeres and telomerase activity accompany immortalization of Epstein-Barr virus-transformed human B lymphocytes. J Virol. 1994;68(5):3410–4.

Culver DA, Dahan A, Bajorunas D, Jeziorska M, van Velzen M, Aarts L, Tavee J, Tannemaat MR, Dunne AN, Kirk RI, et al. Cibinetide improves corneal nerve Fiber abundance in patients with sarcoidosis-associated small nerve Fiber loss and neuropathic pain. Invest Ophthalmol Vis Sci. 2017;58(6):BIO52–60.

Davis SM, Pennypacker KR. The role of the leukemia inhibitory factor receptor in neuroprotective signaling. Pharmacol Ther. 2018;183:50–7.

Diem R, Molnar F, Beisse F, Gross N, Druschler K, Heinrich SP, Joachimsen L, Rauer S, Pielen A, Suhs KW, et al. Treatment of optic neuritis with erythropoietin (TONE): a randomised, double-blind, placebo-controlled trial-study protocol. BMJ Open. 2016;6(3):e010956.

Digicaylioglu M, Garden G, Timberlake S, Fletcher L, Lipton SA. Acute neuroprotective synergy of erythropoietin and insulin-like growth factor I. Proc Natl Acad Sci USA. 2004;101(26):9855–60.

Ehrenreich H, Fischer B, Norra C, Schellenberger F, Stender N, Stiefel M, Siren AL, Paulus W, Nave KA, Gold R, et al. Exploring recombinant human erythropoietin in chronic progressive multiple sclerosis. Brain. 2007;130(Pt 10):2577–88.

Emery B, Cate HS, Marriott M, Merson T, Binder MD, Snell C, Soo PY, Murray S, Croker B, Zhang JG, et al. Suppressor of cytokine signaling 3 limits protection of leukemia inhibitory factor receptor signaling against central demyelination. Proc Natl Acad Sci U S A. 2006;103(20):7859–64.

Esser S, Gopfrich L, Bihler K, Kress E, Nyamoya S, Tauber SC, Clarner T, Stope MB, Pufe T, Kipp M, et al. Toll-like receptor 2-mediated glial cell activation in a mouse model of Cuprizone-induced demyelination. Mol Neurobiol. 2018;55(8):6237–49. https://doi.org/10.1007/s12035-017-0838-2.

Franklin RJ, Blakemore WF. Glial-cell transplantation and plasticity in the O-2A lineage--implications for CNS repair. Trends Neurosci. 1995;18(3):151–6.

Franklin RJ, Gallo V. The translational biology of remyelination: past, present, and future. Glia. 2014;62(11):1905–15.

Green AJ, Gelfand JM, Cree BA, Bevan C, Boscardin WJ, Mei F, Inman J, Arnow S, Devereux M, Abounasr A, et al. Clemastine fumarate as a remyelinating therapy for multiple sclerosis (ReBUILD): a randomised, controlled, double-blind, crossover trial. Lancet. 2017;390(10111):2481–9.

Gresle MM, Butzkueven H, Perreau VM, Jonas A, Xiao J, Thiem S, Holmes FE, Doherty W, Soo PY, Binder MD, et al. Galanin is an autocrine myelin and oligodendrocyte trophic signal induced by leukemia inhibitory factor. Glia. 2015;63(6):1005–20.

Gyetvai G, Hughes T, Wedmore F, Roe C, Heikal L, Ghezzi P, Mengozzi M. Erythropoietin increases myelination in oligodendrocytes: gene expression profiling reveals early induction of genes involved in lipid transport and metabolism. Front Immunol. 2017;8:1394.

Hassouna I, Ott C, Wustefeld L, Offen N, Neher RA, Mitkovski M, Winkler D, Sperling S, Fries L, Goebbels S, et al. Revisiting adult neurogenesis and the role of erythropoietin for neuronal and oligodendroglial differentiation in the hippocampus. Mol Psychiatry. 2016;21(12):1752–67.

Huang da W, Sherman BT, Lempicki RA. Systematic and integrative analysis of large gene lists using DAVID bioinformatics resources. Nat Protoc. 2009;4(1):44–57.

Ishibashi T, Dakin KA, Stevens B, Lee PR, Kozlov SV, Stewart CL, Fields RD. Astrocytes promote myelination in response to electrical impulses. Neuron. 2006;49(6):823–32.

Kahn MA, De Vellis J. Regulation of an oligodendrocyte progenitor cell line by the interleukin-6 family of cytokines. Glia. 1994;12(2):87–98.

Kang YJ, Digicaylioglu M, Russo R, Kaul M, Achim CL, Fletcher L, Masliah E, Lipton SA. Erythropoietin plus insulin-like growth factor-I protects against neuronal damage in a murine model of human immunodeficiency virus-associated neurocognitive disorders. Ann Neurol. 2010;68(3):342–52.

Kremer D, Kury P, Dutta R. Promoting remyelination in multiple sclerosis: current drugs and future prospects. Mult Scler. 2015;21(5):541–9.

Lee H, Lee S, Cho IH, Lee SJ. Toll-like receptors: sensor molecules for detecting damage to the nervous system. Curr Protein Pept Sci. 2013;14(1):33–42.

Li XB, Zheng W, Ning YP, Cai DB, Yang XH, Ungvari GS, Ng CH, Wang CY, Xiang YT. Erythropoietin for cognitive deficits associated with schizophrenia, bipolar disorder, and major depression: a systematic review. Pharmacopsychiatry. 2018;51(3):100–4.

Linker RA, Kruse N, Israel S, Wei T, Seubert S, Hombach A, Holtmann B, Luhder F, Ransohoff RM, Sendtner M, et al. Leukemia inhibitory factor deficiency modulates the immune response and limits autoimmune demyelination: a new role for neurotrophic cytokines in neuroinflammation. J Immunol. 2008; 180(4):2204–13.

Louis JC, Magal E, Muir D, Manthorpe M, Varon S. CG-4, a new bipotential glial cell line from rat brain, is capable of differentiating in vitro into either mature oligodendrocytes or type-2 astrocytes. J Neurosci Res. 1992;31(1):193–204.

Marriott MP, Emery B, Cate HS, Binder MD, Kemper D, Wu Q, Kolbe S, Gordon IR, Wang H, Egan G, et al. Leukemia inhibitory factor signaling modulates both central nervous system demyelination and myelin repair. Glia. 2008;56(6):686–98.

Martino G, Pluchino S. The therapeutic potential of neural stem cells. Nat Rev Neurosci. 2006;7(5):395–406.

Mashayekhi F, Salehi Z. Expression of leukemia inhibitory factor in the cerebrospinal fluid of patients with multiple sclerosis. J Clin Neurosci. 2011; 18(7):951–4.

Massaro AR, Soranzo C, Carnevale A. Cerebrospinal-fluid ciliary neurotrophic factor in neurological patients. Eur Neurol. 1997;37(4):243–6.

Mengozzi M, Cervellini I, Villa P, Erbayraktar Z, Gokmen N, Yilmaz O, Erbayraktar S, Manohasandra M, Van Hummelen P, Vandenabeele P, et al. Erythropoietin-induced changes in brain gene expression reveal induction of synaptic plasticity genes in experimental stroke. Proc Natl Acad Sci USA. 2012;109(24):9617–22.

Mengozzi M, Ermilov P, Annenkov A, Ghezzi P, Pearl F. Definition of a family of tissue-protective cytokines using functional cluster analysis: a proof-of-concept study. Front Immunol. 2014;5:115.

Metcalfe SM. LIF and multiple sclerosis: one protein with two healing properties. Mult Scler Relat Disord. 2018;20:223–7.

Miranda-Hernandez S, Baxter AG. Role of toll-like receptors in multiple sclerosis. Am J Clin Exp Immunol. 2013;2(1):75–93.

Nicola NA, Babon JJ. Leukemia inhibitory factor (LIF). Cytokine Growth Factor Rev. 2015;26(5):533–44.

Ott C, Martens H, Hassouna I, Oliveira B, Erck C, Zafeiriou MP, Peteri UK, Hesse D, Gerhart S, Altas B, et al. Widespread expression of erythropoietin receptor in brain and its induction by injury. Mol Med. 2015;21(1):803–15. https://doi.org/10.2119/molmed.2015.00192.

Park SK, Solomon D, Vartanian T. Growth factor control of CNS myelination. Dev Neurosci. 2001;23(4–5):327–37.

Philips T, Rothstein JD. Oligodendroglia: metabolic supporters of neurons. J Clin Invest. 2017;127(9):3271–80.

Piccinini AM, Midwood KS. DAMPening inflammation by modulating TLR signalling. Mediat Inflamm. 2010;2010:672395. https://doi.org/10.1155/2010/672395.

Robinson S, Winer JL, Chan LAS, Oppong AY, Yellowhair TR, Maxwell JR, Andrews N, Yang Y, Sillerud LO, Meehan WP 3rd, et al. Extended erythropoietin treatment prevents chronic executive functional and microstructural deficits following early severe traumatic brain injury in rats. Front Neurol. 2018;9:451.

Ruckh JM, Zhao JW, Shadrach JL, van Wijngaarden P, Rao TN, Wagers AJ, Franklin RJ. Rejuvenation of regeneration in the aging central nervous system. Cell Stem Cell. 2012;10(1):96–103.

Sargin D, Friedrichs H, El-Kordi A, Ehrenreich H. Erythropoietin as neuroprotective and neuroregenerative treatment strategy: comprehensive overview of 12 years of preclinical and clinical research. Best Pract Res Clin Anaesthesiol. 2010;24(4):573–94.

Sasaki A, Yasukawa H, Shouda T, Kitamura T, Dikic I, Yoshimura A. CIS3/SOCS-3 suppresses erythropoietin (EPO) signaling by binding the EPO receptor and JAK2. J Biol Chem. 2000;275(38):29338–47.

Schreiber K, Magyari M, Sellebjerg F, Iversen P, Garde E, Madsen CG, Bornsen L, Romme Christensen J, Ratzer R, Siebner HR, et al. High-dose erythropoietin in patients with progressive multiple sclerosis: a randomized, placebo-controlled, phase 2 trial. Mult Scler. 2017;23(5):675–85.

Siren AL, Knerlich F, Poser W, Gleiter CH, Bruck W, Ehrenreich H. Erythropoietin and erythropoietin receptor in human ischemic/hypoxic brain. Acta Neuropathol. 2001;101(3):271–6.

Slaets H, Hendriks JJ, Stinissen P, Kilpatrick TJ, Hellings N. Therapeutic potential of LIF in multiple sclerosis. Trends Mol Med. 2010;16(11):493–500.

Sloane JA, Batt C, Ma Y, Harris ZM, Trapp B, Vartanian T. Hyaluronan blocks oligodendrocyte progenitor maturation and remyelination through TLR2. Proc Natl Acad Sci U S A. 2010;107(25):11555–60.

Solly SK, Thomas JL, Monge M, Demerens C, Lubetzki C, Gardinier MV, Matthieu JM, Zalc B. Myelin/oligodendrocyte glycoprotein (MOG) expression is associated with myelin deposition. Glia. 1996;18(1):39–48.

Stankoff B, Aigrot MS, Noel F, Wattilliaux A, Zalc B, Lubetzki C. Ciliary neurotrophic factor (CNTF) enhances myelin formation: a novel role for CNTF and CNTF-related molecules. J Neurosci. 2002;22(21):9221–7.

Steelman AJ, Zhou Y, Koito H, Kim S, Payne HR, Lu QR, Li J. Activation of oligodendroglial Stat3 is required for efficient remyelination. Neurobiol Dis. 2016;91:336–46.

Sugawa M, Sakurai Y, Ishikawa-Ieda Y, Suzuki H, Asou H. Effects of erythropoietin on glial cell development; oligodendrocyte maturation and astrocyte proliferation. Neurosci Res. 2002;44(4):391–403.

Suhs KW, Hein K, Sattler MB, Gorlitz A, Ciupka C, Scholz K, Kasmann-Kellner B, Papanagiotou P, Schaffler N, Restemeyer C, et al. A randomized, double-blind, phase 2 study of erythropoietin in optic neuritis. Ann Neurol. 2012;72(2):199–210.

Takahashi A, Takahashi Y, Matsumoto K, Miyata K. Synergistic effects of insulin-like growth factor II (IGF-II) with leukemia inhibiting factor (LIF) on establishment of rat pluripotential cell lines. J Vet Med Sci. 1995;57(3):553–6.

Tauheed AM, Ayo JO, Kawu MU. Regulation of oligodendrocyte differentiation: insights and approaches for the management of neurodegenerative disease. Pathophysiology. 2016;23(3):203–10.

Ulich TR, Fann MJ, Patterson PH, Williams JH, Samal B, Del Castillo J, Yin S, Guo K, Remick DG. Intratracheal injection of LPS and cytokines. V. LPS induces expression of LIF and LIF inhibits acute inflammation. Am J Phys. 1994;267(4 Pt 1):L442–6.

Vanderlocht J, Hellings N, Hendriks JJ, Vandenabeele F, Moreels M, Buntinx M, Hoekstra D, Antel JP, Stinissen P. Leukemia inhibitory factor is produced by myelin-reactive T cells from multiple sclerosis patients and protects against tumor necrosis factor-alpha-induced oligodendrocyte apoptosis. J Neurosci Res. 2006;83(5):763–74.

Vela L, Caballero I, Fang L, Liu Q, Ramon F, Diez E, de Los Frailes M. Discovery of enhancers of the secretion of leukemia inhibitory factor for the treatment of multiple sclerosis. J Biomol Screen. 2016;21(5):437–45.

Virard I, Coquillat D, Bancila M, Kaing S, Durbec P. Oligodendrocyte precursor cells generate pituicytes in vivo during neurohypophysis development. Glia. 2006;53(3):294–303.

Visser L, Melief MJ, van Riel D, van Meurs M, Sick EA, Inamura S, Bajramovic JJ, Amor S, Hintzen RQ, Boven LA, et al. Phagocytes containing a disease-promoting toll-like receptor/nod ligand are present in the brain during demyelinating disease in primates. Am J Pathol. 2006;169(5):1671–85.

Willson TA, Metcalf D, Gough NM. Cross-species comparison of the sequence of the leukaemia inhibitory factor gene and its protein. Eur J Biochem. 1992; 204(1):21–30.

Wullschleger A, Kapina V, Molnarfi N, Courvoisier DS, Seebach JD, Santiago-Raber ML, Hochstrasser DF, Lalive PH. Cerebrospinal fluid interleukin-6 in central nervous system inflammatory diseases. PLoS One. 2013;8(8):e72399.

Yasukawa H, Ohishi M, Mori H, Murakami M, Chinen T, Aki D, Hanada T, Takeda K, Akira S, Hoshijima M, et al. IL-6 induces an anti-inflammatory response in the absence of SOCS3 in macrophages. Nat Immunol. 2003;4(6):551–6.

Zekki H, Feinstein DL, Rivest S. The clinical course of experimental autoimmune encephalomyelitis is associated with a profound and sustained transcriptional activation of the genes encoding toll-like receptor 2 and CD14 in the mouse CNS. Brain Pathol. 2002;12(3):308–19.

Zhang X, Tao Y, Chopra M, Dujmovic-Basuroski I, Jin J, Tang Y, Drulovic J, Markovic-Plese S. IL-11 induces Th17 cell responses in patients with early relapsing-remitting multiple sclerosis. J Immunol. 2015;194(11):5139–49.

13

The interplay between AR, EGF receptor and MMP-9 signaling pathways in invasive prostate cancer

Anna Mandel[1], Per Larsson[1], Martuza Sarwar[2], Julius Semenas[1], Azharuddin Sajid Syed Khaja[1] and Jenny L. Persson[1,2]*

Abstract

Background: Metastatic Prostate cancer (PCa) cells have gained survival and invasive advantages. Epidermal growth factor (EGF) receptor is a receptor tyrosine kinase, which may mediate signalling to promote progression and invasion of various cancers. In this study, we uncovered the molecular mechanisms underlying the interconnection among the androgen receptor (AR), matrix metalloproteinase-9 (MMP9) and EGFR in promoting PCa progression.

Methods: Immunohistochemical analysis of the tissue microarrays consisting of primary and metastatic PCa tissues was performed. The clinical importance of EGFR and its association with survivals were analyzed using three cohorts from MSKCC Prostate Oncogenome Project dataset (For primary tumors, $n = 181$; for metastatic tumors $n = 37$) and The Cancer Genome Atlas Prostate Adenocarcinoma Provisional dataset ($n = 495$). Targeted overexpression or inhibition of the proteins of interests was introduced into PCa cell lines. Treatment of PCa cell lines with the compounds was conducted. Immunoblot analysis was performed.

Results: We showed that AR, MMP-9 and EGFR are interconnect factors, which may cooperatively promote PCa progression. Altered EGFR expression was associated with poor disease-free survival in PCa patients. Induced overexpression of AR led to an increase in the expression of EGFR, p-GSK-3β and decrease in p27 expression in PCa cell lines in the presence of androgen stimulation. Overexpression of MMP9 significantly induced EGFR expression in PCa cells. Inhibition of PIP5K1α, a lipid kinase that acts upstream of PI3K/AKT greatly reduced expressions of AR, MMP-9 and EGFR.

Conclusions: Our findings also suggest that PCa cells may utilize AR, EGFR and MMP-9 pathways in androgen-dependent as well as in castration-resistant conditions. Our data suggest a new therapeutic potential to block cancer metastasis by targeting AR, EGFR and MMP-9 pathways in subsets of PCa patients.

Keywords: Prostate cancer, Cancer metastasis, Epidermal growth factor receptor, Androgen receptor and androgen

Background

The derivative of the androgen testosterone, dihydrotestosterone (DHT) is the most abundant sex-hormone within the prostate and has a high binding affinity to androgen receptor (AR) (Feldman and Feldman 2001). Prostate cancer (PCa) cells in the initial stages of tumour development are responsive to androgens, however cancer cells often progress to a hormone-refractory state, termed castration-resistant prostate cancer (CRPC) (Denmeade and Isaacs 2002). AR is a transcription factor that regulates a panel of genes controlling the growth of prostate cells. Increased AR expression has been shown to affect the activation of its target genes, thereby promoting proliferation of PCa cells and rendering PCa resistant to androgen deprivation therapy (Hsu et al. 2005; Wang et al. 2005). Elevated level of AR expression is also associated with CRPC metastasis (Grasso et al. 2012; Shen and Abate-Shen 2010). This suggests that overexpression of AR originating from amplification

* Correspondence: jenny_l.persson@med.lu.se; jenny.persson@umu.se
[1]Department of Molecular Biology, Umeå University, 901 87 Umeå, Sweden
[2]Division of Experimental Cancer Research, Department of Translational Medicine, Clinical Research Centre, Lund University, Jan Waldenströms gatan 35, 205 02 Malmö, Sweden

or enhanced phosphorylation may allow PCa cells to circumvent androgen-dependent signaling.

One of the major features of PCa is its heterogeneity. PCa often contains a mixture of heterogeneous populations including cancer cells, stromal cells, fibroblasts and tumor-specific extracellular matrix (ECM) (Joyce and Pollard 2008; Kim et al. 2011). It has become clear that abundant growth factors are not only secreted by cancer cells, but are also produced by tumor-specific stromal cells, fibroblasts, ECM constituents and other cell types. The regulation of growth factors and their receptors is mediated through autocrine- or paracrine-dependent manners (Blume-Jensen and Hunter 2001; Bruzzese et al. 2014; Lemmon and Schlessinger 2010). In PCa, abnormal levels of growth factors are frequently observed in serums and in tumor tissues obtained from PCa patients (Reynolds and Kyprianou 2006). Remarkably, growth factors produced by the bone matrix and bone marrow niche promote growth and proliferation of metastasized PCa cells (Gleave et al. 1991; Kimura et al. 2010). Epidermal growth factor (EGF) family of growth factors interact with their receptors including EGF receptor (also known as ErB-1 or Her 1), Her 2/neu (ErbB-2), Her 3 (ErbB-3) and Her 4 (ErbB-4) (Casaletto and McClatchey 2012). Upon binding to its ligands, EGFR becomes active by formation of homodimers. The homodimers of EGFR phosphorylate and interact with corresponding downstream factors, which regulate fundamental cellular events including proliferation, survival and migration (Chong and Jänne 2013; Wells 1999). Alternatively, EGFR can be activated via hetero-dimerization with other receptors belonging to the epidermal growth factor receptor family of tyrosine kinases (Ono and Kuwano 2006). Similarly to that of their ligands, alterations in the expression and activity of EGFR also occur in PCa (De Miguel et al. 1999). Expression of EGFR is low in normal prostate tissues (Traish and Wotiz 1987), while it is highly expressed in primary and metastatic PCa tissues (Di Lorenzo et al. 2002; Hofer et al. 1991). Furthermore, EGFR and HER-2 have been revealed to play a significant role in metastasis to the bone marrow (Day et al. 2017; Lu and Kang 2010), and these factors exhibited elevated activity in tumour initiating cells (TICs) and circulating tumour cells (CTCs) (Day et al. 2017). Taken together these data suggest a role of EGFR in the development and progression of PCa. Since excess levels of EGF and EGFR are produced by both PCa cells and tumor-specific stromal/fibroblasts, it is likely that EGFR signalling in cancer cells is activated via the production of binding ligands by both cancer cells and tumor-specific stromal/fibroblasts through paracrine and autocrine loops, leading to the growth and survival of PCa cells in the absence of androgens (Di Lorenzo et al. 2002; Traish and Wotiz 1987).

EGFR and its ligands may replace androgens to enhance phosphorylation of AR or act as AR co-regulators to promote activation of its downstream genes. It has been proposed that forced overexpression of HER2 kinase increases AR expression and promotes growth of hormone-refractory PCa cells through AR signaling (Craft et al. 1999; Yeh et al. 1999). Dual repression of EGFR and HER-2 has been shown to impair PCa tumour cell proliferation and survival (Chen et al. 2011; Day et al. 2017). Further, EGFR/ERBB2 kinase activity was revealed to be significantly up-regulated in LNCaP cells co-cultured with osteoblastic cells as determined by multiplex kinase activity profiling. This study hints that EGFR activity is stimulated by tumor-associated bone cells (Bratland et al. 2009). Activation of EGFR is also mediated by type 1 insulin-like growth factor (IGF) and extracellular matrixes, which are produced by the tumor-associated microenvironment during PCa metastases in the bone marrow (Chott et al. 1999). However, the role of EGFR in metastases and the precise mechanisms underlying EGFR activation by the tumor-associated microenvironment are largely unknown.

Matrix metalloproteinase-9 (MMP-9) is involved in degradation of ECM and vascular remodeling during tumor cell invasion (Heissig et al. 2002). It has been shown that MMP-9 produced by fibroblasts promotes mitogenic induction in breast cancer cells by enhancing endothelial cell survival and function in an in vitro co-culture model (Shekhar et al. 2001). MMP-9 may amplify local angiogenesis due to its ability to cleave membrane-bound vascular endothelial growth factor (VEGF), hence elevating the level of functional VEGF in tumors (Bergers et al. 2000). Due to the role of MMP-9 in cancer metastasis, the association between EGFR and MMP-9 is an intriguing target for the investigation of EGFR's involvement in PCa invasion.

During the past years, several new classes of inhibitors against EGFR have been developed and have shown promising effects in targeting metastasized cancers of the lung, breast, colorectal system, and head and neck (Bertotti et al. 2015; Blaszczak et al. 2017; Chong and Jänne 2013; Munagala et al. 2011). The EGFR inhibitors cetuximab, panitumumab and geftinib have been approved by FDA and are currently used for treatment of patients with lung cancer, and head and neck cancers (Blaszczak et al. 2017; Chong and Jänne 2013; Kazandjian et al. 2016). These inhibitors induce apoptosis in cancer cells by blocking multiple EGFR-dependent growth and survival signaling pathways (Chong and Jänne 2013). Third-generation EGFR inhibitors such as rociletinib have been approved for treatment of EGFR-mutated non–small-cell lung cancer (Chabon et al. 2016; Eberlein et al. 2015; Piotrowska et al. 2015). The effects of EGFR inhibitors on CRPC remain to be further investigated in preclinical models and in patient-based clinical trials. A Phase II study in CRPC of lapatinib, an inhibitor of EGFR and human epidermal growth factor receptor 2 (HER2), showed prostate-specific antigen (PSA) response only in a very small number of patients (Whang et al. 2013). Dual inhibition of EGFR and HER2 poses as a promising prospect in terms of PCa therapy (Ahmad et al. 2011; Chen et al. 2011; Day et al. 2017; Sridhar et al. 2010), however to date, trials have been unsuccessful. It is of importance to gain deeper understanding of the cellular mechanisms underlying the interplay between PCa cells and PCa-associated microenvironment during progression of CRPC, and specifically to gain deeper knowledge about the role of EGFR in proliferation, survival and migration of PCa cells and PCa-associated cells during development of CRPC.

The aim of our study was to investigate the mechanisms underlying the interplay between AR and EGFR as well as MMP-9 and EGFR in PCa progression. We found that androgen treatment of both control and AR-overexpressing PCa cells led to a significant increase in the activation of EGFR and its associated activity with PI3K/AKT pathways, thus presumably allowing PCa cells to gain survival and invasive advantages. We also showed that EGFR is likely to be involved in PCa invasive mechanisms via MMP-9 signaling. Our study provides information on clinical and molecular bases suggesting that AR and EGFR are elements of interlinked signalling pathways, which allow PCa cells to use alternative mechanism without consuming large quantities of androgens, thereby bypass androgen-dependent pathways.

Methods
Tissue specimens, tissue microarrays and mRNA expression data
Tissue microarrays (TMAs) containing primary ($n = 17$) and metastatic PCa lesions ($n = 43$) from 14 PCa patients were constructed at Department of Clinical Pathology and Cytology, Skåne University Hospital, Malmö. The tumor tissues were reviewed and selected by two pathologists specialized in urology. The selected tissue cores were collected, paraffin-embedded and sectioned for histological analysis as described (Voduc et al. 2008). For comparison of EGFR between normal prostate free of pathological conditions, primary tumors and metastatic lesions gene expression data from the dataset GDS2545 in the Gene Expression Omnibus (GEO) database at the National Center for Biotechnology Information (NCBI) website was used. The dataset was obtained by performing Affymetrix HG-U95Bv2 oligonucleotide array platform as described (Chandran et al. 2007; Yu et al. 2004). The mean mRNA values of genes of interests from a total 146 human samples in the dataset GDS2546 were used in the present study. The samples included normal

prostate tissues adjacent to tumor ($N = 58$), primary tumor ($N = 64$), and the metastatic lesions ($N = 24$) from liver, para aortic lymph node, para-tracheal lymph node, retroperitoneal lymph node, lung and adrenal gland of 4 patients with CRPC. For mRNA expression and copy number alteration (CNA) data for EGFR, the disease-free survival (DFS) data was extracted from the open-access cBioPortal databases. MSKCC Prostate Oncogenome Project dataset (For primary tumors, $n = 181$; for metastatic tumors $n = 37$) and The Cancer Genome Atlas (TCGA) Prostate Adenocarcinoma Provisional dataset (For tumors taken from primary site $n = 495$) as described (Robinson et al. 2010; Taylor et al. 2010). The follow-up time from diagnosis to disease recurrence known as biochemical recurrence (BCR) ranged from 1 to 60 months was used for analysis of DFS. The study was approved by the Ethics Committee, Lund University, and the Helsinki Declaration of Human Rights was strictly observed.

Immunohistochemistry analysis
Immunohistochemistry on TMAs was performed as previously described (Wegiel et al. 2005). The staining procedure was performed using a semiautomatic staining machine (Ventana ES, Ventana Inc., Tucson, AZ). For immunohistochemical analysis of xenograft mouse organs, tissues or tumors were fixed in 4% paraformaldehyde for 24 h and embedded in paraffin. For histology analysis, the sections were stained with hematoxylin-eosin (H&E) and were subjected to analysis using an Olympus BX51 microscopy. Immunostaining of tumor tissues using antibodies was performed as previously described (Wegiel et al. 2008). The sections were viewed under an Olympus BX51 microscope at magnification of 20× or 40×. The slides were scanned and viewed; microphotographs were taken by using a high resolution scanner (ScanscopeCS, Aperio, Vista, CA). The staining intensity was scored as 0 (negative), 1 (weakly positive or positive), 2 (moderate positive), 3 (strongly or very strongly positive) using an arbitrary semi-quantitative scale.

Cell culturing and treatments
We used VCaP cells that is the "Vertebral-Cancer of the Prostate" cell line, which was established from prostate cancer tissue harvested from a metastatic lesion to a lumbar vertebral body of a patient with hormone refractory prostate cancer. The cells express AR and prostate-specific antigen (PSA). PC-3 cells is the castration-resistant prostate cancer cell line, which does not express AR and is insensitive to androgen stimulation. The cells were purchased from American Type Culture Collection (Manassas, VA, USA). Cells were maintained in RPMI-1640 medium or Ham's F-12 medium supplemented with 10% fetal bovine serum (FBS), 1% penicillin-streptomycin-neomycin (PSN) and

2 mM L-Glutamine. For treatment, cells were grown for 24 h in phenol red-free RPMI-1640 medium containing 10% charcoal stripped-serum and were subsequently treated with agents for 24 h. Dihydrotestosterone (DHT) at a final concentration of 5 nM in 0.1% DMSO, or PIP5K1 alpha inhibitor, a diketopiperazine fused C-1 indol-3-yl substituted 1,2,3,4-tetrahydroisoquinoline derivative, ISA-2011B (Semenas et al. 2014) at a final concentration of 50 μM in 0.1% DMSO, or solvent DMSO 0.1% for 48 h was applied as treatment.

Plasmids transfection

For transient transfection studies, pCMV-AR containing full-length AR and pCMV control vectors were kindly provided by Dr. Yvonne Giwercman at Department of Translational Medicine, Lund University, Sweden. pLX304 (Addgene, MA, USA); pLX304-MMP9 (PlasmID, Harvard Medical School, MA, USA) were used. For introduction of the plasmids, Lipofectamine® 2000/3000 transfection reagent (Life Technologies, Paisley, UK), TransIT-TKO® and TransIT-X2® (Mirus Bio, WI, USA) were used according to the manufacturer's instructions.

Immunoblot analysis and source of antibodies

The cells or tumor tissues were harvested and lysed in ice-cold RIPA buffer. Proteins (20–40 μg) were separated using 10 and 12% SDS-PAGE gels and transferred onto nitrocellulose membranes. Signals were visualized using the Enhanced ChemiLuminescence detection system (Pierce, Rockford, USA) and documented with an AlphaImager CCD system. Densitometric quantification of immunoblots was performed by the ImageJ Image Analysis Software (NIH, Baltimore, USA) and represented as fold change relative to control and were normalized relative to nd GAPDH bands. The following primary antibodies were used in this study: Monoclonal antibodies against estrogen receptor (ER) alpha (Nordic BioSite, Taby, Sweden), MMP-9 (Abcam, Cambridge, UK), EGFR (Abcam, Cambridge, UK), p-GSK-3 beta, p27, AR, GAPDH (Santa Cruz Biotechnology Inc., Santa Cruz, CA). Secondary antibodies used: HRP-conjugated anti-mouse IgG, anti-rabbit IgG (GE Healthcare) and anti-goat (Santa Cruz Biotechnology Inc., Santa Cruz, CA).

Statistical analysis

Student t-test was used for statistical analyses of the experimental data. Spearman rank correlation test was used to establish the level of correlation between mRNA expressions of relevant factors. Distribution of disease-free survival (DFS) was estimated by the method of Kaplan-Meier, with 95% confidence intervals. Differences between survival curves were calculated applying the log-rank test using the statistical program SPSS version 24.0. P-values equal to or less than 0.05 were considered to be statistically significant.

Results

Clinical importance of EGFR expression and its correlation with AR in primary and metastatic PCa tissues from patients

To evaluate clinical importance of EGFR and its correlation with AR expression in PCa patients, we used TMAs consisting of primary PCa ($n = 17$), and PCa metastatic tissues ($n = 43$). The TMAs were immuno-stained with antibodies against EGFR. EGFR was expressed in primary and metastatic lesions including lymph nodes, lungs and bones with bone metastatic TMAs having the highest staining intensity against EGFR protein expression (Fig. 1a). There was a clear trend that EGFR protein expression was higher in metastatic PCa tissues than that in primary PCa tissues, although statistical significance was not achieved, probably due to the small sample size ($p = 0.147$) (Fig. 1b). Pearson correlation test revealed that there was a significantly positive correlation between AR and EGFR protein expression ($r^2 = 0.348$, $p = 0.011$) in primary and metastatic PCa tissues from this patient cohort (Table 1). In order to further examine the clinical relevance of EGFR expression, we compared EGFR mRNA expression between normal prostate tissues adjacent to the prostate tumor tissues, primary PCa tissues, as well as PCa metastatic lesions. We found that EGFR expression was significantly higher in metastatic lesions compared with the normal prostate tissues ($p = 0.05$). There was a trend that EGFR expression was increased in metastatic lesions compared with primary prostate tumors, however, the statistical significance was not achieved (Fig. 1c). This data suggests that EGFR expression was elevated in metastatic PCa.

We next examined EGFR mRNA expression in PCa tissues originating from the primary site ($n = 495$) using The Cancer Genome Atlas (TCGA) Prostate Adenocarcinoma Provisional database. Spearman correlation test revealed that there was a significantly positive correlation between AR and EGFR mRNA expression ($r^2 = 0.756$, $p < 0.001$) in primary PCa tissues ($n = 495$) (Table 2). Alterations in EGFR gene were found in 40% of tumor tissues, alterations in AR gene were detected in 16% of tumors as assessed using the dataset from the MSKCC Prostate cBioportal Database (Fig. 1d). To examine whether alterations in EGFR might be associated with patient outcome, we performed Kaplan-Meier survival analysis. We observed that patients with alterations in EGFR ($n = 70$) suffered poorer DFS as compared to those without alterations ($n = 52$), and

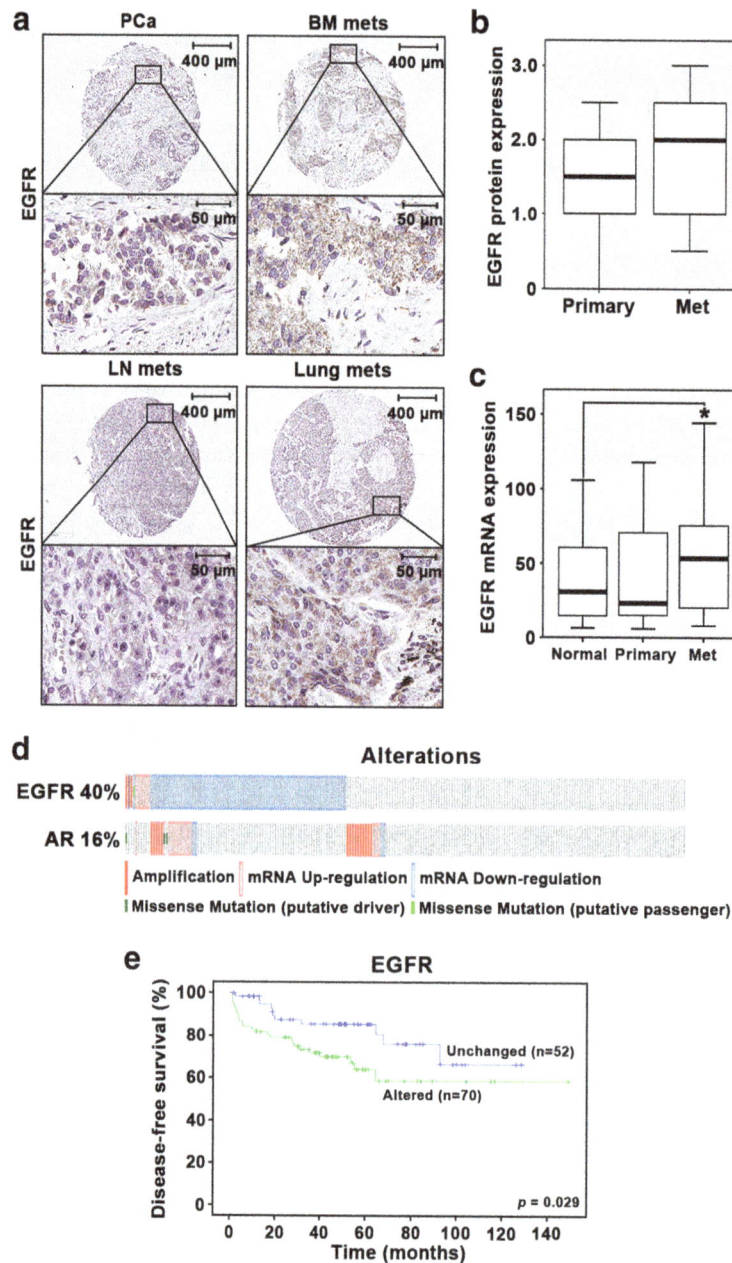

Fig. 1 Evaluation of the clinical importance of EGFR and its correlation with AR in prostate cancer patients. **a** Immunohistochemical analysis of EGFR expression in primary PCa ($n = 17$), and in bone, lymph node and lung metastatic PCa sites ($n = 43$). The TMA staining intensity shows that EGFR protein expression is highest in bone metastatic PCa lesions. **b** Box plot showed the comparison in EGFR protein expression between primary PCa ($n = 17$) and metastatic lesions ($n = 43$) ($p = 0.147$). **c** Box plot showed the comparison in EGFR mRNA expression between normal prostate ($n = 58$), primary PCa ($n = 64$) and metastatic lesions ($n = 24$) ($p = 0.05$). **d** Gene and mRNA alteration profiles of EGFR and AR in PCa patients ($n = 216$) where 40% of patients ($n = 86$) exhibited EGFR alterations on the gene and mRNA level, while 16% of patients ($n = 35$) exhibited discrepancies in AR gene and mRNA expression. MSKCC Prostate Oncogenome Database was used. **e** Kaplan-Meier survival curve revealed that patients with alterations in EGFR ($n = 70$) suffered poorer disease-free survival (DFS) as compared to those without alterations ($n = 52$), and this difference was statistically significant ($p = 0.029$). MSKCC Prostate Oncogenome Database was used

this difference was statistically significant ($p = 0.03$) (Fig. 1e). These data suggested that alterations in both AR and EGFR may be interlinked events and are associated with poor patient outcome in PCa.

The effect of elevated AR expression on EGFR and its associated signaling in VCaP cells

To examine whether AR signaling affects EGFR protein expression, we used VCaP cells derived from metastatic

Table 1 Pearson's correlation of protein expression between AR and EGFR

		EGFR
AR	Correlation coefficient	0.348*
	Significance (p value)	0.011

The analysis implies significant positive correlation between the two factors. The correlation between AR and EGFR is significant at the 0.05 level (*p < 0.05)

Table 2 Spearman's correlation of mRNA expression between AR and EGFR

		EGFR
AR	Correlation coefficient	0.756**
	Significance (p value)	0.000

The analysis implies significant positive correlation between the two factors. The correlation is significant at the 0.001 level (**p < 0.001)

lesions of CRPC. We induced overexpression of AR by transfecting VCaP cells with pCMV-AR or pCMV control vectors. Immunoblot analysis confirmed the overexpression of AR in VCaP cells transfected with pCMV-AR vector compared with the cells transfected with pCMV control vector ($p = 0.04$) (Fig. 2a). To examine whether induction of androgen may further enhance AR expression in VCaP cells, we treated VCaP cells overexpressing AR or transfected with control vector with DHT at 5 nM dose. There was a trend that DHT treatment increased AR expression in VCaP cells expressing control vector, however, statistical significance was not achieved (Fig. 2a). DHT treatment enhanced AR expression in VCaP cells expressing the pCMV-AR vector and this was statistically significant ($p = 0.03$) (Fig. 2a). We next investigated whether elevated level of AR with or without the presence of its ligand androgen may have any effect on EGFR expression. We examined EGFR expression in VCaP cells expressing pCMV-AR or control vector in the presence of absence of 5 nM DHT. DHT stimulation significantly induced an upregulation of EGFR expression in VCaP cells expressing pCMV control vector as determined by immunoblot analysis ($p = 0.01$; Fig. 2b).

Induced overexpression of AR alone had no effect on EGFR expression, however, DHT treatment of VCaP cells that overexpressed AR resulted in a dramatic increase in EGFR expression ($p = 0.01$; Fig. 2b). These data suggest that androgen and the ligand stimulation of AR by androgen have a significant positive effect on EGFR expression.

Since PI3K/AKT axis acts as a mediator between EGFR and AR signaling, we examined the effects of DHT stimulation and AR overexpression on AKT down-stream factors, p-GSK-3β and p27. DHT treatment or AR overexpression alone had no significant effect on p-GSK-3β, however, DHT treatment and AR overexpression additively increased the expression of p-GSK-3β significantly in VCaP cells ($p = 0.003$; Fig. 3a). P27 is a key cell cycle inhibitor, and decreased level of p27 is associated with increased proliferation. We observed that DHT treatment resulted in decreased expression of p27 ($p = 0.01$; Fig. 3b). The combination of DHT treatment and AR overexpression also significantly reduced p27 expression in VCaP cells ($p = 0.01$; Fig. 3b). The findings suggest that there is a functional link between AR/androgen and EGFR and its associated cellular signaling in PCa cells.

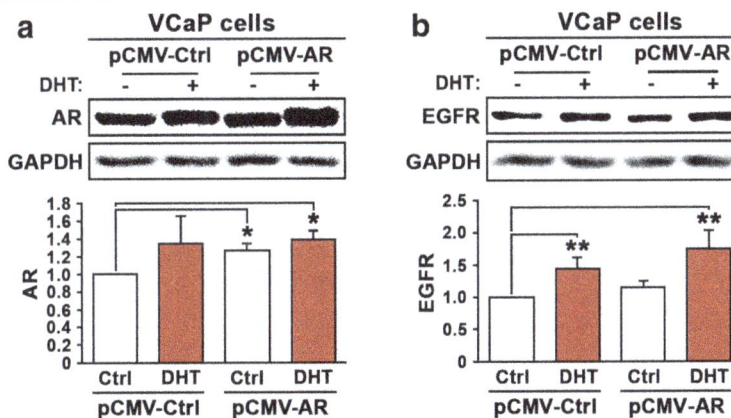

Fig. 2 Evaluation the effect of overexpression of AR and DHT treatment on expression of EGFR in VCaP cells. **a** Immunoblot analysis was performed to examine the expression of AR in VCaP cells that were transfected with pCMV control vector (pCMV-Ctrl) or pCMV-AR vector (pCMVAR) and followed by treatment with DHT or vehicle control. **b** Expression of EGFR protein in VCaP cells that were transfected with pCMV control vector (pCMV-Ctrl) or pCMV-AR vector (pCMVAR) and followed by treatment with DHT or vehicle control. Antibody against GAPDH was used as loading control. Data presented is average of three independent experiments (±SD). $p < 0.05$ is indicated by "*", $p \leq 0.01$ is indicated by "**"

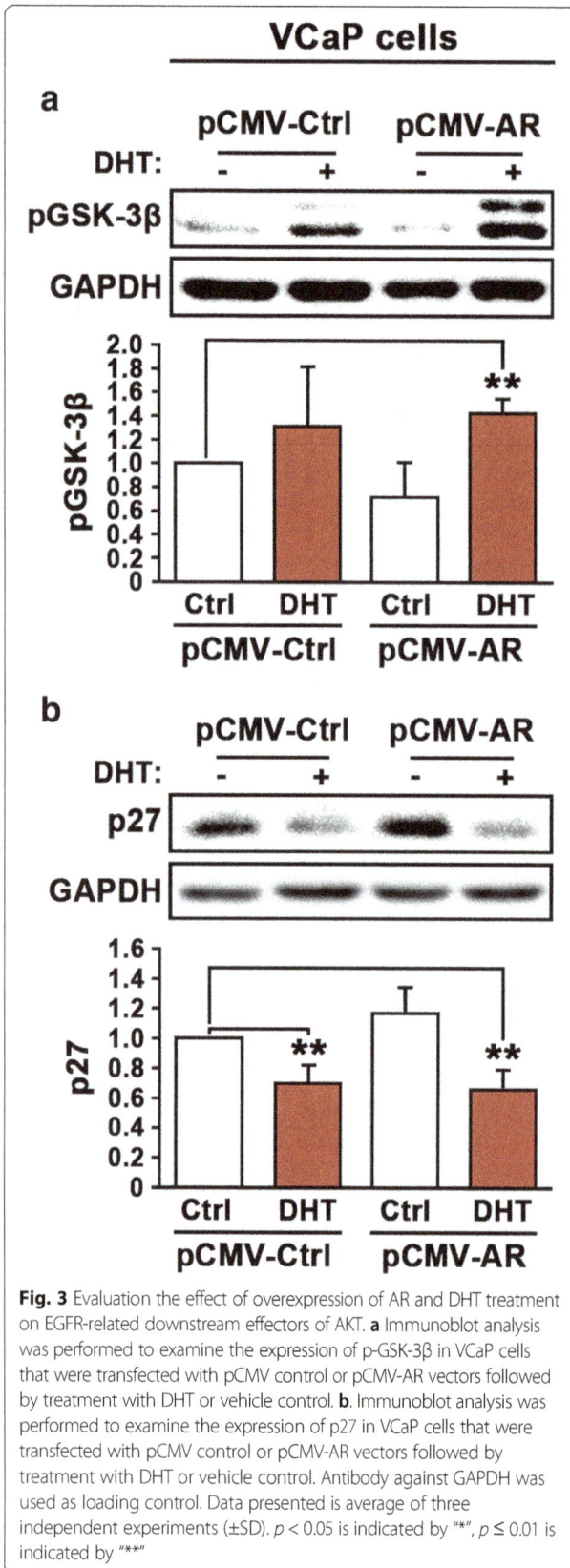

Fig. 3 Evaluation the effect of overexpression of AR and DHT treatment on EGFR-related downstream effectors of AKT. **a** Immunoblot analysis was performed to examine the expression of p-GSK-3β in VCaP cells that were transfected with pCMV control or pCMV-AR vectors followed by treatment with DHT or vehicle control. **b.** Immunoblot analysis was performed to examine the expression of p27 in VCaP cells that were transfected with pCMV control or pCMV-AR vectors followed by treatment with DHT or vehicle control. Antibody against GAPDH was used as loading control. Data presented is average of three independent experiments (±SD). $p < 0.05$ is indicated by "*", $p \leq 0.01$ is indicated by "**"

An association between AR and MMP-9 signaling, and EGFR protein expression in VCaP cell line with invasive phenotype

MMP-9 is a key player in promoting metastatic dissemination and growth of PCa. To further elucidate the functional interlink between AR/EGFR and invasive signaling, we decided to analyze the relationship between AR, MMP-9 and EGFR signaling in PCa cell lines. We first examined whether DHT stimulation and AR overexpression may have any effect on MMP-9 expression in PCa cells. Interestingly, induced overexpression of AR in VCaP cells resulted in a significant increase in MMP-9 expression as compared with the control ($p = 0.001$) (Fig. 4a). However, combined DHT stimulation and AR overexpression did not increase MMP-9 expression (Fig. 4a). Thus AR, in the absence of its ligand androgen, is capable of inducing MMP-9 expression in VCaP cells.

To investigate whether there is a direct link between AR and MMP-9, we employed castration-resistant PC-3 cells, which lack endogenous AR expression. We introduced AR re-expression in PC-3 cells by transfecting the cells with pCMV-AR vector or pCMV control vector, followed by treatment of the transfected cells with DHT at 5 nM. AR expression was successfully induced in PC-3 cells, and DHT treatment further significantly increased AR expression ($p = 0.005$) (Fig. 4b). Similar to what was observed in VCaP cells, induced AR expression in PC-3 cells resulted in a significant increase in MMP-9 expression as compared with the control ($p = 0.05$) (Fig. 4c). However, combined DHT stimulation and AR overexpression did not further increase MMP-9 expression in PC-3 cells (Fig. 4c). These data suggest a direct link between AR and MMP-9 expression occurring independently of androgen.

We next examined EGFR expression in PC-3 cells expressing pCMV control vector or pCMV-AR vector in the absence or presence of DHT at 5 nM concentration. DHT alone showed no effect on EGFR expression in the absence of AR (Fig. 4d). Induced expression of AR alone had no effect on EGFR expression (Fig. 4d). Similar to what was observed in VCaP cells, combined AR expression and DHT treatment resulted in a remarkable increase in EGFR expression ($p = 0.03$) (Fig. 4d). Taken together, these results provide evidence suggesting that there is a positive and direct association between AR pathways and EGFR, and this signaling cascade is independent of stimulation or binding of AR by its ligand androgen.

Having demonstrated that enhanced AR signaling leads to increased expression of EGFR and MMP-9, we next wanted to investigate whether there might be a functional link between MMP-9 and EGFR. To this end, we induced overexpression of MMP-9 by transfecting

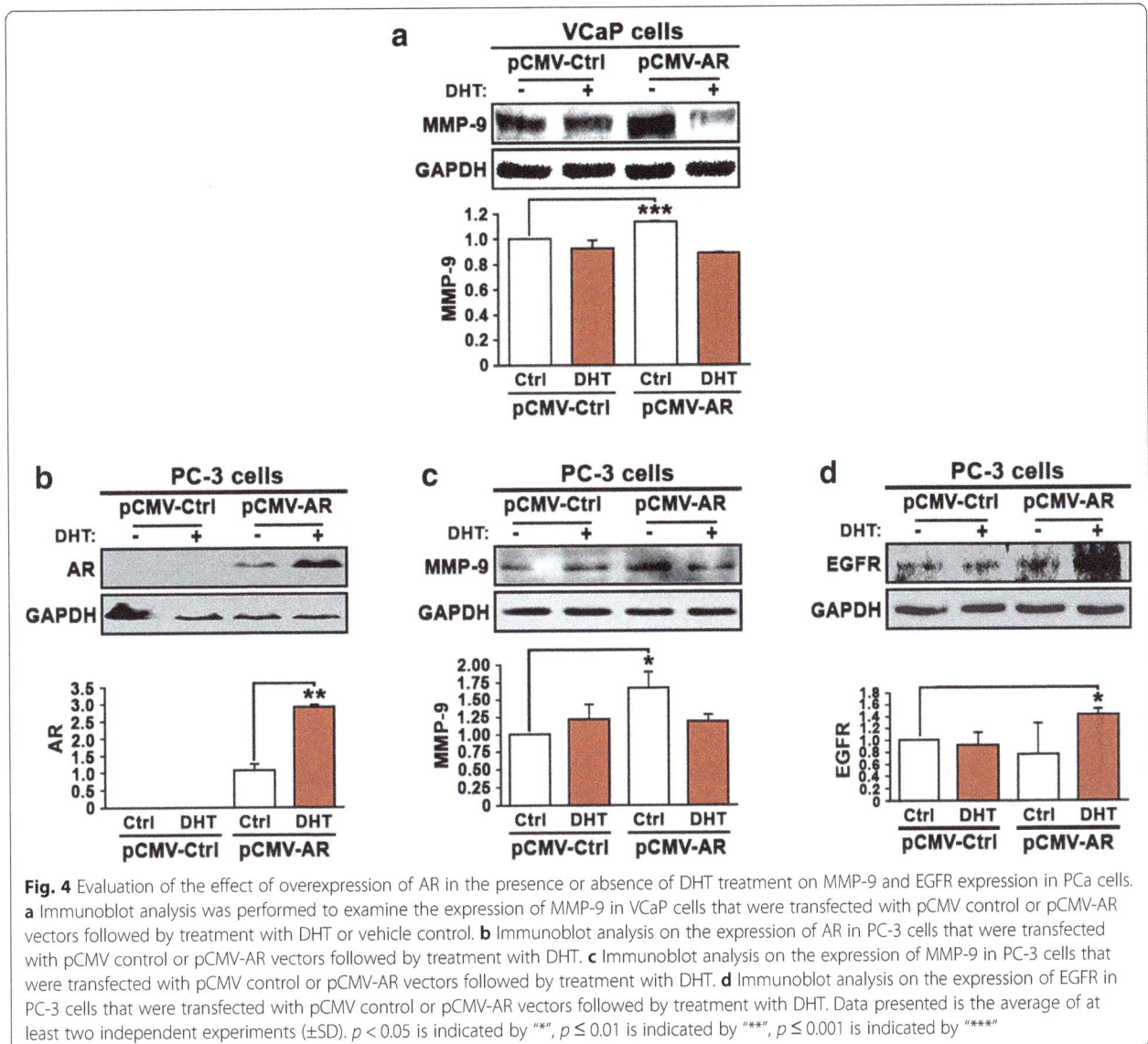

Fig. 4 Evaluation of the effect of overexpression of AR in the presence or absence of DHT treatment on MMP-9 and EGFR expression in PCa cells. **a** Immunoblot analysis was performed to examine the expression of MMP-9 in VCaP cells that were transfected with pCMV control or pCMV-AR vectors followed by treatment with DHT or vehicle control. **b** Immunoblot analysis on the expression of AR in PC-3 cells that were transfected with pCMV control or pCMV-AR vectors followed by treatment with DHT. **c** Immunoblot analysis on the expression of MMP-9 in PC-3 cells that were transfected with pCMV control or pCMV-AR vectors followed by treatment with DHT. **d** Immunoblot analysis on the expression of EGFR in PC-3 cells that were transfected with pCMV control or pCMV-AR vectors followed by treatment with DHT. Data presented is the average of at least two independent experiments (±SD). $p < 0.05$ is indicated by "*", $p \leq 0.01$ is indicated by "**", $p \leq 0.001$ is indicated by "***"

VCaP cells with pLX-MMP-9 or pLX control vector. We found that induced overexpression of MMP-9 in VCaP cells led to a significant increase in EGFR expression ($p = 0.01$) (Fig. 5a). We also examined whether elevated expression of MMP-9 may have any effect on AR in VCaP cells. However, overexpression of MMP-9 had no significant effect on AR expression in VCaP cells (Fig. 5b). Overexpression of MMP-9 did not show significant effect on expression of the downstream targets of AKT including p-GSK-3β and p27 (Fig. 5c and d). Taken together, our results suggest that AR, EGFR and MMP9 are functionally interconnected in PCa cells.

Next, we investigated whether inhibition of PI3K/AKT axis, the upstream regulator of AR signaling may have any effect on MMP-9 and EGFR expression in PCa cells. We employed PC-3 cells expressing control pCMV or

pCMV-AR vectors, which previously provided a model system to examine the direct link between AR, MMP-9 and EGFR. We treated PC-3 cells that expressed pCMV control vector or pCMV-AR vector with ISA-2011B and examined the effect of ISA-2011B on AR expression. ISA-2011B treatment significantly reduced AR expression ($p = 0.05$) (Fig. 6a). Next, we examined the effect of ISA-2011B on MMP-9 expression in the absence or presence of AR expression in PC-3 cells. Interestingly, ISA-2011B treatment resulted in a significant downregulation of MMP-9 in the absence of AR expression ($p = 0.02$) (Fig. 6b). ISA-2011B also significantly decreased MMP-9 expression in PC-3 cells expressing AR ($p = 0.03$) (Fig. 6c). Thus, MMP-9 expression can be inhibited by PIP5K1α inhibitor acting upstream the PI3K/AKT axis in the presence or absence of AR expression. Similar to what was observed in case of

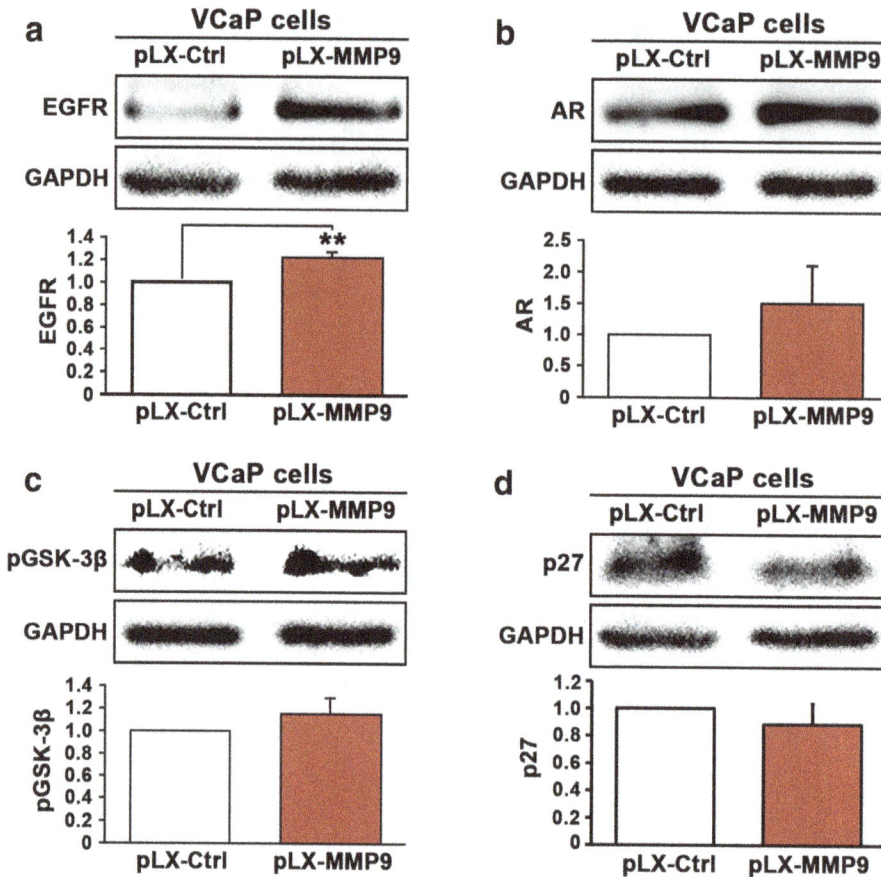

Fig. 5 The effect of overexpression of MMP9 on the expression of EGFR, AR, p-GSK-3β and p27 in VCaP cells. **a** Immunoblot analysis was performed to examine the expression of EGFR in VCaP cells that were transfected with pLX-control vector (PLX-Ctrl) or pLX-MMP9 vector (PLX-MMP9). **b** Expression of AR in VCaP cells that were transfected with pLX-control vector (PLX-Ctrl) or pLX-MMP9 vector (PLX-MMP9). **c** and **d** Expression of p-GSK-3β and p27 in VCaP cells that were transfected with pLX-control vector (PLX-Ctrl) or pLX-MMP9 vector (PLX-MMP9). Data presented is average of two independent experiments (±SD). $p < 0.05$ is indicated by "*", $p \leq 0.01$ is indicated by "**"

MMP-9, ISA-2011B treatment resulted in significant downregulation of EGFR expression in PC-3 cells in the absence or presence of AR expression (For EGFR in the absence of AR, $p = 0.003$, for EGFR in the presence of AR, $p = 0.03$) (Fig. 6d). This data further reinforces the hypothesis that the PI3K/AKT axis plays a fundamental role in mediating signaling between EGFR and AR in CRPC.

Discussion

Under the castration-resistant state, despite the minimal levels of androgens, PCa cells are capable of growing rapidly and obtaining survival and invasive advantages (Semenas et al. 2012). AR is a transcriptional factor, which regulates a panel of genes controlling the growth of prostate cells. However, whether AR may be functionally linked to the EGFR and MMP-9 invasion pathways in the presence or absence of its ligand androgen remains poorly understood.

In this study, we investigated the clinical importance and link between AR, EGFR and MMP-9 in prostate cancer by using clinical tissues from prostate cancer patients and prostate cancer cell lines. One of our important new findings revealed that EGFR expression was elevated in metastatic PCa tissues. PCa patients with altered levels of EGFR mRNA expression in their primary or metastatic tumors suffered poorer DFS compared to those without alterations in EGFR expression. This suggests that elevated level of EGFR expression is associated with poor patient outcome in PCa patients. It is possible to hypothesize that EGFR protein up-regulation in advanced PCa may have either occurred from alterations at transcriptional level or alterations at post-translational level. Increasing evidence suggests that AR cross-talks with the EGFR axis and renders PCa cells independent of androgen (Brizzolara et al. 2017; Craft et al. 1999; Jathal et al. 2016; Pignon et al. 2009). In the present study, we investigated the association and interplay between AR and EGFR in PCa progression. We also found that there was a significant correlation between AR

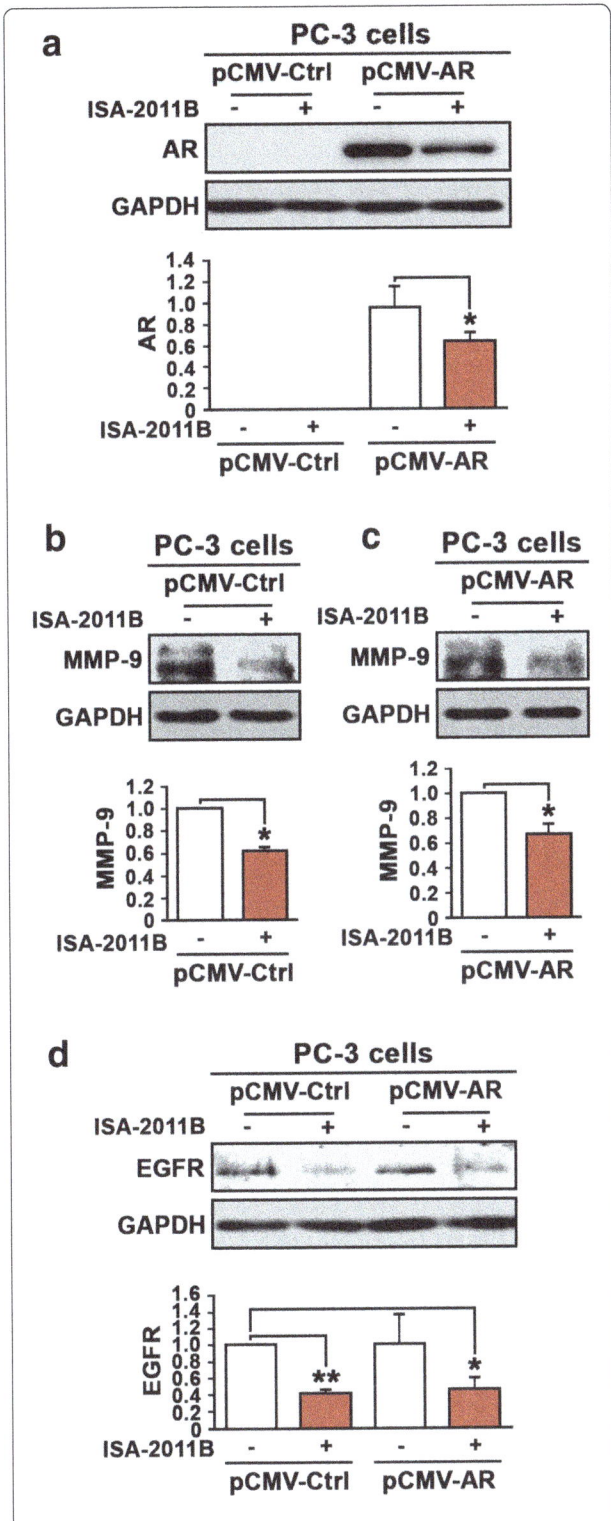

Fig. 6 The effect of inhibition of the PI3K/AKT/AR axis on the expression of AR, MMP-9 and EGFR in PC-3 cells. **a** Immunoblot analysis on the expression of AR in PC-3 cells that were transfected with pCMV control or pCMV-AR vectors followed by treatment with PIP5K1α/AKT inhibitor ISA-2011B. **b** Immunoblot analysis on the expression of MMP-9 in PC-3 cells that were transfected with pCMV control vector followed by treatment with ISA-2011B. **c** Immunoblot analysis on the expression of MMP-9 in PC-3 cells that were transfected with pCMV-AR vector followed by treatment with ISA-2011B. **d** Immunoblot analysis on the expression of EGFR in PC-3 cells that were transfected with pCMV control or pCMV-AR vectors followed by treatment with ISA-2011B. Data presented is the average of at least two independent experiments (±SD). $p < 0.05$ is indicated by "*", $p \leq 0.01$ is indicated by "**", $p \leq 0.001$ is indicated by "***"

and EGFR mRNA expression in a large patient cohort obtained from public dataset. Further, there was a significant correlation between AR and EGFR protein expression in the patient cohort collected by our laboratory.

We found that DHT stimulation and AR overexpression significantly increased the level of EGFR in VCaP cells. Furthermore, simultaneous DHT treatment and AR overexpression increased the level of EGFR somewhat more pronouncedly than DHT treatment alone. These data shows that EGFR expression may be regulated by AR upon stimulation of androgen. We further showed that AR overexpression alone had no significant effect on p-GSK-3β or p27, however, DHT treatment and AR overexpression additively induced significant up-regulation of p-GSK-3β and significant down-regulation of p27 in VCaP cells. These data suggest that constitutive activation of elevated AR through its ligand DHT may further activate pathways downstream of EGFR including PI3K/AKT pathways, thus presumably allowing PCa cells to gain survival and invasive advantages. It has been revealed that EGFR-mediated activation of AKT occurs in part through dimerization of EGFR with HER3 or alternatively, through enhanced HER3 activity and in part via interaction of EGFR with the intracellular adaptor protein (Craft et al. 1999; Di Lorenzo et al. 2002; Turke et al. 2012). Simultaneous occurrence of EGFR and phosphatase and tensin homolog (PTEN) alterations as well as an interplay between these two factors can be observed in various cancers such as cancers of the brain, lung and prostate (Bratland et al. 2009; Chott et al. 1999; Wozniak et al. 2017). Our data provides evidence suggesting that AR is functionally linked to EGFR and its associated AKT pathways. EGFR and its ligands may enhance phosphorylation of AR or act as AR co-regulators to promote activation of its downstream genes in the presence of androgen. Our findings suggest that PCa with elevated expression of AR and EGFR may have increased survival and invasive ability of PCa cells.

MMP-9 is one of the key factors, which promote cancer metastasis and it is also a transcriptional target of AR, commonly present in metastatic PCa (Hu et al. 2016; Semenas et al. 2014). In the present study, we showed that induced AR expression increased MMP-9 expression in VCaP in the absence of DHT. To further investigate whether there is a direct association between AR and MMP-9, we used PC-3 cells, which lack endogenous AR expression. Induced AR expression led to a significant increase in MMP-9 expression in PC-3 cells in the absence of DHT treatment. These results suggest that there is a direct link between AR and MMP-9 in PCa cells, and that AR acts on MMP-9 independently of androgen.

In the present study, we showed that MMP-9 overexpression significantly increased EGFR expression in VCaP cells. Our finding that EGFR is up-regulated in MMP-9 overexpressing cells further reinforces the relationship between EGFR and AR signaling and the involvement of EGFR in invasion promoting signaling networks. MMP-9 as an extracellular matrix factors may be served as ligand to bind to and enhance EGFR protein stability. Alternatively, as shown in the reported studies, MMP9 enhance EGFR expression via PI3K/AKT pathways in cancers of the lung, ovaries, breast and brain (Chen et al. 2016; Comamala et al. 2011; Elbaz et al. 2015; Garrido et al. 2017; Pei et al. 2014). This hypothesis is further supported by the previous published studies suggesting that EGFR cascades of pathways may be associated with MMP-9 during dissemination of PCa cells PCa (Lue et al. 2011; Xiao et al. 2012; Zhu et al. 2013). Our results suggest that upon ligand stimulation, AR increases EGFR expression, which in turn acts on AKT pathways to promote cancer cell survival and invasiveness. In parallel, elevated level of AR increased MMP-9 expression, which also positively stimulated EGFR at an androgen-independent fashion. Our data provides new information suggesting that AR, EGFR and MMP-9 are interconnected and may play important roles during cancer progression from androgen-dependent state to castration-resistant state.

We investigated whether inhibition of PI3K/AKT axis, the upstream of AR signaling may have any effect on MMP9 and EGFR expression in PCa cells. ISA-2011B treatment significantly reduced AR expression. Next, we examined the effect of ISA-2011B on MMP9 expression in the absence or presence of AR expression in PC-3 cells. Interestingly, ISA-2011B treatment resulted in a significant down-regulation of MMP9 in the presence and absence of AR expression. This suggests that MMP-9 expression is influenced not only by AR signal-ing, but also by PI3K/AKT pathways. Thus, elevated level of MMP-9 may be inhibited by blocking PIP5K1α/PI3K/AKT survival pathways, which is in part related to AR in PCa cells. Similar to what was observed for MMP9, ISA-2011B treatment resulted in significantly down regulation of EGFR expression in PC-3 cells in the absence or presence of AR expression. Our data further provided new information on that elevated level of EGFR may be inhibited by blocking both PIP5K1α/PI3K/AKT and AR-androgen pathways in subsets of PCa patients with elevated levels of AR and EGFR in their tumors.

Conclusions

In conclusion, our study provides an insight into the potential role of EGFR in advanced and invasive PCa possibly by acting as an upstream regulator of AR via the PI3K/AKT axis in growth and survival while likely acting through distinct pathways in invasive mechanisms. The study also provides a clue about the communication between the EGFR/AR axis and MMP-9, which might be a crucial component of tumor dissemination and establishment at the metastatic sites.

Abbreviations
AR: Androgen receptor; BCR: Biochemical recurrence; CNA: Copy-number alteration; CRPC: Castration-resistant prostate cancer; CTCs: Circulating tumor cells; DFS: Disease-free survival; DHT: Dihydrotestosterone; ECM: Extracellular matrix; EGFR: Epidermal growth factor receptor; ER: Estrogen receptor; FBS: Fetal bovine serum; HER-2: Human epidermal growth factor receptor-2; IGF: Insulin-like growth factor; MMP-9: Matrix metalloproteinase-9; PCa: Prostate cancer; p-GSK-3β: Phospho-Glycogen synthase kinase-3-beta; PIP5K1α: Phosphatidylinositol 4-phosphate 5-kinase type-1 alpha; PSA: Prostate-specific antigen; PSN: Penicillin-streptomycin-neomycin; PTEN: Phosphatase and tensin homolog; TICs: Tumor initiating cells; TMAs: Tissue microarrays; VEGF: Vascular endothelial growth factor

Acknowledgements
We sincerely thank Yvonne Lundberg Giwercman (Lund University, Lund) for providing vectors for this study. We also thank Kristina Ekström-Holka for technical help.

Funding
This work was supported by grants from the Swedish Cancer Society, Malmö Cancer Foundation, Malmö Cancer Foundation, the Government Health Innovation Grant, Kempe STF, Umeå University, Medical Faculty Grants to JLP. The Royal Physiographical Foundation to MS.

Authors' contributions
AM: Performed experiments, analyzed the data and wrote the manuscript. PL: Performed experiments and analyzed the data. MS: performed experiments and analyzed the data. JS: performed analysis of the bioinformatics. ASSK: Performed experiments, analysis and wrote the manuscript. JLP: analyzed the data and wrote the manuscript. All authors read and approved the final manuscript.

Competing interests

The authors declare that they have no competing interests.

References

Ahmad I, Patel R, Singh LB, Nixon C, Seywright M, Barnetson RJ, Brunton VG, Muller WJ, Edwards J, Sansom OJ, Leung HY. HER2 overcomes PTEN (loss)-induced senescence to cause aggressive prostate cancer. Proc Natl Acad Sci U S A. 2011;108:16392–7.

Bergers G, Brekken R, McMahon G, Vu TH, Itoh T, Tamaki K, Tanzawa K, Thorpe P, Itohara S, Werb Z, Hanahan D. Matrix metalloproteinase-9 triggers the angiogenic switch during carcinogenesis. Nat Cell Biol. 2000;2:737.

Bertotti A, Papp E, Jones S, Adleff V, Anagnostou V, Lupo B, Sausen M, Phallen J, Hruban CA, Tokheim C, et al. The genomic landscape of response to EGFR blockade in colorectal cancer. Nature. 2015;526:263–7.

Blaszczak W, Barczak W, Wegner A, Golusinski W, Suchorska WM. Clinical value of monoclonal antibodies and tyrosine kinase inhibitors in the treatment of head and neck squamous cell carcinoma. Med Oncol. 2017;34:60.

Blume-Jensen P, Hunter T. Oncogenic kinase signalling. Nature. 2001;411:355.

Bratland Å, Boender PJ, Høifødt HK, Østensen IHG, Ruijtenbeek R, M-y W, Berg JP, Lilleby W, Fodstad Ø, Ree AH. Osteoblast-induced EGFR/ERBB2 signaling in androgen-sensitive prostate carcinoma cells characterized by multiplex kinase activity profiling. Clin Exp Metastasis. 2009;26:485.

Brizzolara A, Benelli R, Vene R, Barboro P, Poggi A, Tosetti F, Ferrari N. The ErbB family and androgen receptor signaling are targets of Celecoxib in prostate cancer. Cancer Lett. 2017;400:9–17.

Bruzzese F, Hägglöf C, Leone A, Sjöberg E, Roca MS, Kiflemariam S, Sjöblom T, Hammarsten P, Egevad L, Bergh A, et al. Local and systemic Protumorigenic effects of cancer-associated fibroblast-derived GDF15. Cancer Res. 2014;74:3408–17.

Casaletto JB, McClatchey AI. Spatial regulation of receptor tyrosine kinases in development and cancer. Nat Rev Cancer. 2012;12:387.

Chabon JJ, Simmons AD, Lovejoy AF, Esfahani MS, Newman AM, Haringsma HJ, Kurtz DM, Stehr H, Scherer F, Karlovich CA, et al. Circulating tumour DNA profiling reveals heterogeneity of EGFR inhibitor resistance mechanisms in lung cancer patients. Nat Commun. 2016;7:11815.

Chandran UR, Ma C, Dhir R, Bisceglia M, Lyons-Weiler M, Liang W, Michalopoulos G, Becich M, Monzon FA. Gene expression profiles of prostate cancer reveal involvement of multiple molecular pathways in the metastatic process. BMC Cancer. 2007;7:64.

Chen L, Mooso BA, Jathal MK, Madhav A, Johnson SD, van Spyk E, Mikhailova M, Zierenberg-Ripoll A, Xue L, Vinall RL, et al. Dual EGFR/HER2 inhibition sensitizes prostate cancer cells to androgen withdrawal by suppressing ErbB3. Clin Cancer Res. 2011;17:6218–28.

Chen W, Zhong X, Wei Y, Liu Y, Yi Q, Zhang G, He L, Chen F, Liu Y, Luo J. TGF-beta regulates survivin to affect cell cycle and the expression of EGFR and MMP9 in Glioblastoma. Mol Neurobiol. 2016;53:1648–53.

Chong CR, Jänne PA. The quest to overcome resistance to EGFR-targeted therapies in cancer. Nat Med. 2013;19:1389.

Chott A, Sun Z, Morganstern D, Pan J, Li T, Susani M, Mosberger I, Upton MP, Bubley GJ, Balk SP. Tyrosine kinases expressed in vivo by human prostate Cancer bone marrow metastases and loss of the type 1 insulin-like growth factor receptor. Am J Pathol. 1999;155:1271–9.

Comamala M, Pinard M, Theriault C, Matte I, Albert A, Boivin M, Beaudin J, Piche A, Rancourt C. Downregulation of cell surface CA125/MUC16 induces epithelial-to-mesenchymal transition and restores EGFR signalling in NIH:OVCAR3 ovarian carcinoma cells. Br J Cancer. 2011;104:989–99.

Craft N, Shostak Y, Carey M, Sawyers CL. A mechanism for hormone-independent prostate cancer through modulation of androgen receptor signaling by the HER-2/neu tyrosine kinase. Nat Med. 1999;5:280.

Day KC, Lorenzatti Hiles G, Kozminsky M, Dawsey SJ, Paul A, Broses LJ, Shah R, Kunja LP, Hall C, Palanisamy N, et al. HER2 and EGFR overexpression support metastatic progression of prostate Cancer to bone. Cancer Res. 2017;77:74–85.

De Miguel P, Royuela M, Bethencourt R, Ruiz A, Fraile B, Paniagua R. Immunohistochemical comparative analysis of transforming growth factor α, epidermal growth factor, and epidermal growth factor receptor in normal, hyperplastic and neoplastic human prostates. Cytokine. 1999;11:722–7.

Denmeade SR, Isaacs JT. A history of prostate cancer treatment. Nat Rev Cancer. 2002;2:389–96.

Di Lorenzo G, Tortora G, D'Armiento FP, De Rosa G, Staibano S, Autorino R, D'Armiento M, De Laurentiis M, De Placido S, Catalano G, et al. Expression of epidermal growth factor receptor correlates with disease relapse and progression to androgen-independence in human prostate cancer. Clin Cancer Res. 2002;8:3438–44.

Eberlein CA, Stetson D, Markovets AA, Al-Kadhimi KJ, Lai Z, Fisher PR, Meador CB, Spitzler P, Ichihara E, Ross SJ, et al. Acquired resistance to the mutant-selective EGFR inhibitor AZD9291 is associated with increased dependence on RAS signaling in preclinical models. Cancer Res. 2015;75:2489–500.

Elbaz M, Nasser MW, Ravi J, Wani NA, Ahirwar DK, Zhao H, Oghumu S, Satoskar AR, Shilo K, Carson WE 3rd, Ganju RK. Modulation of the tumor microenvironment and inhibition of EGF/EGFR pathway: novel anti-tumor mechanisms of Cannabidiol in breast cancer. Mol Oncol. 2015;9:906–19.

Feldman BJ, Feldman D. The development of androgen-independent prostate cancer. Nat Rev Cancer. 2001;1:34.

Garrido P, Shalaby A, Walsh EM, Keane N, Webber M, Keane MM, Sullivan FJ, Kerin MJ, Callagy G, Ryan AE, Glynn SA. Impact of inducible nitric oxide synthase (iNOS) expression on triple negative breast cancer outcome and activation of EGFR and ERK signaling pathways. Oncotarget. 2017;8:80568–88.

Gleave M, Hsieh J-T, Gao C, von Eschenbach AC, Chung LWK. Acceleration of human prostate cancer growth in Vivo by factors produced by prostate and bone fibroblasts. Cancer Res. 1991;51:3753–61.

Grasso CS, Wu Y-M, Robinson DR, Cao X, Dhanasekaran SM, Khan AP, Quist MJ, Jing X, Lonigro RJ, Brenner JC, et al. The mutational landscape of lethal castration-resistant prostate cancer. Nature. 2012;487:239.

Heissig B, Hattori K, Dias S, Friedrich M, Ferris B, Hackett NR, Crystal RG, Besmer P, Lyden D, Moore MAS, et al. Recruitment of stem and progenitor cells from the bone marrow niche requires MMP-9 mediated release of kit-ligand. Cell. 2002;109:625–37.

Hofer DR, Sherwood ER, Bromberg WD, Mendelsohn J, Lee C, Kozlowski JM. Autonomous growth of androgen-independent human prostatic carcinoma cells: role of Transforming growth factor α. Cancer Res. 1991;51:2780–5.

Hsu C-L, Chen Y-L, Ting H-J, Lin W-J, Yang Z, Zhang Y, Wang L, Wu C-T, Chang H-C, Yeh S, et al. Androgen receptor (AR) NH2- and COOH-terminal interactions result in the differential influences on the AR-mediated transactivation and cell growth. Mol Endocrinol. 2005;19:350–61.

Hu S, Li L, Yeh S, Cui Y, Li X, Chang H-C, Jin J, Chang C. Corrigendum to "infiltrating T cells promote prostate cancer metastasis via modulation of FGF11→miRNA-541→androgen receptor (AR)→MMP9 signaling" [Mol Oncol 9 (1) (2015) 44–57]. Mol Oncol. 2016;10:1628–9.

Jathal MK, Steele TM, Siddiqui S, Mooso BA, D'Abronzo LS, Drake CM, Ghosh PM. Abstract 1303: in vivo analysis of EGFR family signalling as a bypass mechanism in prostate cancer. Cancer Res. 2016;76:1303.

Joyce JA, Pollard JW. Microenvironmental regulation of metastasis. Nat Rev Cancer. 2008;9:239.

Kazandjian D, Blumenthal GM, Yuan W, He K, Keegan P, Pazdur R. FDA approval of gefitinib for the treatment of patients with metastatic EGFR mutation-positive non–small cell lung cancer. Clin Cancer Res. 2016;22:1307–12.

Kim J, Roh M, Doubinskaia I, Algarroba GN, Eltoum IEA, Abdulkadir SA. A mouse model of heterogeneous, c-MYC-initiated prostate cancer with loss of Pten and p53. Oncogene. 2011;31:322.

Kimura T, Kuwata T, Ashimine S, Yamazaki M, Yamauchi C, Nagai K, Ikehara A, Feng Y, Dimitrov DS, Saito S, Ochiai A. Targeting of bone-derived insulin-like growth factor-II by a human neutralizing antibody suppresses the growth of prostate Cancer cells in a human bone environment. Clin Cancer Res. 2010;16:121–9.

Lemmon MA, Schlessinger J. Cell signaling by receptor tyrosine kinases. Cell. 2010;141:1117–34.

Lu X, Kang Y. Epidermal growth factor signalling and bone metastasis. Br J Cancer. 2010;102:457–61.

Lue H-W, Yang X, Wang R, Qian W, Xu RZH, Lyles R, Osunkoya AO, Zhou BP, Vessella RL, Zayzafoon M, et al. LIV-1 promotes prostate Cancer epithelial-to-Mesenchymal transition and metastasis through HB-EGF shedding and EGFR-mediated ERK signaling. PLoS One. 2011;6:e27720.

Munagala R, Aqil F, Gupta RC. Promising molecular targeted therapies in breast cancer. Indian J Pharmacol. 2011;43:236–45.

Ono M, Kuwano M. Molecular mechanisms of epidermal growth factor receptor (EGFR) activation and response to Gefitinib and other EGFR-targeting drugs. Clin Cancer Res. 2006;12:7242–51.

Pei J, Lou Y, Zhong R, Han B. MMP9 activation triggered by epidermal growth factor induced FoxO1 nuclear exclusion in non-small cell lung cancer. Tumour Biol. 2014;35:6673–8.

Pignon J-C, Koopmansch B, Nolens G, Delacroix L, Waltregny D, Winkler R. Androgen receptor controls *EGFR* and *ERBB2* gene expression at different levels in prostate cancer cell lines. Cancer Res. 2009;69:2941–9.

Piotrowska Z, Niederst MJ, Karlovich CA, Wakelee HA, Neal JW, Mino-Kenudson M, Fulton L, Hata AN, Lockerman EL, Kalsy A, et al. Heterogeneity underlies the emergence of EGFRT790 wild-type clones following treatment of T790M-positive cancers with a third-generation EGFR inhibitor. Cancer Discov. 2015; 5:713–22.

Reynolds AR, Kyprianou N. Growth factor signalling in prostatic growth: significance in tumour development and therapeutic targeting. Br J Pharmacol. 2006;147:S144–52.

Robinson MD, McCarthy DJ, Smyth GK. edgeR: a bioconductor package for differential expression analysis of digital gene expression data. Bioinformatics. 2010;26:139–40.

Semenas J, Allegrucci C, Boorjian SA, Mongan NP, Persson JL. Overcoming drug resistance and treating advanced prostate cancer. Curr Drug Targets. 2012;13: 1308–23.

Semenas J, Hedblom A, Miftakhova RR, Sarwar M, Larsson R, Shcherbina L, Johansson ME, Härkönen P, Sterner O, Persson JL. The role of PI3K/AKT-related PIP5K1α and the discovery of its selective inhibitor for treatment of advanced prostate cancer. Proc Natl Acad Sci. 2014;111:E3689–98.

Shekhar MPV, Werdell J, Santner SJ, Pauley RJ, Tait L. Breast Stroma plays a dominant regulatory role in breast epithelial growth and differentiation: implications for tumor development and progression. Cancer Res. 2001;61: 1320–6.

Shen MM, Abate-Shen C. Molecular genetics of prostate cancer: new prospects for old challenges. Genes Dev. 2010;24:1967–2000.

Sridhar SS, Hotte SJ, Chin JL, Hudes GR, Gregg R, Trachtenberg J, Wang L, Tran-Thanh D, Pham NA, Tsao MS, et al. A multicenter phase II clinical trial of lapatinib (GW572016) in hormonally untreated advanced prostate cancer. Am J Clin Oncol. 2010;33:609–13.

Taylor BS, Schultz N, Hieronymus H, Gopalan A, Xiao Y, Carver BS, Arora VK, Kaushik P, Cerami E, Reva B, et al. Integrative genomic profiling of human prostate cancer. Cancer Cell. 2010;18:11–22.

Traish AM, Wotiz HH. Prostatic epidermal growth factor receptors and their regulation by androgens*. Endocrinology. 1987;121:1461–7.

Turke AB, Song Y, Costa C, Cook R, Arteaga CL, Asara JM, Engelman JA. MEK inhibition leads to PI3K/AKT activation by relieving a negative feedback on ERBB receptors. Cancer Res. 2012;72:3228–37.

Voduc D, Kenney C, Nielsen TO. Tissue microarrays in clinical oncology. Semin Radiat Oncol. 2008;18:89–97.

Wang L, Hsu C-L, Chang C. Androgen receptor corepressors: an overview. Prostate. 2005;63:117–30.

Wegiel B, Bjartell A, Ekberg J, Gadaleanu V, Brunhoff C, Persson JL. A role for cyclin A1 in mediating the autocrine expression of vascular endothelial growth factor in prostate cancer. Oncogene. 2005;24:6385–93.

Wegiel B, Bjartell A, Tuomela J, Dizeyi N, Tinzl M, Helczynski L, Nilsson E, Otterbein LE, Harkonen P, Persson JL. Multiple cellular mechanisms related to cyclin A1 in prostate cancer invasion and metastasis. J Natl Cancer Inst. 2008;100:1022–36.

Wells A. EGF receptor. Int J Biochem Cell Biol. 1999;31:637–43.

Whang YE, Armstrong AJ, Rathmell WK, Godley PA, Kim WY, Pruthi RS, Wallen EM, Crane JM, Moore DT, Grigson G, et al. A phase II study of lapatinib, a dual EGFR and HER-2 tyrosine kinase inhibitor, in patients with castration-resistant prostate cancer. Urol Oncol. 2013;31:82–6.

Wozniak DJ, Kajdacsy-Balla A, Macias V, Ball-Kell S, Zenner ML, Bie W, Tyner AL. PTEN is a protein phosphatase that targets active PTK6 and inhibits PTK6 oncogenic signaling in prostate cancer. Nat Commun. 2017;8:1508.

Xiao LJ, Lin P, Lin F, Liu X, Qin W, Zou HF, Guo L, Liu W, Wang SJ, Yu XG. ADAM17 targets MMP-2 and MMP-9 via EGFR-MEK-ERK pathway activation to promote prostate cancer cell invasion. Int J Oncol. 2012;40:1714–24.

Yeh S, Lin H-K, Kang H-Y, Thin TH, Lin M-F, Chang C. From HER2/Neu signal cascade to androgen receptor and its coactivators: a novel pathway by induction of androgen target genes through MAP kinase in prostate cancer cells. Proc Natl Acad Sci. 1999;96:5458–63.

Yu YP, Landsittel D, Jing L, Nelson J, Ren B, Liu L, McDonald C, Thomas R, Dhir R, Finkelstein S, et al. Gene expression alterations in prostate Cancer predicting tumor aggression and preceding development of malignancy. J Clin Oncol. 2004;22:2790–9.

Zhu C, Li J, Ding Q, Cheng G, Zhou H, Tao L, Cai H, Li P, Cao Q, Ju X, et al. miR-152 controls migration and invasive potential by targeting TGFα in prostate cancer cell lines. Prostate. 2013;73:1082–9.

14

Microarray analysis of human keratinocytes from different anatomic sites reveals site-specific immune signaling and responses to human papillomavirus type 16 transfection

Mohd Israr[1], David Rosenthal[1], Lidia Frejo-Navarro[2], James DeVoti[1], Craig Meyers[3] and Vincent R. Bonagura[1*]

Abstract

Background: Stratified human keratinocytes (SHKs) are an essential part of mucosal innate immune response that modulates adaptive immunity to microbes encountered in the environment. The importance of these SHKs in mucosal integrity and development has been well characterized, however their regulatory immunologic role at different mucosal sites, has not. In this study we compared the immune gene expression of SHKs from five different anatomical sites before and after HPV16 transfection using microarray analyses.

Methods: Individual pools of human keratinocytes from foreskin, cervix, vagina, gingiva, and tonsils (HFKs, HCKs, HVKs, HGKs and HTLKs) were prepared. Organotypic (raft) cultures were established for both normal and HPV16 immortalized HFKs, HCKs, HVKs, HGKs and HTLKs lines which stably maintained episomal HPV16 DNA. Microarray analysis was carried out using the HumanHT-12 V4 gene chip (Illumina). Immune gene expression profiles were obtained by global gene chip (GeneSifter) and Ingenuity pathway analysis (IPA) for each individual site, with or without HPV16 transfection.

Results: We examined site specific innate immune response gene expression in SHKs from all five different anatomical sites before and after HPV16 transfection. We observed marked differences in SHK immune gene repertoires within and between mucosal tracts before HPV 16 infection. In addition, we observed additional changes in SHKs immune gene repertoire patterns when these SHKs were productively transfected with HPV16. Some immune response genes were similarly expressed by SHKs from different sites. However, there was also variable expression of non-immune response genes, such as keratin genes, by the different SHKs.

Conclusions: Our results suggest that keratinocytes from different anatomical sites are likely hard wired in their innate immune responses, and that these immune responses are unique depending on the anatomical site from which the SHKs were derived. These observations may help explain why select HPV types predominate at different mucosal sites, cause persistent infection at these sites, and on occasion, lead to HPV induced malignant and benign tumor development.

Keywords: Immune responses, Immune pathways, HPV, Keratinocytes, Microarrays

* Correspondence: VBonagura@northwell.edu

Mohd Israr, David Rosenthal and Lidia Frejo-Navarro are shared co-first authors.

Craig Meyers and Vincent R. Bonagura are shared senior authors

[1]The Feinstein Institute for Medical Research, Manhasset, NY, USA; Division of Allergy and Immunology, Department of Pediatrics, Donald and Barbara Zucker School of Medicine at Hofstra/Northwell, Great Neck, NY, USA

Full list of author information is available at the end of the article

Background

Stratified human keratinocytes (SHKs) are important immunologic components of both healthy and diseased mucosal surfaces in addition to their established role as physical epithelial barriers to infection. Accumulating evidence shows that SHKs from various mucosal tracts are important in mucosal development, inflammation, and HPV-induced cancer development (Wu et al. 2011; Saenz et al. 2008; Swamy et al. 2010; Nestle et al. 2009; Strid et al. 2009). Responses of SHKs can cause immune dysregulation (Swamy et al. 2010; Nestle et al. 2009; Strid et al. 2009; Albanesi et al. 2005; Tonel and Conrad 2009), however they also support the maintenance of the mucosal microbiome, via defensin expression, and they preserve mucosal homeostasis (Chung and Dale 2004; Frohm et al. 1997). Taken together, the importance of SHKs in both innate and adaptive immunity at mucosal sites is compelling (Swamy et al. 2010). Unresolved is the mechanism(s) that render these cells resistant or permissive to select viruses within a given viral family, such as human papillomaviruses (HPVs).

Towards understanding how oral cavity-derived keratinocytes influence adaptive immunity, Wu et al. (Wu et al. 2011) performed a global gene expression analysis that showed the significant effect of murine oral keratinocytes on adaptive immunity (Wu et al. 2011).

We previously reported that human oral tissues are permissive to HPV16 infection and that HPV replication can spread via the oral cavity (Israr et al. 2016). Here we compared the immune gene expression of SHKs using microarray analyses of pooled human keratinocytes from tonsil, foreskin, uterine cervix, vagina, and gingiva, before and after HPV16 transfection. We also compared immune gene network expression by SHKs taken from each of these anatomical sites to determine how they respond to HPV16 transfection. We observed marked differences in SHK immune gene expression within a given mucosal tract and by those derived from different mucosal tracts. In addition, we observed additional changes in SHK immune gene expression patterns when these SHKs were productively transfected with HPV16.

Methods

SHKs cultures, generation of HPV16 positive cell lines

Individual pools of primary SHKs from foreskin, cervix, vagina, gingiva, and tonsils (HFKs, HCKs, HVKs, HGKs and HTLKs) were grown as previously reported (McLaughlin-Drubin et al. 2004; McLaughlin-Drubin and Meyers 2005). Organotypic (raft) cultures were established as described (Meyers et al. 1997; McLaughlin-Drubin et al. 2005). Each pool of SHKs was prepared from 3 to 5 individual healthy donors. Both normal and HPV16 immortalized HFKs, HCKs, HVKs, HGKs and HTLKs lines which stably maintained episomal HPV16 DNA, and were seeded onto rat tail type 1 collagen matrices with J2 3 T3 feeder cells (Israr et al. 2016).

HPV16 infection of these SHKs could be more closely analogous to a natural infection than transfection. However, HPV16 infection of keratinocytes results in low efficiency and high variability between cell lines. Second, cells often lose more virus during further propagation (i.e.) in raft cultures, while HPV16 transfection provides high uptake efficiency, high cell line consistency, and rare heterogeneity. In addition, during transfection cells stably maintain the HPV genome as an episome, which is a critical step for a productive HPV16 life cycle and persistent HPV infection. Furthermore, integration of the HPV16 genome into keratinocyte DNA suppresses virus expression, and prevents formation of small, circular HPV16 genomes that can be packaged and transmitted to a new host keratinocyte (McBride and Warburton 2017).

RNA isolation and microarrays analysis

Triplicate cultures, of each SHK pool were harvested, and total RNA isolated using an RNeasy mini kit (Qiagen). Microarray analysis was carried out using the HumanHT-12 V4 gene chip (Illumina) containing 47231 probes targeting > 25,000 human genes. Expression data (baseline + HPV infected for each site) was log transformed and normalized to the median. Initial comparisons were performed using GeneSifter software and a volcano plot constructed ($p = 0.05$). Genes with ≥ 2 fold expression changes were considered significant in these analyses.

Comparison of gene expression by SHKs from different mucosae

A list of "immunologic genes" was obtained by querying http://ctdbase.org/ using key words "immu*, interleukin, cytokine, and defensin". Duplicates were removed, resulting in 2576 unique genes. A search for these genes in GeneSifter was done, sorted by expression using Kruskal-Wallis, (p cutoff = 0.02) resulting in 81 differentially expressed genes. A principle component analysis (PCA) was performed (dots = genes; lines with arrows = tissue types; axis 3 principle components) and the tissue types were separated using PC1, PC2, and PC3, to show differential gene expression patterns for these immunologic genes.

We then performed a pairwise analysis (normalized to all medians, p-value cutoff< 0.05) comparing individual SHKs from a single mucosal tract before and after HPV16 transfection. Among all differentially expressed genes (DEGs), a subset of genes known to be involved in immune responses/associated with immune regulation was selected for analysis. Expression data was analyzed using Ingenuity pathway analysis software: (IPA®, QIAGEN Inc., https://www.qiagenbioinformatics.com/products/ingenuitypathway-analysis). Networks were generated using the Core analysis tool (Kramer et al. 2014).

To better visualize the immunological genes uniquely, and/or commonly expressed by SHKs from each of the different anatomical sites, with or without HPV transfection, we applied these data sets to software at http://bioinformatics.psb.ugent.be/webtools/Venn/ to generate a 5 intersection Venn/Euler diagram (Fig. 2e) showing which DEGs were in expressed at each intersection.

Results and discussion

Keratins and immune gene mRNA expression by SHKs with or without HPV16 transfection

First we examined site specific keratins expression in all five different anatomical sites with or without HPV16 transfection that is consistent with published reports (Chu and Weiss 2002). As anticipated, all of the SHKs expressed some of keratin genes, see Additional file 1: Figure S1. However, there was variability in the repertoire of keratin genes that were expressed by different SHKs, suggesting that the cultures of pooled primary keratinocytes grown in rafts maintains the individual gene expression profiles characteristic of the site(s) from which the cells were obtained (Chu and Weiss 2002). As expected, the majority of immune genes having significant levels of expression were expressed at similar levels by all SHK cultures studied, see Fig. 2f. Significantly all 3 GAPDH probe sets, both HPRT-1 probe sets and all 3 B-actin probe sets were detected in all samples at equal levels, as anticipated, since all expression data was normalized prior to analysis. In addition to several keratins present in all tissue types (heat map), IFNAR1 and IFNGR1 and IFNGR2 were detected at equivalent levels in all samples tested, as well as IL-10 and the IL-10RB. Also, both the IL-4R and the IL-13R were expressed by all keratinocytes studied, and the expression of these genes was unaffected by introducing HPV16.

Of note, expression of immune response genes varied by site of SHK origin, see heat map and principal component analysis (Fig. 1a, b). Cluster analysis grouped gingival, vaginal and tonsil cells together, with the latter two being more closely related. Foreskin and cervical cells grouped together, but clearly showed many differences. Within the upper digestive mucosal tract, gingival and tonsil cells also showed differences, for example mRNA expression for individual members of multiple classes of immune genes (CCL-20, CXCL2 and CXCL6, interleukins IL-1, IL-8, and IL1F9 (IL-36γ)), and cell surface receptors/adhesion molecules (IL1RII, IL-13Rα, CD99). Several defensins were expressed by SHKs from these tissues, but not by cervical or foreskin SHKs.

We examined of all of the chemokines and interleukins present on the gene microarray, and found a limited number of immunologic signaling molecules being expressed in our keratinocyte cultures, largely irrespective of the derivation of the SHKs we studied. A single CCL chemokine, specifically CCL-20 was detected in all samples, together with its receptor CCR6. 2 CXC chemokines, CXCL14 and CXCL16 were also expressed by keratinocytes as well as the CXC receptors CXCR1 and CXCR7. IL8 was also expressed by all keratinocytes studied, while IL-23a was absent from both cervical and foreskin cultures. IL1-A and IL1-B were detected in all keratinocytes studied, albeit at varying levels. However, the antagonist of both 1A and 1B, IL1RN, the IL-20 receptor, and the IL17D receptor were highly expressed by all keratinocytes studied. IL-18 was equally expressed by all keratinocytes studied. In contrast, the IL-1 family member IL1F9, now called IL-36γ, and its antagonist IL1F5 were differentially expressed by different keratinocytes obtained from different anatomical sites.

HPV16 transfected cells also showed marked differences between cell types (Fig. 1b). Under these conditions, (cut off significance = 0.02), 92 different genes were identified. Similar to uninfected cells, vaginal and tonsil cells clustered together. However, gingival cell immune gene expression was quite different, while foreskin and cervical cells clustered together, although foreskin and cervical SHKs were quite different from each other. Among the most highly expressed genes by gingiva, vagina, and tonsil cells was IL-36γ. We previously reported that this cytokine was highly expressed by laryngeal papilloma cells (HPV6/11 infected) (DeVoti et al. 2008; DeVoti et al. 2014). Interestingly, IL36γ was not elevated in HPV16$^+$ foreskin and cervical cells. Thus, SHKs from different mucosae show differential immune genes expression before and after HPV transfection.

Comparing SHKs from different sites as a group before or after HPV transfection (Fig. 1c) showed that SHKs before HPV16 transfection behaved more similarly to each other than to their HPV16$^+$ counterparts which also behaved more similarly to each other (Fig. 1c). Two exceptions were noted, HPV16$^+$ SHKs from foreskin did not express a similar repertoire of immune response genes than HPV16$^+$ cells from other anatomical sites expressed, and HPV16$^-$ SHKs vaginal cells expressed similar immune gene profiles as HPV$^+$ cells from other mucosae (Fig. 1c).

Immune gene mRNA networks expressed by SHKs from different sites

We compared mRNA expression of an expanded list of immune genes and regulators by Ingenuity software, at each anatomical site with or without HPV16 transfection (Fig. 2a-e). There were significant differences in gene pathways used by SHKs in response to HPV16 transfection at each site. Differentially expressed genes in these comparisons are show in Additional file 2: Table S1. Fig. 2f (Venn/Euler diagram) shows that there were more

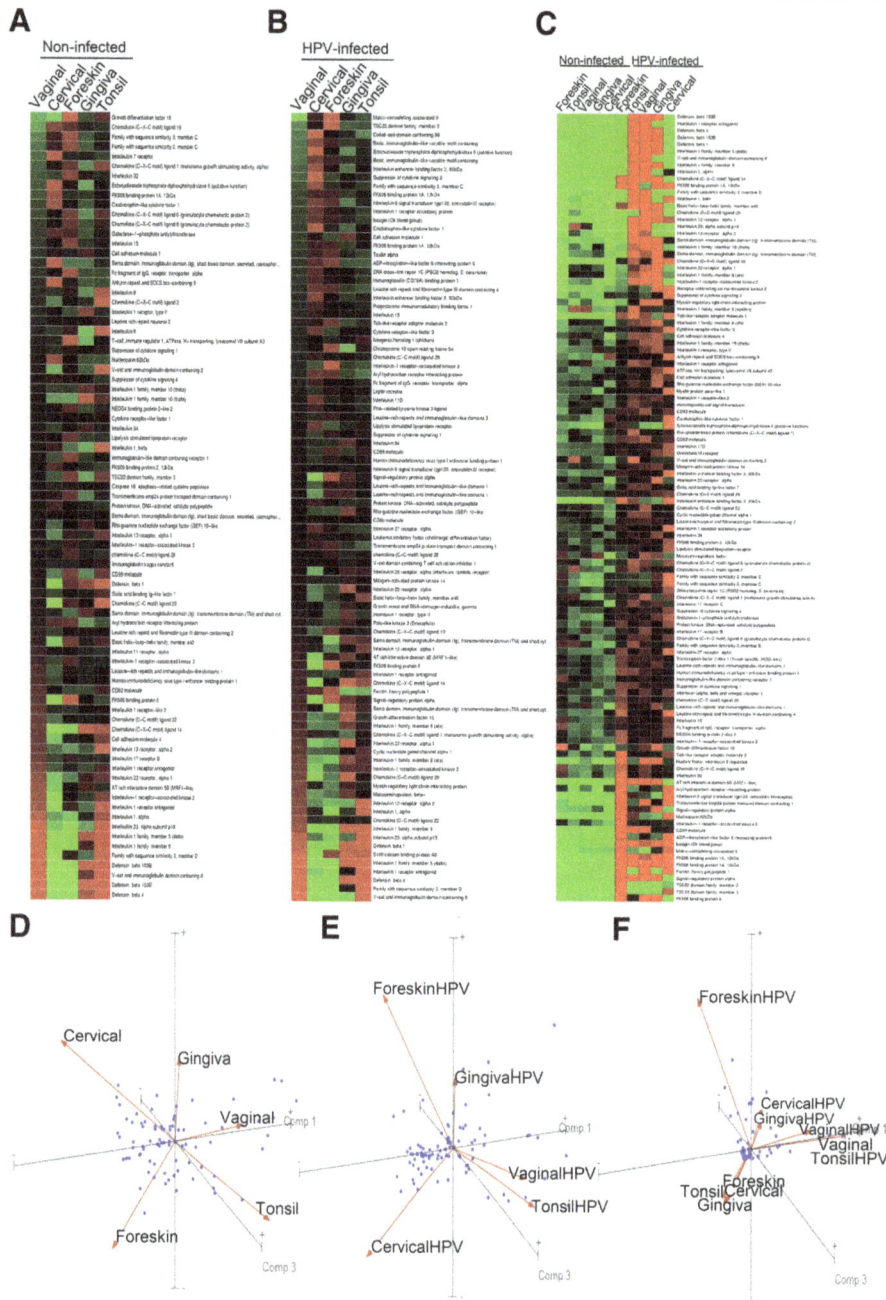

Fig. 1 Immune gene mRNA repertoires of stratified human keratinocytes from different anatomical sites vary significantly. Results are for SHKs grown in organotypic cultures from a pool of 3–5 individuals and represent 3 independent samples of each of the mucosal sites shown (baseline and HPV infected). Data were log transformed, and normalized to the median. Eighty one "immunologic genes" are shown, and a principle component analysis (PCA) performed (dots = genes; lines with arrows = tissue types; axis 3 PCA). Tissue types were separated (PC1, PC2, and PC3), to demonstrate differential genetic expression patterns for these genes. Heat maps and the PCA for SHKs from each site are shown for resting (**a**, **d**), HPV16 transfected (**b**, **e**), and HPV16⁻ or HPV16⁺ keratinocytes from all sites separately grouped together (**c**, **f**)

differences in genes expressed by SHKs from each site, compared to genes expressed in common by SHKs from all sites.

In summary, immune gene expression by SHKs in health and disease has previously been studied predominantly in the oral cavity (gingiva, tonsil), the skin, and the uterine cervix (Wu et al. 2011; Chung and Dale 2004; Frohm et al. 1997; Nees et al. 2001; Adami et al. 2014). In some of these studies, mucosal biopsies from different epithelial tissues contained cells other than keratinocytes, and they showed novel cytokine expression at different anatomical sites (Frohm et al. 1997). However, there is

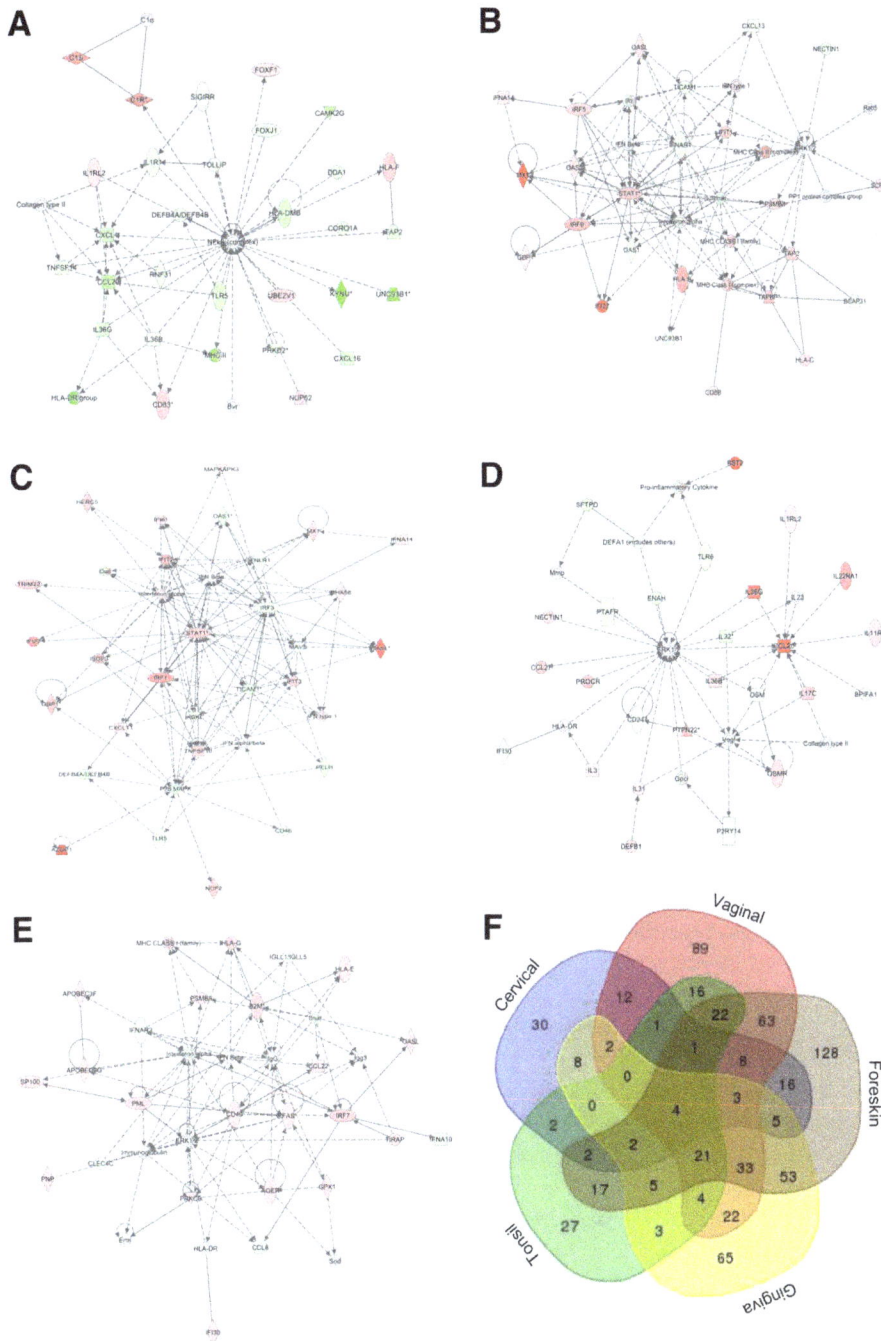

Fig. 2 Immune gene network expression by HPV16[+] stratified human keratinocytes from different anatomical sites vary significantly. Pairwise analysis, normalized to all medians (p-value cutoff < 0.05) was performed individually to comparing SHKs expression at a single mucosal site before and after HPV16 transfection. Differentially expressed genes were selected from a larger list of genes (immune responses/regulation) for the analysis. Data were analyzed using Ingenuity pathway analysis software (IPA®, QIAGEN Inc., https://www.qiagenbioinformatics.com/products/ingenuitypathway-analysis). Networks were generated using the Core analysis tool (**a–e**) (Kramer et al. 2014), and a Venn/Euler diagram was generated (**f**) to visualize common vs. unique gene expression by applying the data sets of SHKs (different sites, resting vs HPV16[+] cells) to software at http://bioinformatics.psb.ugent.be/webtools/Venn/. The number of genes that were uniquely or commonly expressed by cells from each anatomical site are shown within each intersection (**f**)

only a single report of a genome wide analysis of oral mucosa-derived SHKs in mice that demonstrated the essential role of these cells in regulating adaptive immunity (Wu et al. 2011).

Several important points can be drawn from the results presented in this communication. The repertoire of immune response genes expressed by resting SHKs from different mucosal tract show significant differences when compared to each other (Fig. 1). These expression patterns can distinguish one mucosa from another. Even within the same mucosal tract there are marked differences in immune gene expression. These responses are likely to be "hard wired" as SHKs from different sites do not regress to express a common immune gene repertoire in organotypic culture (Fig. 1). HPV16⁻ SHKs from different anatomical sites as a group cluster together and look more similar to each other than do their HPV16+ counterparts, and vice versa. However, there were a few notable exceptions (Fig. 1c). We speculate that the mucosal immune micromilieu at different anatomical sites may influence which immune genes the keratinocytes express as it is likely the stem cells that ultimately differentiate into keratinocytes are the same for all keratinocytes at each site. We have not performed microarrays of naturally infected SHKs from these different anatomical sites, however, our in vitro transfected cervical cell lines showed similar gene expression profiles as previously published in human HPV16 cervical cancers (Nees et al. 2001; Santin et al. 2005; Perez-Plasencia et al. 2007).

Additionally, the immune gene repertoires of HPV16⁺ SHKs from different sites also differ from each other based on the origin of the SHKs (Fig. 1b). Thus, immune gene expression by these cells appears to also be based on mucosal SHK origin (Fig. 1b). Finally, immune gene networks associated with HPV16⁺ SHKs from the different anatomical sites, compared to their HPV16 non-transfected counterparts, was not uniform and significantly varied based on the anatomical origin of origin (Fig. 2a-f). The significant variation in immune gene repertoires and networks (Fig. 2f) may have bearing on why individual members of the large HPV family of DNA viruses predominate as the cause of persistent infection and disease within and between different mucosal tracts (Cubie 2013).

Conclusions

In this study, we identify the differences and similarities in mRNA gene expression made by stratified keratinocytes obtained from five different anatomical sites, grown in organotypic cultures before and after HPV16 transduction. Our results show that keratinocytes within and outside of a given mucosal tract show different immune gene repertoires that are site specific, and that introducing HPV16 into these cells also alters their immune gene expression in a site specific manner. Thus, keratinocytes from different anatomical sites

are likely hard wired in their innate immune responses, before and after the introduction of HPV16, and that these immune responses are unique depending on the anatomical site from which they were derived.

The potential medical significance of understanding and manipulating differential immunologic gene expression by keratinocytes from different mucosal anatomical sites is intriguing. It is known that at some mucosal sites, HPV 16 predominates as a potential pathogen and causes persistent infection leading to malignancy, while others, like HPV6 and 11 rarely if ever cause disease at that mucosal site. For example, tonsil and base of tongue, HPV-induced disease is caused by HPV16, but not HPV6 or 11. In contrast, HPV 6 and 11 commonly cause persist infection and "benign" respiratory papilloma development in the larynx and upper airway, while HPV16 rarely does at this anatomical site. It is interesting to speculate that differential immune gene expression by keratinocytes from a given mucosal site may convey resistance vs. susceptibility to different HPVs dependent on the repertoire of innate immune responses genes they express at a given mucosal site. This may be so given that the keratinocyte HPV receptor appears to be the same for all HPVs (Schafer et al. 2015; Raff et al. 2013). Thus, an explanation of why certain keratinocytes from a given mucosal site are resistant to a some HPVs, but susceptible to others, and vice versa for keratinocytes at different mucosal sites, may be related to the kind of innate immune signaling that a given keratinocyte expresses at a given mucosal site, before and after HPV infection. If this were the case, understanding how keratinocytes confer resistance or susceptibility to a given HPV at a given mucosal site could potentially open a novel preventative and/or therapeutic modality to block a specific HPV from causing persistent infection, and ultimately benign or malignant tumor development at a specificceptible anatomical site. These observations may help explain why select HPV types predominate at different mucosal sites, and can cause persistent infection, that on occasion, can lead to HPV induced malignancy.

Additional files

Additional file 1: Figure S1. Heat map showing the relative gene expression level of keratins among five different stratified human keratinocytes with or without HPV16 transfection. To generate a keratins heat map. All keratin genes, KRT-1 to KRT-86 on the illumina human HT-12v4 expression array were aligned and assigned colors corresponding to the relative expression levels, comparing triplicate cultures of (Strid et al. 2009) types of normal human keratinocytes (NHK) with triplicate cultures from each type transfected with HPV16. KRT-12, − 18, − 20, − 22, KRT-25 to KRT-77, KRT-79, and KRT-82 to KRT-86 were excluded because all 10 triplicates had average expression levels that were below the 95th percentile of all genes on the chip. (XLSX 13 kb)

Additional file 2: Table S1. Genes that are differentially expressed by stratified human keratinocytes from different anatomical sites after HPV16 transfection. (DOCX 16 kb)

Abbreviations
DEGs: Differentially expressed genes; HCKs: Human cervical keratinocytes; HFKs: Human foreskin keratinocytes; HGKs: Human gingival keratinocytes; HPVs: Human papillomaviruses; HTLKs: Human tonsil keratinocytes; HVKs: Human vaginal keratinocytes; IPA: Ingenuity pathway analysis; PCA: Principle component analysis; SHKs: Stratified human keratinocytes

Acknowledgements
We thank Robert Brucklacher, Genome Sciences and Bioinformatics Core, Penn State College of Medicine, Hershey for technical assistance in microarrays.

Funding
Research reported in this publication was supported by the National Institute of Dental and Craniofacial Research (NIDCR) of the National Institutes of Health under Award Numbers DE017227 to Vincent Bonagura and DE018305 to Craig Meyers.

Authors' contributions
MI performed the cell and organotypic cultures and microarrays in Dr. Meyers laboratory before moving to Dr. Bonagura laboratory, DR performed the heat map and principal component data analysis, LF-N performed the Ingenuity analysis. CM conceptualized and supported Dr. Israr's efforts to generate keratinocyte organotypic cultures, and the HPV16 transfection and microarray experiments. VRB conceptualized and supported the experiments that analyzed keratinocyte immune gene expression in the keratinocyte microarray experiments. All authors read and approved the final manuscript.

Competing interests
The authors declare they have no competing interests as defined by Molecular Medicine, or other interests that might be perceived to influence the results and discussion reported in this paper.

Author details
[1]The Feinstein Institute for Medical Research, Manhasset, NY, USA; Division of Allergy and Immunology, Department of Pediatrics, Donald and Barbara Zucker School of Medicine at Hofstra/Northwell, Great Neck, NY, USA. [2]Department of Genomic Medicine, Otology and Neurotology Group CTS495, Centre for Genomics and Oncological Research, Pfizer/Universidad de Granada/Junta de Andalucía (GENYO), Granada, Spain. [3]Department of Microbiology and Immunology, The Pennsylvania State University College of Medicine, Hershey, PA, USA.

References
Adami GR, et al. Gene expression based evidence of innate immune response activation in the epithelium with oral lichen planus. Arch Oral Biol. 2014;59:354–61.

Albanesi C, Scarponi C, Giustizieri ML, Girolomoni G. Keratinocytes in inflammatory skin diseases. Curr Drug Targets Inflamm Allergy. 2005;4:329–34.

Chu PG, Weiss LM. Keratin expression in human tissues and neoplasms. Histopathology. 2002;40:403–39.

Chung WO, Dale BA. Innate immune response of oral and foreskin keratinocytes: utilization of different signaling pathways by various bacterial species. Infect Immun. 2004;72:352–8.

Cubie HA. Diseases associated with human papillomavirus infection. Virology. 2013;445:21–34.

DeVoti JA, et al. Immune dysregulation and tumor-associated gene changes in recurrent respiratory papillomatosis: a paired microarray analysis. Mol Med. 2008;14:608–17.

DeVoti JA, et al. Decreased Langerhans cell responses to IL-36gamma: altered innate immunity in patients with recurrent respiratory papillomatosis. Mol Med. 2014;20:372–80.

Frohm M, et al. The expression of the gene coding for the antibacterial peptide LL-37 is induced in human keratinocytes during inflammatory disorders. J Biol Chem. 1997;272:15258–63.

Israr M, Biryukov J, Ryndock EJ, Alam S, Meyers C. Comparison of human papillomavirus type 16 replication in tonsil and foreskin epithelia. Virology. 2016;499:82–90.

Kramer A, Green J, Pollard J, Tugendreich S Jr. Causal analysis approaches in ingenuity pathway analysis. Bioinformatics. 2014;30:523–30.

McBride AA, Warburton A. The role of integration in oncogenic progression of HPV-associated cancers. PLoS Pathog. 2017;13(4):e1006211.

McLaughlin-Drubin ME, Bromberg-White JL, Meyers C. The role of the human papillomavirus type 18 E7 oncoprotein during the complete viral life cycle. Virology. 2005;338:61–8.

McLaughlin-Drubin ME, Christensen ND, Meyers C. Propagation, infection, and neutralization of authentic HPV16 virus. Virology. 2004;322:213–9.

McLaughlin-Drubin ME, Meyers C. Propagation of infectious, high-risk HPV in organotypic "raft" culture. Methods Mol Med. 2005;119:171–86.

Meyers C, Mayer TJ, Ozbun MA. Synthesis of infectious human papillomavirus type 18 in differentiating epithelium transfected with viral DNA. J Virol. 1997;71:7381–6.

Nees M, et al. Papillomavirus type 16 oncogenes downregulate expression of interferon-responsive genes and upregulate proliferation-associated and NF-kappaB-responsive genes in cervical keratinocytes. J Virol. 2001;75:4283–96.

Nestle FO, Di Meglio P, Qin JZ, Nickoloff BJ. Skin immune sentinels in health and disease. Nat Rev Immunol. 2009;9:679–91.

Perez-Plasencia C, et al. Genome wide expression analysis in HPV16 cervical cancer: identification of altered metabolic pathways. Infect Agent Cancer. 2007;2:16.

Raff AB, et al. The evolving field of human papillomavirus receptor research: a review of binding and entry. J Virol. 2013;87:6062–72.

Saenz SA, Taylor BC, Artis D. Welcome to the neighborhood: epithelial cell-derived cytokines license innate and adaptive immune responses at mucosal sites. Immunol Rev. 2008;226:172–90.

Santin AD, et al. Gene expression profiles of primary HPV16- and HPV18-infected early stage cervical cancers and normal cervical epithelium: identification of novel candidate molecular markers for cervical cancer diagnosis and therapy. Virology. 2005;331:269–91.

Schafer G, Blumenthal MJ, Katz AA. Interaction of human tumor viruses with host cell surface receptors and cell entry. Viruses. 2015;7:2592–617.

Strid J, Tigelaar RE, Hayday AC. Skin immune surveillance by T cells–a new order? Semin Immunol. 2009;21:110–20.

Swamy M, Jamora C, Havran W, Hayday A. Epithelial decision makers: in search of the 'epimmunome'. Nat Immunol. 2010;11:656–65.

Tonel G, Conrad C. Interplay between keratinocytes and immune cells–recent insights into psoriasis pathogenesis. Int J Biochem Cell Biol. 2009;41:963–8.

Wu T, et al. Genome-wide analysis reveals the active roles of keratinocytes in oral mucosal adaptive immune response. Exp Biol Med (Maywood). 2011;236:832–43.

15

Changes in expression profiles of internal jugular vein wall and plasma protein levels in multiple sclerosis

Giovanna Marchetti[1]* [iD], Nicole Ziliotto[2], Silvia Meneghetti[2], Marcello Baroni[2], Barbara Lunghi[2], Erica Menegatti[3], Massimo Pedriali[4], Fabrizio Salvi[5], Ilaria Bartolomei[5], Sofia Straudi[6], Fabio Manfredini[1], Rebecca Voltan[3], Nino Basaglia[1], Francesco Mascoli[7], Paolo Zamboni[3] and Francesco Bernardi[2]

Abstract

Background: Multiple sclerosis (MS) is an inflammatory, demyelinating and degenerative disorder of the central nervous system (CNS). Several observations support interactions between vascular and neurodegenerative mechanisms in multiple sclerosis (MS). To investigate the contribution of the extracranial venous compartment, we analysed expression profiles of internal jugular vein (IJV), which drains blood from CNS, and related plasma protein levels.

Methods: We studied a group of MS patients ($n = 19$), screened by echo-color Doppler and magnetic resonance venography, who underwent surgical reconstruction of IJV for chronic cerebrospinal venous insufficiency (CCSVI). Microarray-based transcriptome analysis was conducted on specimens of IJV wall from MS patients and from subjects undergoing carotid endarterectomy, as controls. Protein levels were determined by multiplex assay in: i) jugular and peripheral plasma from 17 MS/CCSVI patients; ii) peripheral plasma from 60 progressive MS patients, after repeated sampling and iii) healthy individuals.

Results: Of the differentially expressed genes (≥ 2 fold-change, multiple testing correction, $P < 0.05$), the immune-related *CD86* (8.5 fold-change, $P = 0.002$) emerged among the up regulated genes ($N = 409$). Several genes encoding HOX transcription factors and histones potentially regulated by blood flow, were overexpressed. Smooth muscle contraction and cell adhesion processes emerged among down regulated genes ($N = 515$), including the neuronal cell adhesion *L1CAM* as top scorer (5 fold-change, $P = 5 \times 10^{-4}$).

Repeated measurements in jugular/peripheral plasma and overtime in peripheral plasma showed conserved individual plasma patterns for immune-inflammatory (CCL13, CCL18) and adhesion (NCAM1, VAP1, SELL) proteins, despite significant variations overtime (SELL $P < 0.0001$). Both age and MS disease phenotypes were determinants of VAP1 plasma levels. Data supported cerebral related-mechanisms regulating ANGPT1 levels, which were remarkably lower in jugular plasma and correlated in repeated assays but not between jugular/peripheral compartments.

Conclusions: This study provides for the first time expression patterns of the IJV wall, suggesting signatures of altered vascular mRNA profiles in MS disease also independently from CCSVI. The combined transcriptome-protein analysis provides intriguing links between IJV wall transcript alteration and plasma protein expression, thus highlighting proteins of interest for MS pathophysiology.

Keywords: Gene expression, Jugular vein wall, Multiple sclerosis, Chronic cerebrospinal venous insufficiency, Venous abnormalities, Jugular plasma protein levels, Multiplex protein assay, Chemokines, Adhesion molecules

* Correspondence: mrg@unife.it
[1]Department of Biomedical and Specialty Surgical Sciences, University of Ferrara, via Fossato di Mortara n 74, 44121 Ferrara, Italy
Full list of author information is available at the end of the article

Background

Multiple sclerosis (MS) is an inflammatory demyelinating and degenerative disorder of the central nervous system (CNS) (Noseworthy et al. 2000) for which several genetic, epigenetic and environmental components have been proposed to participate through complex interactions (Amato et al. 2018; Olsson et al. 2017).

Several observations suggest that vascular components are involved in the multifactorial pathogenetic interplay and/ or in disease progression, severity and comorbidities development (Karmon et al. 2012; Spencer et al. 2018; Kappus et al. 2016).

The vascular cerebral system, and particularly the venous compartment, early received attention because of venous thrombosis in the brain of MS patients, and plaques of demyelination development around venules and perivascular infiltrations of inflammatory cells just next small and medium size venous of CNS (Adams 1988).

The condition named chronic cerebrospinal venous insufficiency (CCSVI) provided the possible association of MS with extra-cranial venous abnormalities which impaired venous outflow (Zamboni et al. 2009; Zivadinov et al. 2012).

Although highly debated whether associated with MS, and not leading to a viable treatment option in patients (Zamboni et al. 2018), this condition favors better understanding of the function and role of the extracranial venous system in MS (Zivadinov and Weinstock-Guttman 2018). On the other hand, a perspective of reduced blood supply to the brain (D'haeseleer et al. 2015), further argue for the relevance of the vascular component in the disease.

Findings on these conditions associated to MS foster more investigations of both intracranial and extracranial vascular compartments changes in MS (Zivadinov and Weinstock-Guttman 2018; Belov et al. 2018).

Vascular features associated to MS have been deeply investigated (D'haeseleer et al. 2011; Dolic et al. 2012), with the central vein sign recently proposed as a MRI biomarker of MS (Sati et al. 2016). Studies focusing on circulating and endothelial components, which participate in the complex network of immune-vascular interactions have been reported (Alexander et al. 2013). De-regulated patterns of gene expression have been detected in peripheral whole blood or peripheral blood mononuclear cells (PBMC) of MS patients (Ramanathan et al. 2001; Ratzer et al. 2013; Nickles et al. 2013; Paraboschi et al. 2015; Comabella et al. 2016; Lindsey et al. 2011).

To shed light on vascular gene expression changes in MS with associated CCSVI, we focused on internal jugular vein (IJV), which drains blood from the brain. In particular, we explored gene expression changes by using two informative approaches and their combination, transcriptomic analysis on IJV specimens and specific protein assays on plasma from both jugular and peripheral veins.

Methods
Study populations

The first (1st) study population was represented by a group of 19 Italian subjects with MS and positive screening for CCSVI.

Diagnosis of MS was in accordance to the McDonald criteria (Polman et al. 2005). Patients' screening through flow quantification by means of a combination of validated echo-color Doppler (ECD) model with magnetic resonance venography morphological and flow evaluation protocol, and cerebral perfusion evaluation by SPECT-CT, have been previously detailed (Dolic et al. 2012; Zamboni et al. 2013; Zamboni et al. 2016). The patients presented truncular venous malformation in at least one IJV, in form of segmental hypoplasia, defective valves with incomplete or absent opening of their leaflets, other intraluminal obstacles and muscular compression. The 19 patients belonged to a cohort of patients who were eligible for surgical reconstruction of internal jugular vein by angioplasty and entered the study approved by the Ethical Committee of the S. Anna University-Hospital of Ferrara. The details about enrolment and inclusion/exclusion criteria have been previously described (Zamboni et al. 2016). 1st MS population demographics are reported in Table 1.

The second (2nd) study population included 60 Italian MS patients, who participated in the RAGTIME study (ClinicalTrials.gov ID:NCT02421731) (Straudi et al. 2017). This clinical trial compares robot-assisted gait training versus conventional therapy on mobility in severely disabled progressive MS patients. The demographics and clinical characteristics of the 2nd MS population are reported in Additional file 1: Table S1.

Thirty-four Italian healthy subjects (mean age 41.3 ± 9.0; 21 women and 13 men), who have never diagnosed with MS, neurological disorder or other chronic inflammatory diseases, were recruited for protein level analysis in plasma. Eight healthy subjects were recruited and added to the healthy cohort (total subjects = 42; mean age 41.29 ± 11.4; 26 women and 16 men) as control group for the 2nd MS population.

Jugular wall specimens

IJV specimens were obtained at surgery from patients. In MS patients, the surgical procedure included an unilateral or bilateral supra-clavicular transverse incision of about 5 cm. The IJV was isolated at the junction with the subclavian vein. The latter was tangentially clamped following systemic injection of heparin. An endo-phlebectomy was subsequently performed with complete removal of the jugular valve/septum and of a tiny specimen of jugular wall, followed by a patch angioplasty using the autologous great saphenous vein. Omohyoid muscle section was performed, if the pre-operative finding of extrinsic compression was confirmed in the surgical theatre.

Table 1 First study population demographics

	MS-CCSVI Patients $n = 19$	Healthy subjects $n = 34$
Age, mean ± SD	46.5 ± 8.6	41.3 ± 9
Gender, M/F	10/9	13/21
MS clinical class		
RR	11	–
SP	7	
PP	1	
Disease duration RR, mean ± SD	10 ± 4	–
Disease duration SP – PP, mean ± SD	13 ± 4	–
EDSS, mean ± SD	4 ± 2	–
MRI T1 gadolinium enhancing lesions, n	5/19	–
M-mode IJV defective valves, n	29/38	–

RR relapsing remitting, *SP* secondary progressive, *PP* primary progressive, *EDSS* expanded disability status scale, *M-mode* echo Doppler. Age and disease duration are reported in years

Control IJV specimens were obtained from patients without MS or other neurological diseases, undergoing carotid endarterectomy (CEA) for high-grade carotid stenosis. In these five patients ECD analysis of carotid, vertebral and subclavian arteries, and jugular veins, documented the presence of atherosclerotic plaque, mostly localized at carotid bifurcation, and did not detect jugular vein alterations.

During the CEA procedure, the access to common carotid artery needs to separate the small facial vein, crossing the carotid artery just at the level of bifurcation, from the jugular vein. A very small full thickness specimen of jugular wall was taken during this maneuver.

Written informed consent was obtained from all subjects.

Specimens retrieved at surgery were immediately placed into RNAlater (Ambion Inc., Austin, TX) and then stored at – 80 °C.

Microarray-based transcriptome analysis of jugular vein walls

From homogenized wall specimens (TRIZOL Reagent, Invitrogen Carlsab, CA), total RNA was extracted using the miRNeasy Mini Kit (Quiagen, Hilden, Germany) and its quality was assessed with Agilent 2100 Bioanalyzer (Agilent Technologies, Palo Alto, CA). Labelled cRNA was synthesized from 100 ng of total RNA using the Low RNA Input Linear Amplification Kit (Agilent Technologies) in the presence of cyanine 3-CTP (Perkin-Elmer Life Sciences, Boston, MA). Hybridization on Agilent whole human genome oligo microarray (Cat.No. G4851A, Agilent Technologies), which represents 60,000

unique human transcripts, was performed in accordance to manufacturer's indications.

Microarray raw-data were obtained with Feature Extraction software v.10.7 (Agilent Technologies) and analyzed by using the GeneSpring GX v.14 software (Agilent Technologies) as previously described (Coen et al. 2013a; Marchetti et al. 2015).

cDNA preparation and quantitative real-time polymerase chain reaction (qRT-PCR)

cDNA was obtained from 0.150 µg of total RNA by reverse transcription using M-MLV Reverse Transcriptase (Invitrogen Carlsab, CA) and a mixture of oligo(dT) and random primers.

Aliquots of diluted cDNA were amplified using Sso-Fast EvaGreen Supermix (BioRad, Hercules, CA).

As general approach for qRT-PCR the specific primers were chosen to amplify the regions recognized by oligonucleotide probes in the microarray analysis. Forward and reverse primers are reported in the Additional file 2: Table S2. PCR protocol was: 95 °C for 30 s, then 40 cycles of 10 s at 95 °C and 15 s at 58 °C. Each reaction was performed in triplicate. All qRT-PCRs were performed on an CFX96 Real-Time PCR Detection System instrument (BioRad, Hercules, CA) according to the manufacturer's instructions. The relative levels of mRNAs were calculated by $2^{-\Delta\Delta Ct}$ method using *ACTB* and *B2M* as endogenous controls. Values were expressed as mean fold change ± standard error of the mean.

Plasma samples

For the 1st MS population ($N = 17$ patients) blood samples were drawn during the surgical procedure, before systemic injection of heparin, from both IJV (right or left) and a peripheral vein. At time of blood sampling patients were free of therapy for at least one month. All blood samples were drawn at fasting in citrate tubes.

MS patients from the 2nd population, enrolled in the RAGTIME study, provided blood sampling at four time points: T0) baseline point, prior to the first rehabilitative session; T1) intermediate point, after six training sessions; T2) end of treatment, 12 completed rehabilitative sessions, 1 month after T0; T3) follow-up, after 3 months from the end of training program (30)(Ziliotto et al. 2018).

Peripheral venous blood samples were also collected from the healthy volunteers ($n = 34$, or plus eight subjects $n = 42$, as control group for the 2nd MS population).

All plasma samples were separated by two centrifugations (15 min at 2500 g and 5 min at 11000 g at room temperature), aliquoted and frozen at – 80 °C until use.

Protein antigen levels were quantified by a custom-designed Luminex Screening Assays magnetic bead kits (Luminex R&D Systems Inc., Minneapolis, MN, USA) according to the manufacturer's instructions. Data were acquired using the Luminex® 100 system and analyzed using Bioplex Manager Software version 6.0 (both from Biorad Laboratories, Hercules, CA). Soluble CD86 was measured by an enzyme-linked immunosorbent (ELISA)-based assay according to the manufacturer's protocol (Abcam, Cambridge, UK). The inter assay variability assessed by using coefficients of variation (CV%) were as follows: 1.1 (NCAM1), 1.2 (ANGPT1), 2.1 (CCL13), 2.3 (VAP1), 2.6 (CCL18), 3 (SELL), and 3.2 (CD86).

Statistical analysis

In tissue microarray a filter on low gene expression was used to keep only the probes expressed in at least one sample (flagged as Marginal or Present). Then, samples were grouped in accordance to their disease status (MS and Controls) and compared. To evaluate similarities or differences among each group (MS and Controls) principal component analysis was performed on the normalized data using the GeneSpring GX v.14 software (Agilent Technologies). Differentially expressed genes were selected as having a 2-fold expression difference between their geometrical mean in the two groups and a statistically significant p-value (< 0.05) by a moderate t-test, followed by the application of Benjamini- Hoechberg multiple testing correction.

Differentially expressed genes were employed for Cluster Analysis of samples, using the Manhattan correlation as a measure of similarity. Functional categorization was assigned using Gene Ontology (GO) by free access DAVID Bioinformatics database 6.7. Gene expression levels between MS and control jugular walls in qRT-PCR analysis were compared by means of unpaired t-test.

Protein plasma levels were expressed as mean ± SD. Differences between plasma sample groups were assessed by paired or unpaired Student's t test and by ANCOVA test using age as covariate. A p-value ≤ 0.05 was considered statistically significant. Pearson's test was used to assess correlation between jugular and peripheral plasma levels in MS patients and to assess correlation over time for ANGPT1, CCL13, CCL18, NCAM1, SELL and VAP1 plasma levels. ANOVA for repeated measures was used to test differences across the four time points and, in case of a significant p-value, pairwise comparisons were Bonferroni corrected (q-values). All statistical analyses were performed using IBM® SPSS® Statistics version 24 software (IBM Corp. Armonk, NY, USA).

Results

Analysis of gene expression profiles in jugular vein specimens

To explore the expression pattern of IJV wall of patients with MS as compared to unaffected jugular walls, total RNAs extracted from MS specimens ($n = 4$) and from control specimens ($n = 5$) were subjected to microarray analysis. Using the criteria of at least a 2-fold difference in the expression level (corrected P value < 0.05) between the two groups of RNA samples (see Methods), a total of 924 transcripts were found to be differentially expressed (Additional file 3: Table S3).

Clustering analysis (Fig. 1a) indicated that 409 transcripts were up- and 515 down- regulated in MS J wall. Testing for RNA function in NCBI database showed that up regulation was observed for 300 coding and 109 non-coding or uncharacterized RNAs, whereas down regulation was detected for 429 coding and 86 non-coding RNAs.

To assign a functional annotation to the 924 transcripts/genes, GO analysis by the Functional Annotation Chart Instrument of DAVID Bioinformatics 6.7 was conducted. The most enriched biological processes ($P < 0.05$, Benjamini test) are reported in Fig. 1b. In this selection the highest significance was related to the terms "muscle"/"smooth muscle contraction" ($P = 1.2 \times 10^{-4}$ and $P = 0.008$ respectively) and "biological adhesion" ($P = 0.003$), with the term "smooth muscle contraction" showing the highest fold enrichment (7.35).

When sub-analysing up- and down- regulated transcripts ($P < 0.05$, Benjamini test), the terms "pattern specification process" and "nucleosome organization" were overrepresented among up-regulated genes. The biological process "pattern specification" included several homeobox (HOX) genes (HOXA5, HOXA6, HOXA7, HOXB5, HOXB6, HOXC4 and HOXC5), which encode for transcription factors. The GO term "nucleosome organization" comprised several histone subunit genes, and in particular, three H3 variant genes (HIST1H3D, HIST1H3F and HIST1H3H) were included in the list of the most significantly ($P = 0.002$) up-regulated coding RNAs. Among the down regulated genes, the terms related to smooth muscle contraction showed the highest fold enrichment (12.0). Concerning the enriched adhesion terms, 51 genes were found downregulated, of which L1CAM, encoding for the neural cell adhesion molecule L1, was included among the top 10 most significantly downregulated genes ($P = 5 \times 10^{-4}$).

To gain further insight into functional associations, analysis of KEGG and BIOCARTA pathways by DAVID Bioinformatics resource for the 924 transcripts/genes was performed. The selection for enrichment ($P < 0.05$, Benjamini test) provided the terms "vascular smooth muscle contraction", "dilated cardiomyopathy" and "calcium signaling pathway" (Fig. 1c). Among the up- regulated genes, the only enriched term (fold enrichment 7.0, $P = 3 \times 10^{-4}$) was the "systemic lupus erythematosus" pathway (Fig. 1c).

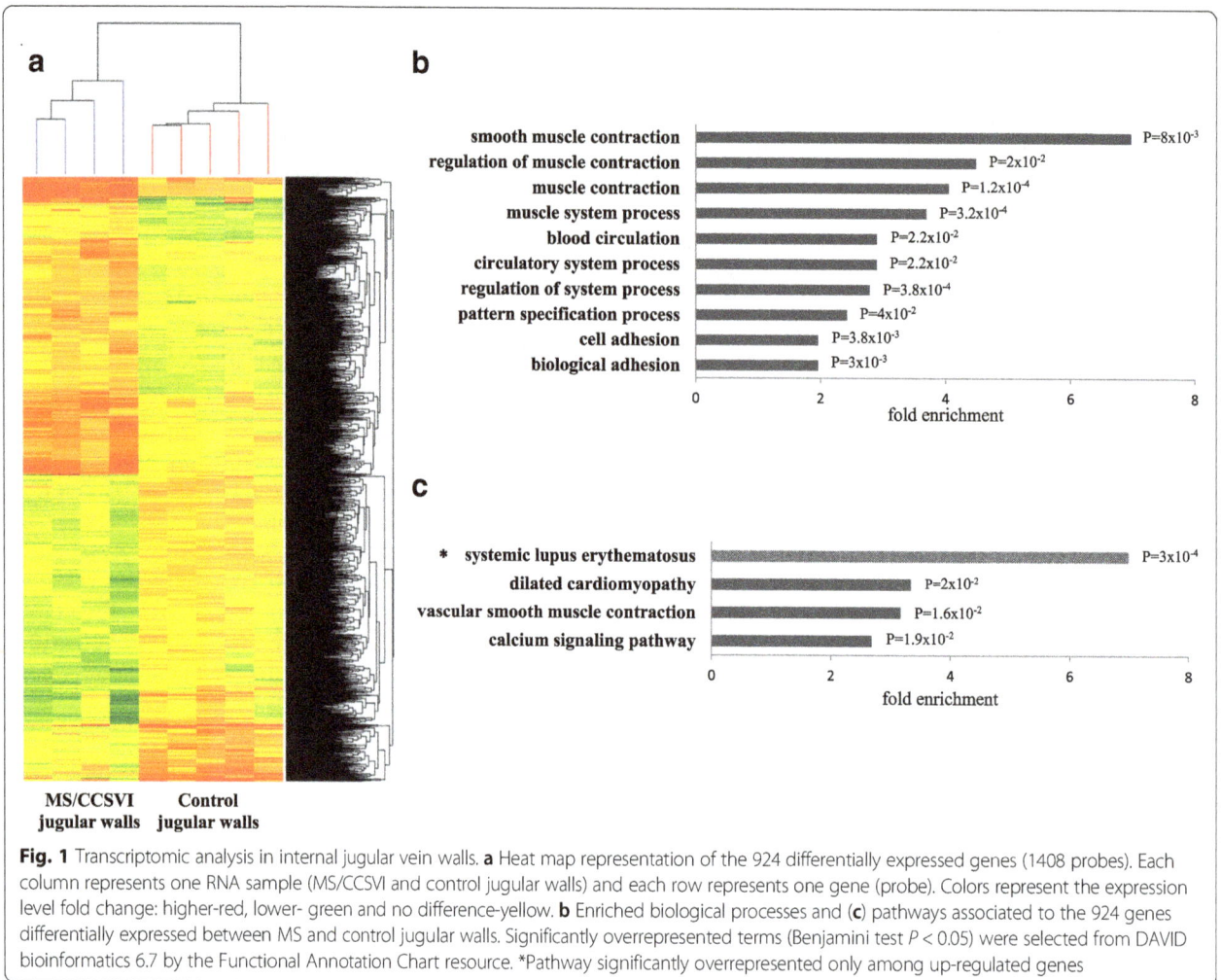

Fig. 1 Transcriptomic analysis in internal jugular vein walls. **a** Heat map representation of the 924 differentially expressed genes (1408 probes). Each column represents one RNA sample (MS/CCSVI and control jugular walls) and each row represents one gene (probe). Colors represent the expression level fold change: higher-red, lower- green and no difference-yellow. **b** Enriched biological processes and (**c**) pathways associated to the 924 genes differentially expressed between MS and control jugular walls. Significantly overrepresented terms (Benjamini test $P < 0.05$) were selected from DAVID bioinformatics 6.7 by the Functional Annotation Chart resource. *Pathway significantly overrepresented only among up-regulated genes

Expression analysis by quantitative real time PCR (qRT-PCR)

Aimed at supporting microarray profiling results by a different assay, qRT-PCR analyses were performed on additional jugular wall samples of MS patients ($N = 7$) and of controls ($N = 4$). Five genes were selected (*ANGPT1*, *AOC3*, *CD86*, *L1CAM* and *SELL*), three of which included in the biological process "adhesion". Three genes were also included in the list of the top ten most significantly up regulated (*CD86*) or down regulated (*L1CAM*, *ANGPT1*) genes (Additional file 3: Table S3).

Significant differences (Additional file 4: Table S4) were observed for *L1CAM* (*ACTB*, $P = 0.0004$; *B2M*, $P = 0.005$) and for *ANGPT1* with *B2M* ($P = 0.013$). For *SELL*, a trend for down regulation was observed with *B2M* ($P = 0.08$) and *ACTB* ($P = 0.11$). For *AOC3*, a trend for down regulation was observed only with *B2M* (P = 0.08). For *CD86*, the significant differences in expression levels revealed by microarray analysis were not detected by qRT-PCR with both *ACTB* and *B2M*. This inconsistency between microarray and qRT-PCR data could derive from the several protein

coding transcripts of *CD86* gene (http://www.ensembl.org/Homo_sapiens/Gene/Summary?db=core;g=ENSG00000114 013;r=3:122055366-122121139), two of which are recognized by the microarray probe in the 3' UTR and six (four additional transcripts) are potentially amplified by the q-PCR primers, bridging the last exons. With the exception of *CD86*, the expression regulation (up or down) in MS- vs control jugular walls indicated by microarray analysis was supported by qRT-PCR analysis (Additional file 3: Tables S3 and Additional file 4: Table S4).

Analysis of protein levels in jugular and peripheral plasma

In order to investigate whether differences in the transcriptome profiles between MS- and control jugular walls would correlate with differences in protein expression levels, we selected genes whose protein products could be measured in plasma, and particularly by using a multiplex detection approach. Ten candidate proteins were eligible (Additional file 5: Table S5). In addition, CD86, in the list of the top ten most significantly up regulated coding genes and showing the highest fold-change, was measured as soluble antigen in plasma by a single ELISA.

The selected proteins mainly participate in adhesion (NCAM1, VAP1, SELL), which was among the most significantly enriched process revealed by jugular wall transcriptome analysis, immune/inflammatory responses (CD86, TNF, TNFRSF6B, CCL3, CCL13, CCL18), angiogenesis (ANGPT1) and cytoskeleton/organelle organization (MAPT).

Protein levels were evaluated in jugular and peripheral plasma from 17 patients (MS 1st population) and in peripheral plasma from 34 healthy subjects (Table 2).

The comparison of peripheral plasma levels between MS patients and healthy subjects showed significant differences for ANGPT1 (3.6 ± 1.7 vs 6.2 ± 2.8 ng/ml, $P = 0.02$). For NCAM1 and VAP1, the P values (0.08 and 0.09 respectively) suggested a trend for differences between patients and healthy subjects.

The lower levels of ANGPT1 and VAP1, and the trend for higher levels of NCAM1in patients, might mimic the RNA expression regulation in the MS jugular wall estimated by transcriptomic analysis (Table 2).

In MS patients, correlation between jugular vein and peripheral plasma concentrations ranged from very high ($r = 0.97$, NCAM1) to virtually absent ($r = 0.04$, ANGPT1) (Fig. 2). Concentrations of ANGPT1, CD86, NCAM1 and SELL were significantly lower (paired t-test) in jugular than in peripheral plasma, with ANGPT1 showing the highest percentage difference ($\Delta = -28.7\%$, Fig. 2).

Four proteins (CCL3, MAPT, TNF and TNFRSF6B) resulted undetectable in the majority of plasma samples in the multiplex assay condition (data not shown).

Analysis of protein levels in peripheral plasma - 2nd MS population

Peripheral plasma levels of ANGPT1, CCL13, CCL18, NCAM1, SELL and VAP1 were further analysed in an independent MS population (2nd study population).

Levels were investigated in 60 patients, grouped by PP-MS and SP-MS clinical phenotypes (Additional file 6: Table S6), and over 4 time points in 56 of them (Table 3). Peripheral plasma protein levels of the 2nd MS population were compared with those of the 1st MS population and of healthy subjects (Table 4).

No differences in plasma protein levels between clinical subgroups, PP-MS and SP-MS were detected either at time 0 (Additional file 6: Table S6) or overtime (data not reported). As significant age differences were present among clinical groups (PP-MS vs SP-MS, $P < 0.001$), ANCOVA adjusted for age was used to evaluate plasma levels, which did not reveal differences (Additional file 6: Table S6).

The comparison between the 2nd MS population and healthy subjects (Table 4) showed, after t-test, significant differences for CCL13, CCL18 and VAP1. However, after correction for age, only NCAM1 showed higher levels in MS patients than healthy subjects (137.3 ± 54.5 ng/mL vs. 124 ± 44 ng/mL; $P = 0.050$).

The comparison between the 1st and 2nd MS populations (Table 4) showed significant differences (t-test) for AGPT1, CCL13, CCL18 and VAP1. After correction for age significant differences were observed for ANGPT1 and VAP1, and as a trend for CCL18 and SELL.

The analysis overtime of plasma protein levels in the 2nd population, aimed at evaluating the stability of protein levels in plasma, detected a significant difference over time only for SELL ($P < 0.0001$). In particular, pairwise analysis revealed differences between several time points (T0-T1, q = 0.023; T0-T2, q = 0.011); T0-T3, q < 0.0001; T1-T3, q = 0.048). High correlation among time points for each protein was observed, ranging from $r = 0.67$ (ANGPT1) to $r = 0.98$, the noteworthy value for NCAM1.

Repeated protein assays in the 1st MS population (jugular and peripheral plasma) and in the 2nd MS population (four time points in peripheral plasma) offered the opportunity to compare, in independent

Table 2 Protein plasma levels in jugular vein (1st MS population) and in peripheral vein (1st MS population and healthy subjects)

PROTEINS	MS/CCSVI JUGULAR PLASMA (n = 17)	P*	MS/CCSVI PERIPHERAL PLASMA (n = 17)	P#	HEALTHY PERIPHERAL PLASMA (n = 34)	mRNA PROFILING
ANGPT1	2.6 ± 0.90	0.016	3.6 ± 1.7	0.02	6.2 ± 2.8	↓
CCL13	87.3 ± 32.8	0.22	79.6 ± 23.2	0.33	89.7 ± 39.6	↓
CCL18	27.2 ± 9.3	0.048	30.4 ± 11.1	0.30	34.7 ± 15.5	↓
CD86	183.9 ± 50.7	0.004	221.3 ± 66.4	0.7	214.2 ± 62.4§	↑
NCAM1	138.2 ± 57	0.005	149.9 ± 58.3	0.08	123.5 ± 44.2	↑
SELL	451.4 ± 97.5	0.002	522.7 ± 117.2	0.16	584.4 ± 158.8	↑
VAP1	223.8 ± 45.6	0.06	241.7 ± 43.5	0.09	272.0 ± 65.8	↓

Proteins: *ANGPT1* angiopoietin 1, *CCL13* chemokine ligand 13, *CCL18* chemokine ligand 18, *CD86* cluster of differentiation 86, *NCAM1* neural cell adhesion molecule 1, *SELL* selectin L, *VAP1(AOC3)* vascular adhesion protein 1(amine oxidase copper containing 3). Protein concentrations are reported in ng/ml, except for CD86 (U/ml). All values are expressed as mean ± standard deviation. Arrows indicate up (↑) or down (↓) mRNA regulation in MS vs non-MS jugular wall. *P values from paired t-test (MS jugular plasma vs MS peripheral plasma). #P value from t-test on peripheral plasma (MS patients vs healthy subjects). § evaluated in 28 plasma controls

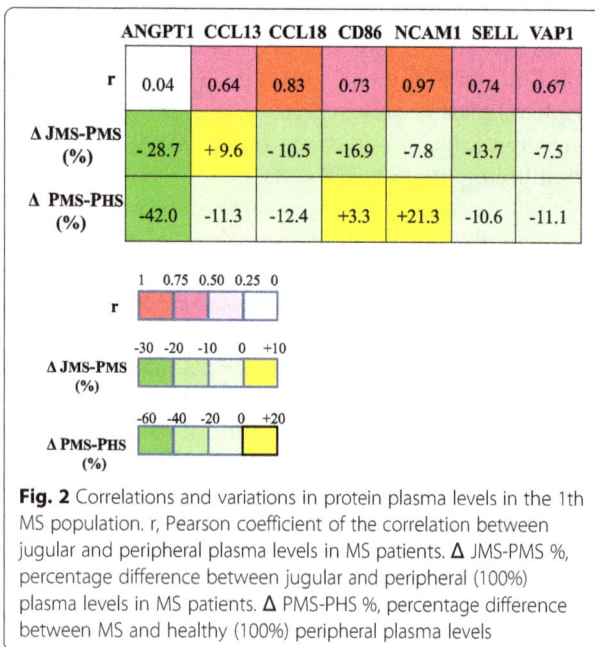

Fig. 2 Correlations and variations in protein plasma levels in the 1th MS population. r, Pearson coefficient of the correlation between jugular and peripheral plasma levels in MS patients. Δ JMS-PMS %, percentage difference between jugular and peripheral (100%) plasma levels in MS patients. Δ PMS-PHS %, percentage difference between MS and healthy (100%) peripheral plasma levels

experiments, concentration variation between vascular bed compartments and overtime. The relation between correlation coefficients is shown in Fig. 3. Interestingly, the r values between jugular and peripheral plasma protein concentrations in the 1st MS population, which ranged from virtually absent ($r = 0.04$, ANGPT1) to very high ($r = 0.97$, NCAM1, Fig. 2), and those observed overtime in the 2nd MS population (Table 3) were highly correlated ($R^2 = 0.96$, $P < 0.001$, r Pearson =0.981, Fig. 3).

Discussion

Early and recent observations (Karmon et al. 2012) suggest interactions between vascular abnormalities and neurodegenerative component in the manifestations of MS, which supports the investigation of both circulating and wall associated factors. We aimed at contributing to these issues, in particular to the involvement of venous compartment, both by transcriptome and plasma protein

investigation in MS patients. Surgical reconstruction of malformed IJV in patients was instrumental for the analysis of transcriptome of the jugular vein wall, which in our knowledge has never been performed.

In transcriptomic profiling, confirmed by qRT-PCR, *L1CAM* emerged as the most significantly downregulated gene, among several coding for proteins participating to adhesion processes. This neural cell adhesion molecule has been shown to function in a variety of dynamic neurological processes and to support adhesion by multiple vascular and platelet integrins (Felding-Habermann et al. 1997) with implication in vascular processes.

Noticeably, transcriptomic data indicated dysregulation of the "pattern specification" and "nucleosome organization" processes, that could be related to the altered features of jugular flow observed in MS patients with associated chronic cerebrospinal venous insufficiency. Several members of the HOX transcription factors family, overexpressed in patients' jugular wall transcriptome and belonging to the "pattern specification" process, are known to regulate embryogenesis, development and also processes in adult tissues, among which vasculature pathways (Gorski and Walsh 2003). In particular, *HOXA5*, and *HOXB5* have been found to be blood flow-sensitive in endothelial cells (Passerini et al. 2004). Disturbed flow conditions have been found to affect also expression of histone genes ("nucleosome organization") in cultured endothelial cells from human carotid artery (Aoki et al. 2016). Our findings link altered transcriptional profiles of the jugular wall in patients to a number of important experimental observations obtained at the gene expression level in cellular and animal models unrelated to MS. Further, the down- regulation of several genes, related to muscle contraction, muscular/cytoskeleton system and members of the large collagen family, might be related to altered features and properties of the internal jugular vein, and particularly anatomy, histology and flow abnormalities (Zamboni et al. 2009; Coen et al. 2013b). However, only the availability of jugular wall expression profiling from MS patients not meeting the

Table 3 Protein plasma levels over four time points in the 2nd MS population

	Time points				P-value	r
	T0	T1	T2	T3		
ANGPT1	6.3 ± 4	5.6 ± 3	6.3 ± 3.5	6.6 ± 4.1	0.186	0.675
CCL13	113.9 ± 53.6	108.2 ± 44.7	111.8 ± 44.4	116.5 ± 50.5	0.266	0.832
CCL18	44.6 ± 20.8	43.6 ± 20.5	44.9 ± 20.5	43.9 ± 21.9	0.568	0.945
NCAM1	137.5 ± 56.3	135.3 ± 54.2	133.4 ± 53.8	135.2 ± 58	0.137	0.980
SELL	553.2 ± 115.4	553 ± 113	527.6 ± 105.2	512.3 ± 103.9	< 0.0001	0.897
VAP1	315.6 ± 84.8	306 ± 81.8	310.5 ± 82.5	310.1 ± 81.4	0.383	0.905

Protein levels were evaluated in 56/60 patients. Protein abbreviations are reported as in Table 2
The P value of ANOVA for repeated measures across time is reported
r = Pearson coefficient of correlations across 4 time points

Table 4 Comparison of protein plasma levels in MS patients (1st and 2nd populations) and healthy subjects

	2nd Population vs 1st Population		2nd Population vs Healthy subjects	
	t-test	ANCOVA	t-test	ANCOVA
ANGPT1	0.021	0.033	0.261	0.330
CCL13	0.021	0.167	0.013	0.690
CCL18	0.004	0.082	0.002	0.302
NCAM1	0.231	0.332	0.204	0.050
SELL	0.241	0.079	0.914	0.161
VAP1	0.001	0.025	0.007	0.389

Protein abbreviations are reported as in Table 2. Protein levels were evaluated in 42 healthy subjects
The P values of t-test and ANCOVA (using age as covariate) are reported

criteria for CCSVI, an unattainable goal, would permit to specifically attribute expression changes to MS or to vascular changes in MS- related CCSVI.

The strong up-regulation in patients' jugular wall transcriptome of CD86, a costimulatory protein involved in several mechanisms of immune response (Jeannin et al. 1999), could be related to immune activation at the level of jugular wall, potentially including immune cells adhering to the vessel surface, coherently with the well-known autoimmune features of MS. Remarkably, overexpression of CD86 transcripts in PBMC at all the stages of MS compared with healthy controls was recently reported (Srinivasan et al. 2017).

Altogether the transcriptome analysis in jugular wall and the transcriptome analysis in PBMC from MS patients (Comabella et al. 2016; Srinivasan et al. 2017; Iglesias et al. 2004) suggest dysregulation of histone, cytoskeleton and CD86 genes as a general signature of altered gene expression in different cells and tissues of MS patients.

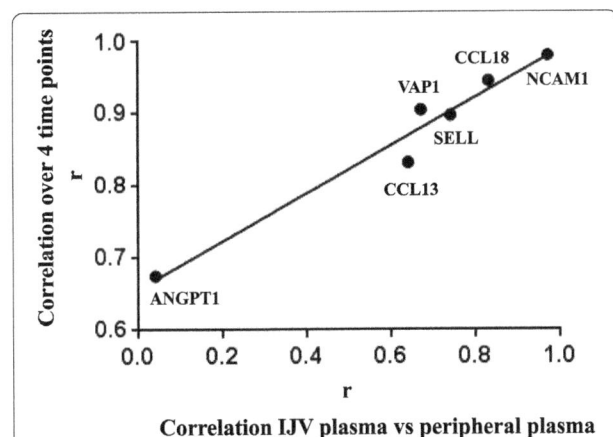

Correlation IJV plasma vs peripheral plasma

Fig. 3 Correlations of protein plasma levels: relation between 1st and 2nd MS population values. X axis: Pearson coefficients (r) of the correlation between jugular and peripheral plasma in 1st MS population. Y axis: Pearson coefficients (r) of the correlation over 4 time points in the peripheral plasma of the 2nd MS population

Investigation of changes observed at RNA level was combined with that in plasma at the protein level, through analysis of molecules acting in immune-inflammatory, in cell adhesion/neuronal cell adhesion and angiogenesis processes, all known to play a role in MS pathogenesis. (Salmi and Jalkanen 2017).

In addition to the 1st population of MS/CCSVI patients a 2nd population with progressive MS phenotypes was analysed for deeper investigation at the plasma protein level and to increase robustness of our study. The repeated measurements help to define particularly conserved plasma patterns, well exemplified by the statistical analysis of CCL18 and VAP-1 values (Table 3).

VAP1, an amine oxidase with also adhesive activities (Salmi and Jalkanen 2017), involved in a rat model of MS in CNS inflammatory lesion development (Elo et al. 2018), was previously found to be significantly lower in RR and in SP patients with absence of MRI active lesions than in controls (Airas et al. 2006). The Finnish cohort mirrors the 1st MS population of our study, in which the majority of patients were free from gadolinium enhancing lesions at preoperative MRI (Table 1), and thus with absence of ongoing inflammatory activity within the brain. Further, the analysis conducted in the 2nd MS population clearly indicated both age and disease phenotypes as important determinants of VAP1 plasma levels.

To further characterize features of the IJV compartment in patients, the concentration of several proteins was analysed in paired jugular and peripheral vein plasma samples. For most molecules, the good to excellent jugular-peripheral correlations, which were highly related to those observed overtime in the 2nd MS population, support the quality of our analysis, conducted by a multiplex assay that prevents most of bias in experimental condition among protein antigens. This approach also permitted to compare variation between vascular compartments with variation over time of specific protein levels. Protein biosynthesis, bio-distribution and stability could participate in producing the different extent of correlation observed for each protein.

Noticeably, significantly lower levels in jugular were assessed for most proteins, with CCL13 being the only exception. The paucity of studies in literature, comparing jugular and peripheral plasma profiles in MS patients, and the unavailability of jugular plasma from healthy individuals limit the interpretation of the observed differences.

Although NCAM1 is thought to be involved in several processes, like neuronal development, organization of synapses and myelination/remyelination process, that take place in MS (Massaro 2002), data concerning plasma levels of NCAM1 in MS patients are not available in literature. In our study, both MS populations showed as a trend higher levels than healthy subjects. Taking into account the tight correlations ($r = 0.97$) between jugular and peripheral plasma levels of NCAM1 and among repeated evaluations over time ($r = 0.98$) performed in the 2nd MS population, which indicate the presence of particularly conserved individual plasma patterns in two MS disease cohorts, our findings suggest that NCAM1 plasma levels could be related to MS disease, independently from the CCSVI status.

Finding significant SELL level variation overtime, in presence of high correlation, could highlight persisting changes dependent on the rehabilitative treatment in patients, as inferred by decreasing SELL concentrations from T0 to T3 time points.

ANGPT1, investigated for the first time in plasma of MS patients, showed remarkably lower levels in the jugular vein than in peripheral plasma. ANGPT1 levels in the 2nd MS population was similar to those in healthy subjects and higher than in the 1st MS population, even after correction for age, which suggests a CCSVI-related association. Further, the absence of correlation between values in jugular/peripheral compartments ($r = 0.04$), compared with the good correlation estimated in repeated overtime measurements ($r = 0.67$), would support the presence of specific mechanisms regulating ANGPT1 levels and, as jugular vein drains blood from brain, cerebral expression/uptake might be candidate. The lower levels of ANGPT1 in plasma from the first MS population might mimic the lower RNA expression in the MS jugular wall estimated by transcriptomic analysis.

Intriguingly, ANGPT1 is thought to play an essential role in microvascular endothelial and blood-brain barrier integrity. Indeed, ANGPT1, produced by endothelial cells, through the Tie-2 receptor is implicated on blood vessel stability and integrity by inhibiting blood vessel leakage, and reducing the infiltration of inflammatory cells (Thurston et al. 2000; Lee et al. 2011). This protective role of ANGPT1 has been suggested in experimental allergic encephalomyelitis studies (Wang et al. 2016), and interestingly mutations in the Tie-2 receptor were

found to be associated with venous malformations (Nätynki et al. 2015).

The "long way" from jugular wall RNA to plasma protein is a remarkable limitation to study the parallel between mRNA and plasma protein concentrations. As a matter of fact, for CD86 several transcripts have been reported and the plasma assay (Wong et al. 2005) is able to detect only the soluble protein form of this membrane receptor, produced either by shedding or by alternative mRNA splicing. These CD86 mRNA and protein features have prevented detection of relation between mRNA and protein expression. Our study presents other limitations. First, the small number of vascular wall specimens undergoing transcriptomic analysis, tiny specimens of internal jugular wall, which represent by necessity very rare samples. Another limitation concerns the "control" CEA samples, being virtually unavailable jugular samples (wall) from MS patients, not meeting criteria for CCSVI, and from healthy individuals. Nevertheless, the analysis of protein levels in peripheral plasma in two independent MS populations, and in addition through repeated assays, favored investigation of MS- related variations.

Conclusions

Our study provides for the first time expression profiles of the IJV wall and suggests signatures of altered vascular mRNA profiles in MS disease. Repeated measurements in plasma indicate conserved plasma patterns for immune-inflammatory and adhesion proteins. The combined transcriptome-protein analysis provides intriguing links between IJV wall transcript alteration and plasma protein expression, thus highlighting proteins of interest for MS pathophysiology.

Additional files

Additional file 1 Table S1. Demographics and clinical characteristics of the 2nd study MS population. (DOCX 16 kb)

Additional file 2 Table S2. qRT-PCR Forward and Reverse Primers. (DOCX 15 kb)

Additional file 3 Table S3. List of 924 transcripts/genes differentially expressed (fold change > or = 2, Benjamini-Hockberg corrected P value < 0.05) in internal jugular vein wall of MS patients (MS-IJW) compared to non-MS controls (C-IJW). (XLSX 207 kb)

Additional file 4 Table S4. qRT-PCR expression levels of selected genes in MS ($n = 7$) vs control ($n = 4$) jugular vein walls. (DOCX 21 kb)

Additional file 5 Table S5. List of genes, differentially expressed in MS jugular vein walls (MS-IJW) compared to control vein walls (C-IJW), selected for protein level analysis in plasma. (DOCX 22 kb)

Additional file 6 Table S6. Plasma protein levels in the 2nd MS population according to clinical phenotypes. (DOCX 18 kb)

Abbreviations

ACTB: Actin beta; ANGPT1: Angiopoietin 1; AOC3 (or VAP-1): Amine oxidase copper containing 3 (or vascular adhesion protein 1); B2M: Beta-2-microglobulin; CCL13: C-C motif chemokine ligand 13; CCL18: C-C motif chemokine ligand 18; CCL3: C-C motif chemokine ligand 3; CCSVI: chronic cerebrospinal venous insufficiency; CD86: Cluster of differentiation 86; EDSS: Expanded disability status scale; GO: Gene ontology; HOX: Homeobox; IJV: Internal jugular vein; L1CAM: Neural cell adhesion molecule L1; MAPT: Microtubule associated protein tau; MRI: Magnetic resonance imaging; MS: Multiple sclerosis; NCAM1: Neural cell adhesion molecule1; PBMCs: Peripheral blood mononuclear cells; PP-MS: Primary progressive multiple sclerosis; RR-MS: Relapsing remitting multiple sclerosis; SELL: Selectin L; SP-MS: Secondary progressive multiple sclerosis; TNF: Tumor necrosis factor; TNFRSF6B: TNF receptor superfamily member 6b

Funding

The study was partially supported by the grant 2010XE5L2R_002 of the Italian Ministry of University and Research and by the grant 1786/2012 from the strategic 2010–2012 Research Program of Emilia Romagna Region.

Authors' contributions

FB, GM and PZ conceived the study design and critically revised the manuscript; GM and FB analysed and interpreted data, and wrote the manuscript; FB supervised the study; PZ, FS and IB, recruited the patients (1st study population), and performed the clinical evaluation of patients; EM collected clinical data and performed instrumental characterization of patients of the 1st MS population; NZ performed transcriptomic analysis, set up and performed protein analyses in plasma and statistical analyses; SM set up and performed transcriptomic analysis, and set up protein analysis in plasma; MB and BL performed protein analyses in plasma; FM participated to the study design, performed instrumental characterization of patients, provided and evaluated the surgical jugular wall specimens and plasma samples; MP performed and interpreted histological analysis of surgical samples; SS, FM and NB recruited patients belonging to the 2nd study population and performed their clinical evaluation; RV collected plasma samples and evaluated pre -analytical variables of the 2nd MS population. All authors approved the final version of the manuscript.

Competing interests

The authors declare that they have no competing interests.

Author details

[1]Department of Biomedical and Specialty Surgical Sciences, University of Ferrara, via Fossato di Mortara n 74, 44121 Ferrara, Italy. [2]Department of Life Science and Biotechnology, University of Ferrara, Ferrara, Italy. [3]Department of Morphology, Surgery and Experimental Medicine, University of Ferrara, Ferrara, Italy. [4]Department of Experimental and Diagnostic Medicine, Sant'Anna University- Hospital, Ferrara, Italy. [5]Center for Immunological and Rare Neurological Diseases, Bellaria Hospital, IRCCS of Neurological Sciences, Bologna, Italy. [6]Department of Neurosciences and Rehabilitation, Sant'Anna University- Hospital, Ferrara, Italy. [7]Unit of Vascular and Endovascular Surgery, S. Anna University-Hospital, Ferrara, Italy.

References

Adams CW. Perivascular iron deposition and other vascular damage in multiple sclerosis. J Neurol Neurosurg Psychiatry. 1988;51:260–5.

Airas L, Mikkola J, Vainio JM, Elovaara I, Smith DJ. Elevated serum soluble vascular adhesion protein-1 (VAP-1) in patients with active relapsing remitting multiple sclerosis. J Neuroimmunol. 2006;177:132–5.

Alexander JS, Prouty L, Tsunoda I, Ganta CV, Minagar A. Venous endothelial injury in central nervous system diseases. BMC Med. 2013;11:219–332.

Amato MP, Derfuss T, Hemmer B, Cavalla P, Goretti B, Marrosu MG, et al. Environmental modifiable risk factors for multiple sclerosis: Report from the 2016 ECTRIMS focused workshop. Mult Scler. 2018;24:590–603.

Aoki T, Yamamoto K, Fukuda M, Shimogonya Y, Fukuda S, Narumiya S. Sustained expression of MCP-1 by low wall shear stress loading concomitant with turbulent flow on endothelial cells of intracranial aneurysm. Acta Neuropathol Commun. 2016;4:48–61.

Belov P, Jakimovski D, Krawiecki J, Magnano C, Hagemeier J, Pelizzari L, et al. Lower arterial cross-sectional area of carotid and vertebral arteries and higher frequency of secondary neck vessels are associated with multiple sclerosis. Am J Neuroradiol. 2018;39:123–30.

Coen M, Marchetti G, Palagi PM, Zerbinati C, Guastella G, Gagliano T, et al. Calmodulin expression distinguishes the smooth muscle cell population of human carotid plaque. Am J Pathol. 2013a;183:996–1009.

Coen M, Menegatti E, Salvi F, Mascoli F, Zamboni P, Gabbiani G, et al. Altered collagen expression in jugular veins in multiple sclerosis. Cardiovasc Pathol. 2013b;22:33–8.

Comabella M, Cantó E, Nurtdinov R, Río J, Villar LM, Picón C, et al. MRI phenotypes with high neurodegeneration are associated with peripheral blood B-cell changes. Hum Mol Genet. 2016;25:308–16.

D'haeseleer M, Cambron M, Vanopdenbosch L, De Keyser J. Vascular aspects of multiple sclerosis. Lancet Neurol. 2011;10:657–66.

D'haeseleer M, Hostenbach S, Peeters I, Sankari SE, Nagels G, De Keyser J, et al. Cerebral hypoperfusion: a new pathophysiologic concept in multiple sclerosis? J Cereb Blood Flow Metab. 2015;35:1406–10.

Dolic K, Marr K, Valnarov V, Dwyer MG, Carl E, Karmon Y, et al. Intra- and extraluminal structural and functional venous anomalies in multiple sclerosis, as evidenced by 2 noninvasive imaging techniques. Am J Neuroradiol. 2012;33:16–23.

Elo P, Tadayon S, Liljenbäck H, Teuho J, Käkelä M, Koskensalo K, et al. Vascular adhesion protein-1 is actively involved in the development ofinflammatory lesions in rat models of multiple sclerosis. J Neuroinflammation. 2018;15:128.

Felding-Habermann B, Silletti S, Mei F, Yip PM, Brooks PC, Cheresh DA, et al. A single immunoglobulin-like domain of the human neural cell adhesion molecule L1 supports adhesion by multiple vascular and platelet integrins. J Cell Biol. 1997;139:1567–81.

Gorski DH, Walsh K. Control of vascular cell differentiation by homeobox transcription factors. Trends Cardiovasc Med. 2003;13:213–20.

Iglesias AH, Camelo S, Hwang D, Villanueva R, Stephanopoulos G, Dangond F. Microarray detection of E2F pathway activation and other targets in multiple sclerosis peripheral blood mononuclear cells. J Neuroimmunol. 2004;150:163–77.

Jeannin P, Herbault N, Delneste Y, Magistrelli G, Lecoanet-Henchoz S, Caron G, et al. Human effector memory T cells express CD86: a functional role in naive T cell priming. J Immunol. 1999;162:2044–8.

Kappus N, Weinstock-Guttman B, Hagemeier J, Kennedy C, Melia R, Carl E, et al. Cardiovascular risk factors are associated with increased lesion burden and brain atrophy in multiple sclerosis. J Neurol Neurosurg Psychiatry. 2016;87:181–7.

Karmon Y, Ramanathan M, Minagar A, Zivadinov R, Weinstock-Guttman B. Arterial, venous and other vascular risk factors in multiple sclerosis. Neurol Res. 2012;34:754–60.

Lee SW, Won JY, Lee HY, Lee HJ, Youn SW, Lee JY. Angiopoietin-1 protects heart against ischemia/ reperfusion injury through VE-cadherin dephosphorylation and myocardial integrin-β1/ ERK/caspase 9 phosphorylation cascade. Mol Med. 2011;17:1095–106.

Lindsey JW, Agarwal SK, Tan FK. Gene expression changes in multiple sclerosis relapse suggest activation of T and non-T cells. Mol Med. 2011;17:95–102.

Marchetti G, Girelli D, Zerbinati C, Lunghi B, Friso S, Meneghetti S, et al. An integrated genomic-transcriptomic approach supports a role for the proto-oncogene BCL3 in atherosclerosis. Thromb Haemost. 2015;113:655–63.

Massaro AR. The role of NCAM in remyelination. Neurol Sci. 2002;22:429–35.

Nätynki M, Kangas J, Miinalainen I, Sormunen R, Pietilä R, Soblet J, et al. Common and specific effects of TIE2 mutations causing venous malformations. Hum Mol Genet. 2015;24:6374–89.

Nickles D, Chen HP, Li MM, Khankhanian P, Madireddy L, Caillier SJ, et al. Blood RNA profiling in a large cohort of multiple sclerosis patients and healthy controls. Hum Mol Genet. 2013;22:4194–205.

Noseworthy JH, Lucchinetti C, Rodriguez M, Weinshenker BG. Multiple sclerosis. N Engl J Med. 2000;343:938–52.

Olsson T, Barcellos LF, Alfredsson L. Interactions between genetic, lifestyle and environmental risk factors for multiple sclerosis. Nat Rev Neurol. 2017;13:25–36.

Paraboschi EM, Cardamone G, Rimoldi V, Gemmati D, Spreafico M, Duga S, et al. Meta-analysis of multiple sclerosis microarray data reveals Dysregulation in RNA splicing regulatory genes. Int J Mol Sci. 2015;16:23463–81.

Passerini AG, Polacek DC, Shi C, Francesco NM, Manduchi E, Grant GR, et al. Coexisting proinflammatory and antioxidative endothelial transcription profiles in a disturbed flow region of the adult porcine aorta. Proc Natl Acad Sci U S A. 2004;101:2482–7.

Polman CH, Reingold SC, Edan G, Filippi HP, Hartung L, Kappos L, et al. Diagnostic criteria for multiple sclerosis: 2005 revisions to the "McDonald criteria". Ann Neurol. 2005;58:840–6.

Ramanathan M, Weinstock-Guttman B, Nguyen LT, Badgett D, Miller C, Patrick K, et al. In vivo gene expression revealed by cDNA arrays: the pattern in relapsing-remitting multiple sclerosis patients compared with normal subjects. J Neuroimmunol. 2001;116:213–9.

Ratzer R, Søndergaard HB, Christensen JR, Börnsen L, Borup R, Sørensen PS, et al. Gene expression analysis of relapsing–remitting, primary progressive and secondary progressive multiple sclerosis. Mult Scler. 2013;19:1841–8.

Salmi M, Jalkanen S. Vascular adhesion Protein-1: a cell surface amine oxidase in translation. Antioxid Redox Signal. 2017; https://doi.org/10.1089/ars.2017.7418.

Sati P, Oh J, Constable RT, Evangelou N, Guttmann CR, Henry RG, et al. The central vein sign and its clinical evaluation for the diagnosis of multiple sclerosis: a consensus statement from the north American imaging in multiple sclerosis cooperative. Nat Rev Neurol. 2016;12:714–22.

Spencer JI, Bell JS, DeLuca GC. Vascular pathology in multiple sclerosis: reframing pathogenesis around the blood-brain barrier. J Neurol Neurosurg Psychiatry. 2018;89:42–52.

Srinivasan S, Di Dario M, Russo A, Menon R, Brini E, Romeo M, et al. Dysregulation of MS risk genes and pathways at distinct stages of disease. Neurol Neuroimmunol Neuroinflamm. 2017;4:e337.

Straudi S, Manfredini F, Lamberti N, Zamboni P, Bernardi F, Marchetti G, et al. The effectiveness of robot-assisted gait training versus conventional therapy on mobility in severely disabled progressIve MultiplE sclerosis patients (RAGTIME): study protocol for a randomized controlled trial. Trials. 2017;18:88.

Thurston G, Rudge JS, Ioffe E, Zhou H, Ross L, Croll SD, et al. Angiopoietin-1 protects the adult vasculature against plasma leakage. Nat Med. 2000;6:460–3.

Wang B, Tian KW, Zhang F, Jiang H, Han S. Angiopoietin-1 and C16 peptide attenuate vascular and inflammatory responses in experimental allergic encephalomyelitis. CNS Neurol Disord Drug Targets. 2016;15:496–513.

Wong CK, Lit LC, Tam LS, Li EK, Lam CW. Aberrant production of soluble costimulatory molecules CTLA-4, CD28, CD80 and CD86 in patients with systemic lupus erythematosus. Rheumatology (Oxford). 2005;44:989–94.

Zamboni P, Galeotti R, Menegatti E, Malagoni AM, Tacconi G, Dall'Ara S, et al. Chronic cerebrospinal venous insufficiency in patients with multiple sclerosis. J Neurol Neurosurg Psychiatry. 2009;80:392–9.

Zamboni P, Menegatti E, Cittanti C, Sisini F, Gianesini S, Salvi F, et al. Fixing the jugular flow reduces ventricle volume and improves brain perfusion. J Vasc Surg Venous Lymphat Disord. 2016;4:434–45.

Zamboni P, Sisini F, Menegatti E, Taibi A, Malagoni AM, Morovic S, et al. An ultrasound model to calculate the brain blood outflow through collateral vessels: a pilot study. BMC Neurol. 2013;13:81.

Zamboni P, Tesio L, Galimberti S, Massacesi L, Salvi F, D'Alessandro R, et al. Brave dreams research group. Efficacy and safety of Extracranial vein angioplasty in multiple sclerosis: a randomized clinical trial. JAMA Neurol. 2018;75:35–43.

Ziliotto N, Baroni M, Straudi S, Manfredini F, Mari R, Menegatti E, et al. Coagulation factor XII levels and intrinsic thrombin generation in multiple sclerosis. Front Neurol. 2018;9:245.

Zivadinov R, Alexander SJ, Minagar A. Vascular pathology of multiple sclerosis. Neurol Res. 2012;34:735–7.

Zivadinov R, Weinstock-Guttman B. Extracranial venous angioplasty is ineffective to treat MS. Nat Rev Neurol. 2018;14:129–30.

16

OSMR gene effect on the pathogenesis of chronic autoimmune Urticaria via the JAK/STAT3 pathway

Xiao-Yan Luo[1,2], Qun Liu[3], Huan Yang[1,4], Qi Tan[1,5], Li-Qiang Gan[1,5], Fa-Liang Ren[1] and Hua Wang[1,2,4,5*]

Abstract

Background: Chronic autoimmune urticaria (CAU) is a common skin disease and remains unclear understanding of pathogenesis in the vast majority of cases. In order to explore a new therapy for CAU, the current study was performed to investigate the possible functioning of the Oncostatin M receptor (OSMR) gene in the autoimmunity of CAU via regulation of the JAK/STAT3 signaling pathway.

Methods: CAU skin tissues from 24 CAU patients and normal skin tissues from normal subjects were collected. Hematoxylin-eosin (HE) staining was conducted to count eosinophils, and immunohistochemistry was carried out to detect the positive rate of OSMR expression in two kinds of skin tissues. A total of 72 Kunming (KM) mice were selected, and 60 mice were used for establishing CAU models and later transfected with different plasmids. The expression of inflammatory factors was evaluated by enzyme-linked immunosorbent assays (ELISA). Expressions of janus kinase (JAK), signal transducer and activator of transcription 3 (STAT3), interferon-stimulated gene 15 (ISG15), CT10-regulated kinase (CRK), and interferon regulatory factor 9 (IRF9) were identified using Western blot assay and reverse transcription quantitative polymerase chain reaction (RT-qPCR). Epithelial cell proliferation was assessed by 3-[4,5-dimethylthiazol-2-yl]-2,5-diphenyl tetrazolium bromide (MTT) assay, and cell cycle distribution and cell apoptosis were assessed using flow cytometry.

Results: The findings confirm that OSMR protein expression and histamine release rate are highly elevated in human CAU skin tissues, and the expression of the JAK/STAT3 signaling pathway-related genes (OSMR, JAK2, STAT3, ISG15, CRK and IRF9) was up-regulated. OSMR gene silencing in CAU mice significantly decreases the content of inflammatory factors (IL-1, IL-6, IFN-γ, and IgE), the number of eosinophils, and reduces the expression of the JAK/STAT3 signaling pathway related genes, and further enhances cell proliferation, promotes cell cycle entry and inhibits apoptosis of epithelial cells.

Conclusion: All aforementioned results indicate that OSMR gene silencing inhibits the activation of the JAK/STAT3 signaling pathway, thereby suppressing the development of CAU.

Keywords: OSMR gene, JAK/STAT3 signaling pathway, Chronic autoimmune urticaria, Pathogenesis, Autoimmunity

* Correspondence: huawang@hospital.cqmu.edu.cn
[1]Department of Dermatology, Children's Hospital of Chongqing Medical University, Chongqing 400014, China
[2]Ministry of Education Key Laboratory of Child Development and Disorders, Chongqing 400014, China
Full list of author information is available at the end of the article

Background

Chronic urticaria (CU), an immune-mediated inflammatory disease, is defined as the spontaneous or inducible appearance of hives, angioedema or both lasting at least 6 weeks and presenting with numerous subtypes, all greatly damage patients' quality of life (Bingham 3rd, 2008; Gimenez-Arnau et al., 2015). CU, the potentially debilitating skin condition, is known to affect up to 1% of the general population with different durations, usually several months, but occasionally decades (Ventura et al., 2013). Chronic idiopathic urticaria (CIU) is a common type of CU accounting for over 70% cases of CU, and chronic autoimmune urticaria (CAU), a subgroup of CIU, accounts for more than 30% of CIU. CIU is characterized by severe and persistent wheals accompanied by redness and itching (Goh & Tan, 2009; Abd El-Azim & Abd, 2011). CAU is caused by anti-FcepsilonRI and less normally, by anti-IgE autoantibodies that result in the activation of mast cells and basophils (Goh & Tan, 2009). Currently, clinical suspicion and autologous serum skin test (ASST) are regarded as the basis of CAU diagnosis (Abd El-Azim & Abd, 2011). Previously, the role of omalizumab in treating refractory CAU patients was studied, and proven possible (Al-Ahmad, 2010). In addition, mizoribine was found to be an effective therapy in some CAU patients, and may possibly be effective for patients not responsive to traditional therapy (Hashimoto et al., 2012). CAU patients are poor responders to antihistamine therapy, which leads to the necessity of immunosuppressive therapy (Cherrez Ojeda et al., 2009). Therefore, new genetic methods are required to find the possible ways for the treatment of CAU.

Oncostatin M (OSM), a member of the interleukin 6 (IL-6) family of cytokines, plays important roles in various biological functions, including inflammatory responses and metabolic diseases (Komori et al., 2013). OSM secreted by skin-infiltrating T-lymphocytes is considered to be a potential keratinocyte activator correlated to skin inflammation (Boniface et al., 2007). Oncostatin M receptor (OSMR) gene is located at 5p13.1, and can bind to gp130 to mediate the biological functions of OSM (Hong et al., 2011; Deng et al., 2009). Therapies based on OSMR have been reported for treatment of various cancers including cervical squamous cell carcinoma and lung adenocarcinomas, as well as skin diseases such as familial primary localized cutaneous amyloidosis (Caffarel & Coleman, 2014; Chen et al., 2008; Arita et al., 2008). Janus kinase-signal transducer and activator of transcription (JAK/STAT) transmits information received from extracellular polypeptide signals through transmembrane receptors, directly to the target gene promoters in the nucleus, providing a mechanism for regulation of transcriptional without second messengers (Aaronson & Horvath, 2002). JAKs are required for numerous inflammatory cytokine signaling pathways, and are implicated in the pathogenesis of chronic dermatitis, atopic dermatitis and psoriasis, and JAK inhibitors are thus promising therapeutic candidates for chronic dermatitis (Tanimoto et al., 2018). Additionally, JAK inhibitors, which are also used to inhibit cytokine signaling, are assumed to be a possible mean of treating skin inflammatory disorders such as contact dermatitis (Amano et al., 2016). It has been reported that OSM is released in inflammatory conditions, and it signals primarily via the JAK/STAT pathway by combining with its receptor complex (Hermanns, 2015). The heterodimeric receptor complex combined with gp130 and OSMR could activate a signaling pathway involved in JAKs as well as transcription factors of the STAT family (Hintzen et al., 2008). However, further verification is required in order to explore whether the OSMR gene is involved in the pathogenesis of CAU through the JAK/STAT3 signaling pathway. Therefore, the current study aims to explore the role of OSMR gene silencing in the pathogenesis of CAU and its underlying mechanism involving the JAK/STAT3 signaling pathway.

Methods
Ethics statement
This study was approved by the Ethics Committee of Children's Hospital of Chongqing Medical University, and signed informed consents were obtained from all patients/guardians. In addition, the experiments were in accordance with the ethical standards, and all efforts were made to minimize the suffering of the animals included in the study.

Study subjects
CAU skin tissues from 24 CAU patients of Children's Hospital of Chongqing Medical University were collected, and normal skin tissues from skin grafts of 24 plastic surgery patients were selected as controls. Skin biopsy specimens were rapidly frozen in liquid nitrogen in order to prevent protein denaturation until total RNA was extracted from the specimens. The 24 CAU patients included 11 males and 13 females, with a mean age of 10 years. The average courses of disease of patients were 6.67 months (range 2–16 months). All patients had been treated with antihistaminic agents, and some patients underwent treatment with corticosteroids but with poor efficacy, for 16 of them complained of joint pain, gastrointestinal or respiratory symptoms.

Hematoxylin-eosin (HE) staining
Skin tissues extracted from CAU patients were fixed in 4% paraformaldehyde for 24 h, washed, dehydrated, cleared, waxed, embedded, sectioned, and made into paraffin sections. After that, the sections were stained with hematoxylin for observing the eosinophil infiltration in skin tissue of patients.

Immunohistochemistry

The sections underwent routine dewaxing, dehydration with gradient ethanol, antigen-repair under high pressure for 1.5 min, and cooling under tap water for 10 min. After the remaining tap water on the sections was removed under running water, the sections were added one drop of endogenous peroxidase blocking solution, incubated at room temperature for 10 min, and rinsed with phosphate buffer solution (PBS) (3 min, 3 times). Then, the sections were added with suitable amount of primary antibody, namely rabbit anti human immunoglobulin G (IgG) antibody for incubation overnight at 4 °C, followed by rinsing with PBS after being taken out (3 min, 3 times), and incubation with the biotin-labeled secondary mouse anti rabbit monoclonal antibody IgG/horseradish peroxidase (HRP) (dilution ratio of 1: 1000, ab6759, Abcam, Inc., Cambridge, MA, USA) at 37 °C for 30 min. After incubation with the two types of antibodies, the sections were rinsed with PBS (3 min, 3 times), dealt by streptomyces anti biotin catalase complex for 15 min, colored with 3,3′-diaminobenzidine (DAB), and then rinsed under tap water to terminate the whole reaction. Later, the sections were re-stained with hematoxylin, dehydrated, cleared, and mounted. PBS was used as the negative control instead of the primary antibody. Finally, each section was randomly photographed under a light microscope (at 10× & 40× magnification) to get 5 non-overlapping visual fields. At last, 100 cells were counted in each visual field randomly, and the percentage of positive cells = positive cells/total cells.

CAU animal model establishment

A total of 72 Kunming (KM) mice weighing 18~ 25 g (J018, Better Biotechnology Co., Ltd., Nanjing, China) were selected for the study, amongst which 60 mice were used for the establishment of CAU mouse models, and the other 12 untreated mice were regarded as the normal group. Each intraplantar of mice was treated with 0.05 mL 5% physiological saline solution containing ovalbumin (the total amount of injection for a mouse was 0.1 mL). Meanwhile, each mouse received pertussis vaccines (4×10^9 U) via intraperitoneal injections. After 12–14 d, the mice were sacrificed by using the neck-breaking method and blood was drawn. Mice blood was collected and centrifuged in order to separate the antiserum, which was stored in a refrigerator for later use (mixed antisera was selected from 5 sensitized mice). With the addition of normal saline (dilution ratio of 1: 10), 0.03 m^{1}L antiserum was injected into the abdominal wall of the mice. Subsequently, antigen attack was conducted by injections of 1 mL normal saline (containing 1 mg ovalbumin). The indications of pruritus include systemic pruritus-head scratching by paw, torso scratching by hind claws, and biting all parts of the body by mouth. The number and total duration of pruritus in each mouse was recorded within 30 min of the 1 mL dextran injections through the tail vein. The CAU mouse model was considered to be successfully established if the number and total duration of pruritus were significantly higher than the normal mice (Yagami et al., 2017). A total of 60 mice were successfully established as CAU models which were classified into: the blank group (model mice without any treatment), the negative control group (NC) (model mice transfected with empty vector plasmid), the OSMR-siRNA group (model mice transfected with OSMR-siRNA plasmid), the anti-phospho-STAT3 (Tyr705) + OSMR-siRNA group (model mice transfected with OSMR-siRNA plasmid + the JAK/STAT3 signaling pathway agonist), and the Tyr705 group (model mice treated with the JAK/STAT3 signaling pathway agonist) groups. The plasmids used in the experiments were purchased from Vigene Biotechnology Co., Ltd. (Shandong, China). Then, attention was paid to the number and total duration of pruritus within 30 min. The mice were sacrificed after successful transfection with corresponding plasmids. Then, mice skin specimens with wheal or rash were extracted and stored at − 80 °C. Eosinophil counting was conducted by routine method and the absolute value was recorded.

Isolation and culture of mast cells

The foreskin of children (1–9 years) was extracted by circumcision under aseptic conditions. The skin grafts were incubated in a RPMI 1640 culture medium (containing 100 U/mL penicillin and 100 µg/mL streptomycin) after blood was removed using normal saline. Subcutaneous tissues were isolated and rinsed with modified Tyrode solution (containing 137 mmol/L NaCl, 2.7 mmol/L KCl, 0.4 mmol/L NaH$_2$PO$_4$, 5.6 mmol/L Glucose, 10 mmol/L HEPES, 1 mmol/L CaCl and 1 mmol/L MgCl$_2$). Subsequently, the skin grafts were cut sliced tissue fragments of 1 mm^2, and placed in RPMI 1640 culture medium containing 1.5 mg/mL type I collagenase and 0.5 mg/mL hyaluronidase for 4-h culturing in an incubator containing 5% CO$_2$ in air and saturated humidity at 37 °C. Next, the fragments were isolated in order to a form a cell suspension by repeated blowing and beating of digestive juice with a straw. The suspension was filtrated with a stainless steel filter net. After removal of the tissue fragments and larger cell clusters, the filtrate was collected, rinsed with icy Tyrode solution, re-suspended in a RPMI 1640 culture medium containing 10% fetal bovine serum (FBS) , 100 U/mL penicillin and 100 µg/mL streptomycin, and cultured in a 5% CO$_2$ incubator with saturated humidity at 37 °C for 12 h. Subsequently, the culture medium was collected after gently shaking the culture bottle.

Histamine release test and enzyme linked immunosorbent assay (ELISA)

A total of 75 μL serum samples and normal serum samples obtained from CAU patients and healthy individuals were respectively mixed with 75 μL mast cell suspension, and incubated at 37 °C for 20 min, followed by centrifugation at 1610×g for 15 min, and the supernatant was collected which was used for evaluation of histamine release rate (the compound tube was used for aforementioned evaluation). The histamine release rate in CAU patients and normal individuals was determined by ELISA. Firstly, the test sample and reagent kit (ZK-G7274, Zike Biotechnology Co., Ltd., Shenzhen, China) were subjected to acylation and dilution following the standard and quality control in accordance with the operating procedures. Then, 50 μL test serum samples were obtained from CAU patients and healthy individuals. A total of 50 μL polyclonal anti-histamine antibody, enzyme conjugates and histamine antiserum were added into each well successively, which were mixed evenly and incubated at room temperature for 3 h, followed by plate rinsing five times. After that, the freshly prepared 200 μL 3,3′,5,5′-tetramethylbenzidine (TMB) substrate solution was added into each well for further incubation at room temperature for 20 min, followed by plate rinsing five times, and pat to dry the plate. Later, 100 μL TMB stop solution was added to each well to terminate the reaction, and the absorbance (A) value measured using a microplate reader at the excitation wavelength of 450 nm. Content of histamine in samples was calculated using a standard curve, and the formula was as follows: $X = A \times 50/m$. The histamine spontaneous release rate = histamine spontaneous release/total histamine content × 100%, and histamine release rate of samples = histamine content/total histamine content × 100%. Interleukin-1 (IL-1) ELISA kit (SBJ-M0582), IL-6 ELISA kit (SBJ-M0044), interferon (IFN)-γ ELISA kit (SBJ-M0038), IgE ELISA kit (SBJ-M0499) were used to measure the contents of IL-1, IL-6, IFN-γ and IgE according to the protocols provided by the manufacturer. All the kits were purchased from Nanjing SenBeiJia Biological Technology Co., Ltd. (Nanjing, Jiangsu, China).

Reverse transcription quantitative polymerase chain reaction (RT-qPCR)

Skin tissues (100 mg) were collected from mice in each group, placed into a glass grinder and added with 1 mL tissue lysate (BB-3209, Bestbio Technology, Co., Ltd., Shanghai, China), ground to an even homogenate by ice-bath, and placed on a nucleic acid protein analyzer (Bio-Photometer D30, Eppendorf, Hamburg, Germany) for the detection of absorbance ratio and RNA concentration. The results of optical density (OD) value at 260 nm/ that at 280 nm placed between 1.8~ 2.0 is indicative of highly purified RNA. Total RNA were extracted from 100 mg skin tissues in each group using the Trizol reagent (16,096,020, Invitrogen Inc., Carlsbad, CA, USA) in accordance with the instructions of the manufacturer, and PrimeScript RT Reagent kit (Fermentas, Maryland, NY, USA) was performed for RNA reserve transcription into cDNA. The reserve transcription conditions were as follows: 70 °C for 5 min, ice-bathing for 3 min, 37 °C for 60 min, and 95 °C for 10 min. The cDNA was temporarily preserved at − 20 °C in a refrigerator. Primers of OSMR, JAK2, STAT3, ISG15, CRK, IRF9, and GAPDH were synthesized by Takara (Takara Biotechnology Co., Ltd., Liaoning China). PCR amplification was performed to the target genes with 25 μL reaction system as follows: 300 ng cDNA, 1× PCR buffer solution, 200 μmol/L dNTPs, 80 pmol/L forward and reverse primers, 0.5 U Taq enzyme (S10118, Yuanye Biotechnology Co., Ltd., Shanghai, China) with the reaction system of pre-denaturation at 94 °C for 5 min, denaturation at 94 °C for 30 s, annealing at 54 °C for 30 s, extension at 72 °C for 30 s, all cycles were repeated 30 times with the last reaction at 72 °C for 10 and preserved at 4 °C. The primer sequences of OSMR, janus kinase 2 (JAK2), signal transducer and activator of transcription 3 (STAT3), interferon-stimulated gene 15 (ISG15), CT10-regulated kinase (CRK), and interferon regulatory factor 9 (IRF9), and glyceraldehyde-3-phosphate dehydrogenase (GAPDH) are shown in Table 1, and GAPDH was regarded as the internal control. The relative ratio of genes between experimental group and control group were calculated using the $2^{-\Delta\Delta Ct}$ method with the formula as: $\Delta\Delta CT = \Delta Ct_{experimental\ group} - \Delta Ct_{control\ group}$, among which $\Delta Ct = Ct_{OSMR} - Ct_{GAPDH}$ (Denley et al., 2013). Ct is the amplification cycle number when real time fluorescence intensity reached the set threshold. At such time, the amplification was in logarithmic phase of growth and the experiment was performed in triplicate.

Western blot analysis

Skin tissues (100 mg) of each group were extracted, placed in a glass grinder containing 1 mL tissue lysate (BB-3209, Bestbio Technology, Co., Ltd., Shanghai, China), and were ground to a homogenate by ice-bath, where after protein lysate was added in for tissue splitting at 4 °C for 30 min, centrifuged at 1610×g, 4 °C for 15 min, and the supernatant was collected. A bicinchoninic acid (BCA) kit (2020ES76, Yeasen Company, Shanghai, China) was employed in order to detect the concentration of each tissue samples. Firstly, deionized water was added to adjust the sample quantity of 30 μg protein lane. Then, 10% sodium dodecyl sulfate (SDS) separating glue and concentration glue was prepared. The sample tissues were mixed with the sample buffer, heated to a boil for 5 min, ice-bathed, centrifuged before

Table 1 RT-qPCR primer sequences

Genes	Sequences
OSMR	F: 5'-AGAAACTGGCACACCATCCT-3'
	R: 5'-ACTGCCCTAATGACCAGTGC-3'
STAT3	F: 5'-GCCACGTTGGTGTTTCATAATC-3'
	R: 5'-TTCGAAGGTTGTGCTGATAGAG-3'
JAK2	F: 5'-TGCTGTCCAGACAAGAATGC-3'
	R: 5'-TCCTTCTCTGCCAACGTCTT-3'
ISG15	F: 5'-CACAGTCCTGCTGGTGG-3'
	R: 5'-GGCGATACTGCGACCCT – 3'
CRK	F: 5'-GGCAGGGTAGTGGAGTGAT-3'
	R: 5'-AGGCTGTCTTGTCGTAGGC-3'
IRF9	F: 5'-TGCTTCCTCCAGAGCCAGAC-3'
	R: 5'-CACAAGGCGGCAATCCAG-3'
GAPDH	F: CCACCCATGGCAAATTCCATGGCA
	R: TCTAGACGGCAGGTCAGGTCCAC

RT-qPCR reverse transcription quantitative polymerase chain reaction, *OSMR* oncostatin M receptor, *STAT3* signal transducer and activator of transcription 3, *JAK2* janus kinase 2, *ISG15* interferon-stimulated gene 15, *CRK* CT10-regulated kinase, *IRF9* interferon regulatory factor 9, *GAPDH* glyceraldehyde-3-phosphate dehydrogenase, *F* forward, *R* reverse

being added into each lane with a micropipette for lectrophoretic separation. After that, the proteins on the membrane were transferred onto a nitrocellulose membrane (ZY-160FP, Zeye Biology, Shanghai, China), blocked with 5% skimmed power at 4 °C overnight. Later, diluted primary antibody, namely rabbit anti human polyclonal antibodies (dilution ratio of 1: 500), including OSMR (11226-R007, dilution ratio of 1: 400, Sino Biological Inc., Beijing, China), JAK2 (ab32101, dilution ratio of 1: 1000, Abcam Inc., Cambridge, MA, USA), STAT3 (ab68153, dilution ratio of 1: 1000, Abcam Inc., Cambridge, MA, USA), ISG15 (LS-C211809, dilution ratio of 1: 1000, Littleton, Colorado, USA), IRF9 (PAB28499, dilution ratio of 1: 400, Lianshuo Biological Technology, Wuhan, Hubei, China) and p-STAT3 (sc-56,747, Univ-bio, Shanghai, China) were added into the membrane for overnight incubation, followed by rinsing with PBS (5 mins, 3 times). The secondary antibody mouse anti rabbit IgG/HRP (Huabio Inc., Hangzhou, Zhejiang, China) was added for rocking incubation at 37 °C for 1 h, followed by rinsing with PBS at room temperature (5 mins, 3 times). At room temperature, the membrane was reacted with enhanced chemiluminescence (ECL) solution for 1 min, after which the membrane was amounted using cling-film with the liquid removed, and observed under an X-ray instrument (36209ES01, Qianchen Bioteachnology, Shanghai, China). GAPDH was regarded as the internal reference, and the grey value ratio of target band and GAPDH band was taken as the relative expression of sample protein. Each experiment was conducted three times.

3-(4,5-Dimethylthiazol-2-yl)-2,5-Diphenyltetrazolium bromide (MTT) assay

Skin tissues were extracted from mice in order to obtain keratinocytes after detachment, isolation and culture. The cells were allowed to reach around 80% confluence, and were rinsed with PBS two times, and detached by trypsin in order to prepare a single cell suspension. After counting, the cells were seeded into a 96-well plate at a density of $3 \times 10^3 \sim 6 \times 10^3$ cells/well, with the cell volume in each well maintained to 0.2 mL. A total of 6 duplicate wells were set, and the cells were cultured in an incubator. At the 30 min, 1 h, 6 h, 12 h, 24 h, and 48 h time periods during the incubation, the culture plate was taken out and the original culture medium was replaced with 5 g/L 10% MTT solution (GD-Y1317, Guduo Biotechnology Co., Ltd., Shanghai, China) for further 4-h incubation. Later, 100 μL dimethyl sulphoxide (DMSO) (D5879-100ML, Sigma-Aldrich Chemical Company, St Louis, MO, USA) were added in, and gently oscillated for uniform mixing for 10 min. After formazan crystals produced by living cells were dissolved with DMSO, the cell plate was placed onto a microplate reader for detecting the OD value of each well at the excitation wavelength of 490 nm. The experiment was repeated three times and the time point was set as the abscissa and the OD value as the ordinate in order to plot the CAU cell activity graph.

Scratch test

The mouse keratinocytes in the logarithmic phase of growth were selected, and isolated and cultured for 48 h. The cells were seeded in a 6-well plate at a density of 1×10^6 cells in each well and cultured in a 5% CO_2 incubator at 37 °C until cell confluence reached 95%. Then, a vertical linear scratch was drawn using a 20 μl micropipette, and then serum-free medium was added to the wells after the 6-well plate was washed with D-hanks solution. Sample cells were collected after scratching at 0 h and 36 h time periods with 3 visual fields at 100X magnification were photographed under a phase contrast microscope in order to compare the different scratch lanes. The healing rate of the scratch line was regarded as the cell migration and healing ability.

Flow cytometry

The mouse keratinocytes were collected for detachment with 0.25% trypsin solution after isolation and culture for 48 h. The number of cell samples was adjusted to 1×10^6 mL^{-1}. Then, 1 mL cells were centrifuged at 402×g for 10 min with the supernatant discarded and the cells collected. Per mL of the collected cells were added with 2 mL PBS before undergoing centrifugation. The supernatant was discarded, and the cells were fixed with 70% pre-cooled ethanol solution at 4 °C overnight. The following day, the fixed cells were rinsed with PBS two times, and a cell suspension of 100 μL (containing more than 10^6 mL^{-1}) was selected, added with 1 mL 50 mg/L propidium iodide (PI) solution (containing RNAase) for 30-min incubation avoiding light exposure. After that, the cells were filtered with nylon net (300 mesh), and the cell cycle was analyzed using flow cytometry at an excitation wavelength of 488 nm.

Cell apoptosis was assessed using the Annexin V-fluorescein isothiocyanate (FITC)/PI double staining, and the cells were underwent the same process of cell cycle. The cells were cultured at 37 °C in an incubator containing 5% CO_2 in air, and then were collected. After rinsing with PBS two times, the cells were centrifuged and re-suspended in 200 μL binding buffer, followed by the addition of fully-mixed 10 μL Annexin V-FITC and 5 μL PI for 15-min reaction avoiding light exposure at room temperature. Later, the cells were added with 300 μL binding buffer and placed onto the flow cytometry (6HT, Cellwar Bio-technology Co., Ltd., Wuhan, Hubei, China) for cell apoptosis detection at the excitation wavelength of 488 nm.

Statistical analysis

Statistical analyses were performed using the SPSS 22.0 software (IBM Corp. Armonk, NY, USA). Measurement data were expressed as mean ± standard deviation. Differences between two groups were compared using the t test, and differences among multiple groups were analyzed

using one-way analysis of variance (ANOVA). $p < 0.05$ was considered to be statistically significant.

Results

Elevated histamine releasing rate in CAU model mice signifies the successful model establishing

In order to observe the histopathological changes of skin tissues after the occurrence of CAU, 24 CAU patients and 12 model mice (blank group) were recruited in the current study. As shown in Fig. 1a, all CAU specimens exhibited vasodilation, mild dermal edema and a perivascular or interstitial infiltrate composed of neutrophils, eosinophil and lymphocyte, while there were no telangiectasia and congestion in addition to lymphocytic and eosinophil infiltration around the dermal vessels in normal tissues. The observation results of skin tissues obtained from CAU mice were in accordance with the aforementioned findings (Fig. 1b).

According to results of the histamine releasing by mast cells, the release rates of histamine by normal human serum activated mast cells were all negative, while 10 positive cases and 14 negative cases of histamine release out of human CAU serum were observed with the release rate of $(21.35 ± 8.40)\%$ which was higher than the normal subjects $(9.08 ± 3.42)\%$ ($p < 0.05$) (Fig. 1c). In CAU model mice, CAU mice with no transfection had a histamine release rate of $(26 ± 5.20)\%$ compared with normal mice which was $(8.16 ± 4.28)\%$, signifying a highly

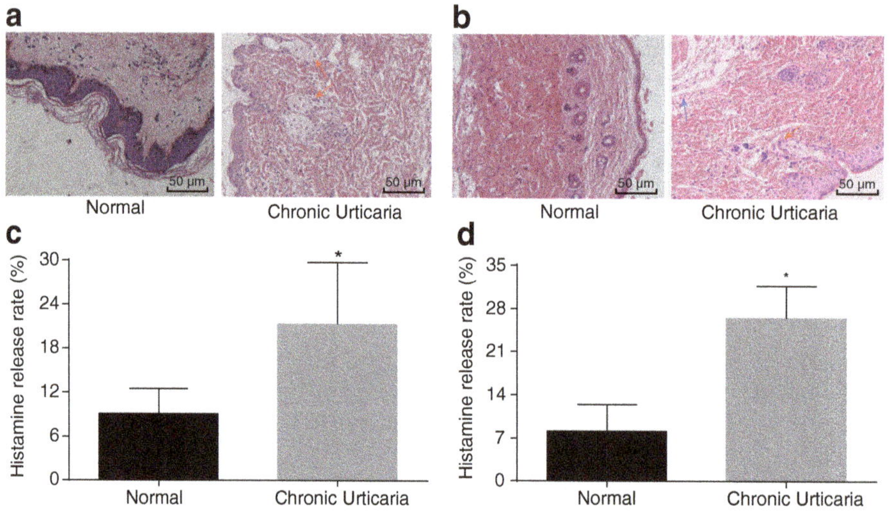

Fig. 1 Deteriorated pathological changes and elevated histamine release rate in CAU revealed by HE staining and Histamine Release ($\times$ 200). Note: **a** normal skin tissues and CAU tissues in patients with CAU after HE staining, with the red arrows indicating towards the dermal vascular wall and the surrounding neutrophils and eosinophil infiltration ($\times$ 200); **b** normal skin tissues and CAU tissues in CAU mice after HE staining, with the red arrows indicating towards the dermal vascular wall and the surrounding neutrophils and eosinophil infiltration, and the blue arrow indicating towards the small amount of lymphocytic infiltration surrounding the dermal vascular wall ($\times$ 200); **c** histamine release experiment of human serum activated mast cells ($n = 24$); **d** histamine release experiment of mice serum activated mast cells in normal and CAU tissues ($n = 12$); *, $p < 0.05$ compared with the normal group; CAU, chronic autoimmune urticaria; HE, hematoxylin-eosin

increased histamine release rate in CAU model mice and successful establishment of CAU models (Fig. 1d).

Higher OSMR positive expression rate and elevated expression of the JAK/STAT3 signaling pathway-related genes in CAU skin tissues

In order to better investigate the expression of OSMR in CAU skin tissues, CAU and normal skin tissues were observed under the light microscope. The findings indicate that OSMR positive cells were primarily located in the superficial and middle dermis, surrounding the blood vessels and appendages in CAU skin tissues, with the positive granule largely located inside the epithelial cells. The OSMR positive expression rate in CAU skin tissues was 34.00%. However, a relatively small number of OSMR positive cells were observed in normal skin tissues with an OSMR positive expression rate of 8.50%, indicating that the OSMR positive expression rate in CAU skin tissues was significantly higher than normal skin tissues ($p < 0.05$) (Fig. 2a, b).

As OSMR plays a vital role in CAU skin tissues, RT-qPCR and Western blot assay were conducted in order to elucidate the relationship between OSMR and the JAK/STAT3 signaling pathway. The results (Fig. 2c) reveal that the mRNA expression of OSMR and the JAK/ STAT3 signaling pathway-related genes, including JAK2, STAT3, ISG15, CRK and IRF9, were evidently elevated in CAU skin tissues ($p < 0.05$), and the same was confirmed by the Western blot analysis ($p < 0.05$) (Fig. 2d). All aforementioned findings indicate that CAU exhibits increased expression of OSMR and the activated JAK/ STAT3 signaling pathway.

Inhibited expression of CAU inflammatory factors as a result of OSMR silencing

The ELISA assay was employed to determine the levels of inflammatory factors such as IL-1, IL-6 and IFN-γ in CAU skin tissues. As shown in Fig. 3a, the inflammatory factors were found to be increased in CAU skin tissues. Mice models with different vectors transfection were established in order to testify the function of OSMR. Results of the ELISA assay (Fig. 3b) show that compared with the normal skin tissues, CAU tissues with no transfection and transfected with blank plasmids exhibited increased levels of IL-1, IL-6 and IFN-γ. Compared with CAU tissues with no transfection and transfected with blank plasmids, CAU tissues transfected with OSMR-siRNA exhibited decreased levels of IL-1, IL-6 and IFN-γ, with an opposite trend observed in CAU skin tissues transfected with Tyr705. Interestingly, there was no

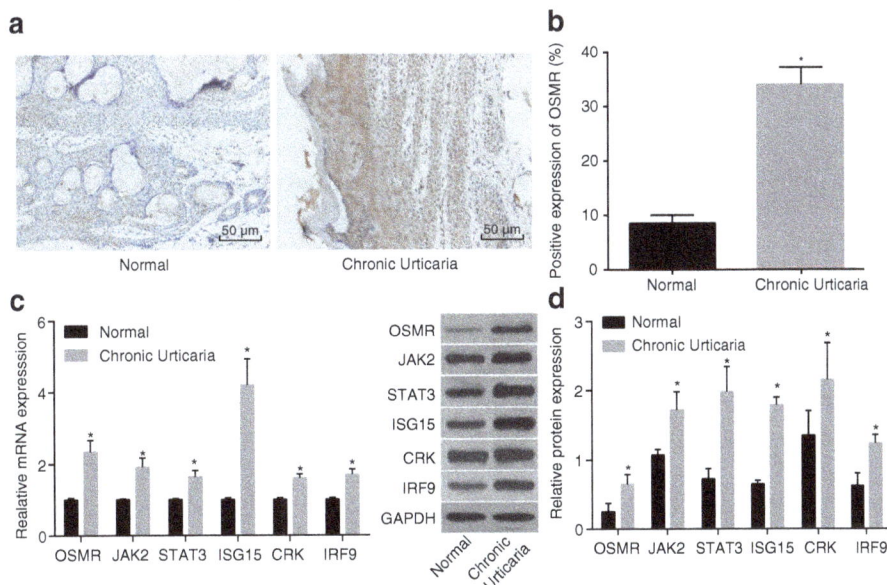

Fig. 2 Increased protein and mRNA expressions of OSMR and JAK/STAT3 signaling pathway-related factors in skin tissues of CAU patients revealed by RT-qPCR assay and Western blot analysis (n = 24). Note: **a** OSMR protein expression in human CAU tissues and normal skin tissues under microscope (× 200); **b** comparison of OSMR protein expression rate in human CAU tissues and normal skin tissues revealed that OSMR protein expression was significantly higher in CAU tissues than the normal skin tissues; **c** mRNA expression of OSMR, JAK2, STAT3, ISG15, CRK and IRF9 was significantly higher in CAU tissues than those in normal skin tissues detected by RT-qPCR; **d** Western blot assay revealed increased protein expression of OSMR, JAK2, STAT3, ISG15, CRK and IRF9 in CAU tissues than those in normal skin tissues; *, $p < 0.05$ when compared with the normal skin tissues; CAU, chronic autoimmune urticaria; RT-qPCR, reverse transcription quantitative polymerase chain reaction; OSMR, Oncostatin M receptor; JAK2, janus kinase 2; STAT3, signal transducer and activator of transcription 3; ISG15, interferon-stimulated gene 15; CRK, CT10-regulated kinase; IRF9, interferon regulatory factor 9

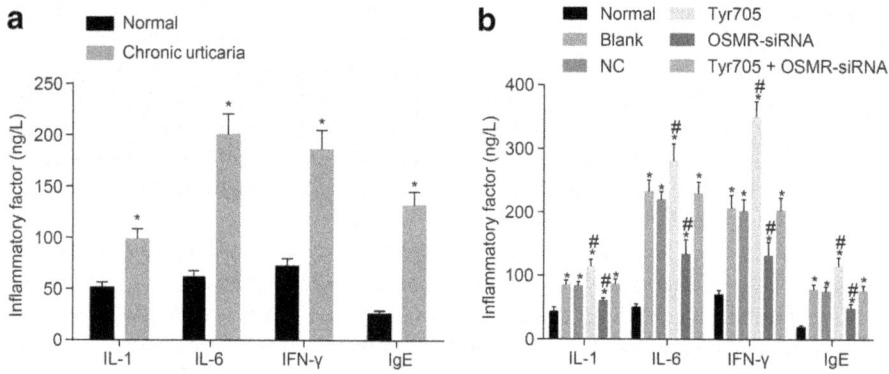

Fig. 3 Decreased inflammatory factor content after transfection with OSMR-siRNA but increased by activation of the JAK/STAT3 signaling pathway. Notes: **a** inflammatory factor expression in serum of CAU patients (n = 24); **b** inflammatory factor expression in serum of CAU mouse tissues with different transfection (n = 12); *, $p < 0.05$ compared with the normal group; #, $p < 0.05$ compared with the blank group; CAU, chronic autoimmune urticaria; OSMR, Oncostatin M receptor; JAK, janus kinase; STAT, signal transducer and activator of transcription

significant differences among CAU skin tissues with no transfection and transfected with blank plasmids, and those transfected with OSMR-siRNA + Tyr705 ($p > 0.05$). The aforementioned findings demonstrate that OSMR silencing inhibited while the activation of the JAK/STAT3 signaling pathway promoted the expression of inflammatory factors.

Pathological reaction of CAU relieved and eosinophil number decreased after transfection with OSMR silencing

As CAU is characterized by pruritus and flare reaction in skin with an increase in eosinophils, the pathological morphology in each group was observed under the microscope, and the number and duration of pruritus in CAU mice was accordingly analyzed and recorded. As shown by Table 2 and Fig. 4, the recorded number and duration of pruritus, and the eosinophils counting number were found to be increased in CAU mice ($p < 0.05$). Compared to the CAU mice with no transfection and transfected with blank plasmids, CAU mice tissues transfected with OSMR-siRNA exhibited significantly decreased number and duration of pruritus and eosinophils counting number, whereas the results were opposite in the CAU mice tissues transfected with Tyr705 ($p < 0.05$). Thereby, it can be concluded that OSMR silencing and

JAK/STAT3 inhibition relieved CAU pathological reaction and decreased the eosinophils counting number.

Enhanced proliferation of epithelial cells after transfected with OSMR silencing and the JAK/STAT3 signaling pathway inhibition

Cell cycle and cell apoptosis are two essential elements for assessing cell growth and death, thus, flow analysis was performed in order to explore the alterations in cell cycle and cell apoptosis after different transfection. As showed by Fig. 5, cell proliferation was found to be decreased significantly with the decreasing condition remained for 6 h ($p > 0.05$). At transfection periods of 12, 24, and 48 h, cells transfected with OSMR-siRNA exhibited increases cell proliferation, while those transfected with Tyr705 had the lowest cell proliferation ($p < 0.05$). The findings reveal that OSMR silencing increased cell proliferation, while activation of the JAK/STAT3 signaling pathway inhibited cell proliferation.

As results of the flow analysis demonstrate, compared with the normal group, epithelial cells had prolonged G0/G1 phases but diminished S phases, along with increased cell apoptosis ($p < 0.05$). Compared to the cells with no transfection or transfected with blank plasmids, cells transfected with OSMR-siRNA demonstrated diminished

Table 2 The number and duration of pruritus ratios in each group

Group	n	Number of pruritus (time)	Duration of pruritus (min)
Normal	12	0	0
Blank	12	57.15 ± 6.72[*]	28.00 ± 4.10[*]
NC	12	55.23 ± 4.38[*]	27.30 ± 3.90[*]
Tyr705	12	92.50 ± 7.80[*#]	40.50 ± 350[*#]
OSMR-siRNA	12	18.40 ± 5.10[*]	17.00 ± 3.35[*]
Tyr705 + OSMR-siRNA	12	56.38 ± 5.20[*#]	29.40 ± 3.40[*#]

[*] $p < 0.05$ compared with the normal group; [#] $p < 0.05$ compared with the blank group; NC negative control, OSMR oncostatin M receptor

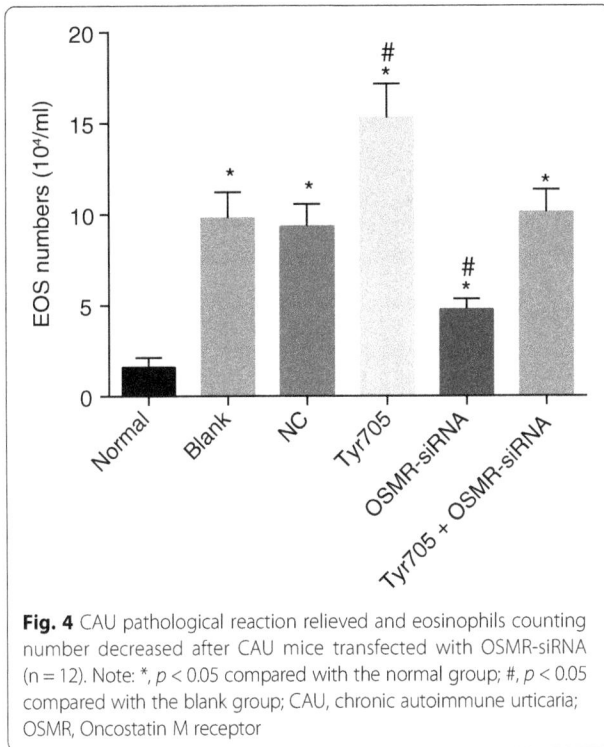

Fig. 4 CAU pathological reaction relieved and eosinophils counting number decreased after CAU mice transfected with OSMR-siRNA (n = 12). Note: *, $p < 0.05$ compared with the normal group; #, $p < 0.05$ compared with the blank group; CAU, chronic autoimmune urticaria; OSMR, Oncostatin M receptor

G0/G1 phases and prolonged S phases, whereas opposite results were observed in the cells transfected with Tyr705 ($p < 0.05$), and the results were not significantly different in cells transfected with Tyr705 + OSMR-siRNA ($p > 0.05$) (Fig. 6a, b). As for changes in cell apoptosis (Fig. 6c, d), decreased cell apoptosis was observed in cells transfected

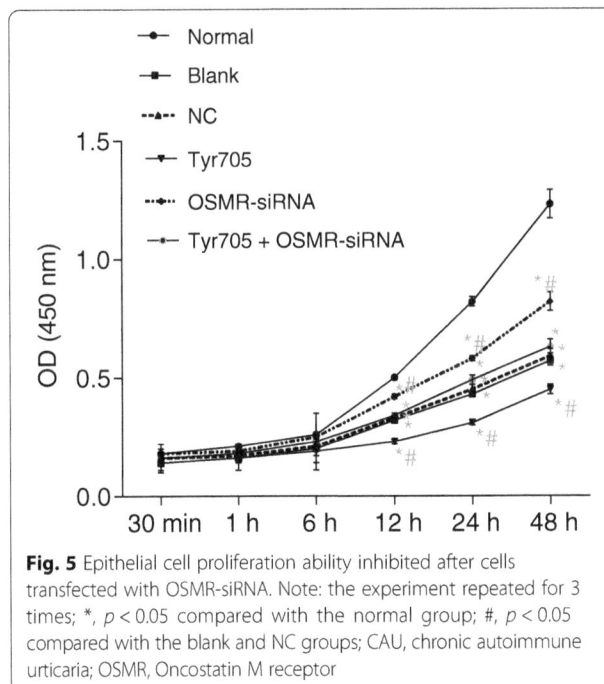

Fig. 5 Epithelial cell proliferation ability inhibited after cells transfected with OSMR-siRNA. Note: the experiment repeated for 3 times; *, $p < 0.05$ compared with the normal group; #, $p < 0.05$ compared with the blank and NC groups; CAU, chronic autoimmune urticaria; OSMR, Oncostatin M receptor

with OSMR-siRNA, whereas it was found to be increased in cells transfected with Tyr705, while there were no significant difference in cells transfected with Tyr705 + OSMR-siRNA ($p > 0.05$). The above results show that OSMR accelerated the apoptosis of epithelial cells by shortening the S phase and prolonging the G0/G1 phase of the cell cycle. Therefore, it can be concluded that OSMR silencing could shorten the G0/G1 phase, prolong the S phase of epithelial cells, thereby inhibiting epithelial cell growth, while down-regulation of the JAK/STAT3 signaling pathway promoted epithelial cell process.

OSMR silencing inhibited the JAK/STAT3 signaling pathway thus suppressed CAU progression

Lastly, in order to assess the relationship between OSMR and the JAK/STAT3 signaling pathway in epithelial cells, RT-qPCR and Western blot assay were performed in order to explore the mRNA and protein expressions of OSMR and the JAK/STAT3 pathway related genes in epithelial cells with different transfection. As shown by Fig. 7a–c, compared to the normal cells, epithelial cells exhibited increased mRNA and protein expressions of OSMR and JAK/STAT3 signaling pathway related genes ($p < 0.05$). Compared with the epithelial cells transfected with blank vectors, epithelial cells transfected with OSMR-siRNA displayed decreased expressions of OSMR and JAK/STAT3 signaling pathway related genes ($p < 0.05$), while those transfected with Tyr705 exhibited elevated levels ($p < 0.05$). Interestingly, epithelial cells transfected with Tyr705 + OSMR-siRNA exhibited decreased OSMR and JAK/STAT3 compared to the epithelial cells transfected with Tyr705, indicating that OSMR could inhibit the JAK/STAT3 signaling pathway.

Discussion

Chronic autoimmune urticaria (CAU), a commonly occurring disease, is accompanied by various symptoms including transient eruption of itchy, edematous swellings of the dermis, and erythematosus, lasting over a duration of 6 weeks (Wardhana, 2012). Recent study has shown that OSMR plays an important role in systemic lupus erythematosus, and further leads to the stimulation of various cytokines and inflammatory substances, such as IL-6 and IL-11 by activating the JAK/STAT pathway and the mitogen-activated protein kinase (MAPK) signaling pathways (Lin et al., 2014). The current study has shown that OSMR gene silencing can restrain the development of CAU, which can be achieved through blocking the JAK/STAT3 signaling pathway.

Initially, it was found that OSMR silencing inhibits the expression of the JAK/STAT3 signaling pathway related-genes (JAK2, STAT3, ISG15, CRK and IRF9). JAK2 is a non-receptor tyrosine kinase responsible for diverse cellular processes via stimulating cytoplasmic signaling

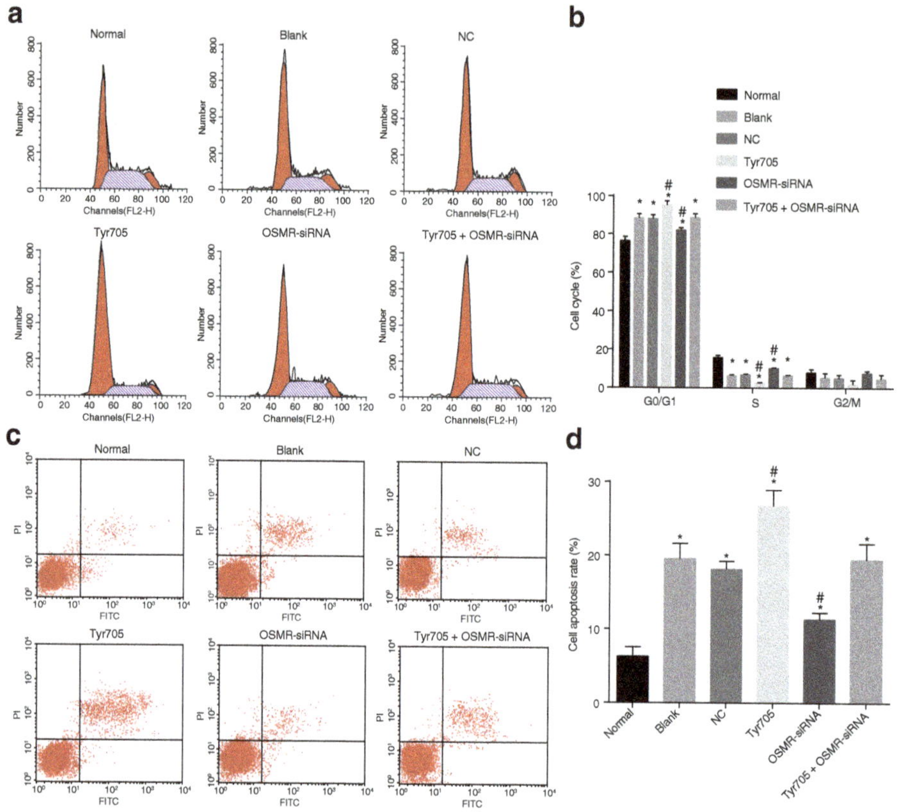

Fig. 6 Shortened epithelial cell cycle and promoted cell apoptosis after cells transfected with OSMR-siRNA thus to inhibit CAU cell growth and promote their apoptosis. Note: **a** flow cytometry image revealed the epithelial cell cycle in different transfection groups; **b** histogram image displayed the epithelial cell cycle in different transfection groups; **c** flow cytometry image revealed the epithelial cell apoptosis in different transfection groups; **d** histogram image displayed the epithelial cell apoptosis in different transfection groups; the experiment repeated 3 times; *, $p < 0.05$ compared with the normal group; #, $p < 0.05$ compared with the blank and NC groups; CAU, chronic autoimmune urticaria; OSMR, Oncostatin M receptor

cascades (Dawson et al., 2009). STAT3, another gene of interest in the current study, is a key member of the JAK/STAT signaling pathway (Yau et al., 2012). ISG15 is an ubiquitin-like protein whose conjugation is involved in the antiviral immune response and regulation of the JAK/STAT signaling pathway (Osiak et al., 2005; Hsiao et al., 2010). CRK belongs to Src homology-2 (SH2) and SH3 domain comprised of proteins that controls the coordinated combination of signaling complexes (Sriram et al., 2015). IRF9 is a crucial factor in the JAK/STAT signaling pathway that stimulates the antiproliferative function of IFN-α (Wu et al., 2017; Tsuno et al., 2009). A previous study found that both type I and type II OSMR activated JAK1, JAK2, and TYK2 receptor-associated tyrosine kinases (Auguste et al., 1997). Recently, OSM has been reported to stimulate ISG genes participating in antigen processing as well as presentation (Hergovits et al., 2017). The OSMR protein has been reported to be capable of heterodimerizing with IL-6 signal transducer (gp130) in order to produce type II OSMR, and when the receptor complexes were taken in, JAK

could be activated, followed by further activation of STAT3 (Hong et al., 2011). Consistently, it has been revealed that the low expression of OSMRβ could decrease atherogenesis by inactivating the JAK2/STAT3 signaling pathway in macrophages (Zhang et al., 2017). The aforementioned findings and evidence suggest that OSMR gene silencing could suppress the JAK/STAT3 signaling pathway.

Additionally, the current findings demonstrate that the contents of IL-1, IL-6, IFN-γ and IgE in serum of mice in the OSMR-siRNA group were significantly reduced, indicating that OSMR gene silencing suppressed the autoimmunity of CAU by blocking the JAK/STAT3 signaling pathway. Notable, it was reported that regulation of IFN-γ-secreting T helper 1 cells could inhibit autoimmunity and immunopathology (Cope et al., 2011). Previous studies have demonstrated that OSMR could increase IL-1 and TNF activity in synovial fibroblasts, which was consistent with the results of the current study (Le Goff et al., 2014). Interestingly, it was reported that inhibition of OSMR results in suppressed IL-31, which was highly expressed in the skin of patients with

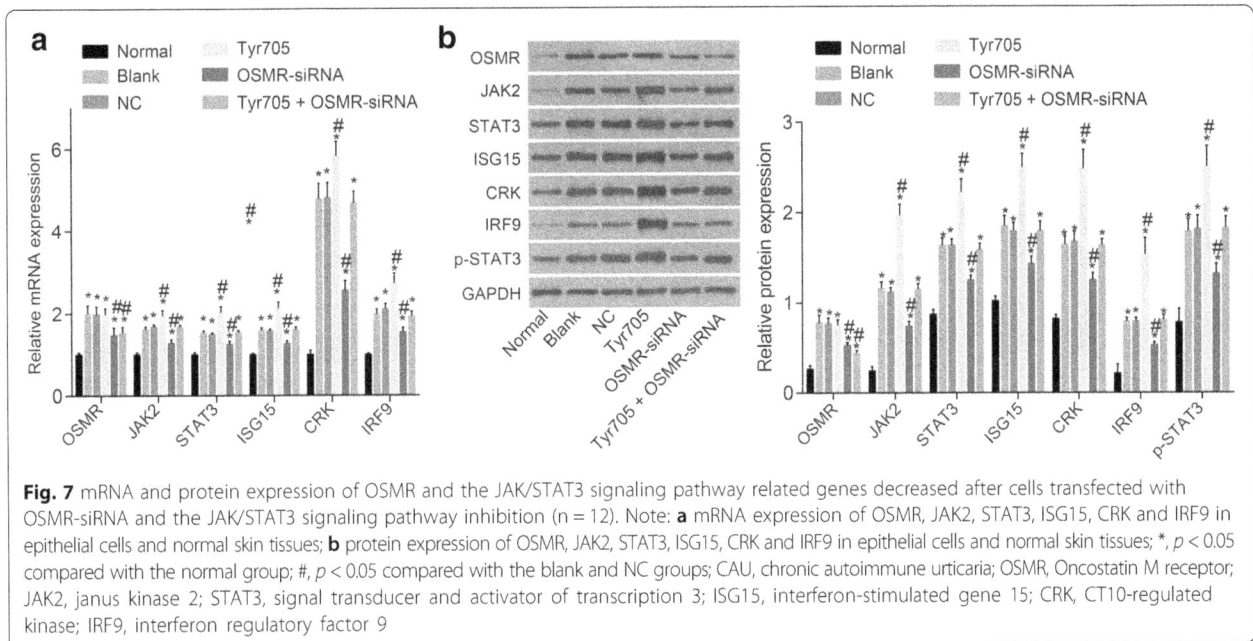

Fig. 7 mRNA and protein expression of OSMR and the JAK/STAT3 signaling pathway related genes decreased after cells transfected with OSMR-siRNA and the JAK/STAT3 signaling pathway inhibition (n = 12). Note: **a** mRNA expression of OSMR, JAK2, STAT3, ISG15, CRK and IRF9 in epithelial cells and normal skin tissues; **b** protein expression of OSMR, JAK2, STAT3, ISG15, CRK and IRF9 in epithelial cells and normal skin tissues; *, $p < 0.05$ compared with the normal group; #, $p < 0.05$ compared with the blank and NC groups; CAU, chronic autoimmune urticaria; OSMR, Oncostatin M receptor; JAK2, janus kinase 2; STAT3, signal transducer and activator of transcription 3; ISG15, interferon-stimulated gene 15; CRK, CT10-regulated kinase; IRF9, interferon regulatory factor 9

chronic spontaneous urticaria and was released from isolated basophils accompanied with anti-IgE activation (Raap et al., 2017). Moreover, it has been reported that inactivation of the JAK/STAT pathway could help in inhibiting the expression of ICAM-1 induced by IFN-γ in HaCaT human keratinocytes (Sung & Kim, 2013). The activated JAK/STAT signaling pathway could stimulate IFNs in order to exert an innate immune response (Cheng et al., 2014). In addition, STAT3 mutations are associated with autosomal dominant-hyper-IgE syndromes (AD-HIES) and this association might allow differentiation of AD-HIES from disorders correlated with elevated serum IgE levels (Schimke et al., 2010).

Consequently, it was revealed that OSMR gene silencing can obstruct the development of CAU by inhibiting the JAK/STAT3 signaling pathway, as increased proliferation, migration and decreased apoptosis of epithelial cells were observed in the OSMR-siRNA group. OSM, is a cytokine capable of modulating cell survival and proliferation, and the over-expression of OSM could result in transdifferentiation of epithelial-myofibroblast (Elbjeirami et al., 2010). In line with the findings of the current study, it was reported that over-expression of OSM in tubular epithelial cells might aggravate mucosal epithelial barrier dysfunction (Pothoven et al., 2015). The JAK/STAT is capable of modulating signaling cascades exerting great effects on proliferation, differentiation, development as well as immune responses (Kim et al., 2011). Additionally, it was reported that acute nitrogen dioxide exposure enhances airway inflammation that both humoral immunity and cellular immunity reaction via modulating Th1/Th2 differentiation and activating the JAK/STAT signaling

pathway (Ji et al., 2015). Therefore, it can be hypothesized that OSMR gene silencing regulates proliferation, migration as well as apoptosis of epithelial cells in CAU by inhibiting the JAK/STAT signaling pathway.

Conclusion

The current study suggested that OSMR gene are highly expressed in human CAU skin tissues, and cause the up-regulation of the JAK/STAT3 signaling pathway-related genes. Additionally, it was demonstrated that OSMR gene silencing significantly decreases the content of inflammatory factors, the number of eosinophils, and reduces the mRNA and protein expressions of JAK/STAT3 signaling pathway-related genes, enhances cell proliferation, migration and inhibits apoptosis of epithelial cells. Thereby, it can be concluded that OSMR gene silencing inhibits autoimmunity in CAU mouse models by inactivating the JAK/STAT3 signaling pathway. These findings may open novel avenues for future CAU therapies and to ultimately, raise the quality of life of CAU patients. However, the limited sample size of the current study remains to be a limitation. Thus, further studies are warranted in order to better the understanding of specific mechanisms.

Acknowledgements

We would like to give our sincere appreciation to the reviewers for their helpful comments on this article.

Funding

This work was supported by the National Natural Science Foundation of China (No. 81301362) and High End Talent Plan of Chongqing Municipal Health and Family Planning Commission.

Authors' contributions

HW and X-YL participated in the conception and design of the study. HW, QL and HY performed the analysis and interpretation of data. HY, QT and L-QG contributed to drafting the article. HW and F-LR revised it critically for important intellectual content. HW is the GUARANTOR for the article who accepts full responsibility for the work and/or the conduct of the study, had access to the data, and oversaw the decision to publish. All authors contributed to the revision and approved the final version of this manuscript.

Competing interests

The authors declare that they have no competing interests.

Author details

[1]Department of Dermatology, Children's Hospital of Chongqing Medical University, Chongqing 400014, China. [2]Ministry of Education Key Laboratory of Child Development and Disorders, Chongqing 400014, China. [3]The Division of Allergy and Clinical Immunology, Johns Hopkins University School of Medicine, Baltimore, MD 21224, USA. [4]China International Science and Technology Cooperation Base of Child Development and Critical Disorders, Chongqing 400014, China. [5]Chongqing Key Laboratory of Pediatrics, No.136, Zhongshan Er Road, Yuzhong District, Chongqing 400014, China.

References

Aaronson DS, Horvath CM. A road map for those who don't know JAK-STAT. Science. 2002;296:1653–5.

Abd El-Azim M, Abd E-AS. Chronic autoimmune urticaria: frequency and association with immunological markers. J Investig Allergol Clin Immunol. 2011;21:546–50.

Al-Ahmad M. Omalizumab therapy in three patients with chronic autoimmune urticaria. Ann Saudi Med. 2010;30:478–81.

Amano W, et al. JAK inhibitor JTE-052 regulates contact hypersensitivity by downmodulating T cell activation and differentiation. J Dermatol Sci. 2016;84:258–65.

Arita K, et al. Oncostatin M receptor-beta mutations underlie familial primary localized cutaneous amyloidosis. Am J Hum Genet. 2008;82:73–80.

Auguste P, et al. Signaling of type II oncostatin M receptor. J Biol Chem. 1997; 272:15760–4.

Bingham CO 3rd. Immunomodulatory approaches to the management of chronic urticaria: an immune-mediated inflammatory disease. Curr Allergy Asthma Rep. 2008;8:278–87.

Boniface K, et al. Oncostatin M secreted by skin infiltrating T lymphocytes is a potent keratinocyte activator involved in skin inflammation. J Immunol. 2007; 178:4615–22.

Caffarel MM, Coleman N. Oncostatin M receptor is a novel therapeutic target in cervical squamous cell carcinoma. J Pathol. 2014;232:386–90.

Chen D, et al. Expression of short-form oncostatin M receptor as a decoy receptor in lung adenocarcinomas. J Pathol. 2008;215:290–9.

Cheng CH, et al. Differential regulation of Tetraodon nigroviridis mx gene promoter activity by constitutively-active forms of STAT1, STAT2, and IRF9. Fish Shellfish Immunol. 2014;38:230–43.

Cherrez Ojeda I, et al. Chronic autoimmune urticaria in children. Allergol Immunopathol (Madr). 2009;37:43–7.

Cope A, Le Friec G, Cardone J, Kemper C. The Th1 life cycle: molecular control of IFN-gamma to IL-10 switching. Trends Immunol. 2011;32:278–86.

Dawson MA, et al. JAK2 phosphorylates histone H3Y41 and excludes HP1alpha from chromatin. Nature. 2009;461:819–22.

Deng G, et al. Unique methylation pattern of oncostatin m receptor gene in cancers of colorectum and other digestive organs. Clin Cancer Res. 2009; 15:1519–26.

Denley SM, et al. Activation of the IL-6R/Jak/stat pathway is associated with a poor outcome in resected pancreatic ductal adenocarcinoma. J Gastrointest Surg. 2013;17:887–98.

Elbjeirami WM, et al. Early differential expression of oncostatin M in obstructive nephropathy. J Interf Cytokine Res. 2010;30:513–23.

Gimenez-Arnau AM, Grattan C, Zuberbier T, Toubi E. An individualized diagnostic approach based on guidelines for chronic urticaria (CU). J Eur Acad Dermatol Venereol. 2015;29(Suppl 3):3–11.

Goh CL, Tan KT. Chronic autoimmune urticaria: where we stand? Indian J Dermatol. 2009;54:269–74.

Hashimoto T, et al. Mizoribine treatment for antihistamine-resistant chronic autoimmune urticaria. Dermatol Ther. 2012;25:379–81.

Hergovits S, Mais C, Haan C, Costa-Pereira AP, Hermanns HM. Oncostatin M induces RIG-I and MDA5 expression and enhances the double-stranded RNA response in fibroblasts. J Cell Mol Med. 2017;21:3087–99.

Hermanns HM. Oncostatin M and interleukin-31: cytokines, receptors, signal transduction and physiology. Cytokine Growth Factor Rev. 2015;26:545–58.

Hintzen C, et al. Box 2 region of the oncostatin M receptor determines specificity for recruitment of Janus kinases and STAT5 activation. J Biol Chem. 2008;283:19465–77.

Hong IK, Eun YG, Chung DH, Kwon KH, Kim DY. Association of the oncostatin m receptor gene polymorphisms with papillary thyroid cancer in the korean population. Clin Exp Otorhinolaryngol. 2011;4:193–8.

Hsiao NW, et al. ISG15 over-expression inhibits replication of the Japanese encephalitis virus in human medulloblastoma cells. Antivir Res. 2010;85:504–11.

Ji X, Han M, Yun Y, Li G, Sang N. Acute nitrogen dioxide (NO2) exposure enhances airway inflammation via modulating Th1/Th2 differentiation and activating JAK-STAT pathway. Chemosphere. 2015;120:722–8.

Kim BH, et al. Benzoxathiol derivative BOT-4-one suppresses L540 lymphoma cell survival and proliferation via inhibition of JAK3/STAT3 signaling. Exp Mol Med. 2011;43:313–21.

Komori T, Tanaka M, Senba E, Miyajima A, Morikawa Y. Lack of oncostatin M receptor beta leads to adipose tissue inflammation and insulin resistance by switching macrophage phenotype. J Biol Chem. 2013;288:21861–75.

Le Goff B, et al. Oncostatin M acting via OSMR, augments the actions of IL-1 and TNF in synovial fibroblasts. Cytokine. 2014;68:101–9.

Lin YZ, et al. Association of OSMR gene polymorphisms with rheumatoid arthritis and systemic lupus erythematosus patients. Autoimmunity. 2014;47:23–6.

Osiak A, Utermohlen O, Niendorf S, Horak I, Knobeloch KP. ISG15, an interferon-stimulated ubiquitin-like protein, is not essential for STAT1 signaling and responses against vesicular stomatitis and lymphocytic choriomeningitis virus. Mol Cell Biol. 2005;25:6338–45.

Pothoven KL, et al. Oncostatin M promotes mucosal epithelial barrier dysfunction, and its expression is increased in patients with eosinophilic mucosal disease. J Allergy Clin Immunol. 2015;136:737–46 e4.

Raap U, et al. Human basophils are a source of - and are differentially activated by - IL-31. Clin Exp Allergy. 2017;47:499–508.

Schimke LF, et al. Diagnostic approach to the hyper-IgE syndromes: immunologic and clinical key findings to differentiate hyper-IgE syndromes from atopic dermatitis. J Allergy Clin Immunol 126. 2010;e1:611–7.

Sriram G, et al. Iterative tyrosine phosphorylation controls non-canonical domain utilization in Crk. Oncogene. 2015;34:4260–9.

Sung YY, Kim HK. Illicium verum extract suppresses IFN-gamma-induced ICAM-1 expression via blockade of JAK/STAT pathway in HaCaT human keratinocytes. J Ethnopharmacol. 2013;149:626–32.

Tanimoto A, et al. A novel JAK inhibitor JTE-052 reduces skin inflammation and ameliorates chronic dermatitis in rodent models: comparison with conventional therapeutic agents. Exp Dermatol. 2018;27:22–9.

Tsuno T, et al. IRF9 is a key factor for eliciting the antiproliferative activity of IFN-alpha. J Immunother. 2009;32:803–16.

Ventura MT, Napolitano S, Menga R, Cecere R, Asero R. Anisakis simplex hypersensitivity is associated with chronic urticaria in endemic areas. Int Arch Allergy Immunol. 2013;160:297–300.

Wardhana DEA. Chronic autoimmune urticaria. Acta Med Indones. 2012;44:165–74.

Wu Z, et al. Interaction of IRF9 and STAT2 synergistically up-regulates IFN and PKR transcription in Ctenopharyngodon idella. Mol Immunol. 2017;85:273–82.

17

Hepatitis B virus downregulates vitamin D receptor levels in hepatoma cell lines, thereby preventing vitamin D-dependent inhibition of viral transcription and production

Neta Gotlieb[1], Irena Tachlytski[1], Yelena Lapidot[1,3], Maya Sultan[1], Michal Safran[1†] and Ziv Ben-Ari[1,2,3*†]

Abstract

Background: Vitamin D is a key immune-modulator that plays a role in the innate and adaptive immune systems. Certain pathogens impair the immune defense by downregulating the vitamin D receptor (VDR) pathway. Low serum levels of vitamin D are associated with increased hepatitis B virus (HBV) replication. Our study aimed to assess the in-vitro relationship between HBV production and Vitamin D signaling pathway and to explore the associated mechanism(s).

Methods: HBV transcription and replication was evaluated by qRT-PCR of the HBV-RNA and covalently closed circular DNA (cccDNA). Furthermore, we have transfected the 1.3 X HBV-Luc plasmid to the cells and measured the Luciferase activity using Luminometer. Vitamin D signaling pathway activation was evaluated by measuring the expression levels of VDR, CYP24A1, Tumor necrosis factor α (TNFα) and cathelicidin (CAMP) by qRT-PCR. All assays were performed on HepG2.2.15, HepG2, and HepAD38 cells treated with or without Vitamin D active metabolite: calcitriol.

Results: Calcitriol did not suppress HBV transcription, cccDNA expression or HBV RNA levels in HepG2.2.15 cells. However, VDR transcript levels in HepG2.215 cells were significantly lower compared to HepG2 cells. Similar results were obtained in HepAD38 cell where VDR expression was down-regulated when HBV transcript level was up-regulated. In addition, calcitriol induced VDR-associated signaling, resulting in upregulation of CYP24A1, TNFα and CAMP expression level in HepG2 cells but not in the HepG2.2.15 cells.

Conclusions: These findings indicate that VDR expression is downregulated in HBV-transfected cells, thereby preventing vitamin D from inhibiting transcription and translation of HBV in vitro. HBV might use this mechanism to avoid the immunological defense system by affecting both TNFα and CAMP signaling pathways.

Keywords: Vitamin D, Hepatitis B virus (HBV), Vitamin D receptor (VDR), Immune system, Downregulation

* Correspondence: ziv.ben-ari@sheba.health.gov.il
†Michal Safran and Ziv Ben Ari contributed equally to this work.
[1]Liver Reaserch Laboratory, Sheba Medical Center, Tel Hashomer, 52620 Ramat Gan, Israel
[2]Liver Disease Center, Sheba Medical Center, Tel Hashomer, 52620 Ramat Gan, Israel
Full list of author information is available at the end of the article

Background

Hepatitis B virus (HBV) infection is a global public health problem, estimated to affect approximately 2 billion people, of whom, 240 million are chronic carriers. About 20–30% of HBV carriers will progress to liver failure, hepatocellular carcinoma (HCC) and eventually, liver transplantation (Seeger & Mason, 2000). Current antiviral HBV therapy regimens dramatically decrease the viral load and thereby inhibit disease progression and complications. However, they do not bring to complete viral clearance in the infected hepatocytes, probably due to the synthesis of nuclear covalently closed circular DNA (cccDNA) and its integration into the hepatocyte genome (Ahmed et al., 2015). Thus, contemporary antiviral treatment (Marcellin et al., 2013) do not fully eliminate the likelihood of progression to cirrhosis and HCC.

Vitamin D exhibits extra-skeletal functions such as immune response, insulin secretion and cellular division (Deluca & Cantorna, 2001; Vanherwegen et al., 2017). Furthermore, Vitamin D deficiency is associated with an increased risk for various autoimmune disorders (Barbalho et al., 2017; Hassanalilou et al., 2017; Knutsen et al., 2017; Sandhya et al., 2017), cancer (Heidari et al., 2017; Hu et al., 2017; Hohaus et al., 2017), metabolic disorders (Wojcik et al., 2017; Schmitt et al., 2018; Lim et al., 2017; Chen et al., 2017)as well infections caused by influenza, rhinovirus, respiratory syncytial virus (RSV) and Human Immunodeficiency Virus (HIV) with high mortality rate from these pathogens (Borella et al., 2014; Pletz et al., 2014; Orkin et al., 2014; Watkins et al., 2015). Calcitriol, the active metabolite of Vitamin D, binds the nuclear Vitamin D receptor (VDR), which is responsible for the biological activity of vitamin D in the cell. VDR is found in a diverse range of tissues, including the liver and immune cells, such as T cells, monocytes and macrophages. After binding its ligand, VDR forms a heterodimer with the X receptor, which binds to vitamin D response elements present on target genes. The complex elicits an extensive biological response via regulation of gene transcription and stimulation of intra-cellular signaling pathways. Evidence of a crucial role played by Vitamin D in defending the body from microbe invasion has recently emerged. It was shown that Vitamin D can induce the expression of antimicrobial peptides (also known as host defense peptides), such as cathelicidin (CAMP), which have been demonstrated to disrupt the integrity of the microbe membrane, resulting in its death (Gombart, 2009). Furthermore, Vitamin D has also been shown to stimulate the expression of several cytokines, such as Tumor Necrosis Factor α (TNFα) (Golovko et al., 2005), that regulate both the recruitment of inflammatory cells to the area of infection and the activation of macrophage and T cell functions. Certain pathogens such as Mycobacterium Tuberculosis and HIV-1, can impair the innate immune defenses by downregulating the VDR pathway (Haug et al., 1994; Haug et al., 1998; Huang et al., 2015). Additionally, a recent meta-analysis showed that VDR polymorphism increases the risk for HBV infection (He et al., 2017).

Studies have shown a high incidence (50–90%) of vitamin D deficiency in patients with chronic liver disease, mainly, nonalcoholic fatty liver disease, cirrhosis and chronic hepatitis C infection. In vitro, vitamin D (3) showed remarkable antiviral activity by inhibiting hepatitis C virus (HCV) production in Huh7.5 hepatoma cells, suggested to be mediated by its active metabolite, calcitriol. Supplementing antiviral treatment in HCV patients with vitamin D significantly increased the odds for cure (sustained virologic response SVR) in patients with HCV genotypes 1, 2 and 3 and in post-transplantation patients (Gutierrez et al., 2011; Villar et al., 2013; Abu-Mouch et al., 2011; Nimer & Mouch, 2012; Bitetto et al., 2011; Kim et al., 2017).

In sharp contrast to HCV, the relationship between vitamin D metabolism and HBV infection is largely elusive. Chan et al. noted a high prevalence of abnormally low vitamin D levels among untreated, active chronic hepatitis B (CHB) patients (Chan et al., 2015). Similarly, in their prospective cohort study, Wong et al. also concluded that vitamin D deficiency is common among patients with CHB and is associated with adverse clinical outcomes, including HCC and increased rated of liver-related deaths (Wong et al., 2015). Farnik et al. (Farnik et al., 2013) demonstrated a correlation between low serum vitamin D levels in chronic HBV patients and high viral replication. Additionally, chronic HBV increased the risk of vitamin D deficiency. However, the researchers failed to detect serum HBsAg, which have been shown to reflect active intrahepatic cccDNA (Martinot-Peignoux & Marcellin, 2016). A recent clinical study found that following long-term treatment with nucleoside/nucleotides analogues the mean level of 25(OH)D3 increased significantly in patients with undetected levels of HBV-DNA (Chen et al., 2015). The current study aimed to determine the relationship between the vitamin D pathway and HBV transcription and replication in vitro.

Methods

Reagents

Calcitriol was purchased from Sigma (St. Louis, MO, USA).

Cell culture and treatment

HepG2 (hepatoma) cell line and HepG.2.215 (HBV-infected hepatoma cells) were generous gift from the lab of Prof. Shaul, Weizmann Institute of Science in Rehovot, Israel. These cells were maintained in Dulbecco's modified Eagle's minimal essential medium (Biological Industries,

Israel), as previously described (Rechtman et al., 2010). Cells were grown to reach near confluence 24 h prior to transfection, which was carried out using the Lipofectamin 2000 reagent (Invitrogen Carlsbad, California USA), according to the manufacture's instructions.

HepAD38 cells were generous gift from the lab of Prof. Seeger, Fox Chase Cancer Center, PA USA, and David Durantel Cancer Research Center of Lyon, France. These cells were cultured in a Dulbecco's modified Eagle's minimal essential medium with 10% FCS with or without 0.3 µg/mL tetracycline (Sigma St. Louis, MO, USA) for 7 days before analyzing the cells.

All cell lines were treated with increasing concentrations of Calcitriol (0–100 nM) (Sigma St. Louis, MO, USA) for 24 h.

Plasmids

The previously described 1.3 X HBV-Luc plasmid (Rechtman et al., 2010), was a generous gift from the lab of Prof. Shaul, Weizmann Institute of Science in Rehovot, Israel.

Luciferase genetic reporter assays

Luciferase assay was performed using the Dual Luciferase Assay System (Promega Madison, WI, USA), according to the manufacturer's instructions. The luminescence levels were determined using a Berthold Technologies luminometer (Titertek-Berthold, Pforzheim,Germany).

RNA purification and quantitative real-time PCR analysis

Total RNA was extracted using TRI-reagent (Sigma St. Louis, MO, USA), followed by treatment with 1 U RNase-free DNase (Roche). Reverse transcription was performed on 2 µg total RNA, using the High Capacity cDNA Reverse Transcription Kit (Applied Biosystems Carlsbad, CA USA), according to the manufacturer's instructions. qRT-PCR was performed on 50 ng cDNA samples, using the SYBR Green Real-Time PCR Kit (Applied Biosystems Carlsbad, CA USA) according to manufacturer's specifications, with gene-specific primers and HPRT as the reference endogenous control (Additional file 1: Table S1).

All reactions were performed in triplicates and relative gene expression was determined using the $2.\delta\delta Ct$ method with ABI Prism 7000 SDS (Applied Biosystems Carlsbad, CA USA).

DNA purification and measurement of cccDNA levels

DNA was extracted using the Q/Amp DNA Mini-kit according to the manufacturer's instructions (QIAGEN Valencia, CA USA). cccDNA expression levels were measured by qRT-PCR analysis (Additional file 1: Table S1).

Western blot analysis

Proteins were extracted using RIPA extraction buffer (Sigma, St. Louis, MI, USA) containing complete, mini-protease inhibitor cocktail tablets (Roche Basel, Switzerland) and phosphatase inhibitors (coktail2&3)(Sigma St. Louis, MO, USA). Protein levels were quantified using a commercial BCA kit (Pierce Appleton, WI USA). Liver protein extracts (40 µg protein/ lane) were separated under reducing conditions on polyacrylamide gels by SDS-PAGE, and then transferred to nitrocellulose membranes. Membranes were soaked for 1 h in a blocking solution, comprised of phosphate buffer saline (PBS), 5% non-fat milk and 0.01% (v/v) Tween-20 (Sigma), and then incubated with anti-VDR antibodies (1:300) (Santa Cruz Dallas, TX USA.) for 1–2 h, at RT. After incubation, the membrane was washed three times with PBST, and then exposed to goat anti-mouse horse radish peroxidase-conjugated antibodies (1:5000 in PBST) (Jackson West Grove, PA, USA) for an additional 1 h. Antibody-antigen complexes were visualized by ECL on an X-ray film.

Statistics

All experiments were done at least three times. Error bars in the graphs present the calculations of standard deviation. Differences between two groups were calculated using 2 tales ttest. Significant result (p) is calculated as < 0.05. Differences between more than two groups were calculated using ANOVA. F represents the statistical result of the ANOVA test. P represent a statistical difference if < 0.05.

Results

HBV transcription, expression and cccDNA levels are not affected by calcitriol treatment

In order to assess the effect of Calcitrol on the expression levels of HBV, HepG2 cells were transfected with the 1.3 X HBV-Luc plasmid HBV construct containing a luciferase ORF under the HBV core promoter. 24 h after the transfection cells were treated with increasing concentrations of Calcitriol for additional 24 h and the levels of Luciferase activity were measured. Treatment with increasing concentrations of Calcitriol did not alter the expression of HBV as demonstrated by the levels of luciferase activity (Fig. 1a (f = 0.937 p = 0 .491). Furthermore, when we have measured the HBV-RNA (B) levels and HBX (C) levels after 24 h of treatment with increasing concentrations of Calcitriol, we found no differences in the levels of these molecules (HBV-RNA,f = 2.364 p = 0.103 HBX f = 0.440 p = 0.815).

In order to further test the functionality of the ongoing viral replication, we then measured the expression level of cccDNA in these HBV-expressing cells. Treatment with

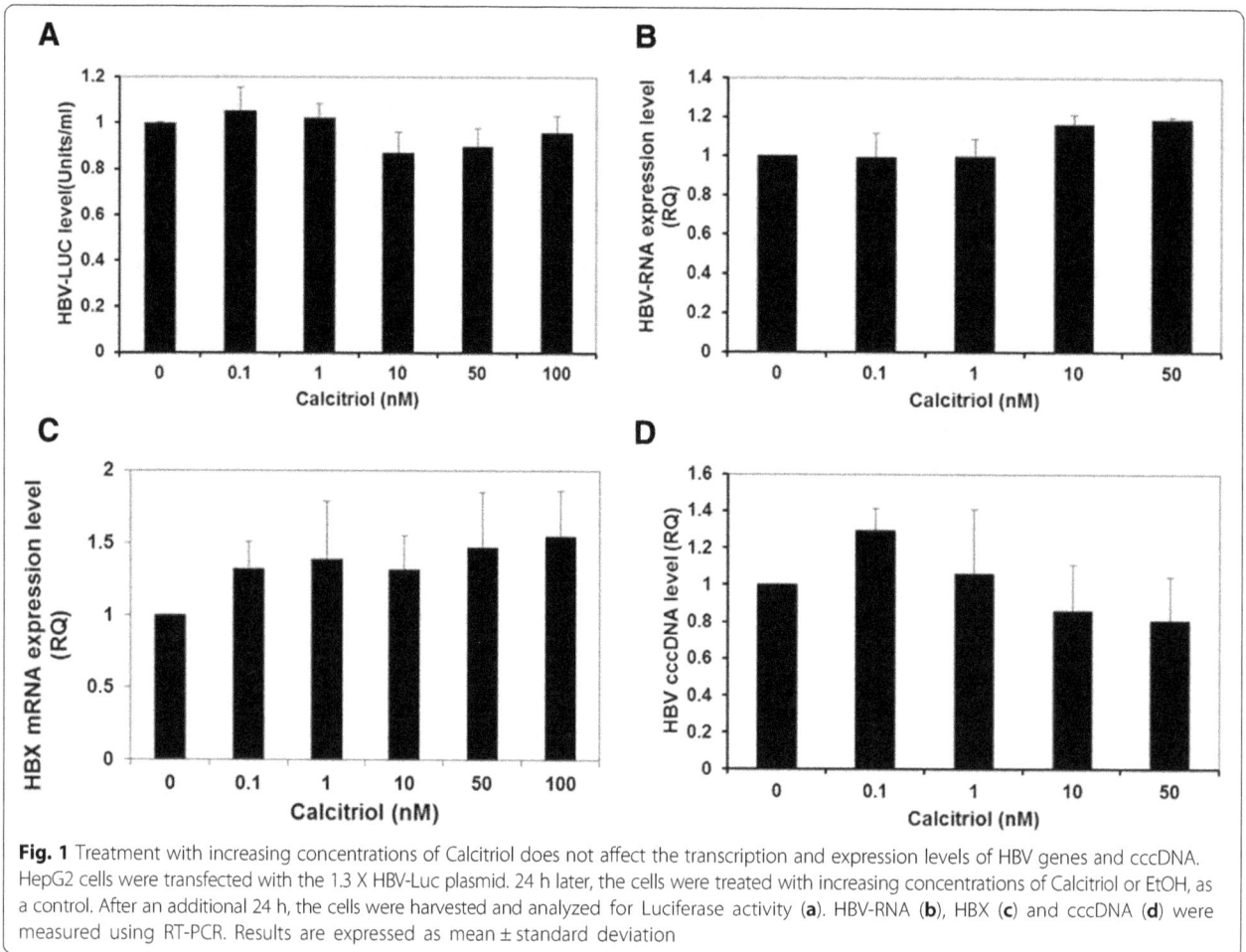

Fig. 1 Treatment with increasing concentrations of Calcitriol does not affect the transcription and expression levels of HBV genes and cccDNA. HepG2 cells were transfected with the 1.3 X HBV-Luc plasmid. 24 h later, the cells were treated with increasing concentrations of Calcitriol or EtOH, as a control. After an additional 24 h, the cells were harvested and analyzed for Luciferase activity (**a**). HBV-RNA (**b**), HBX (**c**) and cccDNA (**d**) were measured using RT-PCR. Results are expressed as mean ± standard deviation

increasing concentrations of Calcitriol did not significantly affect cccDNA, expression levels (Fig. 1d) (P=NS).

VDR transcripts and protein expression levels are repressed by HBV

Since our results demonstrated that vitamin D does not affect HBV levels, we than set to investigate the influence of HBV on the vitamin D pathway. Therefore, we set to compare the vitamin D receptor levels in HepG2.2.15 (HBV-expressing cells) versus HepG2 (non-transfected) cells. VDR transcript and protein levels were significantly lower ($p < 0.001$) in the HBV-infected hepatocytes compared with HepG2 cells (Fig. 2a and b).

HBV represses the expression of VDR in infected cells

Since HepG2 and HepG2.2.15 are two distinct cell lines although they have the same origin, some of the alterations in their transcriptome might not be due to the HBV expression. Hence, we decided to validate these results in another cellular model; HepAD38 cell line. HepAD38 cells, a variant of HepG2 cells, express the HBV genome under the control of a tetracycline. In the presence of the antibiotic, HepAD38 is free of virus due

to the repression of pregenomic (pg) RNA synthesis. Upon removal of tetracycline from the culture medium, HepAD38 express viral pg RNA (Ladner et al., 1997). Therefore, HepAD38 cells were cultured in a medium free of tetracyclin for 7 days and levels of HBV and VDR transcripts were measured. As expected HBV transcript level were up-regulated after tetracycline withdrawal (Fig. 3a). However a significant decrease in the levels of VDR was noted (Fig. 3b) ($p < 0.05$). Measuring the levels of the VDR proteins in those cells with or without tetracycline showed us again lower levels of VDR protein in the cells that express the HBV virus (Fig. 3c).

VDR-induced CYP24A1 expression in calcitriol-treated HepG2 and HepG2.2.15 cells

CYP24A1 is a known regulator of Vitamin D activity. However, CYP24A1 expression is induced by 25(OH)D3 through activation of the VDR. Since HBV-transfected cells do express lower levels of VDR, we have expected that these cells are unable to activate the Vitamin D signal transduction pathway. Therefore, we have measured the expression level of CYP24A1, following 24 h of treatment with increasing concentrations of Calcitriol. In this

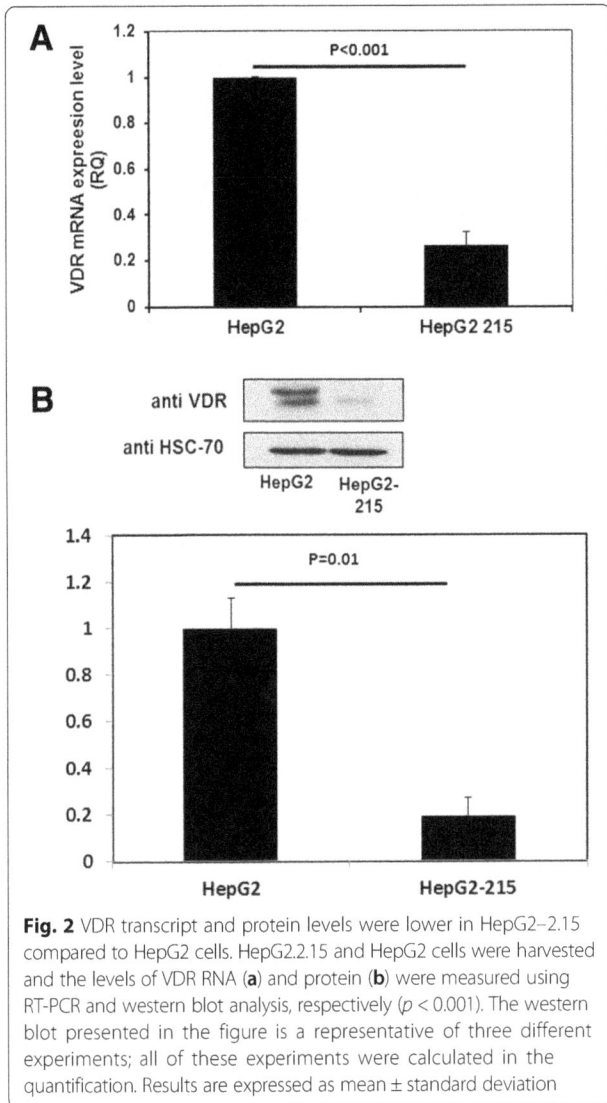

Fig. 2 VDR transcript and protein levels were lower in HepG2–2.15 compared to HepG2 cells. HepG2.2.15 and HepG2 cells were harvested and the levels of VDR RNA (**a**) and protein (**b**) were measured using RT-PCR and western blot analysis, respectively ($p < 0.001$). The western blot presented in the figure is a representative of three different experiments; all of these experiments were calculated in the quantification. Results are expressed as mean ± standard deviation

experiment we have found, as expected, that the expression levels of CYP24A1were significantly higher in HepG2 compared to HepG2.2.15 after treatment with calcitriol (Fig. 4). CYP24A1 transcript levels increased 1036 fold in calcitriol (10 nM)-treated HepG2 cells, compared to only 8-fold in the calcitriol-treated HepG2.2.15 cells.

TNFα expression in HepG2.2.15 and HepG2 cells following treatment with calcitriol

As an immune-modulator, Vitamin D can upregulate the expression of several proteins that play a role in the body's response to microbe invasion, including CAMP, an antimicrobial peptide, and the cytokine TNFα (Gombart, 2009; Golovko et al., 2005). To this end, we analyzed the relationship between the downregulation of VDR in Calcitriol-treated HBV-expressing cells and the activation of CAMP and TNFα. Levels of both TNFα

and CAMP transcripts were significantly lower in the HepG2.2.15 compared to HepG2 cells (Fig. 5, $p = 0.023$ and $p = 0.0373$, respectively) following 24 h of treatment with calcitriol.

Discussion

This study established the relationship between the vitamin D molecular pathway and HBV transcription and replication in vitro. While Calcitriol treatment did not suppress HBV transcription, cccDNA expression and HBV RNA levels in HepG2.2.15 cells, the levels of VDR transcripts in HepG2.2.15 cells was significantly lower compared with non-transfected HepG2 cells. A similar effect was further established using HepAD38 cells where high levels of HBV expression was associated with a decrease in the levels of VDR transcripts and vise versa. Moreover, following the administration of Calcitriol, the expression levels of CYP24A1, an VDR-regulated gene, was significantly lower HepG2.2.15 as compared to HepG2 cells. Finally, the calcitriol-induced VDR signaling pathway, as determined by TNFα and CAMP transcripts levels, was not observed in HepG2.2.15 cells, while significant upregulation was noted in HepG2 cells.

Recently studies (Chan et al., 2015; Wong et al., 2015; Chen et al., 2015) demonstrated a correlation between low serum vitamin D levels in chronic HBV patients and high levels of viral replication. These studies raised the possibility that vitamin D levels inhibit HBV replication. In contrast, our in-vitro study showed that Vitamin D does not affect the rate of HBV replication, and downregulates VDR levels in the presence of the virus, thereby attenuating vitamin D signal transduction.

Vitamin D plays a crucial role in the regulation of genes central to protection against microbe invasion, such as the induction of the expression of antimicrobial peptides (also known as host defense peptides) such as CAMP and defensin. These peptides were demonstrated to disrupt the integrity of the microbe membrane, resulting in its death (Gombart, 2009). In addition, Vitamin D regulates the immune system by managing the expression of TNFα (Golovko et al., 2005), one of the most important pro-inflammatory and pro-immune cytokines. Therefore, downregulation of the vitamin D signaling pathway by viruses, can result in decreased production of antimicrobial peptides and cytokines and as a result, to attenuation of the immune response. Several studies have previously indicated that certain viruses can inhibit the Vitamin D signal transduction. In 2009, Yenamandra et al. demonstrated that VDR mRNA and protein levels were lower in EBV-transformed cells compared with primary B cells (Yenamandra et al., 2009). A few years earlier, Haug et al. reported a marked decrease in serum Calcitriol levels in human immunodeficiency virus (HIV)-infected patients, that correlated with the degree

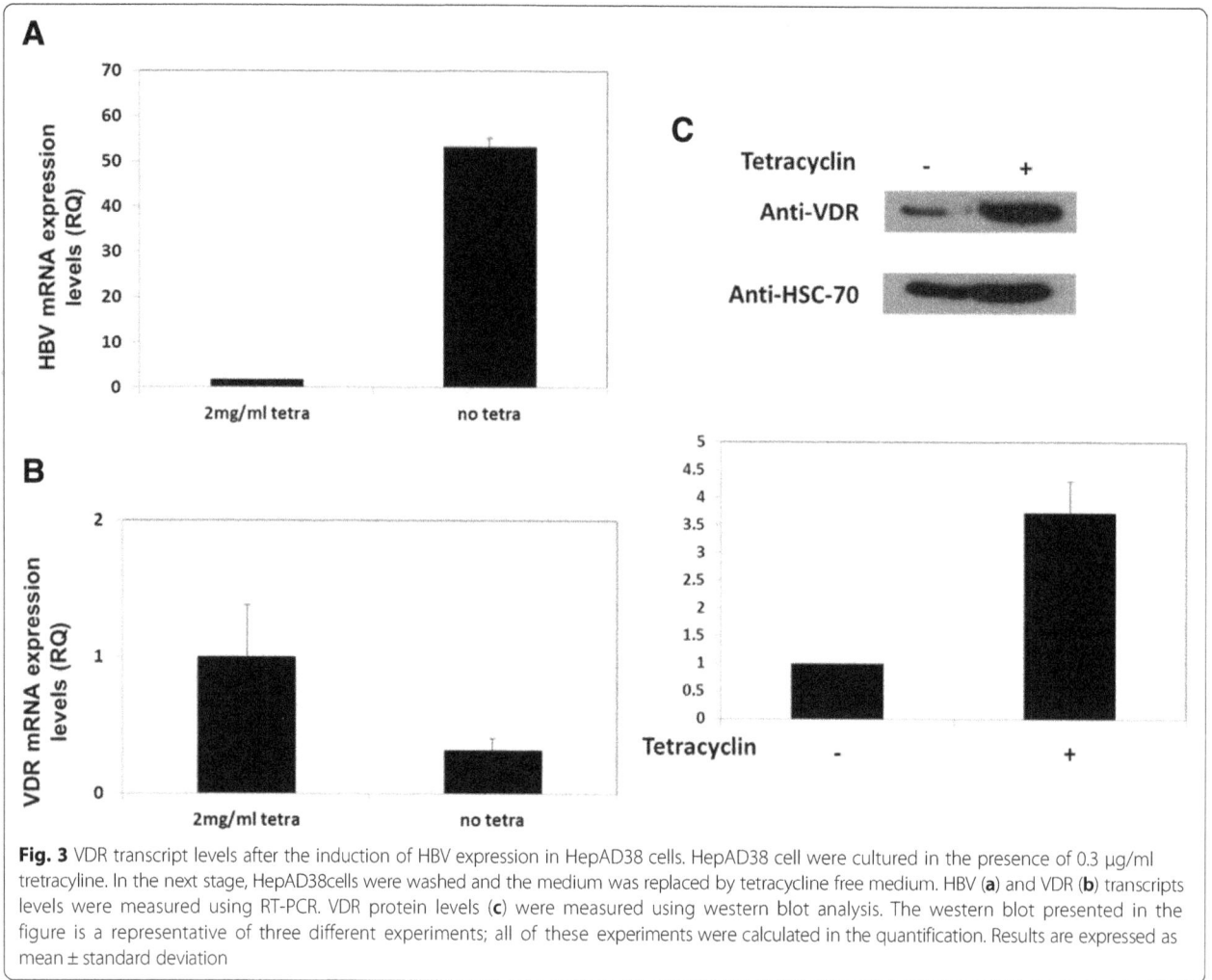

Fig. 3 VDR transcript levels after the induction of HBV expression in HepAD38 cells. HepAD38 cell were cultured in the presence of 0.3 µg/ml tretracyline. In the next stage, HepAD38cells were washed and the medium was replaced by tetracycline free medium. HBV (**a**) and VDR (**b**) transcripts levels were measured using RT-PCR. VDR protein levels (**c**) were measured using western blot analysis. The western blot presented in the figure is a representative of three different experiments; all of these experiments were calculated in the quantification. Results are expressed as mean ± standard deviation

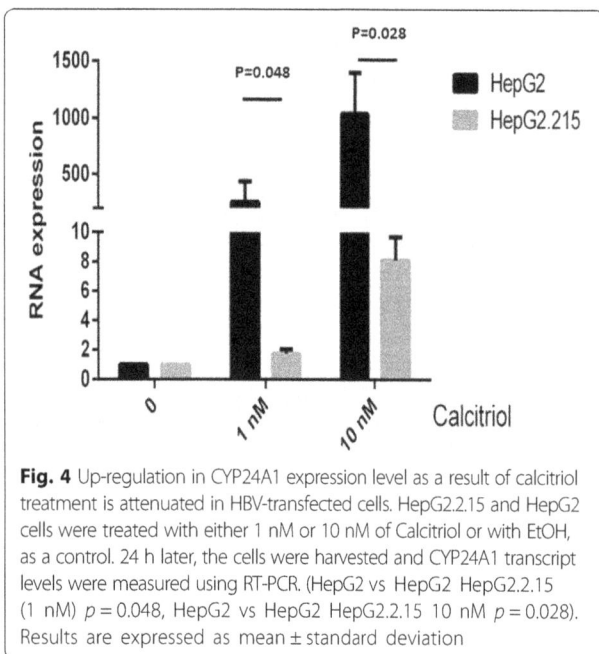

Fig. 4 Up-regulation in CYP24A1 expression level as a result of calcitriol treatment is attenuated in HBV-transfected cells. HepG2.2.15 and HepG2 cells were treated with either 1 nM or 10 nM of Calcitriol or with EtOH, as a control. 24 h later, the cells were harvested and CYP24A1 transcript levels were measured using RT-PCR. (HepG2 vs HepG2 HepG2.2.15 (1 nM) $p = 0.048$, HepG2 vs HepG2 HepG2.2.15 10 nM $p = 0.028$). Results are expressed as mean ± standard deviation

of immunodeficiency and patient survival (Haug et al., 1994). Therefore, in this study, we compared the activation of both TNFa and CAMP in HepG2 cell versus HepG2.2.15 cells following Cacitriol stimulation. Indeed, while the addition of Calcitriol upregulates both CAMP and TNFα expression in HepG2 cells, significantly less transcription of these genes was observed in HepG2.2.15 cells. These findings suggest that HBV can repress the activation of the immune system by downregulating the vitamin D signaling pathway.

Several signaling pathways may be involved in the inhibition of VDR expression following HBV infection. HBx is a 17-kD protein encoded by the X open reading frame of HBV, that complexes with cellular proteins and transactivates virus gene expression and replication (Keasler et al., 2007). Furthermore, HBx protects virus-infected cells from immune-mediated destruction (Arzumanyan et al., 2013). However, we did not detect a correlation between HBx expression level and the administration of calcitriol. Moreover, a relationship between HBx and Vitamin D is yet to be established.

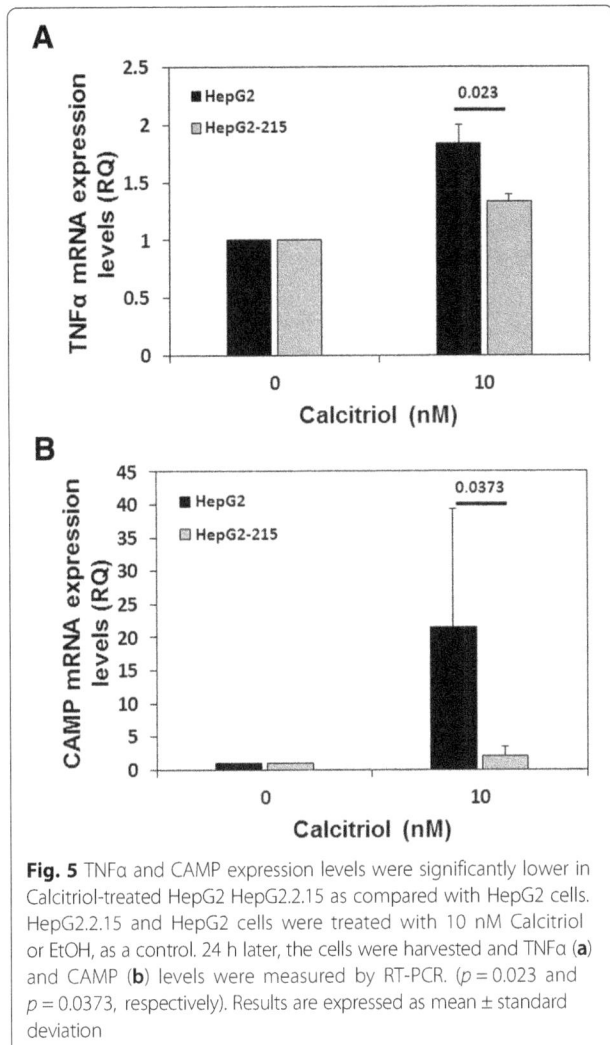

Fig. 5 TNFα and CAMP expression levels were significantly lower in Calcitriol-treated HepG2 HepG2.2.15 as compared with HepG2 cells. HepG2.2.15 and HepG2 cells were treated with 10 nM Calcitriol or EtOH, as a control. 24 h later, the cells were harvested and TNFα (**a**) and CAMP (**b**) levels were measured by RT-PCR. ($p = 0.023$ and $p = 0.0373$, respectively). Results are expressed as mean ± standard deviation

Alternatively, HBV polymerase may be involved in the inhibition of VDR expression (Wu et al., 2007). Further studies will be necessary to identify the factors inhibiting VDR expression following viral infection.

Conclusions

In this study, we have shown that HBV downregulates the expression levels of Vitamin D receptor in the HBV-infected HepG2 cell line, thereby preventing the effect of Vitamin D on viral transcription and production. Furthermore, these findings suggest that HBV might use this mechanism to avoid the immunological defense system, by affecting the expression of immune-modulators such as CAMP and TNFα. The precise mechanisms regulating the innate and adaptive immune response in these cells remain to be further investigated.

Abbreviations
cccDNA: Closed circular DNA; HBV: Hepatitis B virus; HCC: Hepatocellular carcinoma; HCV: Hepatitis C virus; HIV: Human immunodeficiency virus; RSV: Respiratory syncytial virus; TNFα: Tumor necrosis factor α; VDR: Vitamin D receptor

Acknowledgements
The authors would like to thank Prof. Yosef Shaul for the generous gifts of the HepG2.2.15 and 1.3 X HBV-Luc plasmid. Furthermore, we would like to thank Prof. Christoph Seeger and Prof. David Durantel for providing us the HepAD38 cells.

Authors' contributions
NG, TI, LY, SM, SM preformed the experiments, analyzed and interpreted the data. NG, SM, SM and BAZ are major contributors in writing the manuscript. All authors read and approved the final manuscript.

Competing interests
The authors declare that they have no competing interests.

Author details
[1]Liver Reaserch Laboratory, Sheba Medical Center, Tel Hashomer, 52620 Ramat Gan, Israel. [2]Liver Disease Center, Sheba Medical Center, Tel Hashomer, 52620 Ramat Gan, Israel. [3]The Sackler School of Medicine, Tel Aviv University, Tel Aviv, Israel.

References
Abu-Mouch S, et al. Vitamin D supplementation improves sustained virologic response in chronic hepatitis C (genotype 1)-naive patients. World J Gastroenterol. 2011;17(47):5184–90.
Ahmed M, et al. Targeting the Achilles heel of the hepatitis B virus: a review of current treatments against covalently closed circular DNA. Drug Discov Today. 2015;20(5):548–61.
Arzumanyan A, Reis HM, Feitelson MA. Pathogenic mechanisms in HBV- and HCV-associated hepatocellular carcinoma. Nat Rev Cancer. 2013;13(2):123–35.
Barbalho SM, Goulart RA, Gasparini RG. Associations between inflammatory bowel diseases and vitamin D. Crit Rev Food Sci Nutr. 2017:1–10.
Bitetto D, et al. Vitamin D supplementation improves response to antiviral treatment for recurrent hepatitis C. Transpl Int. 2011;24(1):43–50.
Borella E, et al. Vitamin D: a new anti-infective agent? Ann N Y Acad Sci. 2014; 1317:76–83.
Chan HL, et al. Association of baseline vitamin D levels with clinical parameters and treatment outcomes in chronic hepatitis B. J Hepatol. 2015;63(5):1086–92.
Chen EQ, et al. Sustained suppression of viral replication in improving vitamin D serum concentrations in patients with chronic hepatitis B. Sci Rep. 2015;5:15441.
Chen FH, et al. Association of Serum Vitamin D Level and Carotid Atherosclerosis: a systematic review and meta-analysis. J Ultrasound Med. 2018;37(6):1293–1303.
Deluca HF, Cantorna MT. Vitamin D: its role and uses in immunology. FASEB J. 2001;15(14):2579–85.
Farnik H, et al. Low vitamin D serum concentration is associated with high levels of hepatitis B virus replication in chronically infected patients. Hepatology. 2013;58(4):1270–6.
Golovko O, Nazarova N, Tuohimaa P. Vitamin D-induced up-regulation of tumour necrosis factor alpha (TNF-alpha) in prostate cancer cells. Life Sci. 2005;77(5):562–77.
Gombart AF. The vitamin D-antimicrobial peptide pathway and its role in protection against infection. Future Microbiol. 2009;4(9):1151–65.
Gutierrez JA, Parikh N, Branch AD. Classical and emerging roles of vitamin D in hepatitis C virus infection. Semin Liver Dis. 2011;31(4):387–98.
Hassanalilou T, et al. Role of vitamin D deficiency in systemic lupus erythematosus incidence and aggravation. Auto Immun Highlights. 2017;9(1):1.
Haug C, et al. Subnormal serum concentration of 1,25-vitamin D in human immunodeficiency virus infection: correlation with degree of immune deficiency and survival. J Infect Dis. 1994;169(4):889–93.
Haug CJ, et al. Severe deficiency of 1,25-dihydroxyvitamin D3 in human immunodeficiency virus infection: association with immunological

hyperactivity and only minor changes in calcium homeostasis. J Clin Endocrinol Metab. 1998;83(11):3832–8.

He Q, et al. Association between vitamin D receptor polymorphisms and hepatitis B virus infection susceptibility: a meta-analysis study. Gene. 2018; 645:105–112.

Heidari Z, et al. Vitamin D deficiency associated with differentiated thyroid carcinoma: a case- control study. Asian Pac J Cancer Prev. 2017;18(12):3419–22.

Hohaus S, et al. Vitamin D deficiency and supplementation in patients with aggressive B-cell lymphomas treated with immunochemotherapy. Cancer Med. 2018;7(1):270–281.

Hu K, et al. Circulating Vitamin D and Overall Survival in Breast Cancer Patients: A Dose-Response Meta-Analysis of Cohort Studies. Integr Cancer Ther. 2018; 17(2):217–225.

Huang L, et al. Vitamin D receptor gene FokI polymorphism contributes to increasing the risk of tuberculosis: an update meta-analysis. Medicine (Baltimore). 2015;94(51):e2256.

Keasler VV, et al. Enhancement of hepatitis B virus replication by the regulatory X protein in vitro and in vivo. J Virol. 2007;81(6):2656–62.

Kim HB, et al. Efficacy of vitamin D supplementation in combination with conventional antiviral therapy in patients with chronic hepatitis C infection: a meta-analysis of randomised controlled trials. J Hum Nutr Diet. 2018;31(2):168–177.

Knutsen KV, et al. Effect of vitamin D on thyroid autoimmunity: a randomized, double-blind, controlled trial among ethnic minorities. J Endocr Soc. 2017; 1(5):470–9.

Ladner SK, et al. Inducible expression of human hepatitis B virus (HBV) in stably transfected hepatoblastoma cells: a novel system for screening potential inhibitors of HBV replication. Antimicrob Agents Chemother. 1997;41(8): 1715–20.

Lim HS, et al. Relationship between serum 25-hydroxy-vitamin D concentration and risk of metabolic syndrome in patients with fatty liver. J Bone Metab. 2017;24(4):223–8.

Marcellin P, et al. Regression of cirrhosis during treatment with tenofovir disoproxil fumarate for chronic hepatitis B: a 5-year open-label follow-up study. Lancet. 2013;381(9865):468–75.

Martinot-Peignoux M, Marcellin P. Virological and serological tools to optimize the management of patients with chronic hepatitis B. Liver Int. 2016;36(Suppl 1):78–84.

Nimer A, Mouch A. Vitamin D improves viral response in hepatitis C genotype 2-3 naive patients. World J Gastroenterol. 2012;18(8):800–5.

Orkin C, et al. Vitamin D deficiency in HIV: a shadow on long-term management? AIDS Rev. 2014;16(2):59–74.

Pletz MW, et al. Vitamin D deficiency in community-acquired pneumonia: low levels of 1,25(OH)2 D are associated with disease severity. Respir Res. 2014;15:53.

Rechtman MM, et al. Curcumin inhibits hepatitis B virus via down-regulation of the metabolic coactivator PGC-1alpha. FEBS Lett. 2010;584(11):2485–90.

Sandhya P, et al. Vitamin D levels and associations in Indian patients with primary Sjogren's syndrome. J Clin Diagn Res. 2017;11(9):OC33–6.

Schmitt EB, et al. Vitamin D deficiency is associated with metabolic syndrome in postmenopausal women. Maturitas. 2018;107:97–102.

Seeger C, Mason WS. Hepatitis B virus biology. Microbiol Mol Biol Rev. 2000;64(1): 51–68.

Vanherwegen AS, Gysemans C, Mathieu C. Regulation of immune function by vitamin D and its use in diseases of immunity. Endocrinol Metab Clin N Am. 2017;46(4):1061–94.

Villar LM, et al. Association between vitamin D and hepatitis C virus infection: a meta-analysis. World J Gastroenterol. 2013;19(35):5917–24.

Watkins RR, Lemonovich TL, Salata RA. An update on the association of vitamin D deficiency with common infectious diseases. Can J Physiol Pharmacol. 2015;93(5):363–8.

Wojcik M, et al. The potential impact of the hypovitaminosis D on metabolic complications in obese adolescents - preliminary results. Ann Agric Environ Med. 2017;24(4):636–9.

Wong GL, et al. Adverse effects of vitamin D deficiency on outcomes of patients with chronic hepatitis B. Clin Gastroenterol Hepatol. 2015;13(4):783–90 e1.

Wu M, et al. Hepatitis B virus polymerase inhibits the interferon-inducible MyD88 promoter by blocking nuclear translocation of Stat1. J Gen Virol. 2007;88(Pt 12): 3260–9.

Yenamandra SP, et al. Expression profile of nuclear receptors upon Epstein -- Barr virus induced B cell transformation. Exp Oncol. 2009;31(2):92–6.

18

Attenuation of diet-induced hypothalamic inflammation following bariatric surgery in female mice

Mary K. Herrick[1,2], Kristin M. Favela[1], Richard B. Simerly[3], Naji N. Abumrad[4] and Nathan C. Bingham[1*] ⓘ

Abstract

Background: Exposure of rodents to chronic high-fat diet (HFD) results in upregulation of inflammatory markers and proliferation of microglia within the mediobasal hypothalamus. Such hypothalamic inflammation is associated with metabolic dysfunction, central leptin resistance, and maintenance of obesity. Bariatric surgeries result in long-term stable weight loss and improved metabolic function. However, the effects of such surgical procedures on HFD-induced hypothalamic inflammation are unknown. We sought to characterize the effects of two bariatric surgical procedures, Roux-en-Y gastric bypass (RYGB) and biliary diversion (BD-IL), in female mice with particular emphasis on HFD-induced hypothalamic inflammation and microgliosis.

Methods: RYGB and BD-IL were performed on diet-induced obese (DIO) mice. Quantitative RT-PCR and fluorescent microscopy were used to evaluate hypothalamic inflammatory gene expression and microgliosis. Results were compared to lean (CD), DIO sham-surgerized mice (DIO-SHAM), and dietary weight loss (DIO-Rev) controls.

Results: In female mice, RYGB and BD-IL result in normalization of hypothalamic inflammatory gene expression and microgliosis within 8 weeks of surgery, despite ongoing exposure to HFD. Paralleling these results, the hypothalamic expression levels of the orexigenic neuropeptide *Agrp* and the anorexic response of surgical mice to exogenous leptin were comparable to lean controls (CD). In contrast, results from DIO-Rev mice were comparable to DIO-SHAM mice, despite transition back to standard rodent show and normalization of weight.

Conclusion: Bariatric surgery attenuates HFD-induced hypothalamic inflammation and microgliosis and restores leptin sensitivity, despite ongoing exposure to HFD.

Keywords: Obesity, Bariatric surgery, Hypothalamus, Inflammation, Microglia

Background

It is well established, in human and rodent models, that caloric excess and the ensuing diet-induced obesity (DIO), result in a state of chronic, low-grade inflammation and accumulation of professional immune cells such as macrophages in metabolic tissues including liver, adipose and muscle. This inflammatory state is often termed 'metaflammation' (metabolically induced inflammation) to distinguish it from the more acute and high-grade inflammation associated with injury and infection that more often results in appetite suppression and weight loss. In peripheral tissues, metaflammation has been linked to metabolic dysfunction including insulin resistance (Hotamisligil et al. 1993; Kern et al. 1995). More recent work has shown a similar condition occurring in the mediobasal hypothalamus (MBH), an important center of neuronal control of energy homeostasis. With exposure to high-fat diet (HFD), hypothalamic inflammatory pathways, such as NF-κB, are activated and the expression of pro-inflammatory mediators, including canonical proinflammatory cytokines, *Il-1β* and *Tnfα* are upregulated (De Souza et al. 2005; Zhang et al. 2008). Comparable to that observed in peripheral tissues, hypothalamic metaflammation is accompanied by accumulation of microglia, the resident immune cells of the central nervous system (Thaler et al. 2012a). Such

* Correspondence: nathan.bingham@vanderbilt.edu
[1]Department of Pediatrics, Vanderbilt University Medical Center, 1500 21 st. Ave South, Suite 1514, Nashville, TN 37212, USA
Full list of author information is available at the end of the article

reactive microgliosis is generally a response to central nervous system injury and is associated with a transition of microglia from a resting or surveillance state to a more active state accompanied by the production of immune response molecules (Streit et al. 1999). Importantly, hypothalamic metaflammation and microglial activation contribute to hypothalamic resistance to peripheral anorexic hormones such as leptin, thus increasing the threshold for leptin's catabolic effects and contributing to an elevated level of homeostatically defended body weight (Zhang et al. 2008). Both pharmacologic and genetic experimental interventions that inhibit hypothalamic inflammatory pathways reduce food intake and body weight and improve the response of obese animals to exogenous leptin (Zhang et al. 2008). These findings suggest that therapies designed to abrogate hypothalamic metaflammation may prove valuable in the treatment of obesity.

Currently, bariatric surgery has emerged as the most effective obesity treatment available in both magnitude and durability of its effects (Mingrone et al. 2012; Schauer et al. 2017). Roux-en-Y gastric bypass (RYGB), one of the most effective and commonly performed procedures, involves creation of a smaller stomach pouch while diverting nutrient flow to varying distal segments of the intestine. Studies from the past 10–15 years have shown that RYGB, while initially designed to produce weight loss through a combination of gastric restriction and malabsorption, clearly has metabolic benefits independent from these intended mechanisms of action (Albaugh et al. 2016). Importantly, there is mounting evidence that bariatric surgeries result in a downward shift in the level of homeostatically defended body weight. In humans, RYGB leads to a decrease in hunger and preference for calorically-dense foods despite the significant decrease in serum leptin levels, an environment that should generally induce hyperphagia (Laurenius et al. 2013; Ullrich et al. 2013; Beckman et al. 2010). Following bariatric surgery, rodents that are induced to gain weight via pharmacologic blockade of central melanocortin receptors, rapidly return to their stable, post-operative body weight after removal of the blockade. Similar results are seen in female mice following pregnancy (Grayson et al. 2013; Munzberg et al. 2015). These studies demonstrate that despite the physical ability to increase food intake following bariatric surgery, rodents choose to eat less and defend a lower body weight. Given the known effects of hypothalamic metaflammation on hypothalamic leptin resistance, these studies raise the possibility that bariatric surgery may improve hypothalamic metaflammation contributing to a lower set point of defended body weight.

In this study, we use two mouse models to investigate the effects of bariatric surgery on hypothalamic metaflammation. In addition, given that the large majority of bariatric surgery patients are female (Pratt et al. 2009) we evaluated these effects in female mice, an underutilized model. We demonstrate that HFD-induced hypothalamic metaflammation and microgliosis persist in DIO mice, even after reverting back to a low-fat diet and loss of excess weight, while bariatric surgery results in a rapid normalization of both parameters.

Methods
Animals and diets
Female C57BL/6J and CX3CR1^GFP mice, on a C57BL/6J background (> 12 generations) were obtained from Jackson Laboratory (Stock no. 000664 and 005582, respectively). A cohort of CX3CR1^GFP mice were used for microglial quantification, while all other experiments were performed using wild-type C57BL/6J mice. All experimental mice were bred in-house and housed at 23 °C on a 12-h light cycle. From birth until 6 weeks of age, mice were given free access to a standard rodent chow (PicoLab® Laboratory Rodent Diet 5L0D, 13.4% kcal from fat; Land O'Lakes Inc., St. Louis, MO, USA). Beginning at 6 weeks of age, mice were randomly allocated to each of five experimental groups 1) control diet (CD), 2) diet-induced obese sham (DIO-SHAM), 3) diet-induced obese reversal (DIO-Rev), 4) Roux-en-Y gastric bypass (RYGB), or 5) biliary diversion to the ileum (BD-IL). At that time, all groups, except for CD controls, were transitioned to a HFD (60% kcal from fat, Research Diets, D12492, New Brunswick, NJ) for 12 weeks. At 18 weeks of age, surgical groups underwent their respective surgical procedures and remained on HFD. DIO-Rev animals were transitioned back to the standard rodent chow while CD animals remained on standard rodent chow (Fig. 1c). All mice were weighed weekly and fed ad libitum for an additional 8 weeks before being sacrificed for analysis.

Bariatric surgery
RYGB, BD-IL, and sham surgical procedures were performed at 18 weeks of age under isoflurane anesthesia using a 12-15X microsurgical scope as previously described (Flynn et al. 2015; Yin et al. 2011). Briefly, for RYGB, the stomach was ligated between the gastric fundus (forestomach) and glandular portion while the jejunum was transected 4 cm from the Ligament of Treitz. The distal jejunum was subsequently anastomosed to the forestomach with GI continuity maintained via a jejuno-jejunostomy 6 cm distal from the initial transection (Fig. 1a). BD-IL was performed by ligating the common bile duct and creating a gallbladder to ileum anastomosis 4 cm proximal to the ileo-cecal valve (Fig. 1b). The sham surgical procedure was performed in parallel to RYGB with similar abdominal incision, physical manipulation of stomach and intestine (without transection or re-anastomosis), and suturing.

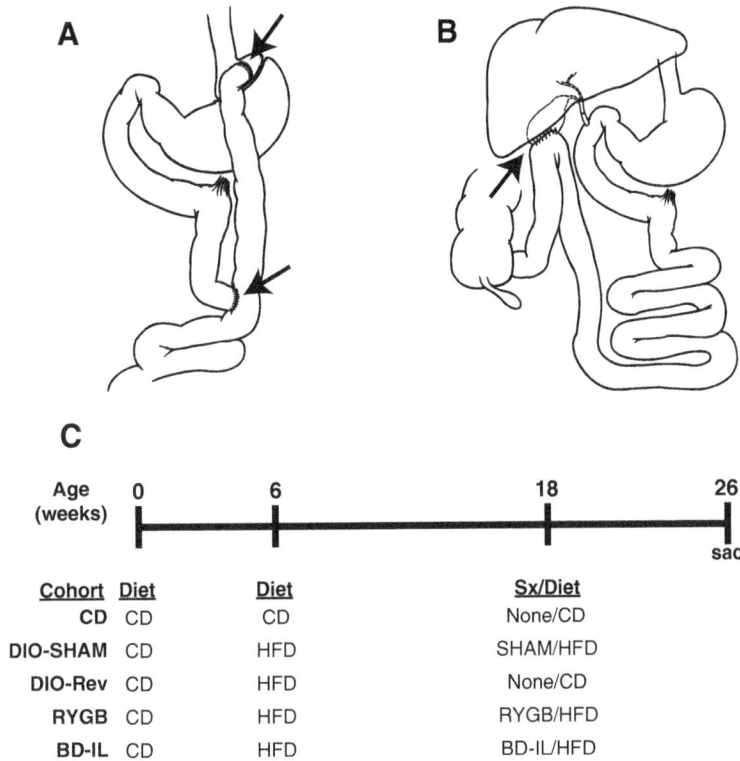

Fig. 1 Models of murine bariatric surgery and experimental design. **a** For Roux-en-Y gastric bypass (RYBG) procedure, the stomach was ligated between the gastric fundus (forestomach) and glandular portion while the jejunum was transected 4 cm from the Ligament of Treitz. The distal jejunum was subsequently anastomosed to the forestomach (top arrow) with GI continuity being maintained via a jejuno-jejunostomy 6 cm distal from the initial transection (lower arrow). Image modified from (Albaugh et al. 2016). **b** For the biliary diversion procedure (BD-IL), the common bile duct was ligated proximal to the pancreatic duct and the gallbladder anastomosed to the ileum 4 cm proximal to the ileo-cecal valve. Image modified from (Albaugh et al. 2016). **c** Experimental design. Age of mice shown in weeks with time of dietary changes and surgical procedures (Sx) shown at 6 and 18 weeks. All mice were sacrificed at 26 weeks of age

Body weight and composition

Body mass was measured using mq10 NMR analyzer (Bruker Optics Inc., Billerica, MA) following 2 h of fasting. Fat and muscle mass were calculated in grams.

Glucose tolerance tests

After a 6 h fast, mice were given a 1.5 mg/g dose of glucose by oral gavage. Blood glucose was measured using a hand-held glucometer (Accu-chek, Roche Diagnostic Corporation, Indianapolis, IN) at 0, 15, 30, 60 and 120 min.

Intraperitoneal leptin treatment

Mice were individually housed and sham injected for 5 days with intraperitoneal (i.p.) saline prior to drug treatment. Subsequently, mice received i.p. injections of recombinant murine leptin (Peprotech, 2.0 µg/g body weight) for 3 days. Food intake was measured daily. Caloric intake during the 72 h after first leptin injection was compared to the last 72 h of saline injections.

Microglial quantification

Female heterozygous CX3CR1^{GFP} mice were allocated to surgical and control groups as described above. Deeply anesthetized mice were transcardially perfused with ~ 10–15 ml of 0.1 M PBS (pH 7.4) followed by 50 ml of ice-cold 4% paraformaldehyde (PFA) in 0.1 M PBS at 4 °C. Brains were carefully dissected and post-fixed overnight in 4% PFA at 4 °C then equilibrated for 24-48 h with 30% sucrose in 0.1 M PBS. Twenty-five micron sections were obtained using a sliding microtome (Leica Microsystems, Deerfield, IL) with frozen stage set at – 18 °C (Physitemp, Clifton, NJ). Sections were stored free-floating at – 20 °C in cryoprotectant (30% ethylene glycol, 30% glycerol, in 0.1 M PBS). Subsequently, sections were washed in PBS and counterstained with DAPI before being mounted onto Superfrost Plus microscope slides (Fisher Scientific, Walham, MA) and coverslipped using Prolong Gold antifade mounting media (Invitrogen, La Jolla, CA).

Four to five mice were used from each experimental cohort with two to three sections from the mediobasal hypothalamus used for analysis (Bregma – 1.6 to – 1.9.

Slides were scanned using a Leica Aperio Scanscope FL with 20X magnification. Bilateral arcuate (ARC), ventro-medial (VMH), and dorsomedial (DMH) nuclei were manually outlined and annotated using Aperio Image-Scope software. Bilateral areas of the retrosplenial cortex, just lateral to the longitudinal fissure, were used as nonhypothalamic control areas. GFP+ microglia in each area were quantified using the CytoNuclear algorithm (v1.4, Indica Laboratories) within the Aperio eSlide Manager platform and the number of positive cells was normalized to the area of each annotated region. Representative images of HFD-induced ARC microgliosis were obtained using a laser-scanning confocal microscope (Leica TCS SPE confocal microscope) equipped with a 40x oil-corrected objective. Image stacks (20 μm thick) were collected through the z-axis at a frequency of 0.5 μm.

Quantitative real-time PCR

Female C57BL/6J mice were allocated to surgical and control groups as described above. Deeply anesthetized mice were transcardially perfused with ~ 10–15 ml of 0.1 M PBS (pH 7.4) at 4 °C and brains were carefully dissected. Using a brain matrix (Braintree Scientific, Braintree, MA), a 1 mm coronal section was obtained and the mediobasal hypothalamus removed under dissecting microscope. Hypothalami where placed directly in tissue lysis solution and snap frozen on dry ice. Samples were kept at − 80 °C until RNA extraction using a commercially available kit according to manufacturer specifications (RNAqueous-Micro Kit; Ambion). RNA was amplified and reverse transcribed using the Ovation RNA amplification kit (Nugen). Semiquantitive PCR was performed on a QuantStudio 3 Real-Time PCR System (Applied Biosystems, Foster City, CA) using gene-specific Taqman probes (Applied Biosystems). The transcripts assayed with their NCBI reference sequence and Taqman assay IDs (RefSeq, ID) are as follows: *Gapdh*, (NM_001289726.1, Mm99999915_g1); *Rn18s* (NR_003278.3 m, Mm03928990_g1); *Tnf* (NM_013693.3, Mm00443258_m1); *Il1b* (NM_008361.3, Mm00434228_m1); *Ccl2* (NM_011333.3, Mm00441242_m1); *Pomc* (NM_001278584.1, Mm00435874_m1); *Agrp* (NM_007427.3, Mm00475829_g1). Expression levels of each gene were normalized to reference genes (*Gapdh* and *18S*) and expressed relative to DIO-controls using the ΔΔCT method.

Statistics

Statistical analysis was performed using Prism Statistical Software (v6.07, GraphPad Software, La Jolla, CA). Means were analyzed by either unpaired t test or analysis of variance (ANOVA) and appropriate post hoc analyses. All data are expressed as mean ± SEM with $P < 0.05$ considered significant.

Results

Biliary diversion to the ileum (BD-IL), roux-en-Y gastric bypass (RYGB), and diet-induced obesity reversal (DIO-rev) result equivalent weight loss and improved glucose tolerance

Both BD-IL and RYGB have been shown to effectively induce and maintain weight loss in male DIO mice (Flynn et al. 2015). To evaluate the ability of these procedures to ameliorate metabolic parameters in female mice, we compared surgical mice to DIO sham-surgerized (DIO-SHAM) and lean controls (CD), as well as DIO mice transitioned from high-fat diet to standard chow diet (DIO-Rev) (Fig. 1a). All mice, except for CD mice, were transitioned to HFD at 6 weeks of age. After 12 weeks of HFD feeding, HFD mice weighed approximately 8 g more than the CD controls (Fig. 2b), with the excess weight entirely accounted for by increased adipose mass (Fig. 2c). DIO mice were then randomly assigned to a surgical (BD-IL, RYGB, or DIO-SHAM) or the diet reversal (DIO-Rev) cohort. All surgical mice were continued on their pre-surgical high-fat diet while DIO-Rev mice were transitioned back to standard rodent chow fed ad libitum (Fig. 1c).

Following surgery, BD-IL and RYGB mice rapidly normalized their body weight and were statistically similar to CD controls within one week (Fig. 2a). Both surgical groups maintained a stable, lower body weight, equivalent to CD controls, through the end of the study (Fig. 2a,b) without any significant (< 5%) mortality outside of the immediate post-operative period (10 days). DIO-Rev animals also normalized their body weight, albeit at a slower rate than their surgical counterparts, reaching statistical equivalency to the CD controls after ~ 4 weeks post diet reversal (Fig. 2a). To assure a stable, steady-state weight, mice were maintained for an additional 4 weeks before further testing or analysis. At the end of the study, DIO-SHAM mice were approximately 16 g heavier than their surgical or control counterparts. Body composition analysis showed that neither surgical procedure resulted in a loss of lean body mass and differences in weight between groups was again almost entirely accounted for by adipose mass, with no statistical difference in lean body mass seen between cohorts (Fig. 2c).

Eight weeks following surgery all cohorts were subjected to oral glucose tolerance tests (Fig. 2d-f). DIO-SHAM animals demonstrated significant glucose intolerance with both elevated fasting and glucose area under the curve. DIO-Rev animals normalized their glucose tolerance while BD-IL surgical animals showed a significant decrease in both fasting and stimulated glucose levels well below that of CD controls. Interestingly, after a six hour fast, RYGB animals had glucose levels similar to DIO-SHAM animals, although their glucose dynamics where significantly

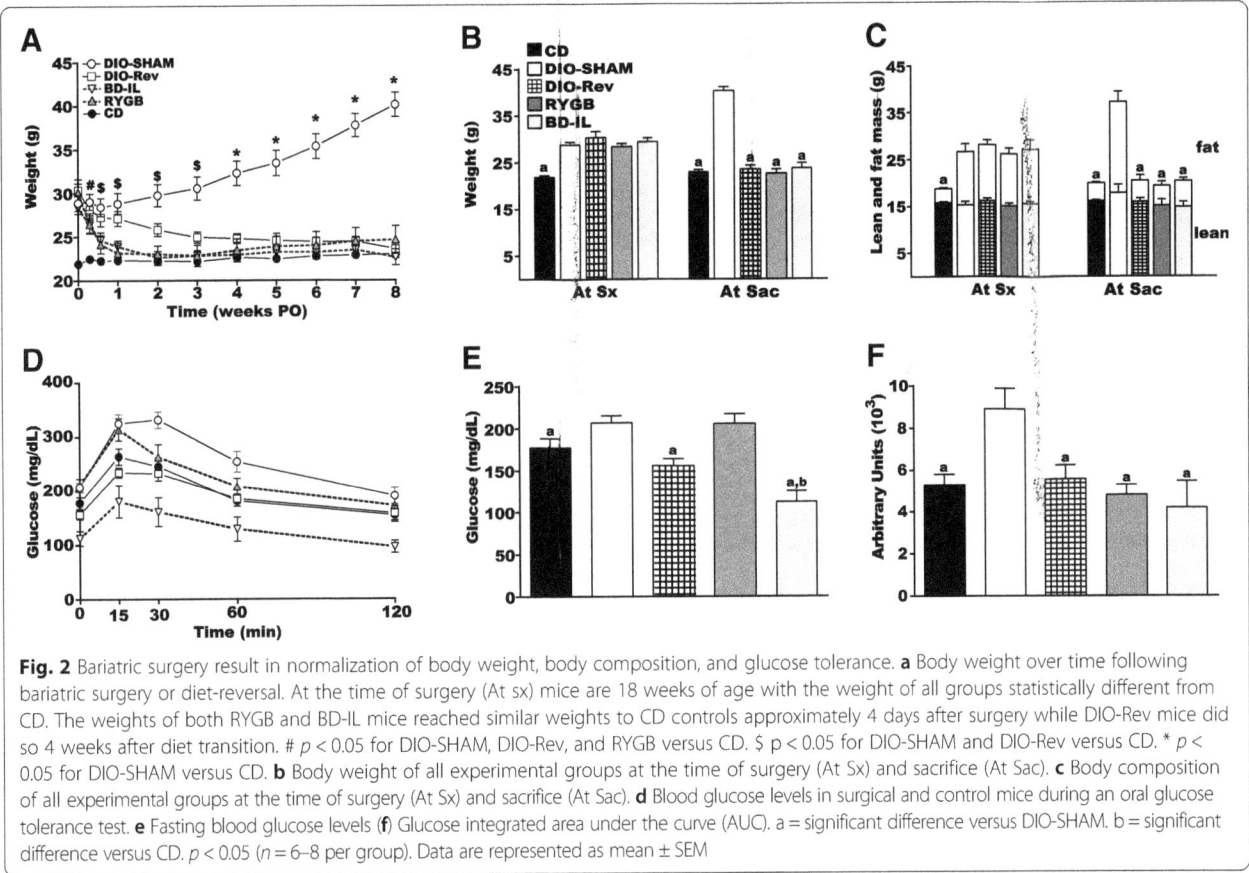

Fig. 2 Bariatric surgery result in normalization of body weight, body composition, and glucose tolerance. **a** Body weight over time following bariatric surgery or diet-reversal. At the time of surgery (At sx) mice are 18 weeks of age with the weight of all groups statistically different from CD. The weights of both RYGB and BD-IL mice reached similar weights to CD controls approximately 4 days after surgery while DIO-Rev mice did so 4 weeks after diet transition. # $p < 0.05$ for DIO-SHAM, DIO-Rev, and RYGB versus CD. \$ $p < 0.05$ for DIO-SHAM and DIO-Rev versus CD. * $p < 0.05$ for DIO-SHAM versus CD. **b** Body weight of all experimental groups at the time of surgery (At Sx) and sacrifice (At Sac). **c** Body composition of all experimental groups at the time of surgery (At Sx) and sacrifice (At Sac). **d** Blood glucose levels in surgical and control mice during an oral glucose tolerance test. **e** Fasting blood glucose levels (**f**) Glucose integrated area under the curve (AUC). a = significant difference versus DIO-SHAM. b = significant difference versus CD. $p < 0.05$ ($n = 6$–8 per group). Data are represented as mean ± SEM

improved. Following, administration of glucose, RYGB animals demonstrated a brisk rise in glucose levels with a peak similar to that of DIO-SHAM. However, this was followed by rapid return to baseline levels, such that the glucose area under the curve was similar to CD fed animals.

BD-IL and RYGB bariatric surgeries normalize HFD-induced hypothalamic microgliosis

Chronic exposure to HFD results in a reactive microgliosis and increased inflammatory gene expression within the mediobasal hypothalamus of (Thaler et al. 2012a), a condition associated with central leptin resistance (Flynn et al. 2015). Given that BD-IL and RYGB animals maintain a stable normal level of body weight and adiposity without hyperphagia, despite continued exposure to HFD, we hypothesized that these surgeries might improve or resolve hypothalamic metaflammation. Following the same experimental structure (12-week HDF feeding, surgery, and sacrifice at 8 weeks post-operative), we first evaluated the effects of RYGB and BD-IL surgeries on HFD-induced microgliosis. To facilitate identification and visualization of hypothalamic microglia, we used CX3CR1[GFP/+] mice, a model that uses the CX3CR1 promoter to drive GFP expression in

microglia. Using fluorescent microscopy, we found that, consistent with previous reports, chronic HFD-feeding resulted in a significant increase in arcuate microglia numbers (Thaler et al. 2012a; Valdearcos et al. 2014). Both RYGB and BD-IL surgical procedures resulted in a complete normalization of arcuate nucleus microglial cell counts, comparable to CD controls (Fig. 3a,b). Surprisingly, while we observed a trend towards decreased arcuate microglia numbers following diet reversal, this was not statistically different from that of DIO-SHAM animals. In comparison to the ARC, we did not observe any effects of HFD-feeding on microglial counts within nearby hypothalamic nuclei (VMH, DMH) or in the cortex (Fig. 3c). Using multi-comparisons analysis, we did note a decrease of microglia within the VMH of BD-IL animals, which was statistically lower than DIO-SHAM animals.

BD-IL and RYGB bariatric surgeries normalize HFD-induced hypothalamic metaflammation

Given the improvement in microgliosis, we next evaluated hypothalamic proinflammatory gene expression in wild-type C57BL/6J mice following bariatric surgery. At baseline, we found the expression levels of the proinflammatory genes assayed, including *Tnfα*, *Il-1β*, and *Ccl2*, to be extremely low in hypothalamus of the CD

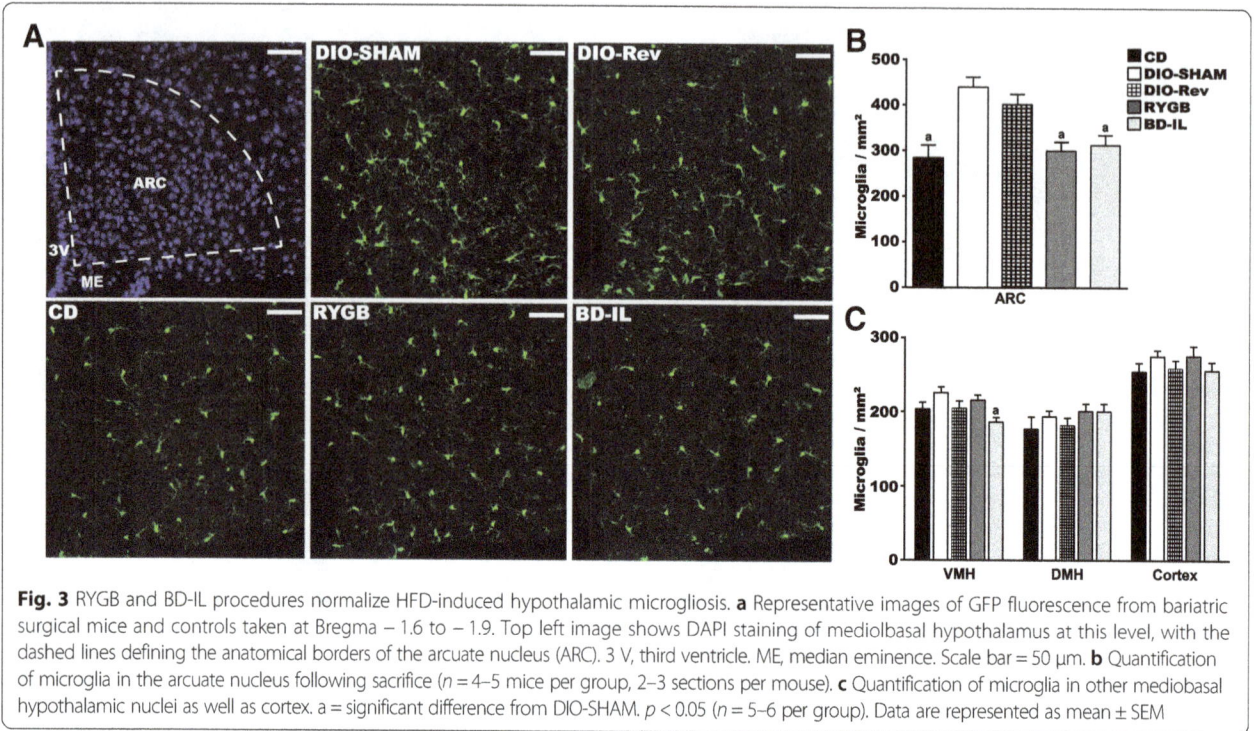

Fig. 3 RYGB and BD-IL procedures normalize HFD-induced hypothalamic microgliosis. **a** Representative images of GFP fluorescence from bariatric surgical mice and controls taken at Bregma − 1.6 to − 1.9. Top left image shows DAPI staining of mediolbasal hypothalamus at this level, with the dashed lines defining the anatomical borders of the arcuate nucleus (ARC). 3 V, third ventricle. ME, median eminence. Scale bar = 50 μm. **b** Quantification of microglia in the arcuate nucleus following sacrifice (n = 4–5 mice per group, 2–3 sections per mouse). **c** Quantification of microglia in other mediobasal hypothalamic nuclei as well as cortex. a = significant difference from DIO-SHAM. $p < 0.05$ (n = 5–6 per group). Data are represented as mean ± SEM

control animals, with most samples failing to reach a cycle threshold (Ct) using specific Taqman probes to the genes of interest. In contrast, all assays run on DIO-SHAM samples readily amplified and detected all three genes assayed. Consistent with the pattern seen in microgliosis, hypothalamic proinflammatory gene expression from bariatric surgical samples resembled that of CD controls, with very low detection. We found that weight loss resulting from diet reversal (DIO-Rev) alone did not significantly reduce, but surprisingly led to a general increase in the levels of hypothalamic proinflammatory gene expression, although we saw broad variation. In order to more readily compare hypothalamic gene expression levels between experimental groups, expression levels of each gene were normalized to a reference gene (*Gapdh*) and expressed relative to DIO-controls using the ∆∆CT method, with undetectable samples assigned a Ct value of 35, the latest threshold value seen across all samples assayed. These results suggest that both RYGB and BD-IL procedures promote an anti-inflammatory profile within the hypothalamus of HFD-fed mice while weight loss alone, at least in the time frame assayed here, does not result in resolution of hypothalamic inflammation (Fig. 4a).

BD-IL and RYGB bariatric surgeries normalize expression of hypothalamic orexigenic gene expression and restores the anorexic response to exogenous leptin

Because hypothalamic metaflammation is associated with leptin resistance within the MBH (Zhang et al. 2008;

Milanski et al. 2009; Posey et al. 2009), we hypothesized that the improved hypothalamic inflammatory profile might be associated with changes in the expression of leptin-responsive genes and an improved response to exogenous leptin. We found that expression of the orexigenic neuropeptide *Agrp* was significantly upregulated in the DIO-SHAM animals compared to CD controls (Fig. 5a). Similar to previous reports, we found that weight loss associated with diet reversal was also associated with increased expression of *Agrp* (Yu et al. 2009). However, following both RYGB and BD-IL, expression

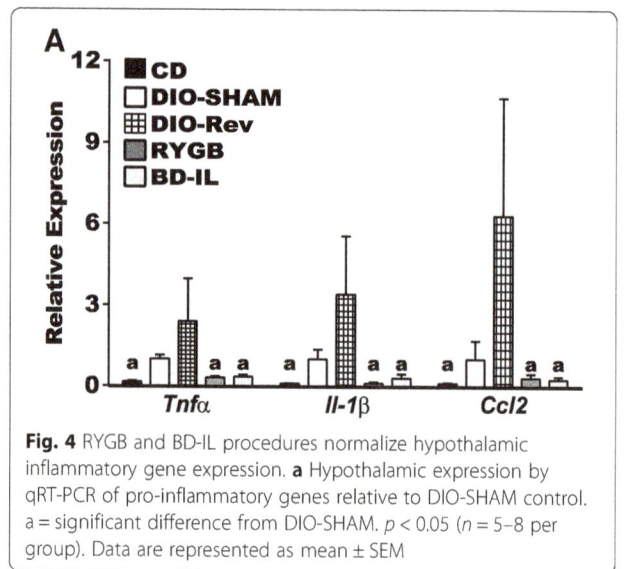

Fig. 4 RYGB and BD-IL procedures normalize hypothalamic inflammatory gene expression. **a** Hypothalamic expression by qRT-PCR of pro-inflammatory genes relative to DIO-SHAM control. a = significant difference from DIO-SHAM. $p < 0.05$ (n = 5–8 per group). Data are represented as mean ± SEM

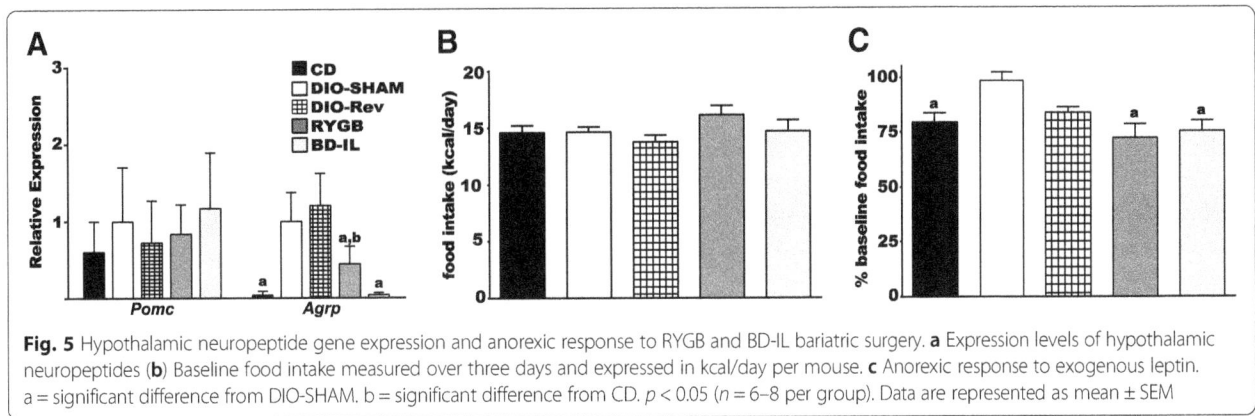

Fig. 5 Hypothalamic neuropeptide gene expression and anorexic response to RYGB and BD-IL bariatric surgery. **a** Expression levels of hypothalamic neuropeptides (**b**) Baseline food intake measured over three days and expressed in kcal/day per mouse. **c** Anorexic response to exogenous leptin. a = significant difference from DIO-SHAM. b = significant difference from CD. $p < 0.05$ ($n = 6$–8 per group). Data are represented as mean ± SEM

levels of hypothalamic *Agrp* were normalized to similar levels found in CD controls. Evaluation of *Pomc* levels, the pro-gene of the anorexigenic neuropeptide α-MSH, showed no significant difference between any of the experimental groups (Fig. 5a). Taken together these results indicate a shift towards a more anorexigenic profile in the hypothalamus and suggest an improved sensitivity to endogenous leptin in HFD-fed mice following bariatric surgery.

Finally, we assayed the response of bariatric surgical animals to exogenous leptin. All animal cohorts where given 3 days of vehicle injections followed by three days of leptin (2 mg/kg) and food intake measured daily. Consistent with previous reports, DIO-SHAM animals proved to be generally resistant to the anorexic effects of leptin, with little reduction of food intake in response to treatment (Fig. 5b). Both the surgical and CD cohorts, however, reduced their intake by 20–25%, while the DIO-Rev again showed an intermediate phenotype. In response to leptin treatment, DIO-Rev animals showed a clear trend towards reduction of food intake (~ 15%), however analysis of variance with multiple comparisons did not show a significant difference between DIO-SHAM and DIO-Rev animals, nor a difference between CD and DIO-Rev animals.

Discussion

The induction of hypothalamic metaflammation and microgliosis in rodents following chronic HFD-feeding, has been extensively documented and confirmed by our studies here (De Souza et al. 2005; Zhang et al. 2008; Thaler et al. 2012a; Milanski et al. 2009; Posey et al. 2009). Importantly, hypothalamic metaflammation and microglial activation have been associated with hypothalamic resistance to peripheral anorexic signals, including leptin, and inhibition of hypothalamic inflammatory pathways reduces food intake and body weight of DIO animals (Zhang et al. 2008; Milanski et al. 2009; Posey et al. 2009). In addition, recent evidence suggests that depletion or inhibition of hypothalamic microglia prevents

HFD-induced metaflammation and protects against DIO (Valdearcos et al. 2014; Andre et al. 2017; Thaler et al. 2012b; Valdearcos et al. 2017). Diet-induced obese rodents tend to reduce their body weight when switched to a less palatable diet (Myers Jr. et al. 2010). We have shown here that following transition back to standard chow diet, DIO mice normalize their weight, at mass, and glucose tolerance comparable to CD-fed controls. However, it is apparent from our results, as well as work done by others, that despite such weight loss hypothalamic metaflammation is slow to resolve (Wang et al. 2012; Enriori et al. 2007). Thus, while hypothalamic metaflammation is insufficient to maintain the full obesity phenotype in DIO animals in the absence of the primary precipitant (palatable high-calorie chow), persistent hypothalamic metaflammation and its ensuing leptin resistance could explain the accelerated weight gain and exacerbated metabolic derangements seen after weight cycling in rodent models (Barbosa-da-Silva et al. 2012; Thaiss et al. 2016), while in human obesity such mechanisms may contribute to the difficulty that most individuals have in achieving sustained weight loss in an environment with easy access to calorically-dense highly palatable foods (Anastasiou et al. 2015).

In contrast to the lingering hypothalamic metaflammation following dietary weight loss, our results show that hypothalamic metaflammation and the associated microgliosis are quick to resolve following two different bariatric surgical procedures, RYGB and BD-IL, despite ongoing exposure to HFD. The rapidity of these changes when compared to the DIO-Rev model suggests that these bariatric surgeries may elicit anti-inflammatory mediators that attenuate hypothalamic metaflammation and inhibit microglial activation, allowing for a reset of defended body weight to a new and lower level. Further studies are needed to assess the role, if any, the immediate post-operative anorexia and acute weight loss plays in the resolution of hypothalamic inflammation. It may be that following diet-reversal such inflammation may resolve given the same amount of time at a normal weight. However, other studies have shown that exposure to high-fat diet, and not obesity itself, rapidly induces hypothalamic inflammation (Yi et al. 2012).

In the setting of HFD-feeding, one would anticipate expression of hypothalamic anorexigenic genes, such as *Pomc*, to be upregulated while expression of orexigenic genes, such as *Agrp*, to be downregulated, reducing appetite, enhancing metabolism, and attenuating weight gain. Previous reports have demonstrated, however, that the expression levels of these hypothalamic leptin-responsive genes often counter the maintenance of homeostasis in the setting of DIO and increased serum leptin (Guan et al. 1998; Bergen et al. 1999; Huang et al. 2003), suggesting a degree of leptin resistance in the hypothalamic neurocircuitry. Consistent with these reports, we have observed that DIO-SHAM mice exhibit elevated hypothalamic expression of *Agrp* with no change in the expression of *Pomc* compared to CD-fed controls. We found that DIO-Rev mice exhibit a similar pattern of hypothalamic gene expression, although this pattern might be expected from animals who have recently lost weight (Yu et al. 2009). However, it also suggests that these animals continue to defend a higher body weight and would rapidly regain weight if returned to a more obesogenic environment (Barbosa-da-Silva et al. 2012; Thaiss et al. 2016). In contrast, the normalization of *Agrp* gene expression following both bariatric surgeries implies a state of homeostasis and is consistent with a reduced level of homeostatically defended body weight despite continued exposure to the same HFD as DIO-SHAM mice and a similar weight loss as DIO-Rev mice. Interestingly, hypothalamic AGRP neurons appear to be particularly sensitive to changes in the inflammatory environment and suppression of inflammatory pathways specifically in this neuronal population protects against DIO (Zhang et al. 2008), suggesting a mechanistic link between improved inflammation and *Agrp* levels.

Our results, while observational, generate important hypotheses regarding the relationship between hypothalamic metaflammation and the efficacy of bariatric surgery to induce sustainable weight loss. Changes in the anatomy and delivery of nutrients to the distal intestine following RYGB increase secretion of a number of metabolically active hormones and metabolites, some of which have anti-inflammatory properties which may act on hypothalamic cell types via direct or indirect mechanisms (le Roux et al. 2006). Recently, serum bile acids have emerged as important regulators of energy balance and possible mediators of bariatric surgery's metabolic benefits (Kuipers and Bloks 2014; Albaugh et al. 2017). A number of studies in both human and animal models have shown increased serum bile acid concentrations following RYGB (Ahmad et al. 2013; De Giorgi et al. 2015; Pournaras et al. 2012; Bhutta et al. 2015;

Spinelli et al. 2016). The BD-IL model of bariatric surgery, developed to investigate the effects of increased serum bile acids independent of surgical rearrangement of nutrient flow, results in weight loss and a reversal of DIO metabolic dysregulation, similar to that of RYGB (Flynn et al. 2015). Pertinent to our observations here, bile acids have potent anti-inflammatory effects via the G protein-coupled bile acid receptor GPBAR1 (Kawamata et al. 2003; Perino et al. 2014; Pols et al. 2011; Wang et al. 2011). Further, *Gpbar1* is expressed by microglia and GPBAR1 agonists have been shown to reduce neuroinflammation in several neurodegenerative diseases including models of multiple sclerosis, hepatic encephalopathy, and stroke (Lewis et al. 2014; Mano et al. 2004; Parry et al. 2010; McMillin et al. 2015; Rodrigues et al. 2002). Thus, we propose that bile acids may similarly mediate the anti-inflammatory effects of bariatric surgery on metabolically-induced hypothalamic inflammation. Further studies will be needed to define the cellular and molecular mechanisms underlying these effects, but such studies are likely to reveal important insights into the nature of hypothalamic inflammation and uncover novel targets for the non-surgical treatment of obesity.

Conclusion

In summary, chronic high-fat diet (HFD) results in upregulation of inflammatory markers and proliferation of microglia within the mediobasal hypothalamus. We have shown here that two different models of bariatric surgery have an ameliorating effect on HFD-induced hypothalamic metaflammation and microgliosis while normalizing hypothalamic *Agrp* expression and the anorexigenic response to exogenous leptin, despite ongoing exposure to HFD. In contrast, animals that lost weight by transitioning back to a low-fat diet, continued to show evidence of hypothalamic inflammation and leptin resistance. These results suggest that bariatric surgeries may elicit anti-inflammatory mediators that counter the inflammatory effects of HFD and may be one reason for the efficacy of bariatric surgery in long-term weight loss. A better understanding of the mechanisms behind these effects may provide insight into novel therapies for obesity.

Abbreviations

Agrp: Agouti-related peptide; ARC: Arcuate nucleus; BD-IL: Biliary diversion to the ileum; Ccl2: Chemokine (C-C motif) ligand 2; CD: Control diet; CX3CR1: Chemokine (C-X3-C motif) receptor 1; DAPI: 4′,6-Diamidine-2′-phenylindole dihydrochloride; DIO: Diet-induced obesity; DMH: Dorsomedial nucleus; GFP: Green fluorescent protein; GPBAR1: G protein-coupled bile acid receptor 1; HFD: High-fat diet; Il-1β: Interleukin 1 beta; MBH: Mediobasal hypothalamus; NF-κB: Nuclear factor kappa B; NMR: Nuclear magnetic

resonance; PBS: Phosphate-buffered saline; PFA: Paraformaldehyde; Pomc:
Pro-opiomelanocortin; RYGB: Roux-en-Y gastric bypass; SEM: Standard error of
the mean; Tnfα: Tumor necrosis factor alpha; VMH: Ventromedial nucleus;
αMSH: Alpha-melanocyte-stimulating hormone

Acknowledgements

We would like to recognize technical assistance given by the Vanderbilt
Metabolic Physiology Shared Resource (MPSR). Bariatric surgical procedures
were performed through the Body Weight Regulation Core of the Vanderbilt
Mouse Metabolic Phenotyping Center which is supported by NIH grants
DK059637 (Vanderbilt Mouse Metabolic Phenotyping Center), DK020593
(Vanderbilt Diabetes Research and Training Center), and DK058404
(Vanderbilt Digestive Disease Research Center). We would like to thank Drs.
Owen McGuinness, Robb Flynn, Kevin Niswender as well as other members
of the Abumrad lab for helpful discussions and support.

Funding

This study was supported by the NIH (K12 HD087023 to NCB).

Author's contributions

MKH and NCB designed the study. MKH, KMF, and NCB carried out experiments
and carried out data analysis. NCB, MKH, RBS, NNA contributed to drafting the
initial manuscript. All authors read and approved the final manuscript.

Competing interests

The authors declare that they have no competing interests.

Author details

[1]Department of Pediatrics, Vanderbilt University Medical Center, 1500 21 st.
Ave South, Suite 1514, Nashville, TN 37212, USA. [2]Present address:
Department of Physiology, Emory University School of Medicine, Atlanta, GA
30322, USA. [3]Department of Molecular Physiology and Biophysics, Vanderbilt
University Medical Center, Nashville, TN 37232, USA. [4]Department of Surgery,
Vanderbilt University Medical Center, Nashville, TN 37232, USA.

References

Ahmad NN, Pfalzer A, Kaplan LM. Roux-en-Y gastric bypass normalizes the
blunted postprandial bile acid excursion associated with obesity. Int J Obes.
2013;37(12):1553–9.

Albaugh VL, Banan B, Ajouz H, Abumrad NN, Flynn CR. Bile acids and bariatric
surgery. Mol Aspects Med. 2017;56:75–89.

Albaugh VL, Flynn CR, Tamboli RA, Abumrad NN. Recent advances in metabolic and
bariatric surgery. F1000Res. 2016;5:978. https://doi.org/10.12688/f1000research.7240.1.

Anastasiou CA, Karfopoulou E, Yannakoulia M. Weight regaining: from statistics and
behaviors to physiology and metabolism. Metabolism. 2015;64(11):1395–407.

Andre C, Guzman-Quevedo O, Rey C, Remus-Borel J, Clark S, Castellanos-
Jankiewicz A, et al. Inhibiting microglia expansion prevents diet-induced
hypothalamic and peripheral inflammation. Diabetes. 2017;66(4):908–19.

Barbosa-da-Silva S, Fraulob-Aquino JC, Lopes JR, Mandarim-de-Lacerda CA, Aguila
MB. Weight cycling enhances adipose tissue inflammatory responses in male
mice. PLoS One. 2012;7(7):e39837.

Beckman LM, Beckman TR, Earthman CP. Changes in gastrointestinal hormones
and leptin after roux-en-Y gastric bypass procedure: a review. J Am Diet
Assoc. 2010;110(4):571–84.

Bergen HT, Mizuno T, Taylor J, Mobbs CV. Resistance to diet-induced obesity is
associated with increased proopiomelanocortin mRNA and decreased
neuropeptide Y mRNA in the hypothalamus. Brain Res. 1999;851(1–2):198–203.

Bhutta HY, Rajpal N, White W, Freudenberg JM, Liu Y, Way J, et al. Effect of roux-
en-Y gastric bypass surgery on bile acid metabolism in normal and obese
diabetic rats. PLoS One. 2015;10(3):e0122273.

De Giorgi S, Campos V, Egli L, Toepel U, Carrel G, Cariou B, et al. Long-term
effects of roux-en-Y gastric bypass on postprandial plasma lipid and bile
acids kinetics in female non diabetic subjects: a cross-sectional pilot study.
Clin Nutr. 2015;34(5):911–7.

De Souza CT, Araujo EP, Bordin S, Ashimine R, Zollner RL, Boschero AC, et al.
Consumption of a fat-rich diet activates a proinflammatory response and
induces insulin resistance in the hypothalamus. Endocrinology. 2005;146(10):
4192–9.

Enriori PJ, Evans AE, Sinnayah P, Jobst EE, Tonelli-Lemos L, Billes SK, et al. Diet-
induced obesity causes severe but reversible leptin resistance in arcuate
melanocortin neurons. Cell Metab. 2007;5(3):181–94.

Flynn CR, Albaugh VL, Cai S, Cheung-Flynn J, Williams PE, Brucker RM, et al. Bile
diversion to the distal small intestine has comparable metabolic benefits to
bariatric surgery. Nat Commun. 2015;6:7715.

Grayson BE, Schneider KM, Woods SC, Seeley RJ. Improved rodent maternal
metabolism but reduced intrauterine growth after vertical sleeve
gastrectomy. Sci Transl Med. 2013;5(199):199ra12.

Guan XM, Yu H, Trumbauer M, Frazier E, Van der Ploeg LH, Chen H. Induction of
neuropeptide Y expression in dorsomedial hypothalamus of diet-induced
obese mice. Neuroreport. 1998;9(15):3415–9.

Hotamisligil GS, Shargill NS, Spiegelman BM. Adipose expression of tumor
necrosis factor-alpha: direct role in obesity-linked insulin resistance. Science.
1993;259(5091):87–91.

Huang XF, Han M, South T, Storlien L. Altered levels of POMC, AgRP and MC4-R
mRNA expression in the hypothalamus and other parts of the limbic system
of mice prone or resistant to chronic high-energy diet-induced obesity. Brain
Res. 2003;992(1):9–19.

Kawamata Y, Fujii R, Hosoya M, Harada M, Yoshida H, Miwa M, et al. A G protein-
coupled receptor responsive to bile acids. J Biol Chem. 2003;278(11):9435–40.

Kern PA, Saghizadeh M, Ong JM, Bosch RJ, Deem R, Simsolo RB. The expression
of tumor necrosis factor in human adipose tissue. Regulation by obesity, weight
loss, and relationship to lipoprotein lipase. J Clin Invest. 1995;95(5):2111–9.

Kuipers F, Bloks VW. Groen AK. Nat Rev Endocrinol: Beyond intestinal soap-bile
acids in metabolic control; 2014.

Laurenius A, Larsson I, Melanson KJ, Lindroos AK, Lonroth H, Bosaeus I, et al.
Decreased energy density and changes in food selection following roux-en-Y
gastric bypass. Eur J Clin Nutr. 2013;67(2):168–73.

le Roux CW, Aylwin SJ, Batterham RL, Borg CM, Coyle F, Prasad V, et al. Gut
hormone profiles following bariatric surgery favor an anorectic state, facilitate
weight loss, and improve metabolic parameters. Ann Surg. 2006;243(1):108–14.

Lewis ND, Patnaude LA, Pelletier J, Souza DJ, Lukas SM, King FJ, et al. A GPBAR1
(TGR5) small molecule agonist shows specific inhibitory effects on myeloid
cell activation in vitro and reduces experimental autoimmune encephalitis
(EAE) in vivo. PLoS One. 2014;9(6):e100883.

Mano N, Goto T, Uchida M, Nishimura K, Ando M, Kobayashi N, et al. Presence of
protein-bound unconjugated bile acids in the cytoplasmic fraction of rat
brain. J Lipid Res. 2004;45(2):295–300.

McMillin M, Frampton G, Tobin R, Dusio G, Smith J, Shin H, et al. TGR5 signaling
reduces neuroinflammation during hepatic encephalopathy. J Neurochem.
2015;135(3):565–76.

Milanski M, Degasperi G, Coope A, Morari J, Denis R, Cintra DE, et al. Saturated
fatty acids produce an inflammatory response predominantly through the
activation of TLR4 signaling in hypothalamus: implications for the
pathogenesis of obesity. J Neurosci. 2009;29(2):359–70.

Mingrone G, Panunzi S, De Gaetano A, Guidone C, Iaconelli A, Leccesi L, et al.
Bariatric surgery versus conventional medical therapy for type 2 diabetes. N
Engl J Med. 2012;366(17):1577–85.

Munzberg H, Laque A, Yu S, Rezai-Zadeh K, Berthoud HR. Appetite and body
weight regulation after bariatric surgery. Obes Rev. 2015;16(Suppl 1):77–90.

Myers MG Jr, Leibel RL, Seeley RJ, Schwartz MW. Obesity and leptin resistance:
distinguishing cause from effect. Trends Endocrinol Metab. 2010;21(11):643–51.

Parry GJ, Rodrigues CM, Aranha MM, Hilbert SJ, Davey C, Kelkar P, et al. Safety,
tolerability, and cerebrospinal fluid penetration of ursodeoxycholic acid in
patients with amyotrophic lateral sclerosis. Clin Neuropharmacol. 2010;33(1):
17–21.

Perino A, Pols TW, Nomura M, Stein S, Pellicciari R, Schoonjans K. TGR5 reduces
macrophage migration through mTOR-induced C/EBPbeta differential
translation. J Clin Invest. 2014;124(12):5424–36.

Pols TW, Nomura M, Harach T, Lo Sasso G, Oosterveer MH, Thomas C, et al. TGR5
activation inhibits atherosclerosis by reducing macrophage inflammation and
lipid loading. Cell Metab. 2011;14(6):747–57.

Posey KA, Clegg DJ, Printz RL, Byun J, Morton GJ, Vivekanandan-Giri A, et al.
Hypothalamic proinflammatory lipid accumulation, inflammation, and insulin
resistance in rats fed a high-fat diet. Am J Physiol Endocrinol Metab. 2009;
296(5):E1003–12.

Pournaras DJ, Glicksman C, Vincent RP, Kuganolipava S, Alaghband-Zadeh J, Mahon D, et al. The role of bile after roux-en-Y gastric bypass in promoting weight loss and improving glycaemic control. Endocrinology. 2012;153(8): 3613–9.

Pratt GM, Learn CA, Hughes GD, Clark BL, Warthen M, Pories W. Demographics and outcomes at American Society for Metabolic and Bariatric Surgery Centers of excellence. Surg Endosc. 2009;23(4):795–9.

Rodrigues CM, Spellman SR, Sola S, Grande AW, Linehan-Stieers C, Low WC, et al. Neuroprotection by a bile acid in an acute stroke model in the rat. J Cereb Blood Flow Metab. 2002;22(4):463–71.

Schauer PR, Bhatt DL, Kirwan JP, Wolski K, Aminian A, Brethauer SA, et al. Bariatric surgery versus intensive medical therapy for diabetes - 5-year outcomes. N Engl J Med. 2017;376(7):641–51.

Spinelli V, Lalloyer F, Baud G, Osto E, Kouach M, Daoudi M, et al. Influence of roux-en-Y gastric bypass on plasma bile acid profiles: a comparative study between rats, pigs and humans. Int J Obes. 2016;40(8):1260–7.

Streit WJ, Walter SA, Pennell NA. Reactive microgliosis. Prog Neurobiol. 1999;57(6): 563–81.

Thaiss CA, Itav S, Rothschild D, Meijer M, Levy M. Moresi C, et al. Nature: Persistent microbiome alterations modulate the rate of post-dieting weight regain; 2016.

Thaler JP, Yi CX, Guyenet S, Hwang B, Matsen M, Nguyen H, et al. Microglial Inactivation during HFD Feeding Promotes Weight Gain. Houston: ENDO 2012; 2012b.

Thaler JP, Yi CX, Schur EA, Guyenet SJ, Hwang BH, Dietrich MO, et al. Obesity is associated with hypothalamic injury in rodents and humans. J Clin Invest. 2012a;122(1):153–62.

Ullrich J, Ernst B, Wilms B, Thurnheer M, Schultes B. Roux-en Y gastric bypass surgery reduces hedonic hunger and improves dietary habits in severely obese subjects. Obes Surg. 2013;23(1):50–5.

Valdearcos M, Douglass JD, Robblee MM, Dorfman MD, Stifler DR, Bennett ML, et al. Microglial inflammatory signaling orchestrates the hypothalamic immune response to dietary excess and mediates obesity susceptibility. Cell Metab. 2017;26(1):185–97 e3.

Valdearcos M, Robblee MM, Benjamin DI, Nomura DK, Xu AW, Koliwad SK. Microglia dictate the impact of saturated fat consumption on hypothalamic inflammation and neuronal function. Cell Rep. 2014;9(6):2124–38.

Wang X, Ge A, Cheng M, Guo F, Zhao M, Zhou X, et al. Increased hypothalamic inflammation associated with the susceptibility to obesity in rats exposed to high-fat diet. Exp Diabetes Res. 2012;2012:847246.

Wang YD, Chen WD, Yu D, Forman BM, Huang W. The G-protein-coupled bile acid receptor, Gpbar1 (TGR5), negatively regulates hepatic inflammatory response through antagonizing nuclear factor kappa light-chain enhancer of activated B cells (NF-kappaB) in mice. Hepatology. 2011;54(4):1421–32.

Yi CX, Tschop MH, Woods SC, Hofmann SM. High-fat-diet exposure induces IgG accumulation in hypothalamic microglia. Dis Model Mech. 2012;5(5):686–90.

Yin DP, Gao Q, Ma LL, Yan W, Williams PE, McGuinness OP, et al. Assessment of different bariatric surgeries in the treatment of obesity and insulin resistance in mice. Ann Surg. 2011;254(1):73–82.

Yu Y, Deng C, Huang XF. Obese reversal by a chronic energy restricted diet leaves an increased arc NPY/AgRP, but no alteration in POMC/CART, mRNA expression in diet-induced obese mice. Behav Brain Res. 2009;205(1):50–6.

Zhang X, Zhang G, Zhang H, Karin M, Bai H, Cai D. Hypothalamic IKKbeta/NF-kappaB and ER stress link overnutrition to energy imbalance and obesity. Cell. 2008;135(1):61–73.

MicroRNAs 143 and 150 in whole blood enable detection of T-cell immunoparalysis in sepsis

P Möhnle[1†], S Hirschberger[1,2†], L C Hinske[1], J Briegel[1], M Hübner[1,2], S Weis[3,4,5], G Dimopoulos[6], M Bauer[3,4], E J Giamarellos-Bourboulis[7] and S Kreth[1,2*]

Abstract

Background: Currently, no suitable clinical marker for detection of septic immunosuppression is available. We aimed at identifying microRNAs that could serve as biomarkers of T-cell mediated immunoparalysis in sepsis.

Methods: RNA was isolated from purified T-cells or from whole blood cells obtained from septic patients and healthy volunteers. Differentially regulated miRNAs were identified by miRNA Microarray ($n = 7$). Validation was performed via qPCR ($n = 31$).

Results: T-cells of septic patients revealed characteristics of immunosuppression: Pro-inflammatory miR-150 and miR-342 were downregulated, whereas anti-inflammatory miR-15a, miR-16, miR-93, miR-143, miR-223 and miR-424 were upregulated. Assessment of T-cell effector status showed significantly reduced mRNA-levels of IL2, IL7R and ICOS, and increased levels of IL4, IL10 and TGF-β. The individual extent of immunosuppression differed markedly. MicroRNA-143, − 150 and − 223 independently indicated T-cell immunoparalysis and significantly correlated with patient's IL7R-/ICOS-expression and SOFA-scores. In whole blood, composed of innate and adaptive immune cells, both traits of immunosuppression and hyperinflammation were detected. Importantly, miR-143 and miR-150 − both predominantly expressed in T-cells − retained strong power of discrimination also in whole blood samples.

Conclusions: These findings suggest miR-143 and miR-150 as promising markers for detection of T-cell immunosuppression in whole blood and may help to develop new approaches for miRNA-based diagnostic in sepsis.

Keywords: Sepsis, Immunoparalysis, T-cells, T cell exhaustion, miRNA, Biomarker

Background

Sepsis has long been viewed as a disease with sequentially proceeding phases of hyperinflammation and immunoparalysis. Currently, it has become increasingly clear that sepsis is more a complex syndrome than a disease: Recent studies have indicated that states of hyperinflammation, largely driven by innate immune cells, and immunosuppression, mainly affecting adaptive immunity, can occur at any time, sequentially or even simultaneously (Boomer et al. 2014; Xiao et al. 2011). Immunoparalysis, however, has been identified as the major clinical problem leading to death in a large number of patients (Boomer et al. 2011). In this situation, effective tools for early detection and consecutive monitoring of immunosuppression are lacking, which reduces therapeutic.

success and hampers development of new strategies targeting immune dysfunction. Commonly used biomarkers in sepsis, e.g. C-reactive Protein, Interleukin-6, and Procalcitonin, lack sensitivity and specificity and cannot indicate immunosuppression (Samraj et al. 2013). Very recent attempts to assess an impaired immune status based on quantification of cell surface markers (HLA-DR3) or mRNAs (IL-10, CD74) have not yet made their way into clinical practice, as these strategies either rely on flow cytometric analysis, which is technically

* Correspondence: simone.kreth@med.uni-muenchen.de
[†]P Möhnle and S Hirschberger contributed equally to this work.
[1]Department of Anaesthesiology and Intensive Care Medicine, University Hospital, Ludwig Maximilian University (LMU), Marchioninistraße 15, 81377 Munich, Germany
[2]Walter-Brendel-Center of Experimental Medicine, Ludwig Maximilian University (LMU), Munich, Germany
Full list of author information is available at the end of the article

highly demanding, or on quantification of mRNA transcripts, which is always threatened by the mRNA's intrinsic instability (Landelle et al. 2010; Peronnet et al. 2017). MiRNAs might bear the potential to fill this gap.

MicroRNAs are small non-coding RNAs acting as key regulators in gene expression networks, thus playing a pivotal role in almost all cellular processes (Bartel 2009). By base-pairing to the 3′-untranslated region (3'UTR) of their respective target genes, miRNAs posttranscriptionally repress gene expression (Bartel 2004). MicroRNAs display regulatory potential in a wide range of human diseases including cardiovascular conditions, degenerative processes, systemic inflammation and cancer (Pencheva and Tavazoie 2013; Hata 2013; Jung and Suh 2014; O'Connell et al. 2012; Hirschberger et al. 2018). In addition, identification and validation of miRNAs as biomarkers is an emerging field in medicine, given their tissue- and disease-specific expression and high stability even when released into the circulation (Weiland et al. 2012). In sepsis, recent publications reported altered expression of specific miRNAs. The authors suggested individual or sets of miRNAs as biomarkers to enable an early diagnosis, to differentiate different sepsis severity grades, and/or to predict survival (reviewed in (Kreth et al. 2017)). Results of these studies, however, were remarkably heterogeneous, and a consensus with respect to actually suitable biomarkers has not been reached so far. Disparate findings of these studies were most likely due to varying study aims, small sample sizes, and use of different sample types (either plasma/ serum or whole blood or peripheral blood mononuclear cells) (Benz et al. 2016; Ho et al. 2016; Kingsley and Bhat 2017). The latter is of particular importance as different blood cell types exhibit highly specific transcriptomes and, naturally, differ considerably in miRNA expression profiles (Ecker et al. 2017; Leidinger et al. 2014; Palmer et al. 2006). Taking into consideration the fact that innate and adaptive immune cells may be regulated in a diametrically opposed way during sepsis (Boomer et al. 2014; Xiao et al. 2011; Cavaillon and Annane 2006; Tang et al. 2010), a more specific approach for the detection of immunosuppression is needed.

We hypothesized that specific miRNAs are capable to detect and to characterize sepsis-associated immunoparalysis. As particularly lymphocytes represent the suppressed adaptive immune response, we first set out to identify suitable miRNAs in T-cells and then – to facilitate clinical application – transferred our findings to whole blood samples. We here present a pilot study using miRNAs to specifically assess immunosuppression in sepsis.

Methods
Blood sampling
After obtaining informed consent, blood samples were withdrawn from healthy volunteers and from patients diagnosed with either sepsis or septic shock (by fulfilling the criteria SIRS + infection, according to the American College of Chest Physicians/Society of Critical Care Medicine consensus conference (Bone et al. 1992)). Retrospective evaluation showed that all patients were meeting the Sepsis-3 definitions (Singer et al. 2016). Patient analysis and microRNA evaluation was performed between 2011 and 2017, controls have been sampled from 2010 to 2016. For whole blood analysis a second, independent patient/ control group was analysed. The study protocol was approved by the Institutional Ethics Committees of the Ludwig-Maximilian-University Munich, Germany (No. 107–11 and No. 287–13; approved in 2006), of the University Hospital of Jena (No.2007–004333-42, local amendment for Munich University Hospital 2242–03/08), and by the Ethics Committee of ATTIKON University Hospital (approval 5/2008). Research was performed in accordance to the Declaration of Helsinki (ethical principles for medical research involving human subjects). Samples of sepsis patients were withdrawn immediately after diagnosis of sepsis and admission to the intensive care unit and before induction of an antibiotic and/or steroid treatment. History of malignant diseases, immunodeficiency, age younger than 18 years, and previous corticosteroid or antibiotic therapy were exclusion criteria. Patient characteristics are listed in Tables 1, 2, 3, 4 and 5.

Blood cell isolation
After isolation of peripheral blood mononuclear cells (PBMCs) by density centrifugation (Histopaque 1077, Sigma-Aldrich, St. Louis, MO), T-cells were purified using an AutoMACS Pro Separator (Cat. # 130–092-545, Miltenyi Biotec, Bergisch-Gladbach, Germany) and magnetic cell separation (Pan T Cell Isolation Kit, Cat. # 130–096-535, Miltenyi Biotec, Bergisch Gladbach, Germany), as to the manufacturer's recommendations. Cell number and viability were assessed using a ViCell analyzer (Beckman Coulter, Fullerton, CA). Only experiments exhibiting a cell viability of more than 90% were included in our analyses. By applying untouched negative selection, binding of isolation beads to T-cells and potential T-cell activation was avoided. Succesful T-cell isolation was confirmed by flow cytometry analysis using a FTIC anti-human CD3 antibody (Cat. # 344804, BioLegend, San Diego, CA, USA). whole blood

Table 1 miRNA Microarray: Characteristics of Sepsis Patients

n	7
Gender (male/female)	3/4 (42.9%/ 57.1%)
Age, years (mean ± SD)	65.1 (± 13.4)
Septic Shock	4 (57.1%)
Sequential organ failure score (mean ± SD)	14.1 (± 3.5)
Nonsurvivors	3 (42.9%)

Table 2 T-cell samples: Characteristics of Sepsis Patients

n	31
Gender (male/female)	19/12 (61.2%/38.7%)
Age, years (mean ± SD)	57.2 (± 17.8)
Septic shock	14 (45.2%)
Sequential organ failure score (mean ± SD)	10.4 ± 5.4
Nonsurvivors	11 (35.5%)

Table 4 Whole blood samples: Characteristics of Sepsis Patients

n	20
Gender (male/female)	13/7 (65%/35%)
Age, years (mean ± SD)	76.4 ± 6.0
Septic shock	11 (55%)
APACHE II Score (mean ± SD)	23,4 ± 7,9
Nonsurvivors	10 (50%)

analysis, PAXgene Blood RNA Tubes (PreAnalytiX, Hombrechtikon, Switzerland) were used according to the manufacturer's instructions.

RNA-isolation

Total RNA was isolated from primary T-cells using the mirVana miRNA Isolation Kit (Thermo Fisher Scientific, Waltham, MA, USA) with subsequent DNase treatment (Turbo DNase, Thermo Fisher Scientific, Waltham, MA, USA). Total RNA from whole blood samples was purified using the PAXgene Blood RNA Kit (PreAnalytiX, Hombrechtikon, Switzerland). The respective isolation procedures followed the manufacturer's instructions. Quantity of total RNA was measured using a NanoDrop 2000 spectrophotometer (Thermo Fisher Scientific, Waltham, MA, USA), quality was verified by an Agilent 2100 Bioanalyzer. No differences in RNA quality/ quantity related to the age of RNA samples could be detected. Storage of RNA has been performed at − 80 °C. To further ensure stability of miRNA over time, the same RNA samples independently transcribed and analyzed in RT-qPCR in 2011, 2013 and 2017 have been depicted in Additional file 1: Figure S5.

miRNA microarray

RNA from seven patients and from seven controls was used for miRNA microarray analysis (miRCURY LNA™ microRNA Array, Exiqon A/S, Vedbaek, Denmark), as to the manufacturer's recommendations.

Quantification of mRNA and miRNA expression

Expression of mRNAs and miRNAs was determined using a LightCycler 480 instrument (Roche Diagnostics, Mannheim, Germany) as described in (van der Heide et al. 2016). In all reactions, equal amounts of RNA were used (for miRNA transcription 6 ng of total RNA, for mRNA transcription 1000 ng of total RNA). TaqMan assays and specifications for qPCR primer and probes are given in Tables 6 and 7. Mean Target/Reference and

Target/Reference standard deviation has been calculated for each miRNA/mRNA Target. Expression levels of septic patients are depicted relative to healthy control subjects. Determination of quantification cycles has been performed by the LightCycler software using the second derivative maximum method. Quantification cycle (Cq) cut-offs have been defined for miRNA (Cq 40) and mRNA (Cq 35) quantification. Cq values beyond cut-offs have been considered unspecific. For further validation of microRNA expression, both miR-143 and miR-150 in Pan T-cells and in whole blood cells have been assessed using additional internal controls U44 and U48; results are depicted in Additional file 2: Figure S1, Additional file 3: Figure S2, Additional file 4: Figure S3 and Additional file 5: Figure S4.

Statistical analysis

Student's *t*-test or Mann-Whitney U tests, as appropriate, served for comparisons. Normal distribution was tested using the Kolmogorov-Smirnov test. The quantified array signals were background corrected (Normexp with offset value 10 - Convolution model described by Ritchie et al. (Ritchie et al. 2007)) and normalized using the global Lowess (LOcally WEighted Scatterplot Smoothing) regression algorithm. The obtained values were further analyzed using two-sided Student's t-test and corrected via Benjamini-Hochberg False Discovery Rate (Benjamini and Hochberg 1995). A false discovery value of less than 5% was considered significant.

Statistical analysis was performed using the statistical software R (Developement Core Team 2008) and GraphPad Prism 5.01 (GraphPad Software, Inc., USA). R 3.2.4 was used for predictive modeling and Area-under-the-ROC -curve (AUC) generation. All miRNAs that yielded significant expression differences in T-cells were selected for predictive modeling. R's step-function was used for step-wise backward logistic regression on T-cell samples. AUCs were visualized and generated using the R-package pROC, with

Table 3 T-cell samples: Healthy controls

n	20
Gender (male/female)	12/8 (60%/40%)
Age, years (mean ± SD)	40.5 (± 5.5)

Healthy volunteers were all nonsmokers, without suspect of any acute or chronical disease, blood count and electrolytes within normal limits

Table 5 Whole blood samples: Healthy controls

n	10
Gender (male/female)	6/4 (60%/40%)
Age, years (mean ± SD)	77,8 ± 7,7

Healthy volunteers were age-matched ambulatory patients before elective minor surgeries without suspect of severe chronical disease

Table 6 TaqMan miRNA assays

Target	Assay Nr.
U44	001094
U47	001223
U48	001006
hsa-mir-15a	000389
hsa-mir-16	000391
hsa-mir-93	001090
hsa-mir-143	002249
hsa-mir-150	000473
hsa-mir-223	002295
hsa-mir-342	002260
hsa-mir-424	000604

standard settings for bootstrapping. Vector artwork has been designed using Adobe Illustrator CS5.1 (Adobe Systems Inc., San Jose, CA, USA). Data are depicted as median, 25th and 75th percentile and outliers, if not stated otherwise. P values of less than 0.05 were defined as statistically significant ($*p < 0.05$; $**p < 0.001$).

Results

T-cells of septic patients exhibit a specific miRNA signature pointing to immunoparalysis

To investigate if miRNAs could serve as biomarkers indicative of immunoparalysis in sepsis, we performed a

Table 7 qPCR primer and probes

Target/ Probe/ primer direction	Primer sequence
SDHA #132 FW	5'-GAG GCA GGG TTT AAT ACA GCA-3'
SDHA #132 RV	5'-CCA GTT GTC CTC CTC CAT GT-3'
TBP #87 FW	5'-GAA CAT CAT GGA TCA GAA CAA CA-3'
TBP #87 RV	5'-ATA GGG ATT CCG GGA GTC AT-3'
IL-1β #41 FW	5'GAG GCA CAA GGC ACA ACA G-3'
IL-1β #41 RV	5'-CCA TGG CTG CTT CAG ACA C-3'
IL-2 #65 FW	5'-AAG TTT TAC ATG CCC AAG AAG G-3'
IL-2 #65 RV	5'-AAG TGA AAG TTT TTG CTT TGA GCT A-3'
IL-4 #38 FW	5'-TGC CTC ACA TTG TCA CTG C-3'
IL-4 #38 RV	5'-GCA CAT GCT AGC AGG AAG AAC-3'
IL-10 #67 FW	5'-TGC CTT CAG CAG AGT GAA GA-3'
IL-10 #67 RV	5'-GCA ACC CAG GTA ACC CTT AAA-3'
IL-7R #9 FW	5'-GCT TTT GAG GAC CCA GAT-3'
IL-7R #9 RV	5' AGG CAC TTT ACC TCC ACG-3'
ICOS #2 FW	5'-TTC TGC TTG CGC ATT AAA GTT-3'
ICOS #2 RV	5'-CAT CTC ATA ATT GGC AGA ACC A-3'
TGF-β #31 FW	5'-ACT ACT ACG CCA AGG AGG TCA C-3'
TGF-β #31 RV	5'-TGC TTG AAC TTG TCA TAG ATT TCG-3'

FW forward primer, *RV* reverse primer; # probe number

miRNA microarray using RNA isolated from T-cells of septic patients and from healthy individuals. As depicted in Fig. 1a, 35 miRNAs were identified as being differentially regulated in sepsis versus controls. Out of these, eight miRNAs revealed p-values < 0.01. Importantly, for all of them, a role in immunological processes has previously been described. The direction of regulation in our array analysis strongly points towards immunosuppression: miR-150 and miR-342 - both regulators of pro-inflammatory processes (Robertson et al. 2016; Roderburg et al. 2013) - were downregulated. Conversely, miR-15a, miR-16, miR-93, miR-143, miR-223 and miR-424 - all involved in anti-inflammatory signaling networks (Goodwin et al. 2015; Haneklaus et al. 2013; Honardoost et al. 2015; Liu et al. 2016; Zhao et al. 2014) - showed increased expression levels.

To validate our findings, we analyzed the expression levels of these miRNAs in a larger cohort of septic patients and healthy controls using TaqMan miRNA assays, which confirmed the initial array analysis (Fig. 1b): The expression of pro-inflammatory miR-150 and miR-342 was significantly reduced in septic T-cells, whereas anti-inflammatory miR-15a, miR-16, miR-93, miR-143, miR-223 and miR-424 showed markedly elevated levels (for fold induction analysis see also Additional file 6: Table S1). Taken together, our analysis of T-cells from sepsis patients identified a signature of eight differentially regulated miRNAs that - due to their biological functions - might indicate an immunosuppressive state.

Cytokine expression profile of septic T-cells indicates immunoparalysis

To substantiate our assumption that the observed alterations in miRNA expression patterns are associated with immunoparalysis, we analyzed the expression of a set of characteristic pro- and anti-inflammatory cytokines as well as immune receptors relevant for T-cell immunity in the same set of T-cell samples. Compared to healthy controls, T-cells from septic patients showed significantly reduced expression levels of T-cell growth and survival factor interleukin 2 (IL-2), pro-inflammatory cytokine receptor interleukin 7 receptor (IL-7R) and inducible T-cell co-stimulator (ICOS) (Fig. 2a-c). Transcripts of T_{H2}-cytokines interleukin 4 (IL-4) and interleukin 10 (IL-10) as well as T_{reg}-differentiation promoting transforming growth factor beta (TGF-β) were markedly increased in sepsis samples (Fig. 2d-f). Collectively, we found expression patterns of cytokines, inflammatory mediators and immune receptors that suggest a state of immunoparalysis in T-cells of sepsis patients. These results were in line with the observed miRNA pattern.

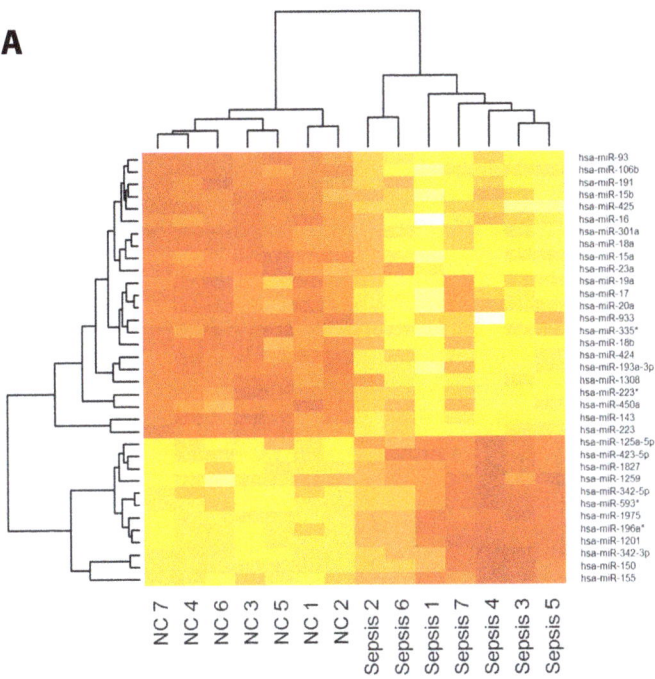

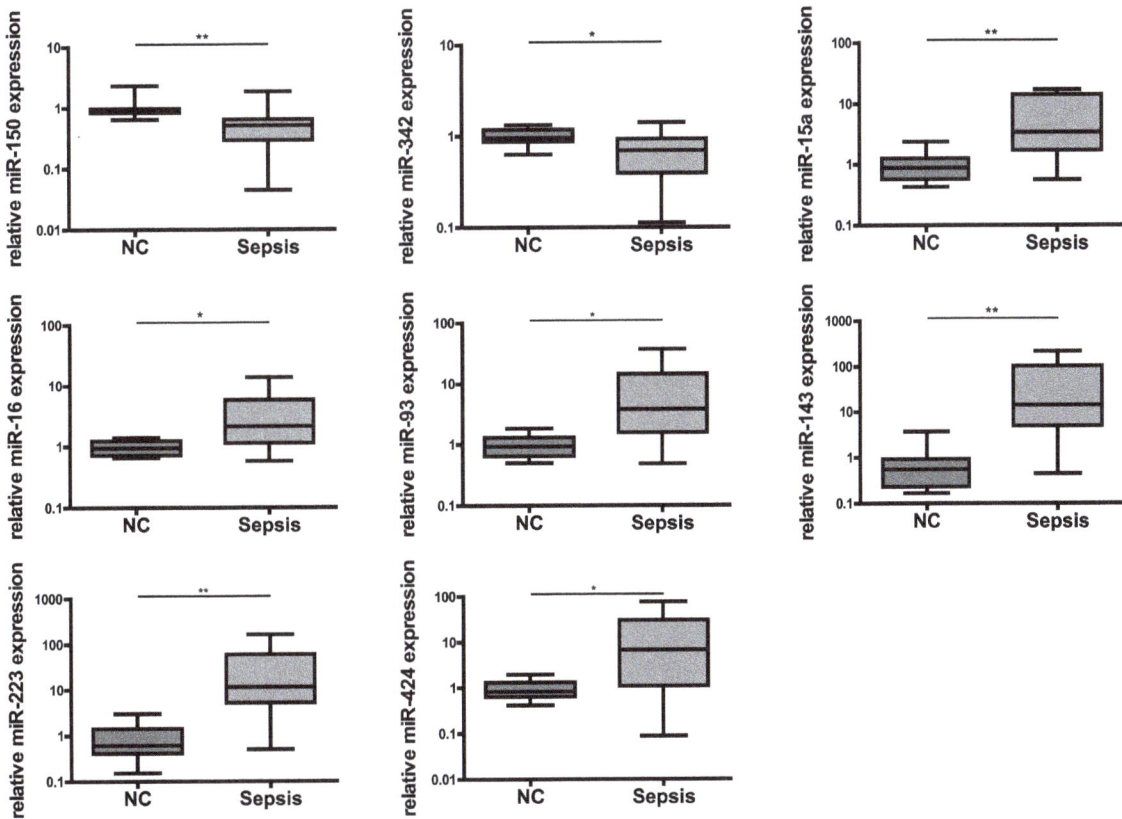

Fig. 1 (See legend on next page.)

(See figure on previous page.)

Fig. 1 Differential expression of miRNA in septic T-cells. **a** MicroRNA Microarray analysis. Heat map showing the differentially expressed miRNAs in sepsis patients as compared to healthy controls, n = 7/7 (NC/Sepsis). RNA was isolated and miRNA array analysis was performed. Yellow colour indicates upregulation of miRNA expression, red colour indicates decreased miRNA levels. **b** MiRNAs in human Pan T-cells of septic patients as compared to healthy controls. Expression levels of miR-150, miR-342, miR-15a, miR-16, miR-93, miR-143, miR-223 and miR-424 in Pan T-cells of septic patients and healthy controls were measured by TaqMan miRNA assays relative to U47. Data are shown as median, 25th and 75th percentile and outliers, n = 10/20 (NC/Sepsis), performed in duplicates. Values represent expression relative to controls, *p < 0.05, **p < 0.001. Quantification cycle (Cq) values for the single miRNAs were in the range of 21 (NC) and 23 (Sepsis) for miR-150, 24 (NC) and 26 (Sepsis) for miR-342, 30 (NC) and 29 (Sepsis) for miR-15a, 23 (NC) and 22 (Sepsis) for miR-16, 30 (NC) and 28 (Sepsis) for miR-93, 34 (NC) and 29 (Sepsis) for miR-143, 26 (NC) and 22 (Sepsis) for miR-223, 36 (NC) and 34 (Sepsis) for miR-424, respectively

MicroRNA-223, microRNA-150 and microRNA-143 are markers of immunosuppression in T-cells

To facilitate a potential clinical use, we next set out to evaluate, whether single miRNAs out of the signature might serve as surrogate marker for detection of sepsis-associated immunosuppression in T-cells. To this end, we used a variable selection procedure, focusing on those miRNAs exhibiting the highest significance with respect to differential expression in sepsis versus healthy controls (miR-223, miR-150 and miR-143). The best model for discrimination in T-cell samples displayed miR-223 with an excellent area under the curve (AUC) of 0.96 (95% CI: 0.9–1.0, Fig. 3). With AUCs of 0.91 (95% CI: 0.8–1.0) and 0.95 (95% CI: 0.88–1.0), miR-150 and miR-143 also revealed as very well performing markers. We next crosschecked whether these three

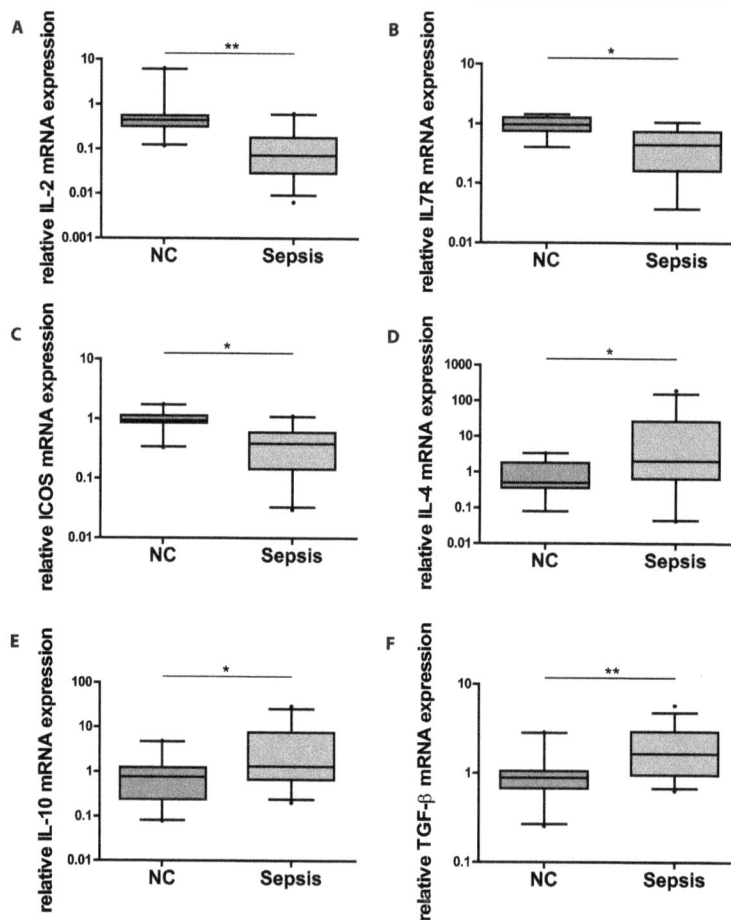

Fig. 2 T-cell immunoparalysis in sepsis. Cytokine and immune receptor expression in T-cells of septic patients as compared to healthy controls. mRNA levels of (**a**) IL-2, (**b**) IL-7R (**c**) ICOS, (**d**) IL-4, (**e**) IL-10 and (**f**) TGF-ß in Pan T-cells of septic patients and healthy controls, respectively, were measured by qPCR relative to reference genes SDHA and TBP. Data are presented as median, 25th and 75th percentile and outliers, measurements were performed in duplicates. Values represent expression relative to controls, *p < 0.05, **p < 0.001. Quantification cycle (Cq) values for the single cytokines and receptors were in the range of 34 (NC) and 36 (Sepsis) for IL-2, 24 (NC) and 25 (Sepsis) for IL7R, 32 (NC) and 33 (Sepsis) for ICOS, 35 (NC) and 32 (Sepsis) for IL-4, 35 (NC) and 33 (Sepsis) for IL-10, 25 (NC) and 24 (Sepsis) for TGF-ß, respectively

miRNAs actually indicate impairment of adaptive immune functions and found highly significant correlations between the expression levels of these three miRNAs and the T-cell specific markers of immunosuppression IL7R and ICOS (miR-143: $r = -0.95$ and -0.78, $p < 0.0005$, miR-150: $r = 0.87$ and 0.66, $p < 0.005$, miR-223: $r = -0,78$ and $-0,64$ $p < 0.05$), and, importantly, with SOFA-scores (miR-143: 0.65, miR-150: -0.7, miR-223: 0.57, $p < 0.01$; see also Table 8) Thus, we suggest that determination of these miRNAs in T-cells provides a useful method to assess immunoparalysis in sepsis.

T-cell specific expression profiles are largely masked in whole blood samples

Purification of T-cells may be difficult to implement into a clinical setting. A widely used approach to obtain patient's immune cell samples for gene expression analysis is the use of whole blood filter systems. While fast and easy to handle, they contain a mixture of cells of innate and adaptive immunity. It is therefore not clear, if T-cell related immunosuppression can be detected in these specimens.

We thus aimed to test, whether those miRNAs identified as markers of T-cell immunosuppression might also perform sufficiently in whole blood samples. We first characterized PAXgene samples of 20 sepsis patients and ten healthy controls with respect to expression of the "immunosuppressive" miRNA signature and mRNA-levels of anti-inflammatory IL4, IL10, TGF-ß and pro-inflammatory "master cytokine" interleukin 1 beta (IL-1β). As shown in Fig. 4a, pro-inflammatory miRNAs miR-150 and miR-342 in Paxgene samples were also diminished in patients with sepsis as compared to healthy controls. Regarding anti-inflammatory miRNAs, only for miR-143 significant up-regulation could be detected, whereas miR-16 and miR-93 exhibited markedly reduced levels and miR-15a, miR-223 and miR-424 showed no relevant alterations at all. Analysis of cytokine expression (Fig. 4b) revealed significant upregulation of pro-inflammatory IL-1β but also of anti-inflammatory TGF-β. T_{H2}-cytokines showed disparate results as well: IL-4 was downregulated, while IL-10 was upregulated.

Taken together, neither a distinct pro- nor anti-inflammatory miRNA/cytokine signature could be detected

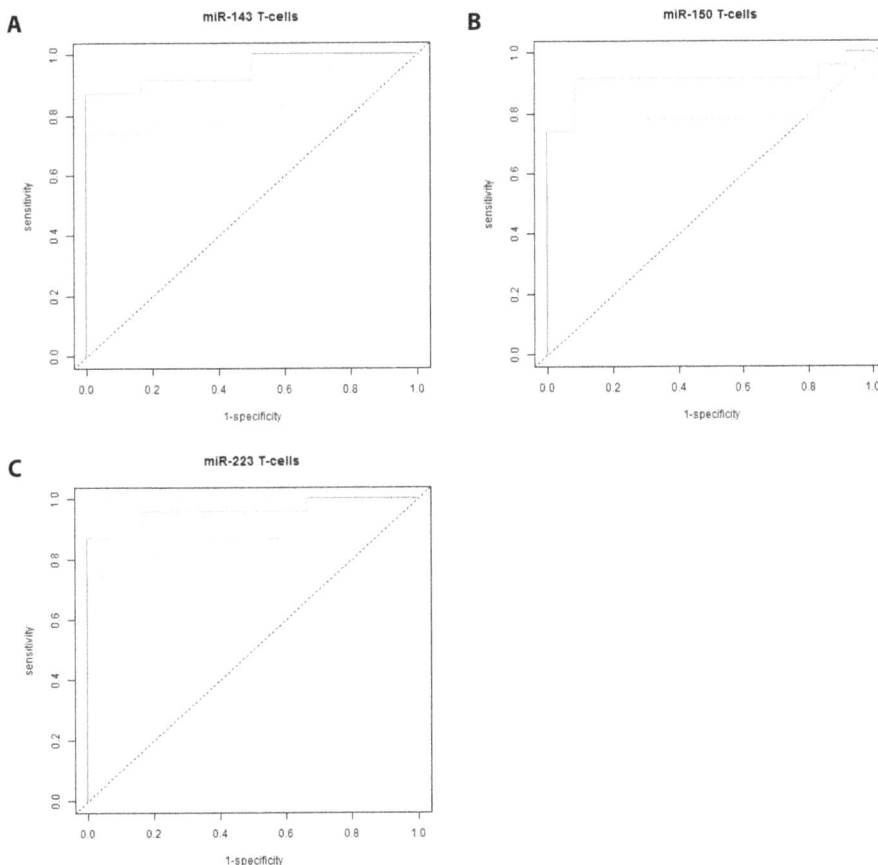

Fig. 3 Discriminatory power of miR-143, miR-150 and miR-223 in T-cells. Predictive modeling and Area-under-the-ROC-curve generation. Candidate miRNAs were selected for predictive modeling: (**a**) miR-143, (**b**) miR-150 and (**c**) miR-223 in T-cells of septic patients as compared to healthy controls, $n = 10/20$ (NC/Sepsis). The shadowed areas denote the confidence interval for the area under the curve

Table 8 correlation analysis miR-143, −150, −223

	ICOS		IL7R		SOFA	
	r	p	r	p	r	p
miR-143	−0,78	< 0,0005	−0,95	< 0,0005	0,65	< 0,01
miR-150	0,66	< 0,005	0,87	< 0,005	−0,7	< 0,01
miR-223	−0,64	< 0,05	−0,78	< 0,05	0,57	< 0,01

in whole blood samples. Since whole blood consists of a mixture of innate and adaptive immune cells - with neutrophils and lymphocytes accounting for a share of approximately 50% and 40%, respectively - miRNA and cytokine expression is likely to represent a net result of simultaneously occurring hyper- and hypoinflammation evoked by both innate and adaptive immunity.

In whole blood samples, miR-143 and miR-150 can serve as markers of T-cell immunosuppression

Still aiming to use whole blood samples for detection of immunosuppression, we hypothesized that it might be a promising approach to focus on miRNAs that i.) are differentially regulated in the same direction in both sample types, and ii.) exhibit markedly lower expression levels in PAXgene samples than in T-cells. In these cases, polymorphonuclear cells (PMN) would not significantly contribute to the expression level of the respective miRNA in whole blood samples. Consequently, the effect seen in T-cells would – albeit diluted – be visible also in whole blood.

These criteria were met by miR-143, miR-150 and miR-342 (Figs. 4a and 5b). Using a variable selection procedure, miR-143 and miR-150 revealed a strong discriminative power (AUCs 0.88 (95% CI: 0.74–1.0) and 0.95 (95% CI: 0.9–1.0), Fig. 5a). MiR-223, the best performing marker in T-cells, was not differentially regulated and – as a typical innate miRNA – was found to be strongly expressed in PAXgene samples. Consequently, the resulting AUC was 0.66 (95% CI: 0.44–0.87, Fig. 5a), thus revealing miR-223 being not suitable as a biomarker for immunoparalysis in whole blood samples.

In summary, we suggest that whole blood analysis of miR-143 and miR-150 might be a promising strategy for the detection of T-cell immunosuppression in sepsis.

Discussion

The dynamics of immune reactions during sepsis has long been regarded as a linear sequence of an initial hyperinflammatory phase followed by prolonged immunosuppression. Recent research, however, has revealed a more complex immunopathology: It is clear now that sepsis is a condition of constant immune dysfunction with alternating periods of pro- and anti-inflammatory predominance (Boomer et al. 2014), where hyperinflammation is mainly driven by innate immune cells, whereas immunoparalysis

is a characteristic reaction of the adaptive immune system (Xiao et al. 2011; Hotchkiss et al. 2013). Immunosuppression has turned out the leading cause of death in sepsis (Boomer et al. 2011). While modern treatment concepts of sepsis are often capable to control hyperinflammation, therapy of immunoparalysis remains difficult and reliable methods allowing its early detection are lacking. In this situation, identification of miRNAs that are suitable to serve as biomarkers of a compromised immunity might be a promising approach.

We here identified a miRNA signature of eight differentially expressed miRNAs in T-cells of sepsis patients, which are indicative of sepsis-associated immunoparalysis. Of these miRNAs, miR-143 and miR-150 also performed well in whole blood samples: With AUCs of 0.88 (95% CI: 0.74–1.0) and 0.95 (95% CI: 0.9–1.0), respectively, they may even serve as surrogate biomarkers to assess septic T-cell immunoparalysis in a clinical setting, where the selection of T-cells is not feasible. These findings may open up new diagnostic perspectives for septic immune dysfunction.

MiRNAs offer unique features, which render them attractive as clinical biomarkers: They are expressed in disease-specific patterns, they are remarkably stable – even when released extracellularly – and they can easily be detected in virtually all tissues and body fluids (Benz et al. 2016). A considerable number of studies investigating miRNAs as biomarker in sepsis have been published in the last few years. In these studies, the expression of miRNAs was profiled in various tissue samples (plasma/serum/whole blood/purified blood cells) (Ho et al. 2016). Results, however, were heterogeneous with significant differences in expression profiles, e.g. miR-15/−16 (Goodwin et al. 2015; Wang et al. 2012a; Wang et al. 2014a; Wang et al. 2015; Wang et al. 2012b; Wang et al. 2012c; Wang et al. 2014b), miR-146 (Wang et al. 2010; Wu et al. 2014; Wang et al. 2013), miR-150 (Roderburg et al. 2013; Vasilescu et al. 2009; Ma et al. 2013) and miR-223 (Wang et al. 2012a; Wang et al. 2015; Wang et al. 2012c; Wang et al. 2010). Thus, commonly accepted sepsis biomarkers are yet to be identified, in particular with respect to the discrimination between the hyperinflammatory and the immunoparalytic phase of the syndrome. As different types of human immune cells express cell-type-specific "miRNomes" (Leidinger et al. 2014; Ludwig et al. 2016; Wang et al. 2012d), evaluation of miRNAs as sepsis biomarkers in whole blood samples, serum, plasma or PBMCs is likely to yield mixtures of expression patterns. Moreover, a potential release of different miRNA signatures by acute or chronic co-morbidities may further hamper the diagnostic values of these approaches (Chen et al. 2008).

We aimed at avoiding such confounders by directly assessing the miRNA expression profile in T-cells using

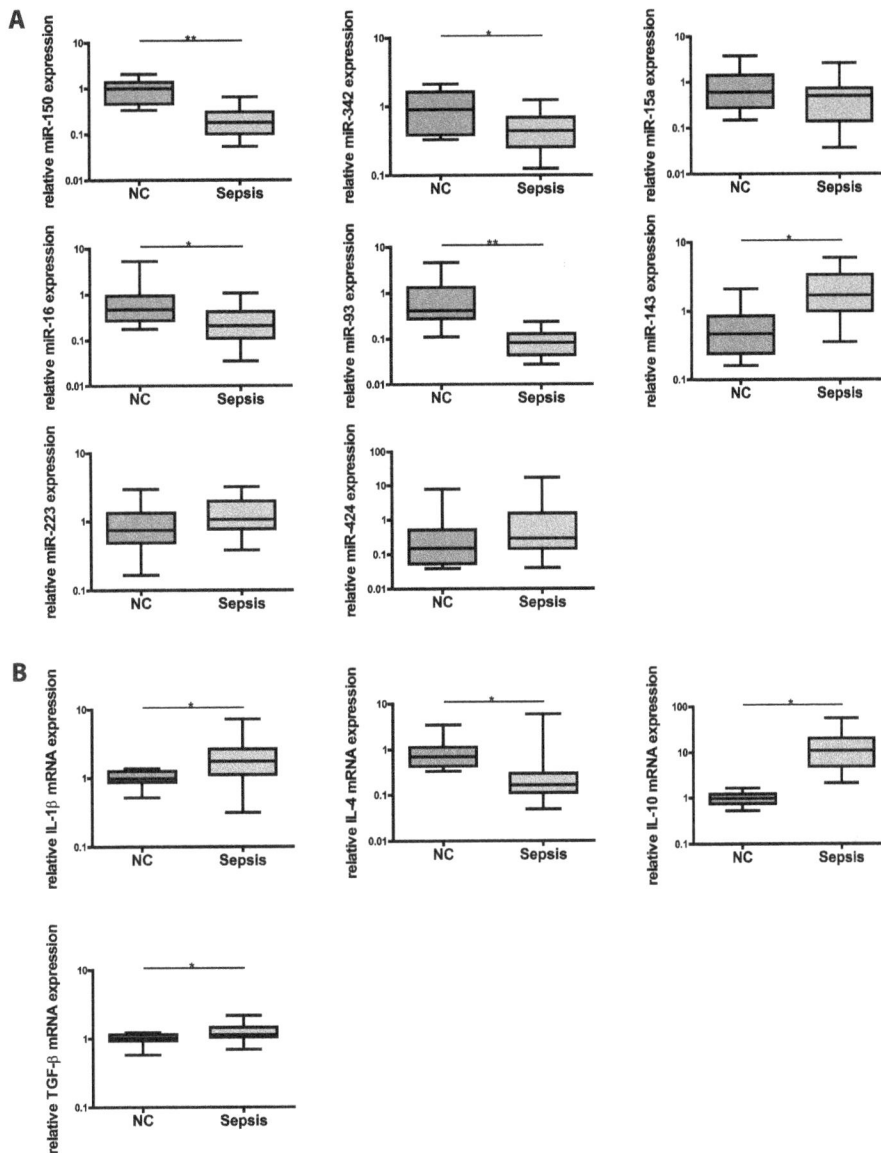

Fig. 4 Simultaneous hyper- and hypoinflammation in whole blood of septic patients. **a** MiRNA expression in human whole blood obtained from septic patients as compared to healthy controls. Expression levels of miR-150, miR-342, miR-15a, miR-16, miR-93, miR-143, miR-223 and miR-424 were assessed by TaqMan miRNA assays relative to U47. Data are shown as median, 25th and 75th percentile and outliers, n = 10/20 (NC/Sepsis) performed in duplicates. Values represent expression relative to controls, *$p < 0.05$, **$p < 0.001$. Quantification cycle (Cq) values for the single miRNAs were in the range of 24 (NC) and 26 (Sepsis) for miR-150, 26 (NC) and 27 (Sepsis) for miR-342, 30 (NC) and 31 (Sepsis) for miR-15a, 21 (NC) and 23 (Sepsis) for miR-16, 26 (NC) and 29 (Sepsis) for miR-93, 34 (NC) and 33 (Sepsis) for miR-143, 21 (NC and Sepsis) for miR-223, 40 (NC) and 39 (Sepsis) for miR-424, respectively. **b** Cytokine expression in human whole blood obtained from septic patients as compared to healthy controls. mRNA levels of IL-4, IL-1β, IL-10 and TGF-β were measured by qPCR relative to reference genes SDHA and TBP. Data are shown as median, 25th and 75th percentile and outliers, n = 10/20 (NC/Sepsis) performed in duplicates. Values represent expression relative to controls, *p < 0.05, **$p < 0.001$. Quantification cycle (Cq) values for the single cytokines and receptors were in the range of 32 (NC) and 35 (Sepsis) for IL-4, 27 (NC and Sepsis) for IL-1β, 35 (NC) and 32 (Sepsis) for IL-10, 24 (NC) and 25 (Sepsis) for TGF-β, respectively

a whole transcriptome approach, and detected eight highly differentially expressed miRNAs, which were subsequently validated in a larger cohort of sepsis patients by qPCR. The observed miRNA expression strongly indicates a state of immunosuppression: MiR-150 and miR-342, both exerting proinflammatory action, were markedly downregulated. While miR-150 targets IL-10 and IL-18 in leukocytes, microRNA-342 contributes to broad host cell immunity against infection (Robertson et al. 2016). Also, low serum levels of miR-150 in critically ill patients have been associated with an unfavourable outcome, and miR-150has been discusssed as prognostic

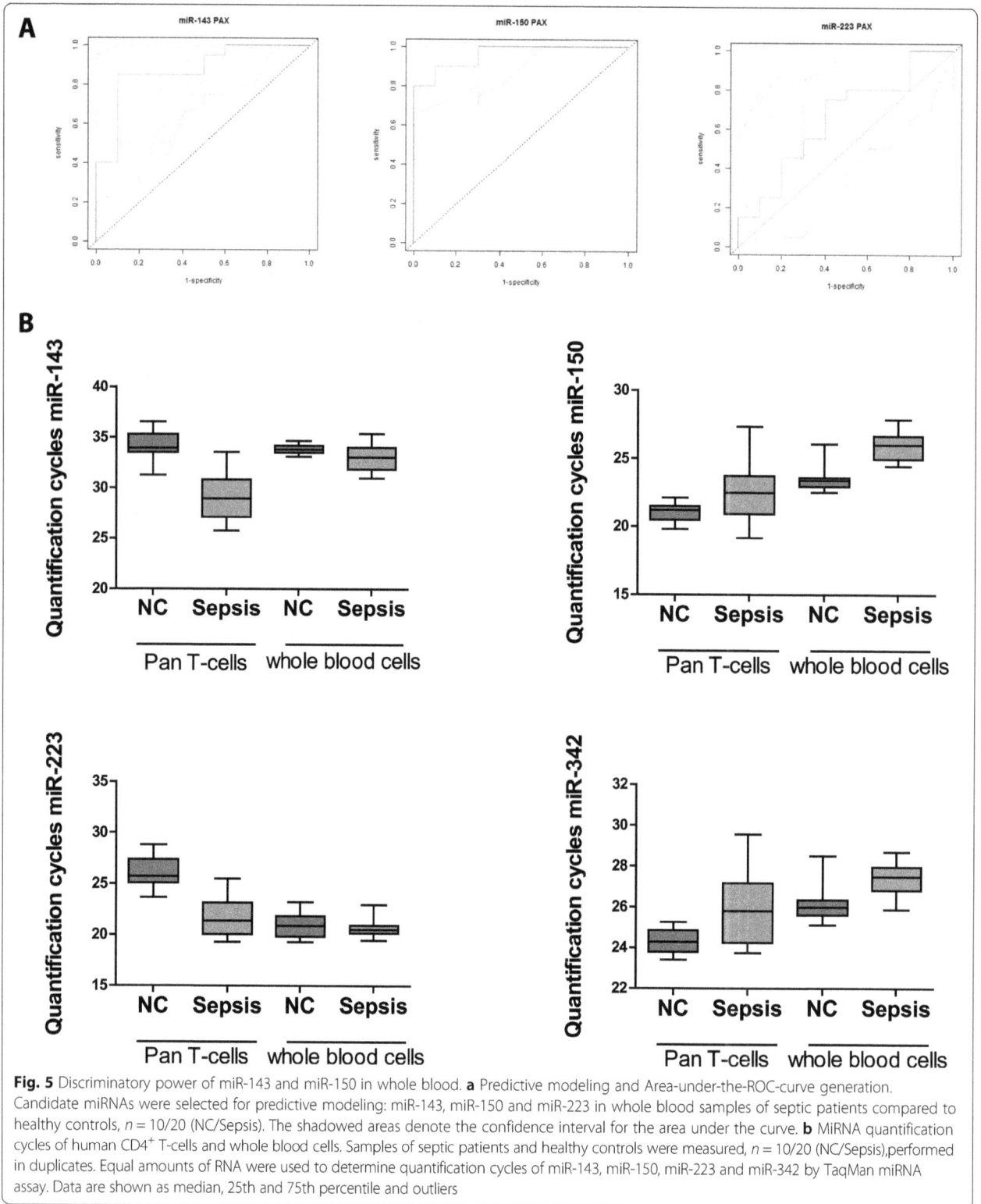

Fig. 5 Discriminatory power of miR-143 and miR-150 in whole blood. **a** Predictive modeling and Area-under-the-ROC-curve generation. Candidate miRNAs were selected for predictive modeling: miR-143, miR-150 and miR-223 in whole blood samples of septic patients compared to healthy controls, n = 10/20 (NC/Sepsis). The shadowed areas denote the confidence interval for the area under the curve. **b** MiRNA quantification cycles of human CD4[+] T-cells and whole blood cells. Samples of septic patients and healthy controls were measured, n = 10/20 (NC/Sepsis),performed in duplicates. Equal amounts of RNA were used to determine quantification cycles of miR-143, miR-150, miR-223 and miR-342 by TaqMan miRNA assay. Data are shown as median, 25th and 75th percentile and outliers

marker (leukocytes and plasma) and for discrimination between sepsis and SIRS (whole blood) (Roderburg et al. 2013; Vasilescu et al. 2009; Ma et al. 2013). The detected downregulation of both miRNAs thus may lead to a restriction of

T-cell effector functions. Six further miRNAs – miR-15a, miR-16, miR-93, miR-143, miR-223 and miR-424, mainly exhibiting anti-inflammatory or anti-proliferative functions – were upregulated in septic T-cells. MiR-15a and miR-16 have been shown to downregulate NF-κB signaling pathways and to reduce pro-inflammatory cytokine production in T-cells via downregulation of CXCL10 (Goodwin et al. 2015; Liu et al. 2016). Moreover, they are known to exert pro-apoptotic effects in lymphocytes and granulocytes (Precone et al. 2013). MiR-93 is proposed to suppress T_{H17}-cells (Honardoost et al. 2015), whereas miR-143 was reported to exhibit immunosuppressive functions via targeting COX-2 and TAK-1 (Zhao et al. 2014) and has been suggested as biomarker to distinguish between sepsis and SIRS (Han et al. 2016). (Zhao et al. 2014). MicroRNA-223 is interfering with several important inflammatory pathways, e.g. STAT1/3,NF-κB, and controls the NLRP3 inflammasome (Haneklaus et al. 2013). Collectively, upregulation of these miRNAs is likely to contribute to an immunosuppressive state.

Hallmarks of immunosuppression during sepsis have been defined in recent studies (Hamers et al. 2015): Lymphocytes express altered cytokine expression profiles with reduced levels of pro-inflammatory cytokines, enhanced production of anti-inflammatory cytokines (e.g. IL-10 and TGF-β), and receptor expression patterns favoring inhibitory receptors (Boomer et al. 2012; Gogos et al. 2000). Moreover, increased apoptosis rates, diminished IL-7 receptor expression and low levels of IL-2, indicating a reduced proliferative potential, have been found (Lang et al. 2005; Wherry and Kurachi 2015). In line with these data, we detected increased levels of anti-inflammatory cytokines IL-4, IL-10 and TGF-β as well as a reduction of IL-7R in isolated T-cells of sepsis patients, indicating a compromised T-cell immune status. Also, a substantial loss of IL-2 mRNA and diminished levels of T-cell inflammatory response regulation factor ICOS clearly suggest reduced survival and activity of effector T-cells (Boomer et al. 2014; Hotchkiss et al. 2013; Wikenheiser and Stumhofer 2016). Thus, in all sepsis patients, signs of immunoparalysis within the adaptive immunity could be detected. The extent, however, was inter-individually different and quantification of immunosuppression may provide valuable information to assess the actual state of the individual patient - also during the course of the disease - and to define optimal treatment strategies. In this dynamic situation, our miRNA signature could be a fast and reliable tool.

As requirement for simultaneous quantification of eight miRNAs might impede the clinical use of our approach, we next aimed at identifying key markers of immunosuppression. Indeed, miR-223, miR-143 and miR-150 exhibited an outstanding predictive power with AUCs of 0.96, 0.95 and 0.90. Importantly, these miRNAs significantly correlated with T-cell specific markers of immunosuppression and with SOFA scores. Therefore,

all three miRNAs might be potential candidates to evaluate T-cell associated immunoparalysis in sepsis.

Even when limited to measurement of single miRNAs with sufficient discriminatory power, a T-cell-based approach may not be feasible in a clinical routine situation. In this setting, the commonly applied method is the use of filter systems, enabling a fast and easy-to-handle approach to obtain patient's blood samples for gene expression analyses. It has to be kept in mind, however, that these filters retain a mixture of both innate and adaptive immune cells (with PMN, T-cells, and Monocytes making up for the largest shares of cells with 50%, 40%, and 10%) and it therefore is not clear, whether T-cell immunoparalysis is assessable in these samples. In our analyses, indeed, cytokine and miRNA expression profiles exhibited signs of both immune activation and suppression, which is likely to represent the net result of simultaneously occurring but divergent activation patterns of innate and adaptive immune cells, thereby masking T-cell specific effects. These findings are in line with previous studies showing that human leukocytes during sepsis do not express distinct pro- or anti-inflammatory profiles (Tang et al. 2010). Notwithstanding that, we assumed that innate immune cells would not significantly impair the diagnostic use of T-cell specific miRNAs in whole blood samples, if the expression levels of the respective miRNAs in PMN and Monocytes were markedly lower compared to T-cells. Indeed, we identified miR-143 and miR-150 as extremely well performing markers indicative of T-cell immunosuppression not only in T-cells but also in PAXgene samples: They were differentially regulated in the same direction in both sample types, they exhibited low expression levels in innate cells and - after applying a variable selection procedure - they showed excellent discriminatory power with AUCs of 0.88 and 0.95, respectively, also in PAXgene samples. Nevertheless, biases caused by larger shifts in lymphocyte numbers may occur when using PAXgene. As we included both immunosuppressive (upregulated) miR-143 and proinflammatory (downregulated) miR-150 into our analyses, such distortions could easily be detected. In our series, however, this phenomenon was not observed.

Medical and ethical restriction have limited the spectrum of possible molecular analyses of this pilot study:

1. We could only analyze mRNA and miRNA expression levels, additional analysis of protein levels or quantification of T-cell surface markers was not possible. However, as reported in a recent study, mRNA levels of the most relevant cytokines in activated T cells are translated into comparable protein levels (Mohnle et al. 2015).

2. We were only able to investigate Pan T-cells, which did not allow specifying septic T-cell immunoparalysis with respect to T-cell subsets. However, relatively stable CD4/CD8 ratios and unaltered CD4+ proportions in peripheral blood during sepsis have been described in several studies (Francois et al. 2018; Inoue et al. 2014).

3. Both patient groups differ in age, since the samples have been provided from ICUs of different countries and with different clinical focus. However, we analyzed the study cohorts independently with respect to the validity of our T cell miRNA markers. Remarkably, despite different age-distributions, both miR-143 and miR-150 performed comparably well in either group thus indicating age-independency.

4. Sampling of patients was performed over a long course of time. However, as microRNA is known for its outstanding stability (Jung et al. 2010; Mraz et al. 2009), bias due to sample degradation is unlikely. Furthermore, storage has been performed properly, RNA analysis showed no major differences in quality or quantity related to the age of RNA samples and additional RT-qPCR analyses revealed no significant alterations in microRNA level over time (Additional file 1: Figure S5).

Conclusions

Efficient therapeutic interventions in septic patients are currently hampered by a lack of reliable biomarkers for diagnosis of sepsis-associated immune dysfunction. Our pilot study identifies miR-143 and miR-150 as candidate markers for detection of T-cell immunosuppression and thus contributes to the development of innovative strategies using miRNAs as biomarkers of a compromised immune status during sepsis. Importantly, these markers can be determined in whole blood samples, which facilitates a future clinical use. Large-scale, multicenter, prospective evaluations are now required to further elaborate our diagnostic approach and to enable its implementation into clinical routine.

Additional files

Additional file 1: Figure S5. U47 Quantification cycles for samples analyzed in 2011, 2013 and 2017. Quantification cycles of U47 in (A) healthy controls and (B) septic patients were measured by TaqMan miRNA assays. The same RNA samples have been used for independent transcription and RT-qPCR analysis in the years 2011, 2013 and 2017, all experiments performed in duplicates. (EPS 1313 kb)

Additional file 2: Figure S1. Expression of microRNA-143 in T-cell samples using additional internal controls. Expression levels of miR-143 in Pan T-cells of septic patients and healthy controls were measured by TaqMan miRNA assays relative to (A) U44, (B) U47, (C) U48 and (D) U44/U47/U48. Data are shown as median, 25th and 75th percentile and outliers, $n = 5/10$ (NC/Sepsis), performed in duplicates. Values represent expression relative to controls, $*p < 0.05$, $**p < 0.001$. (EPS 747 kb)

Additional file 3: Figure S2. Expression of microRNA-150 in T-cell samples using additional internal controls. Expression levels of miR-150 in Pan T-cells of septic patients and healthy controls were measured by TaqMan miRNA assays relative to (A) U44, (B) U47, (C) U48 and (D) U44/U47/U48. Data are shown as median, 25th and 75th percentile and outliers, $n = 5/10$ (NC/Sepsis), performed in duplicates. Values represent expression relative to controls, $*p < 0.05$, $**p < 0.001$. (EPS 749 kb)

Additional file 4: Figure S3. Expression of microRNA-143 in whole blood samples using additional internal controls. Expression levels of miR-143 in whole blood cells of septic patients and healthy controls were measured by TaqMan miRNA assays relative to (A) U44, (B) U47, (C) U48 and (D) U44/U47/U48. Data are shown as median, 25th and 75th percentile and outliers, $n = 5/10$ (NC/Sepsis), performed in duplicates. Values represent expression relative to controls, $*p < 0.05$, $**p < 0.001$. (EPS 746 kb)

Additional file 5: Figure S4. Expression of microRNA-150 in whole blood samples using additional internal controls. Expression levels of miR-150 in whole blood cells of septic patients and healthy controls were measured by TaqMan miRNA assays relative to (A) U44, (B) U47, (C) U48 and (D) U44/U47/U48. Data are shown as median, 25th and 75th percentile and outliers, $n = 5/10$ (NC/Sepsis), performed in duplicates. Values represent expression relative to controls, $*p < 0.05$, $**p < 0.001$. (EPS 734 kb)

Additional file 6: Table S1. Fold difference miRNA expression in T-cells of septic patients compared to healthy controls. **Table S2.** Positive and negative predictive values for miR-143/– 150/ -223. **Table S3.** Benjamini–Hochberg correction: p-value and false discovery rate. (DOCX 19 kb)

Acknowledgements

The authors thank Jessica Rink, Gaby Gröger and Gudrun Prangenberg for their expert technical assistance.

Funding

This work has been funded by the Charles-Evans-Foundation, New Jersey, USA. Sebastian Weis and Michael Bauer are supported by the Integrated Research and Treatment Center - Center for Sepsis Control and Care (CSCC) at the Jena University Hospital. The CSCC is funded by the German Ministry of Education and Research (BMBF No. 01EO1002; 01EO1502). The collection of the Greek cohort was funded by the Hellenic Institute for the Study of Sepsis.

The sponsors had no role in study design or collection, analysis and interpretation of data, nor in writing or submission of this manuscript.

Authors' contributions

MP, HS and KS designed the study, analyzed the data and wrote the manuscript. HC performed all bioinformatics and statistical analyses. HM and BJ participated in study design, experimental analyses, and interpretation of data.WS, DG, BM and GB collected data, and participated in interpretation of all experiments. All authors have read and approved the final manuscript.

Competing interests

The authors declare that they have no competing interests.

Author details

Department of Anaesthesiology and Intensive Care Medicine, University Hospital, Ludwig Maximilian University (LMU), Marchioninistraße 15, 81377 Munich, Germany. [2]Walter-Brendel-Center of Experimental Medicine, Ludwig Maximilian University (LMU), Munich, Germany. [3]Department of

Anaesthesiology and Intensive Care Medicine, Friedrich-Schiller University, Jena, Germany. [4]Center for Sepsis Control and Care, Jena University Hospital, Jena, Germany. [5]Center for Infectious Disease and Infection Control, Jena University Hospital, Jena, Germany. [6]2nd Department of Critical Care Medicine, ATTIKON University Hospital, National and Kapodistrian University of Athens, Athens, Greece. [7]4th Department of Internal Medicine, ATTIKON University Hospital, National and Kapodistrian University of Athens, Athens, Greece.

References

Bartel DP. MicroRNAs: genomics, biogenesis, mechanism, and function. Cell. 2004; 116:281–97.

Bartel DP. MicroRNAs: target recognition and regulatory functions. Cell. 2009;136: 215–33.

Benjamini Y, Hochberg Y. Controlling the false discovery rate: a practical and powerful approach to multiple testing. J R Stat Soc Ser B Methodol. 1995;57: 289–300.

Benz F, Roy S, Trautwein C, Roderburg C, Luedde T. Circulating MicroRNAs as biomarkers for Sepsis. Int J Mol Sci. 2016;17:78.

Bone RC, Sprung CL, Sibbald WJ. Definitions for sepsis and organ failure. Crit Care Med. 1992;20:724–6.

Boomer JS, Green JM, Hotchkiss RS. The changing immune system in sepsis: is individualized immuno-modulatory therapy the answer? Virulence. 2014;5:45–56.

Boomer JS, Shuherk-Shaffer J, Hotchkiss RS, Green JM. A prospective analysis of lymphocyte phenotype and function over the course of acute sepsis. Crit Care. 2012;16:R112.

Boomer JS, et al. Immunosuppression in patients who die of sepsis and multiple organ failure. JAMA. 2011;306:2594–605.

Cavaillon JM, Annane D. Compartmentalization of the inflammatory response in sepsis and SIRS. J Endotoxin Res. 2006;12:151–70.

Chen X, et al. Characterization of microRNAs in serum: a novel class of biomarkers for diagnosis of cancer and other diseases. Cell Res. 2008;18:997–1006.

Developement Core Team R. R: a language and environment for statistical computing. Vienna: R Foundation for Statistical Computing; 2008.

Ecker S, et al. Genome-wide analysis of differential transcriptional and epigenetic variability across human immune cell types. Genome Biol. 2017;18:18.

Francois B, et al. Interleukin-7 restores lymphocytes in septic shock: the IRIS-7 randomized clinical trial. JCI Insight. 2018;3:5.

Gogos CA, Drosou E, Bassaris HP, Skoutelis A. Pro- versus anti-inflammatory cytokine profile in patients with severe sepsis: a marker for prognosis and future therapeutic options. J Infect Dis. 2000;181:176–80.

Goodwin AJ, et al. Plasma levels of microRNA are altered with the development of shock in human sepsis: an observational study. Crit Care. 2015;19:440.

Hamers L, Kox M, Pickkers P. Sepsis-induced immunoparalysis: mechanisms, markers, and treatment options. Minerva Anestesiol. 2015;81:426–39.

Han Y, Dai QC, Shen HL, Zhang XW. Diagnostic value of elevated serum miRNA-143 levels in sepsis. J Int Med Res. 2016;44:875–81.

Haneklaus M, Gerlic M, O'Neill LA, Masters SL. miR-223: infection, inflammation and cancer. J Intern Med. 2013;274:215–26.

Hata A. Functions of microRNAs in cardiovascular biology and disease. Annu Rev Physiol. 2013;75:69–93.

Hirschberger S, Hinske LC, Kreth S. MiRNAs: dynamic regulators of immune cell functions in inflammation and cancer. Cancer Lett. 2018;431:11–21.

Ho J, et al. The involvement of regulatory non-coding RNAs in sepsis: a systematic review. Crit Care. 2016;20:383.

Honardoost MA, Naghavian R, Ahmadinejad F, Hosseini A, Ghaedi K. Integrative computational mRNA-miRNA interaction analyses of the autoimmune-deregulated miRNAs and well-known Th17 differentiation regulators: an attempt to discover new potential miRNAs involved in Th17 differentiation. Gene. 2015;572:153–62.

Hotchkiss RS, Monneret G, Payen D. Sepsis-induced immunosuppression: from cellular dysfunctions to immunotherapy. Nat Rev Immunol. 2013;13:862–74.

Inoue S, et al. Persistent inflammation and T cell exhaustion in severe sepsis in the elderly. Crit Care. 2014;18:R130.

Jung HJ, Suh Y. Circulating miRNAs in ageing and ageing-related diseases. J Genet Genomics. 2014;41:465–72.

Jung M, et al. Robust microRNA stability in degraded RNA preparations from human tissue and cell samples. Clin Chem. 2010;56:998–1006.

Kingsley SM, Bhat BV. Role of microRNAs in sepsis. Inflamm Res. 2017;66(7):553–69.

Kreth S, Hubner M, Hinske LC. MicroRNAs as clinical biomarkers and therapeutic tools in perioperative medicine. Anesth Analg. 2017;126(2):670–81.

Landelle C, et al. Low monocyte human leukocyte antigen-DR is independently associated with nosocomial infections after septic shock. Intensive Care Med. 2010;36:1859–66.

Lang KS, et al. Inverse correlation between IL-7 receptor expression and CD8 T cell exhaustion during persistent antigen stimulation. Eur J Immunol. 2005;35:738–45.

Leidinger P, Backes C, Meder B, Meese E, Keller A. The human miRNA repertoire of different blood compounds. BMC Genomics. 2014;15:474.

Liu XF, et al. MiR-15a contributes abnormal immune response in myasthenia gravis by targeting CXCL10. Clin Immunol. 2016;164:106–13.

Ludwig N, et al. Distribution of miRNA expression across human tissues. Nucleic Acids Res. 2016;44:3865–77.

Ma Y, et al. Genome-wide sequencing of cellular microRNAs identifies a combinatorial expression signature diagnostic of sepsis. PLoS One. 2013;8:e75918.

Mohnle P, et al. MicroRNA-146a controls Th1-cell differentiation of human CD4+ T lymphocytes by targeting PRKCepsilon. Eur J Immunol. 2015;45:260–72.

Mraz M, Malinova K, Mayer J, Pospisilova S. MicroRNA isolation and stability in stored RNA samples. Biochem Biophys Res Commun. 2009;390:1–4.

O'Connell RM, Rao DS, Baltimore D. microRNA regulation of inflammatory responses. Annu Rev Immunol. 2012;30:295–312.

Palmer C, Diehn M, Alizadeh AA, Brown PO. Cell-type specific gene expression profiles of leukocytes in human peripheral blood. BMC Genomics. 2006;7:115.

Pencheva N, Tavazoie SF. Control of metastatic progression by microRNA regulatory networks. Nat Cell Biol. 2013;15:546–54.

Peronnet E, et al. Association between mRNA expression of CD74 and IL10 and risk of ICU-acquired infections: a multicenter cohort study. Intensive Care Med. 2017;43:1013–20.

Precone V, et al. Different changes in mitochondrial apoptotic pathway in lymphocytes and granulocytes in cirrhotic patients with sepsis. Liver Int. 2013;33:834–42.

Ritchie ME, et al. A comparison of background correction methods for two-colour microarrays. Bioinformatics. 2007;23:2700–7.

Robertson KA, et al. An interferon regulated MicroRNA provides broad cell-intrinsic antiviral immunity through multihit host-directed targeting of the sterol pathway. PLoS Biol. 2016;14:e1002364.

Roderburg C, et al. Circulating microRNA-150 serum levels predict survival in patients with critical illness and sepsis. PLoS One. 2013;8:e54612.

Samraj RS, Zingarelli B, Wong HR. Role of biomarkers in sepsis care. Shock. 2013; 40:358–65.

Singer M, et al. The third international consensus definitions for Sepsis and septic shock (Sepsis-3). JAMA. 2016;315:801–10.

Tang BM, Huang SJ, McLean AS. Genome-wide transcription profiling of human sepsis: a systematic review. Crit Care. 2010;14:R237.

van der Heide V, Mohnle P, Rink J, Briegel J, Kreth S. Down-regulation of MicroRNA-31 in CD4+ T cells contributes to immunosuppression in human Sepsis by promoting TH2 skewing. Anesthesiology. 2016;124:908–22.

Vasilescu C, et al. MicroRNA fingerprints identify miR-150 as a plasma prognostic marker in patients with sepsis. PLoS One. 2009;4:e7405.

Wang H, Yu B, Deng J, Jin Y, Xie L. Serum miR-122 correlates with short-term mortality in sepsis patients. Crit Care. 2014b;18:704.

Wang H, et al. Serum microRNA signatures identified by Solexa sequencing predict sepsis patients' mortality: a prospective observational study. PLoS One. 2012a;7:e38885.

Wang H, et al. Evidence for serum miR-15a and miR-16 levels as biomarkers that distinguish sepsis from systemic inflammatory response syndrome in human subjects. Clin Chem Lab Med. 2012b;50:1423–8.

Wang HJ, et al. Four serum microRNAs identified as diagnostic biomarkers of sepsis. J Trauma Acute Care Surg. 2012c;73:850–4.

Wang HJ, et al. Serum miR-122 levels are related to coagulation disorders in sepsis patients. Clin Chem Lab Med. 2014a;52:927–33.

Wang JF, et al. Serum miR-146a and miR-223 as potential new biomarkers for sepsis. Biochem Biophys Res Commun. 2010;394:184–8.

Wang K, et al. Comparing the MicroRNA spectrum between serum and plasma. PLoS One. 2012d;7:e41561.

Wang L, et al. Differential expression of plasma miR-146a in sepsis patients compared with non-sepsis-SIRS patients. Exp Ther Med. 2013;5:1101–4.

Wang X, et al. miR-15a/16 are upreuglated in the serum of neonatal sepsis patients and inhibit the LPS-induced inflammatory pathway. Int J Clin Exp Med. 2015;8:5683–90.

Weiland M, Gao XH, Zhou L, Mi QS. Small RNAs have a large impact: circulating microRNAs as biomarkers for human diseases. RNA Biol. 2012;9:850–9.

Wherry EJ, Kurachi M. Molecular and cellular insights into T cell exhaustion. Nat Rev Immunol. 2015;15:486–99.

Wikenheiser DJ, Stumhofer JS. ICOS co-stimulation: friend or foe? Front Immunol. 2016;7:304.

Wu Y, et al. Relationship between expression of microRNA and inflammatory cytokines plasma level in pediatric patients with sepsis. Zhonghua Er Ke Za Zhi. 2014;52:28–33.

Xiao W, et al. A genomic storm in critically injured humans. J Exp Med. 2011;208:2581–90.

Zhao X, et al. The toll-like receptor 3 ligand, poly(I:C), improves immunosuppressive function and therapeutic effect of mesenchymal stem cells on sepsis via inhibiting MiR-143. Stem Cells. 2014;32:521–33.

Permissions

The contributors of this book come from diverse backgrounds, making this book a truly international effort. This book will bring forth new frontiers with its revolutionizing research information and detailed analysis of the nascent developments around the world.

We would like to thank all the contributing authors for lending their expertise to make the book truly unique. They have played a crucial role in the development of this book. Without their invaluable contributions this book wouldn't have been possible. They have made vital efforts to compile up to date information on the varied aspects of this subject to make this book a valuable addition to the collection of many professionals and students.

This book was conceptualized with the vision of imparting up-to-date information and advanced data in this field. To ensure the same, a matchless editorial board was set up. Every individual on the board went through rigorous rounds of assessment to prove their worth. After which they invested a large part of their time researching and compiling the most relevant data for our readers.

The editorial board has been involved in producing this book since its inception. They have spent rigorous hours researching and exploring the diverse topics which have resulted in the successful publishing of this book. They have passed on their knowledge of decades through this book. To expedite this challenging task, the publisher supported the team at every step. A small team of assistant editors was also appointed to further simplify the editing procedure and attain best results for the readers.

Apart from the editorial board, the designing team has also invested a significant amount of their time in understanding the subject and creating the most relevant covers. They scrutinized every image to scout for the most suitable representation of the subject and create an appropriate cover for the book.

The publishing team has been an ardent support to the editorial, designing and production team. Their endless efforts to recruit the best for this project, has resulted in the accomplishment of this book. They are a veteran in the field of academics and their pool of knowledge is as vast as their experience in printing. Their expertise and guidance has proved useful at every step. Their uncompromising quality standards have made this book an exceptional effort. Their encouragement from time to time has been an inspiration for everyone.

The publisher and the editorial board hope that this book will prove to be a valuable piece of knowledge for researchers, students, practitioners and scholars across the globe.

List of Contributors

Zhao Yan, Jinyu Zhu, Lifeng Yu, Dawei Zhang, Yanwu Liu, Chongfei Yang, Qingsheng Zhu and Xiaorui Cao
PLA Institute of Orthopaedics, Xijing Hospital, Fourth Military Medical University, Xi'an 710032, China

Xiaoxi Tian
Emergency department of Tangdu Hospital, Fourth Military Medical University, Xi'an 710038, China

Zifan Lu
State Key Laboratory of Cancer Biology, Department of Pharmacogenomics, Fourth Military Medical University, Xi'an 710032, China

Hong Chen, Wenjun Zhou, Yuting Ruan, Ningning Xu, Rongping Chen, Rui Yang, Jia Sun and Zhen Zhang
Department of Endocrinology, Zhujiang Hospital, Southern Medical University, 253, Gongyedadao Middle, Guangzhou, Guangdong 510282, People's Republic of China

Lei Yang
Department of Nephrology, Zhujiang Hospital, Southern Medical University, 253, Gongyedadao Middle, Guangzhou, Guangdong 510282, People's Republic of China

Mark Simon Stein
The Royal Melbourne Hospital, Parkville, Australia
Department of Diabetes and Endocrinology, The Royal Melbourne Hospital, Parkville, VIC 3050, Australia
Walter and Eliza Hall Institute of Medical Research, Parkville, Australia

Gregory John Ward
Sullivan Nicolaides Pathology, Brisbane, Australia

Helmut Butzkueven
The Royal Melbourne Hospital, Parkville, Australia
Florey Neuroscience Institutes, Parkville, Australia
University of Melbourne, Parkville, Australia
Monash University, Melbourne, Australia

Trevor John Kilpatrick
The Royal Melbourne Hospital, Parkville, Australia

Florey Neuroscience Institutes, Parkville, Australia
University of Melbourne, Parkville, Australia

Leonard Charles Harrison
The Royal Melbourne Hospital, Parkville, Australia
Walter and Eliza Hall Institute of Medical Research, Parkville, Australia
University of Melbourne, Parkville, Australia

Sean F. Monaghan, Chun-Shiang Chung, Joanne Lomas-Neira, Daithi S. Heffernan, William G. Cioffi and Alfred Ayala
Division of Surgical Research, Department of Surgery, Alpert School of Medicine at Brown University and Rhode Island Hospital, 593 Eddy Street, Providence, RI 02903, USA

Debasree Banerjee and Mitchell M. Levy
Division of Pulmonary and Critical Care, Department of Medicine, Alpert School of Medicine at Brown University and Rhode Island Hospital, Providence, RI 02903, USA

Kamil J. Cygan, Christy L. Rhine and William G. Fairbrother
MCB Department, Brown University, Providence, RI 02903, USA

Zhun Wu, Wei Huang, Xuegang Wang, Tao Wang, Yuedong Chen, Bin Chen, Rongfu Liu, Peide Bai and Jinchun Xing
Department of Urology, the First Affiliated Hospital of Xiamen University, No.55 Zhenhai Road, Xiamen 361003, Fujian, China

Agnieszka Sowinska and Helena Erlandsson Harris
Department of Medicine, Rheumatology Unit, Karolinska Institutet, Stockholm, Sweden

Peter Lundback
GE Healthcare Life Sciences, Uppsala, Sweden

Hannah Aucott
Department of Medicine, Rheumatology Unit, Karolinska Institutet, Stockholm, Sweden
Department of Medicine, Rheumatology Unit, Centre for Molecular Medicine (CMM) L8:04, Karolinska Hospital, 17176 Solna, Sweden

Lei Liu, Xin-Lu Pang, Wen-Jun Shang, Hong-Chang Xie, Jun-Xiang Wang and Gui-Wen Feng
Department of Kidney Transplantation, The First Affiliated Hospital of Zhengzhou University, No. 1, Jianshe Road, Erqi District, Zhengzhou 450052, Henan Province, People's Republic of China

Hao Wang, Yu Zhao, Jianguo Wang and Ting C. Zhao
Department of Surgery, Boston University Medical School, Roger Williams Medical Center, 50 Maude Street, Providence, RI 02908, USA

Ling Zhang, Patrycja M. Dubielecka and Shougang Zhuang
Department of Emergency Medicine, Department of Medicine, Rhode Island Hospital, Brown University, Providence, RI, USA

Gangjian Qin
Feinberg Cardiovascular Research Institute, Northwestern University Feinberg School of Medicine, Chicago, USA

Y Eugene Chin
Key Laboratory of Stem Cell Biology, Institutes of Health Sciences, Shanghai Institutes for Biological Sciences, Chinese Academy of Sciences, Shanghai, China

Race L. Kao
Department of Surgery, East Tennessee State University, Johnson City, TN, USA

Hélène Cabanas, Natalie Eaton, Cassandra Balinas, Donald Staines and Sonya Marshall-Gradisnik
School of Medical Science, Griffith University, Gold Coast, QLD, Australia
The National Centre for Neuroimmunology and Emerging Diseases, Menzies Health Institute Queensland, Griffith University, Gold Coast, QLD, Australia

Katsuhiko Muraki
Laboratory of Cellular Pharmacology, School of Pharmacy, Aichi-Gakuin University, Chikusa, Nagoya, Japan

Monowar Aziz, Yasumasa Ode, Mian Zhou and Mahendar Ochani
Center for Immunology and Inflammation, The Feinstein Institute for Medical Research, 350 Community Dr, Manhasset, NY 11030, USA

Nichol E. Holodick and Thomas L. Rothstein
Center for Oncology and Cell Biology, The Feinstein Institute for Medical Research, Manhasset, New York 11030, USA
Present Address: Western Michigan University Homer Stryker M.D. School of Medicine, 1000 Oakland Drive, Kalamazoo, MI 49008, USA

Ping Wang
Center for Immunology and Inflammation, The Feinstein Institute for Medical Research, 350 Community Dr, Manhasset, NY 11030, USA
Department of Surgery and Molecular Medicine, Donald and Barbara Zucker School of Medicine at Hofstra/ Northwell, Manhasset, New York 11030, USA

Antonela Matana, Marijana Popović, Ivana Gunjača, Vesna Boraska Perica, Maja Barbalić and Tatijana Zemunik
Department of Medical Biology, University of Split, School of Medicine, Šoltanska 2, Split, Croatia

Dubravka Brdar, Vesela Torlak and Ante Punda
Department of Nuclear Medicine, University Hospital Split, Spinciceva 1, Split, Croatia

Thibaud Boutin and Caroline Hayward
MRC Human Genetics Unit, University of Edinburgh, Western General Hospital, Crewe Road, Edinburgh, UK

Ivana Kolčić and Ozren Polašek
Department of Public Health, University of Split, School of Medicine Split, Šoltanska 2, Split, Croatia

Georgina Gyetvai, Cieron Roe, Lamia Heikal, Pietro Ghezzi and Manuela Mengozzi
Department of Clinical and Experimental Medicine, Brighton & Sussex Medical School, Brighton BN1 9PS, UK

Anna Mandel, Per Larsson, Julius Semenas and Azharuddin Sajid Syed Khaja
Department of Molecular Biology, Umeå University, 901 87 Umeå, Sweden

Martuza Sarwar
Division of Experimental Cancer Research, Department of Translational Medicine, Clinical Research Centre, Lund University, Jan Waldenströms gatan 35, 205 02 Malmö, Sweden

Jenny L. Persson
Department of Molecular Biology, Umeå University, 901 87 Umeå, Sweden
Division of Experimental Cancer Research, Department of Translational Medicine, Clinical Research Centre, Lund University, Jan Waldenströms gatan 35, 205 02 Malmö, Sweden

Mohd Israr, David Rosenthal, James DeVoti and Vincent R. Bonagura
The Feinstein Institute for Medical Research, Manhasset, NY, USA; Division of Allergy and Immunology, Department of Pediatrics, Donald and Barbara Zucker School of Medicine at Hofstra/ Northwell, Great Neck, NY, USA

Lidia Frejo-Navarro
Department of Genomic Medicine, Otology and Neurotology Group CTS495, Centre for Genomics and Oncological Research, Pfizer/Universidad de Granada/Junta de Andalucía (GENYO), Granada, Spain

Craig Meyers
Department of Microbiology and Immunology, The Pennsylvania State University College of Medicine, Hershey, PA, USA

Giovanna Marchetti, Fabio Manfredini and Nino Basaglia
Department of Biomedical and Specialty Surgical Sciences, University of Ferrara, via Fossato di Mortara n 74, 44121 Ferrara, Italy

Nicole Ziliotto, Silvia Meneghetti, Marcello Baroni, Barbara Lunghi and Francesco Bernardi
Department of Life Science and Biotechnology, University of Ferrara, Ferrara, Italy

Erica Menegatti, Rebecca Voltan and Paolo Zamboni
Department of Morphology, Surgery and Experimental Medicine, University of Ferrara, Ferrara, Italy

Massimo Pedriali
Department of Experimental and Diagnostic Medicine, Sant'Anna University- Hospital, Ferrara, Italy

Fabrizio Salvi and Ilaria Bartolomei
Center for Immunological and Rare Neurological Diseases, Bellaria Hospital, IRCCS of Neurological Sciences, Bologna, Italy

Sofia Straudi
Department of Neurosciences and Rehabilitation, Sant'Anna University- Hospital, Ferrara, Italy

Francesco Mascoli
Unit of Vascular and Endovascular Surgery, S. Anna University-Hospital, Ferrara, Italy

Fa-Liang Ren
1Department of Dermatology, Children's Hospital of Chongqing Medical University, Chongqing 400014, China

Xiao-Yan Luo
Department of Dermatology, Children's Hospital of Chongqing Medical University, Chongqing 400014, China
Ministry of Education Key Laboratory of Child Development and Disorders, Chongqing 400014, China

Qun Liu
The Division of Allergy and Clinical Immunology, Johns Hopkins University School of Medicine, Baltimore, MD 21224, USA

Huan Yang
Department of Dermatology, Children's Hospital of Chongqing Medical University, Chongqing 400014, China
China International Science and Technology Cooperation Base of Child Development and Critical Disorders, Chongqing 400014, China

Qi Tan and Li-Qiang Gan
Department of Dermatology, Children's Hospital of Chongqing Medical University, Chongqing 400014, China
Chongqing Key Laboratory of Pediatrics, No.136, Zhongshan Er Road, Yuzhong District, Chongqing 400014, China

Hua Wang
Department of Dermatology, Children's Hospital of Chongqing Medical University, Chongqing 400014, China
Ministry of Education Key Laboratory of Child Development and Disorders, Chongqing 400014, China
China International Science and Technology Cooperation Base of Child Development and Critical Disorders, Chongqing 400014, China

Chongqing Key Laboratory of Pediatrics, No.136, Zhongshan Er Road, Yuzhong District, Chongqing 400014, China

Neta Gotlieb, Irena Tachlytski, Maya Sultan and Michal Safran
Liver Reaserch Laboratory, Sheba Medical Center, Tel Hashomer, 52620 Ramat Gan, Israel

Yelena Lapidot
Liver Reaserch Laboratory, Sheba Medical Center, Tel Hashomer, 52620 Ramat Gan, Israel
The Sackler School of Medicine, Tel Aviv University, Tel Aviv, Israel

Ziv Ben-Ari
Liver Reaserch Laboratory, Sheba Medical Center, Tel Hashomer, 52620 Ramat Gan, Israel
Liver Disease Center, Sheba Medical Center, Tel Hashomer, 52620 Ramat Gan, Israel
The Sackler School of Medicine, Tel Aviv University, Tel Aviv, Israel

Kristin M. Favela and Nathan C. Bingham
Department of Pediatrics, Vanderbilt University Medical Center, 1500 21 st. Ave South, Suite 1514, Nashville, TN 37212, USA

Mary K. Herrick
Department of Pediatrics, Vanderbilt University Medical Center, 1500 21 st. Ave South, Suite 1514, Nashville, TN 37212, USA
Department of Physiology, Emory University School of Medicine, Atlanta, GA 30322, USA

Richard B. Simerly
Department of Molecular Physiology and Biophysics, Vanderbilt University Medical Center, Nashville, TN 37232, USA

Naji N. Abumrad
Department of Surgery, Vanderbilt University Medical Center, Nashville, TN 37232, USA

P Möhnle, L C Hinske and J Briegel
Department of Anaesthesiology and Intensive Care Medicine, University Hospital, Ludwig Maximilian University (LMU), Marchioninistraße 15, 81377 Munich, Germany

S Hirschberger, M Hübner and S Kreth
Department of Anaesthesiology and Intensive Care Medicine, University Hospital, Ludwig Maximilian University (LMU), Marchioninistraße 15, 81377 Munich, Germany
Walter-Brendel-Center of Experimental Medicine, Ludwig Maximilian University (LMU), Munich, Germany

M Bauer
Department of Anaesthesiology and Intensive Care Medicine, Friedrich-Schiller University, Jena, Germany
Center for Sepsis Control and Care, Jena University Hospital, Jena, Germany

S Weis
Department of Anaesthesiology and Intensive Care Medicine, Friedrich-Schiller University, Jena, Germany
Center for Sepsis Control and Care, Jena University Hospital, Jena, Germany
Center for Infectious Disease and Infection Control, Jena University Hospital, Jena, Germany

G Dimopoulos
2nd Department of Critical Care Medicine, ATTIKON University Hospital, National and Kapodistrian University of Athens, Athens, Greece

E J Giamarellos-Bourboulis
4th Department of Internal Medicine, ATTIKON University Hospital, National and Kapodistrian University of Athens, Athens, Greece

Index

www.ingramcontent.com/pod-product-compliance
Lightning Source LLC
Chambersburg PA
CBHW082038190326
41458CB00010B/3399